ESSENTIAL TISSUE HEALING OF THE FACE AND NECK

ESSENTIAL TISSUE HEALING OF THE FACE AND NECK

DAVID B. HOM MD, FACS
Professor & Director, Division of Facial Plastic & Reconstructive Surgery
Department of Otolaryngology – Head and Neck Surgery
University of Cincinnati, College of Medicine
Cincinnati Children's Hospital
Cincinnati, Ohio

PATRICIA A. HEBDA PHD
Associate Professor of Otolaryngology,and Pathology
University of Pittsburgh School of Medicine
Otolaryngology Wound Healing Research Program Children's Hospital of Pittsburgh
Pittsburgh, Pennsylvania

Editor-in-Chief, Wound Repair and Regeneration

ARUN K. GOSAIN MD, FACS
De Wayne Richey Professor and Vice Chair
Department of Plastic Surgery
Chief, Pediatric Plastic Surgery, Rainbow Babies and Children's Hospital
Case School of Medicine
Cleveland, Ohio

CRAIG D. FRIEDMAN MD, FACS
Facial Plastic Surgeon
Visiting Surgeon, Yale-New Haven Hospital
New Haven, Connecticut

Executive Vice President, Medical Affairs and Technology
Biomerix Inc
New York, New York

2009
BC Decker Inc

PEOPLE'S MEDICAL PUBLISHING HOUSE
SHELTON, CONNECTICUT

People's Medical Publishing House
2 Enterprise Drive, Suite 509
Shelton, CT 06484
Tel: 203-402-0646
Fax:203-402-0854
E-mail: info@pmph-usa.com

 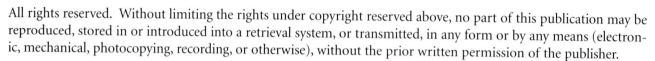

PEOPLE'S MEDICAL PUBLISHING HOUSE

09 10 11 12 13 14 15 / AOP / 9 8 7 6 5 4 3 2 1

ISBN 978-1-60795-007-3

Printed in India by Ajanta Offset and Packagings Limited
Managing Editor: Patricia Bindner; Cover Design: Lisa Mattinson

Sales and Distribution

Canada
McGraw-Hill Ryerson Education
Customer Care
300 Water St.
Whitby, Ontario   L1N 9B6
Tel: 1-800-565-5758
Fax: 1-800-463-5885

Foreign Rights
John Scott & Company
International Publishers' Agency
P.O. Box 878
Kimberton, PA 19442
Tel: 610-827-1640
Fax: 610-827-1671
E-mail: jsco@voicenet.com

Japan
United Publishers Services Limited
1-32-5 Higashi-Shinagawa
Shinagawa-Ku, Tokyo 140-0002
Tel: 03 5479 7251
Fax: 03 5479 7307
Email: kakimoto@ups.co.jp

UK, Europe, Middle East, Africa
McGraw-Hill Education
Shoppenhangers Road
Maidenhead
Berkshire, England SL6 2QL
Tel: 44-0-1628-502500
Fax: 44-0-1628-635895
www.mcgraw-hill.co.uk

*Singapore, Thailand, Philippines,
Indonesia, Vietnam, Pacific Rim, Korea*
McGraw-Hill Education
60 Tuas Basin Link
Singapore 638775
Tel: 65-6863-1580
Fax: 65-6862-3354

Australia, New Zealand
Elsevier Australia
Tower 1, 475 Victoria Avenue
Chatswood NSW 2067
Australia
Tel: 0-9422-8553
Fax: 0-9422-8562
www.elsevier.com.au

Brazil
Tecmedd Importadora E Distribuidora
De Livros Ltda.
Avenida Maurílio Biagi, 2850
City Ribeirão, Ribeirão Preto – SP – Brasil
CEP: 14021-000
Tel: 0800 992236
Fax: (16) 3993-9000
E-mail: tecmedd@tecmedd.com.br

*India, Bangladesh, Pakistan, Sri Lanka,
Malaysia*
CBS Publishers & Distributors
4819/X1 Prahlad Street 24
Ansari Road, Darya
New Delhi-11002, India
Tel: 91-11-23266861/67
Fax: 91-11-23266818
Email: cbspubs@vsnl.com

People's Republic of China
PMPH
Bldg 3, 3rd District, Fangqunyuan
Fangzhuang, Beijing 100078
P.R. China
Tel: 8610-676533423
Fax: 8610-67691034
www.pmph.com

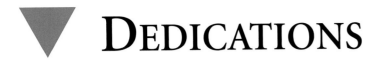

▼ DEDICATIONS

Dedicated to my parents, James and Evelyn Hom for your many years of caring guidance and my wife, Lori, for your constant support.

David B. Hom

To my husband, Jim Morrow, a true partner in life, who has always supported and encouraged me; and to our children, Catherine and James, who have grown to share our passion for biology.

Patricia A. Hebda

To my wife, Smita, and to my children, Sankalp and Sidhi, for helping me to learn how to work with others, and to my patients, for allowing me to work with them.

Arun K. Gosain

To my parents, family, and LS for their support and encouragement and to my patients who have trusted me to heal them and allowed me to learn as well.

Craig D. Friedman

▼ FOREWORD

In the last decade, a steady stream of books have asked: "How can we assure that wounds will heal, and how can we accelerate it?" Here we have a book, written by an excellent group of authors experienced in both practice and theory, that asks, "How can we prevent and/or deal with healing's imperfections in the head and neck?"

Due to the superior perfusion and oxygen supply in the head and neck, healing is usually fast and secure. Resistance to infection is exceptional. However, in this region more than any, we want scars to be invisible, mobile, and free from shrinkage and contracture. Perfection is possible. I bear the "scar" of an incision in my neck that has hosted two surgeons, and I can't see it in my shaving mirror. But, reality so often falls short.

What is to be gained inside this book? First, what you will get is up-to-date attitudes on healing. You'll get theory and practicality in one place. Practicality points to the importance of limiting inflammation. Although inflammatory oxidants are part of the biological basis of healing, too much is a constant threat to perfection. Uncontrolled, inflammation stimulates scarring to excess. However, in the head and neck, healing is so assured that we have the luxury of using anti-inflammatory therapies that we would shun in other areas.

The multi-disciplinary approach in this book is particularly useful. Surgical technique is important! Treatment in the first week influences events the following year. Care of the patient, both pre-and post-operatively influences the final result more than one might think. Many perioperative events enhance inflammation. Only a few are well understood. For instance, for reasons unknown some patients seem to become more inflamed than others. I suspect that medication, such as excessive vitamin A or retinoic acid are "inflammatory." Excessive motion, glove powder, dust, etc. are all potential problems. These details are important in acute wound healing and not discussed in many books that are focused on chronic wounds. Even shear forces enhance inflammation. They introduce electrical fields that generate excessive oxidants.

Here are remedies. We can immobilize the wound, apply heat, antioxidants, silastic sheeting. We can change patterns of physical forces during the critical inflammatory period while the healing wound lacks mechanical compliance, and is vulnerable to shear. How about the idea—of Botulinum toxin in the periwound of facial tissue which is currently being tested. Are timely injections of steroids or other anti-inflammatory agents useful? Many surgeons and dentists seem to think so. The issue needs serious study. One creative idea now under development is to inject new wounds with the anti-inflammatory isoform Transforming Growth Factor (TGF) beta 3. Unfortunately, the expense for an uncertain return is a commercial disincentive. At any rate the best time to discourage unwanted inflammation starts at the end of the operation and lasts for about two weeks.

I am compelled to insert one opinion here. Healing in irradiated tissues, often a problem in the head and neck, poses special issues. I am pleased to see a chapter on radiation damage and one on hyperbaric oxygen. I want to re-enforce the importance of hyperbaric oxygen in treatment of osteoradionecrosis because there will be disagreement. Nests of inflammatory cells that remain in irradiated tissues slowly cause deposition of connective tissue. The inflamed tissue thickens and, almost like a tumor that outgrows its blood supply, often becomes critically ischemic. There is sufficient oxygen for neither endothelial cell movement, i.e. angiogenesis, nor for bacterial killing. The problem will persist or worsen until the oxygen supply is increased. In many cases, hyperbaric oxygen is the only effective therapy. A government panel has recently put hyperbaric therapy for osteoradionecrosis on the "experimental" list for reimbursement! Having developed some of the proof myself, I assure you that despite this perverse ruling, there is no doubt that alternating between hypoxia and hyperoxia is angiogenic! This is not the place to explain the science, but I confidently warn the skeptics to keep an open mind. Your opinions will one day come back to bite you!

Among other notable discussion in the book is the modern view of nutrition. Is there a role for nutrition in the redox (inflammatory) balance? Many head and neck patients are undernourished particularly in respect to antioxidants, and may tend to become inflamed for that reason. Vitamin C acts as a useful (and necessary!) oxidant in human wounds. That poor diet may deplete arginine, for instance, is a sound observation. We are seeing more and more of the value of the oxidant nitric oxide (NO) in healing, and as the chapter says, arginine is its source. However, as in all redox processes, too little is insufficient and too much is harmful. Vitamin A and NO are required necessary. Large doses of both are inflammatory and may promote scarring. How to maintain a productive redox balance is currently one of the major questions in the management of healing.

Basic science is beginning to resolve some of the riddles. For instance, in normal repair, the major stimuli to vascular endothelial growth factor (VEGF) and collagenases (MMPs) in wounds are hydrogen peroxide and lactate, not hypoxia. Angiogenesis requires oxygen and is most competent in hyperoxia. How best to use these new data is still an issue. Perhaps a recent demonstration that hyperbaric oxygen increases stem cells in blood may be a clue. How we might attract stem cells to injured sites may be the next step. Can we induce angiogenesis to reduce ischemia without inducing excessive collagen deposition as well? Can we effectively suppress inflammation locally? Can we even temporarily change patterns of motion until inflammation subsides and mechanical compliance is restored?

This book is, I hope, part of a trend. We have had too much of the "wounds-magically-heal-with-growth-factors" kind of thinking. We need to think more in terms of isolating the components of healing and correcting their excesses as well as their deficiencies. This book, with its combined look at the clinical and the theoretical tends to take that view.

Thomas K. Hunt, MD
Professor of Surgery
University of California, San Francisco
Founder and First President of the Wound Healing Society

For too long, too many surgeons and others concerned with operative and non-operative problems of the head and neck have regarded that area almost exclusively in terms of its anatomy and to a lesser extent its physiology and pathology while ignoring the process of healing of any one or more of its numerous, diverse components. A cynic or realist, depending upon one's viewpoint, might conclude that it is possible to be an effective and successful surgeon above the clavicle without such knowledge, even though it would enlarge the individual's perspective and improve his or her performance, all to the patient's advantage. For those who want to learn about such matters, this text is an excellent opportunity.

The editors, contributors, and publishers have succeeded admirably in producing a book that is unique, needed, and helpful. Seldom does a literary project of this dimension achieve every stated objective as this has. The reader benefits from an integration of the newest information in the basic sciences and the most current practices in clinical management, presented in a clear, non-repetitive style. Why this has been possible is due not just to the expertise and excellence of the authors but to the diversity of their backgrounds and experience.

As this book well illustrates, and as any clinician knows, richness of the blood supply to the head and neck does not guarantee successful healing. One has in this volume the latest data and insights about how and why most wounds do heal satisfactorily but others do not. While these pages contain an abundance of facts, which is an important attribute, perhaps the greater value lies in its stimulating the reader to think about an old problem in a new way, to ponder what wound healing in the future could be.

Getting the most from this book requires more than quick reading; it demands and fortunately encourages study preferably at an unhurried pace, and a willingness to consider the head and neck and healing in this area in ways different from those in the past.

When I was a resident, my former Chief of Plastic Surgery at Pittsburgh, Dr. William L. White, used to say, "You stay young only if you are being stretched intellectually." This book does that and more.

I appreciate the opportunity of writing this Foreword from the perspective of a plastic and reconstructive surgeon. The added pleasure by coincidence is that my friend and classmate at both college and medical school, Tom Hunt, has also furnished a foreword from his perspective.

Robert M. Goldwyn, MD
Clinical Professor of Surgery, Harvard Medical School
Editor Emeritus, Plastic and Reconstructive Surgery

This book is a critical accumulation of current knowledge of wound healing of the face and neck. The editors have gathered a group of experts from several specialties that bring very useful information to the practicing surgeon and advanced information for the research-oriented physician. Having worked primarily in clinical research and in clinical observation during my 57 years of practice, I cannot recommend enough to any surgeon that he know the healing properties of the tissues he works with and what to expect during all phases of healing. Especially the young surgeon should know what to expect at different stages of wound repair. He should see postoperative patients frequently to give them strong reassurance of what is normally expected for that time in healing. This also adds to the surgeon's maturing observation and critique of the material, methods, and techniques he is using.

The oldest surgical document in existence related to healing of the face was written on Papyrus 1700 years ago, which describe treatments on the face 1000 years previously. The treatise written by an ancient Egyptian surgeon describes operations of which magic was listed as the last resort in only one instance. In each case, the surgeon stated his clinical findings and proceeded to appropriately intervene.

Many years later, Tagliacozzi described a facial surgeon's role and the importance of proper healing in his quote, "We restore, repair and make whole those parts of the face which nature has given but which fortune has taken away, not so much that they might delight the eye but that they buoy up the spirit and help the mind of the afflicted."

Essentially, everything starts with the *cell*. Tissue engineering, growth factors, recombinant protein, stem cell research are parts of our increasing knowledge and pose exciting prospects. Molecular biology, biophysics, biomechanics and biophysiology come into play as new materials and methods are developed. Tissue reaction and the healing process must be evaluated for all foreign substances from sutures, modern metallic implants and other synthetic materials. Even in the selection of suture materials, reaction varies. Rapid absorption with greater cellular reaction must be balanced with the length of tissue tensile strength is maintained. Inert materials, even permanent sutures, can be rejected or extruded by the host.

Wound healing of the head and neck is influenced by life style and nature. Considerations would include sun exposure, smoking, alcohol intake, nutrition, diabetes, radiation, chemotherapy, immunosuppression and autoimmune disorders. The difference between adult healing and that of a child should be evaluated as well as with the aging process.

Wound healing is an exacting and fascinating subject and this unique book provides us with a deeper understanding of the process in a comprehensive fashion. In assuming the role of a senior counselor, I urge you to enjoy your practice more and constantly strive to obtain better results- *"Love people and have respect for the tissues."*

Richard T. Farrior, MD, FACS
Clinical Professor Emeritus of Otolaryngology – Head and Neck Surgery
Past President of the American Academy of Facial Plastic & Reconstructive Surgery
Past President of the American Academy of Otolaryngology – Head & Neck Surgery

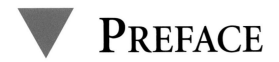

PREFACE

Wound healing is a physiological process essential for survival. It was only a century ago when an infected open wound was a common outcome. Lister's application of antisepsis was the major discovery that completely changed the outcome of healing wounds. Since then, normal healing of acute wounds is expected rather than considered to be a unique result. Over the last 15 years, understanding of the mechanisms of wound healing has increased dramatically among researchers and practitioners.

Several outstanding books have been written about the process of wound healing of the body. However, no recent book has focused on the unique healing properties and wound management challenges of the structures in the face and neck.

The face and neck region is unique from other anatomical areas in that it usually heals faster following surgery due to its higher vascularity. However, post-surgical wound complications continue to occur resulting in significant patient morbidity and mortality. Open to full public view in our society, facial wounds and disfigurement are difficult to conceal and can be mentally devastating to the patient. Wound healing problems on the face and neck decrease quality of life by compromising all of the five senses (sight, hearing, smell, taste and touch).

Over the last decade there has been an explosion of information pertaining to the basic science of wound healing. With the advent of recombinant DNA technology, evaluation of cellular and molecular events during wound repair has greatly been enhanced. However, the potential impact of these discoveries upon head and neck surgery are just beginning to emerge. Recombinant DNA technology has made it possible to produce growth factors in large quantities that may make it possible to improve wound healing among the various tissues in the face and neck area (skin, cartilage, bone, mucosa, nerve, muscle, middle ear and upper airway). Wound management has also improved through extensive research, with sophisticated new materials and biomaterials being fabricated for use as dressings, devices and implants. The application of information learned from the basic science of wound healing to solving difficult problems in face and neck surgery is the basic goal of this book. The end product represents the result of significant efforts made by basic scientists and clinicians in many specialties.

COMMON POST-SURGICAL HEALING PROBLEMS OF THE FACE & NECK

Site	Clinical Presentation
Chronic Cutaneous Wounds	Scarring and Facial Disfigurement Persistent open wound causing exposure of vital structures (vessels, nerves, bone) Wound dehiscence, Fistula formation
Airway Mucosa	Airway stenosis causing airway obstruction
Oral Mucosa	Wound contracture limiting oral mobility for swallowing and articulation
Peripheral Nerve	Poor nerve recovery causing nerve paralysis and synkinesis
Cartilage	Resorption or altered shape causing decreased support and deformity
Bone	Osteomyelitis, nonunion, malunion Abnormal bone growth
Sinus Mucosa	Altered ciliary function increasing sinusitis
Muscle	Fibrosis limiting functional movement in swallowing and articulation with facial disfigurement
Larynx	Airway stricture causing airway obstruction and vocal dysfunction
Esophagus	Stricture causing dysphagia
Tympanic Membrane and Middle Ear	Persistent tympanic membrane perforation or cholesteatoma causing decreased hearing

The goals of our book are to address the contemporary major tissue healing problems of the face and neck, describe current clinical ways to treat them, and discuss future potential therapies.

The chapters in the First Section of the book describe the unique healing aspects of different structures of the face and neck.

The chapters in the Second Section of the book discuss common clinical tissue healing problems encountered, methods to treat them, and future potential techniques.

The chapters in the Third Section of the book address the current and possible future therapies to optimize healing.

The style of the book was written for surgeons, clinicians, and researchers who deal with the tissues of the face and neck. This book attempts to cross specialty boundaries in order to gain a diverse perspective. We would like to thank the authors for their contributions and hope the readers will appreciate and make use of the exciting progress being made to improve the healing of wounds in the face and neck.

In Memoriam

"Dr. George L. Adams (1941- 2006) was a gifted surgeon and generous teacher who over 39 years dedicated his lifetime talent treating cancer patients and their challenging surgical wounds. His knowledge, clinical experience, and surgical skills made a major impact on our specialty for which he also taught numerous residents and fellows as Chairman of the Department of Otolaryngology - Head and Neck Surgery at the University of Minnesota School of Medicine from 1989 to 2006. We are indebted to have had Dr. Adams share his knowledge for his chapter entitled " Irradiated Soft Tissue Wounds" in this book. We will sincerely miss him.

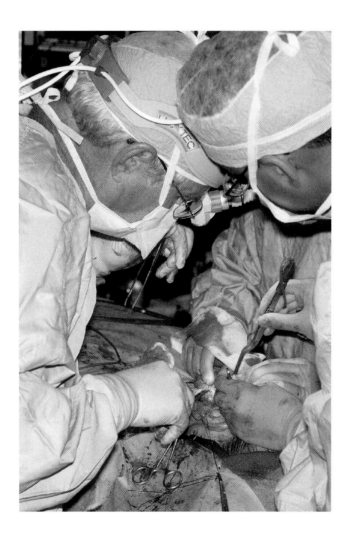

▼ CONTENTS

▼ CONTRIBUTORS

George L. Adams, MD (deceased)
Former Professor, Chairman
Department of Otolaryngology - Head and Neck
Surgery
University of Minnesota School of Medicine
Minneapolis, Minnesota
Irradiated Soft Tissue Wounds

Louis C. Argenta, MD
Bowman-Gray Plastic Surgery
Medical Center Boulevard
Winston-Salem, North Carolina
*Vacuum Assisted Devices for Difficult
  Wounds of the Face and Neck*

Elizabeth Ayello, PhD
Clinical Associate Editor
Advances in Skin & Wound Care Faculty
Excelsior College, School of Nursing
Albany, New York
Wound Débridement

Vishal Banthia, MD
Fellow, Division of Facial Plastic &
Reconstructive Surgery
Department of Otolaryngology-HNS
Stanford University Medical Center
Stanford, California
*Laser Resurfaced Facial Skin: Clinical
  Problems and Issues of Healing Tissues,
  Pearls and Pitfalls*

Adrian Barbul, MD, FACS
Chief, Professor, Division of General Surgery
Department of Surgery
Johns Hopkins Medical Institutions
Sinai Hospital of Baltimore
Baltimore, Maryland
Nutrition and Wound Healing

Pete S. Batra, MD
Assistant Professor
Section of Nasal and Sinus Disorders
Head and Neck Institute
The Cleveland Clinic
Cleveland, Ohio
*Sinonasal Mucosal Wound Healing:
  Implications for Contemporary
  Rhinologic Surgery*

Kofi D.O. Boahene, MD
Assistant Professor
Division of Facial Plastic and
Reconstructive Surgery
Department of Otolaryngology
Johns Hopkins University School of Medicine
Baltimore, Maryland
The Facial Nerve After Injury

Harold Brem, MD
Director, Wound Healing Center
Department of Plastic Surgery
Columbia University College of
Physicians and Surgeons
New York, New York
Wound Débridement

Hilary A. Brodie, MD, PhD
Professor and Chairman
Department of Otolaryngology-HNS
University of California – Davis
Sacramento, California
Irradiated Temporal Bone

Christine D. Brown, MD
Associate Attending
Division of Dermatology
Department of Internal Medicine
Baylor University Medical Center
Dallas, Texas
Choice of Wound Dressings and Ointments

Harvey Chim, MBBS, MRCS (UK), MMed
Resident
Department of Plastic Surgery
Case School of Medicine
Cleveland, Ohio
Keloids and Hypertropic Scarring

Martin J. Citardi, MD
Professor and Chair
Department of Otorhinolaryngology – Head and Neck
Surgery
The University of Texas Medical School at Houston
Houston, Texas
Sinonasal Mucosal Wound Healing:
  Implications for Contemporary
  Rhinologic Surgery

Dipan Das, MD
Resident
Department of Plastic Surgery
Medical College of Wisconsin
Milwaukee, Wisconsin
Burned Facial Skin

Anthony J. DeFranzo, MD
Associate Professor of Surgery
Department of Plastic Surgery
Wake Forest University
School of Medicine
Winston-Salem, North Carolina
Vacuum Assisted Devices for Difficult
  Wounds of the Face and Neck

Joseph E. Dohar, MD, MS
Associate Professor
Division of Pediatric Otolaryngology
Department of Otolaryngology
University of Pittsburgh
School of Medicine
Pittsburgh, Pennsylvania
Clinical Considerations of Wound Healing
  In the Subglottis and Trachea
Wound Healing in the Subglottis and Trachea

Robert C. Dinsmore, MD FACS
Assistant Clinical Professor
Section of Plastic Surgery
Medical College of Georgia
Augusta, Georgia
Facial Bones

Harley S. Dresner, MD
Assistant Professor
Department of Otolaryngology - Head and Neck
Surgery
University of Minnesota
Minneapolis, Minnesota
General Approach to a Poorly Healing
  Problem Wound: Practical and Clinical Overview

John J. Feldmeier, DO
Professor and Chairman
Department of Radiation Oncology
University of Toledo
College of Medicine
Toledo, Ohio
Hyperbaric Oxygen and Wound Healing
  in the Head and Neck

Rebecca E. Fraioli, MD
Resident
Department of Otolaryngology
University of Pittsburgh
School of Medicine
Pittsburgh, Pennsylvania
Controlling Infection

Craig D. Friedman, MD, FACS
Facial Plastic Surgeon
Visiting Surgeon, Yale-New Haven Hospital
New Haven, Connecticut

Executive Vice President
Medical Affairs and Technology
Biomerix Inc.
New York, New York
Craniofacial Cartilage Wound Healing:
  Implications for Facial Surgeons

Arun K. Gosain, MD, FACS
De Wayne Richey Professor and Vice Chair
Department of Plastic Surgery
Chief, Pediatric Plastic Surgery
Rainbow Babies and Children's Hospital
Case School of Medicine
Cleveland, Ohio
Burned Facial Skin

Joseph A. Greco III, MD
Plastic Surgery Research Fellow
Department of Plastic Surgery
Vanderbilt University Medical Center
Nashville, Tennessee
Growth Factors – Modulators of Wound Healing

Ryan M. Greene, MD, PhD
Resident Physician
Department of Otolaryngology-HNS
University of Chicago at Illinois
Chicago, Illinois
Blood Products in Wound Healing

Yoav N. Hahn, MD
Resident
Department of Otolaryngology-HNS
University of California – Davis
Sacramento, California
Irradiated Temporal Bone

Patricia A. Hebda, PhD
Associate Professor
Division of Pediatric Otolaryngology
Department of Otolaryngology
University of Pittsburgh
School of Medicine
Pittsburgh, Pennsylvania
Wound Healing of the Skin
Wound Healing in the Subglottis and Trachea

Sten D.M. Hellström, MD, PhD
Professor and Chairman
Department of Audiology
Karolinska Hospital
Stockholm, Sweden
*Salient Healing Features of the
  Tympanic Membrane*

Vu T. Ho, MD
Fellow, Facial Plastic Surgery
Department of Otorhinolaryngology -
Head and Neck Surgery
University of Michigan Medical Center
Ann Arbor, Michigan
*Irradiated Skin and Its
  Postsurgical Management*

David B. Hom, MD, FACS
Professor, Director, Division of
Facial Plastic & Reconstructive Surgery
Department of Otolaryngology-HNS
University of Cincinnati College of Medicine
Cincinnati Children's Hospital Medical Centers
Cincinnati, Ohio
*General Approach to a Poorly Healing
  Problem Wound: Practical and Clinical Overview*
Irradiated Skin and Its Postsurgical Management

Benjamin C. Johnson, MD
Resident Physician
Department of Otolaryngology
University of Illinois at Chicago
Chicago, Illinois
Blood Products in Wound Healing

Jonas T. Johnson, MD
Professor and Chairman
Department of Otolaryngology
University of Pittsburgh
School of Medicine
Pittsburgh, Pennsylvania
Controlling Infection

Loree K. Kalliainen, MD, FACS
Assistant Professor
Division of Plastic and Reconstructive Surgery
Department of Surgery
University of Minnesota
Minneapolis, Minnesota
*Salient Healing Features of Muscles
  of the Face and Neck*

Adam J. Katz, MD
Assistant Professor
Department of Plastic Surgery
University of Virginia
Charlottesville, Virginia
Adipose Tissue in Stem Cell Biology

Ryan Katz, MD
Division Plastic Surgery
Department of Surgery
Johns Hopkins Hospital
Baltimore, Maryland
Nutrition and Wound Healing

R. James Koch, MD
Director
California Face and Laser Institute
Palo Alto, California
*Laser Resurfaced Facial Skin: Clinical
  Problems and Issues of Healing Tissues,
  Pearls and Pitfalls*

Chung Kyu Kim Lee, MD
Professor
Department of Radiation Oncology
University of Minnesota Medical Center
Minneapolis, Minnesota
*Irradiated Skin and Its Postsurgical
  Management*

Michael T. Longaker, MD, MBA
Deane P. and Louise Mitchell Professor
Division of Plastic and Reconstructive Surgery
Department of Surgery
Stanford University School of Medicine
Palo Alto, California
Cranial Suture Biology and Craniosynostosis

Stephen P. R. MacLeod, BDS, MB, ChB,
FDS RCS (Ed and Eng), FRCS (Ed)
Clinical Assistant Professor
Division of Oral Maxillo Facial Surgery
Department of Developmental and
Surgical Sciences
University of Minnesota School of Dentistry
Minneapolis, Minnesota
*Nonunion of the Mandible and the
  Irradiated Mandible*

John Maddalozzo, MD
Associate Professor
Division of Otolaryngology
Department of Otolaryngology
Northwestern University
Feinberg School of Medicine
Chicago, Illinois
Cervical Esophagus

Hani S. Matloub, MD
Professor of Plastic and
Reconstructive Surgery
Department of Plastic Surgery
Medical College of Wisconsin
Milwaukee, Wisconsin
Perhipheral Nerve

Mark May, MD
Clinical Professor Emeritus
Department of Otolaryngology-HNS
University of Pittsburgh
School of Medicine
Pittsburgh, Pennsylvania
The Facial Nerve After Injury

Melissa Kurtis Micou, PhD
Lecturer
Department of Bioengineering
University of California at San Diego
La Jolla, California
*Craniofacial Cartilage Wound Healing:
  Implications for Facial Surgeons*

Joseph A. Molnar, MD, PhD
Professor, Surgical Sciences –
Plastic, Reconstructive
Associate Director, WFUMBC Burn Unit
Wake-Forest University Baptist Medical Center
Winston-Salem, North Carolina
*Vacuum Assisted Devices for Difficult
  Wounds of the Face and Neck*

Randall P. Nacamuli, MD
Plastic Surgery Fellow
Division of Children's Surgical Research
Department of Surgery
Stanford University School of Medicine
Palo Alto, California
Cranial Suture Biology and Craniosynostosis

Lillian B. Nanney, PhD
Professor of Plastic Surgery
Vanderbilt University School of Medicine
Nashville, Tennessee
Growth Factors – Modulators of Wound Healing

Roy C. Ogle, PhD
Professor
Department of Cell Biology, Neurosurgery,
Plastic Surgery
University of Virginia
Charlottesville, Virginia
Adipose Tissue in Stem Cell Biology

Kevin M. O'Grady, BS, BA
Clinical Research Coordinator
Department of Otolaryngology-HNS
University of Illinois at Chicago
Chicago, Illinois
Blood Products in Wound Healing

Todd D. Otteson, MD
Assistant Professor
Division of Pediatric Otolaryngology
Department of Otolaryngology-HNS
University of Pittsburgh School of Medicine
Pittsburgh, Pennsylvania
*Clinical Considerations of Wound Healing
  in the Subglottis and Trachea*

Aron Parekh, PhD
Postdoctoral Fellow
Department of Bioengineering
McGowan Institute for
Regenerative Medicine
University of Pittsburgh
Pittsburgh, Pennsylvania
*Clinical Considerations of Wound Healing
  in the Subglottis and Trachea*

David J. Rowe, MD
Assistant Professor
Department of Plastic Surgery
Case School of Medicine
Cleveland, Ohio
Peripheral Nerve

Vlad C. Sandulache, PhD
Medical Student
Division of Pediatric Otolaryngology
Department of Otolaryngology
University of Pittsburgh, School of Medicine
Pittsburgh, Pennsylvania
Wound Healing in the Subglottis and Trachea

Robert T. Sataloff, MD, DMA
Professor of Otolaryngology-HNS
Department of Otolaryngology
Thomas Jefferson University
Philadelphia, Pennsylvania
Vocal Fold Scar

Henning Schliephake, DDS, PhD
Professor
Department of Oral and Maxillofacial Surgery
Georg-August-University of Goettingen
Goettingen, Germany
Salient Features of the Oral Mucosa

Gregory S. Schultz, PhD
Professor
Department of Obstetrics and Gynecology
University of Florida
Gainesville, Florida
Wound Débridement

Stefan Schultze-Mosgau, MD, DDS PhD
Professor, Head and Chairman
Department of Oral and Cranio Maxillofacial
Surgery/Plastic Surgery
Freidrich Schiller University of Jena
Jena, Germany
Salient Features of the Oral Mucosa

Taha Z. Shipchandler, MD
Resident
Head and Neck Institute
Cleveland Clinic Foundation
Cleveland, Ohio
*Sinonasal Mucosal Wound Healing:
  Implications for Contemporary
    Rhinologic Surgery*

William T. Stoeckel, MD
Chief Resident
Department of Plastic and Reconstructive Surgery
Wake Forest Medical Center
Winston-Salem, North Carolina
*Vacuum Assisted Devices for Difficult
  Wounds of the Face and Neck*

Cecille G. Sulman, MD
Assistant Professor
Division of Pediatric Otolaryngology
Department of Otolaryngology and
Communication Sciences
Medical College of Wisconsin
Milwaukee, Wisconsin
Cervical Esophagus

Mark Boon Yang Tang, MBBS, MRCP,
MMed, FAMS
Consultant(attending) Dermatologists
National Skin Center, Singapore
Keloids and Hypertrophic Scarring

Susan L. Thibeault, PhD
Assistant Professor
Division of Otolarlyngology-HNS
University of Wisconsin at Madison
Madison, Wisconsin
Wound Healing of the Larynx

Sunil S. Tholopady, MS, MD, PhD
Resident
Department of Plastic Surgery
University of Virginia
Charlottesville, Virginia
Adipose Tissue in Stem Cell Biology

Dean M. Toriumi, MD
Professor, Division of Facial Plastic
and Reconstructive Surgery
Department of Otolaryngology-HNS
University of Illinois at Chicago
Chicago, Illinois
Blood Products in Wound Healing

Derrick C. Wan, MD
Division of Children's Surgical Research
Department of Surgery
Stanford University School of Medicine
Palo Alto, California
Cranial Suture Biology and Craniosynostosis

Falk Wehrhan, MD, DDS
Clinic of Oral and Maxillofacial Surgery
University of Erlagen – Nuremberg
Nuremberg, Germany
Salient Features of the Oral Mucosa

Jack Yu, MD
Milford B. Hatcher Chair, Professor
and Chief, Section of Plastic Surgery
Department of Plastic Surgery
Medical College of Georgia
Augusta, Georgia
Facial Bones

John A. Zitelli, MD
Clinical Associate Professor of
Dermatology and Otolaryngology
Department of Dermatology
University of Pittsburgh Medical Center
Pittsburgh, Pennsylvania
Choice of Wound Dressings and Ointments

Wound Healing of the Skin

Patricia A. Hebda, PhD

OVERVIEW

The skin is the most extensively studied organ with respect to the wound healing response, and research in this area has led to many advances in the clinical management of cutaneous wounds. Lessons learned in the skin may be applicable to similar tissues in other organs, such as mucosal tissues of the head and neck, but there is also evidence of tissue specificity, which argues for a rigorous analysis of healing in other tissues. This chapter attempts to provide an overview of the events of cutaneous wound healing. Given the extensive literature, this chapter provides a basic synopsis of salient features, with references provided for more extensive exploration. In addition, more recent areas of research have been included to bring the reader to a current perspective of this subject. Some of these areas are discussed in subsequent chapters of this book.

Wound healing is a complex, dynamic process dependent on the coordinated activities of multiple cell types in the epithelium, the connective tissue, and the vasculature. Essential features of this process can be described using a simplified paradigm of three basic cellular functions, migration, mitosis, and maturation, which are delineated as they apply to the three main components of the skin: epidermis, dermal connective tissue, and dermal vasculature. For the purposes of discussion, these events are dealt with individually, but it should be emphasized that not only are these processes occurring simultaneously, there is also coordination and crosstalk among the responding cells in each compartment.

Some recently emerging areas of research build on the extensive body of literature to find new, biologically driven approaches for improving the wound healing response. Exploration of more regenerative healing, as is observed in fetal skin, is a potentially promising area, as is the possibility of using stem cell–based therapies for more regenerative healing. Later chapters focus on clinical problems and therapeutic approaches for better management of cutaneous wounds. Therefore, this first chapter lays the foundation for what is to follow.

THE SKIN

At the interface between the organism and the environment, the skin is at risk of exposure to injury from a variety of agents. In addition to injury through trauma or disease processes, the skin may be wounded as a necessary part of surgical and other invasive medical procedures. Fortunately, the skin has a great inherent capacity for healing, and, through several basic mechanisms, the skin of the face and neck will normally achieve wound closure and restoration of barrier function. However, the wound healing process is less than perfect and the skin's response to injury results in repair, or scar formation, rather than regeneration of the component tissue structures. Therefore, a basic understanding of the wound healing response in the skin, including its capacity for restoration and its limits of repair, is essential for optimal wound care and management.

ANATOMY AND HISTOLOGY

The skin is the largest organ of the body, composed of two layers, an outer epidermis and inner dermis, with an underlying layer of adipose tissue forming the hypodermis. The structural features of the skin reflect its functional properties, mainly protection from without and maintenance of homeostasis within. The skin also performs important immunologic functions through a complex of skin-associated lymphatic tissue (SALT).[1] The diagram in Figure 1 shows an overview of basic anatomic features of the skin. The skin of the head and neck has additional structural features, including skeletal muscles inserting into the facial dermis; modified hair follicles and glands associated with the eyes, ears, and scalp; and margins with mucosal tissues of the eyes, nose, and mouth.[2]

Epidermis

The outer layer of skin, the epidermis, is a stratified squamous keratinized epithelium with important barrier and immune functions. The predominant cell type in the epidermis is the keratinocyte, which is committed to a program of

NORMAL SKIN

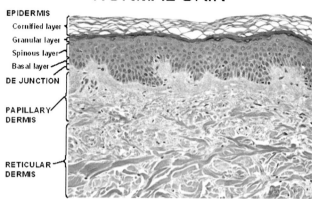

Figure 2. Histology of the skin: cross section stained with hematoxylin and eosin (×10 original magnification).

terminal differentiation and thus is normally undergoing a process of continuous renewal as cells transit from the basal layer of the epidermis, entering the spinous layer first and then the granular layer and finally forming the uppermost keratinized or cornified layer, a process that takes about 3 to 6 weeks (Figure 2).[3,4] Keratinocytes form numerous cell–cell contacts called desmosomes, which contribute to epidermal integrity. During terminal differentiation, the keratinocyte produces intracellular keratins and lipid-filled granules (membrane-coating granules), whereas

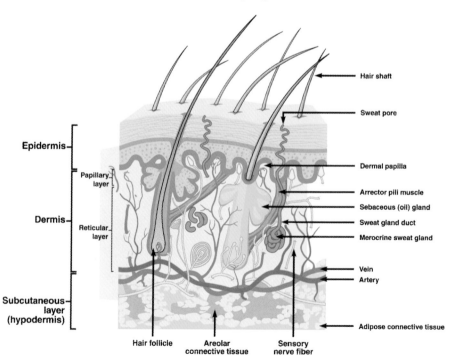

Figure 1. Anatomy of the skin.

its cell nucleus becomes inactive and condensed. The dead cells of the cornified layer are composed of cell membranes, keratin proteins, and complex lipids, which form the major barrier against water loss and microbial or chemical invasion. Dead cells, or squames, are gradually shed or sloughed from the surface and replaced from below, through a process called desquamation. The basal layer is maintained by cell mitosis, but once a cell leaves the basal layer, it is committed to the differentiation pathway and is no longer capable of cell division.[4] The basal keratinocyte is the primary cell involved in the epidermal wound healing response.

Other cells residing in the epidermis are the melanocyte, which produces pigment to provide protection against ultraviolet radiation; the Merkel cell, a neuroendocrine cell; Langerhans' cell, an antigen-presenting immune cell of macrophage lineage; and the dendritic epithelial T cell (DETC), a specialized subset of T cells that express the $\gamma\delta$-T-cell receptor.[5] Activated DETCs produce keratinocyte growth factors and chemokines, raising the possibility that DETCs play a role in wound repair. In experimental wounds in mouse skin, the absence of wild-type DETCs produced defects in keratinocyte proliferation and tissue reepithelialization.[6] It has been proposed that DETCs recognize antigens expressed by injured keratinocytes and produce factors that directly affect healing.[7] A potential active role in wound healing has not been ascribed to the other minor cellular components of the epidermis; over time, they repopulate the healed epidermis.

Epidermal appendages are specialized structures that arise from the epidermis during a defined stage of embryonic development by means of dermal-epidermal induction.[8,9] In the skin of the head and neck, these structures include the hair follicle or sebaceous gland (also called the pilosebaceous unit), eccrine sweat glands and ducts, and specialized apocrine glands of the eyes and ears.[10] Experimental evidence indicates that epidermal stem cells reside in the bulge region of the hair follicle and contribute to renewal of basal keratinocytes and follicular epithelium.[11] During wound healing, cells from epidermal appendages and basal keratinocytes contribute to wound reepithelialization.[12,13]

Basement Membrane Zone or Dermal-Epidermal Junction

The border between the epidermis and the dermis is called the cutaneous basement membrane zone or the dermal-epidermal junction (DEJ). It is a specialized assemblage of basal keratinocyte structures and extracellular matrix (ECM) components, including the basal lamina and anchoring filaments and fibrils.[14,15] The structural integrity of this region is achieved by a series of linked components starting from keratin tonofilaments in the cytoplasm of basal epithelial cells, to hemidesmosomes in the basal cell membrane, to anchoring filaments within the basal lamina, to anchoring fibrils below the basal lamina, to anchoring plaques on collagen type I fibrils in the papillary dermis (Figure 3). Anchoring filaments, thread-like structures that traverse the lamina lucida, are composed of laminin type 5 and several other ECM molecules. At the lower portion of basal lamina, anchoring fibrils, composed predominantly of collagen type VII, extend from the lamina densa to the papillary dermis,

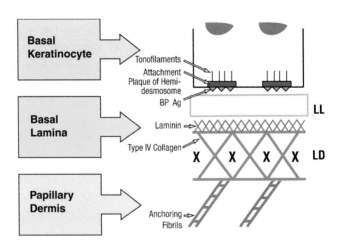

Figure 3. The cutaneous basement membrane zone (BMZ) or dermal-epidermal junction (DEJ). The region between the epidermis and dermis is composed of an assembly of extracellular matrix molecules. The linkage of structural elements in the basal keratinocyte, the lamina lucida (LL) and lamina densa (LD) of the basal lamina, and the papillary dermis contribute to close adherence and structural integrity of the two layers.

where they are associated with basement membrane–like structures, named anchoring plaques, which, in turn, are adherent to interstitial collagen type I.[14,15] Most of the components of the DEJ are synthesized by epithelial cells and must be reproduced during wound healing.[9,13,16] In the absence of this linkage network, the skin is susceptible to mechanical shearing and separation of the epidermis from the dermis, leading to reinjury through blistering and sloughing.[17]

Another feature of the DEJ is its irregular border, composed of ridges and invaginations of the papillary dermis (see Figures 2 and 3). These formations, called rete ridges, increase the surface area, which also helps maintain adherence between the two layers. In a newly healed wound, the DEJ is flat and therefore more susceptible to shear forces, which may result in separation between the two layers and blistering.[12] Over time, the rete ridge pattern is restored during the remodeling phase of healing, accompanied by greater integrity between the layers. Newly reepithelialized skin should be protected from mechanical stress to allow for reestablishment of the morphology and structures of the DEJ.

Dermis

The dermis is a dense irregular connective tissue populated by fibroblasts and other connective tissue cells residing in an ECM composed of collagen, elastic fibers, glycosaminoglycans (GAGs), proteoglycans (PGs), and other minor components.[18] It is designed to maintain its integrity under an onslaught of physical forces and to provide metabolic and communicative support for the epidermis. Collagen types I and III and elastic fibers provide the skin with its tensile strength and elasticity, respectively, whereas GAGs and PGs bind water molecules to help create interfibrillar spaces for the transit of cells and molecules. More recent immunohistochemical studies and electron microscopic studies have revealed less abundant but structurally significant connective tissue components, including fibrillin and minor collagens and laminins.[19,20]

A vascular network runs through the dermis, with capillary loops terminating just below the basement membrane zone (see Figure 1).[21] Similarly, afferent sensory nerves and specialized nerve endings, end-bulbs or corpuscles, form an intricate network within the dermis (see Figure 1). There are also efferent autonomic nerve branches in all layers of the skin.[22] The dermis also harbors and supports epidermal appendages. Hair follicles have specialized vasculature and smooth muscle, the arrector pili muscle, as part of their dermal component. Facial skin is unique in that it has skeletal muscle and associated motoneurons in defined anatomic niches for voluntary movement and facial expression. The complex architecture of the dermis, established during embryonic development, is not readily regenerated after wounding and thus heals by an imperfect reparative process.[23,24]

Extracellular Matrix

Collagen types I and III, forming cross-linked fibrils of high tensile strength, are the predominant components of the dermis, with collagen types VI and VII and minor fibril-associated collagens comprising a small but functionally critical constituent.[19,25] Under normal conditions, collagen is a highly stable molecule with relatively low turnover, but following injury, it is synthesized by dermal fibroblasts through a complex intracellular and extracellular biosynthetic pathway, including post-translational modifications to facilitate cross-linking, to repair the connective tissue and restore structural integrity.[25] Elastic fibers, composed of elastin and other complex glycoproteins, make up a relatively small percentage of the dermis, about 2% of the total protein, but provide the skin with its elastic properties.[26] Elastin, like collagen, is a very stable molecule but, unlike collagen, is not readily resynthesized following injury or with aging; thus, scars are stiffer and exhibit less elasticity than normal skin.[27] Elastin production diminishes in adult skin and elastin is denatured by ultraviolet irradiation; thus, aging or photoaged (sun damaged) skin is less resilient owing to loss of dermal elastic fibers.[28]

GAGs and PGs form the ground substance of the dermis. GAGs are complex carbohydrates with sulfated and nonsulfated sugar components; PGs are composed of a protein core with GAG side chains. This family of macromolecules binds water and provides a gel-like environment between fibrillar matrix components. In skin, hyaluronic acid is the predominant free GAG, with chondroitin sulfate, dermatan sulfate, heparin, and heparin sulfate forming the GAG side chains of dermal PGs.[4] Versican and decorin are the major PGs in human skin, with GAG side chains of chondroitin sulfate and dermatan sulfate, respectively.[18–20] In addition to binding water and helping to regulate interfibrillar spatial architecture, these complex carbohydrates sequester several key growth factors important in the regulation of wound healing.[27]

Connective Tissue Cells

Fibroblasts are the predominant cell type in normal dermis, with resident mast cells and tissue macrophages being minor components.[4] As part of its barrier function, the skin is an immunologically active organ with SALT, composed of loosely organized aggregates of B and T lymphocytes.[1,29] During inflammatory processes, including the wound healing response, circulating leukocytes, primarily neutrophils and macrophages, rapidly enter the connective tissue by passing through the walls of postcapillary venules by a process called diapedesis.[30] Circulating fibrocytes, a distinct population of bloodborne cells of uncertain lineage, also enter the connective tissue by this route to participate in the wound healing response.[31,32]

Nerve Endings in the Skin

The skin has an important sensory and mechanoreceptor function with several specialized nerve endings and corpuscles, some of which are associated with hair follicles and sweat glands.[33] Motoneurons in the skin supply sweat glands, the arrector pili muscle of hair follicles, and adventitia of the microvasculature, as well as innervating facial skeletal muscles.[4,2]

Hypodermis

In humans, there is a layer of adipose tissue beneath the dermis, called the subcutis or hypodermis (see Figure 1). This soft tissue is a type of connective tissue composed primarily of adipocytes in close approximation with individual fibroblasts residing in the septa between adipocytes.[4] This layer provides a cushion and separates the dermis from underlying fascia, muscle, cartilage, and bone. There is experimental evidence that mesenchymal stem cells reside in adipose tissue and may be recruited to participate in dermal wound healing.[34] Adipocytes do not readily undergo mitosis, and the hypodermis is not regenerated following injury but is replaced by fibroblast-generated collagenous (scar) tissue, adding to the limitations of wound healing of connective tissue and compounding functional impairment.

WOUND HEALING

Cells from different layers of the skin respond to injury according to their regenerative capacity. Among the responding cells, there is a parallel, complex, and coordinated wound healing response, as summarized in the flow diagram in Figure 4. Tissue response to injury is a very important mechanism for survival. This wound healing response is achieved through basic cellular processes of cell movement, cell replication, and restoration of specialized function, which establish a new tissue equilibrium.

Tissue injury causes drastic changes in the local environment. Cells and ECM are damaged or lost, the blood supply is disturbed or disrupted, and there is at least a partial loss of function; in the case of skin, the barrier is compromised. These changes are detected by cells in the adjacent tissue. In response to injury, there is an orchestrated sequence of events:

Migration Cell movement or recommitment

Mitosis Cell proliferation

Maturation Restoration of specialized function

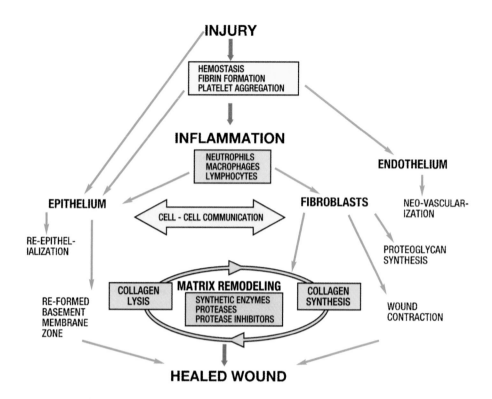

Figure 4. Schematic concept of wound healing. Following injury, the cells of the skin exhibit a complex but coordinated response in which the various tissue components, inflammatory cells, epithelium, connective tissue, and vasculature, become activated to counteract damage and restore function. Although this model was established by experimental and clinical studies in the skin, more recent evidence has shown that this basic scheme applies to wound healing in other organs with these tissue components. Adapted from Hunt TK et al.[23]

Epidermal Wound Healing

Basal keratinocytes are continually renewing under normal conditions. In response to injury, they have the capacity to regenerate by a regulated sequence of migration, mitosis, and maturation (Figure 5 and Table 1).

Epidermal migration is triggered by cytokines, growth factors, and other wound signals acting on basal keratinocytes in wound margins and within remnants of epidermal appendages, such as hair follicles and sweat glands.[12] Migrating epidermal cells undergo structural and functional changes to facilitate motility while retaining cell–cell associations to move as an epithelial sheet.[35] As healing progresses, some cells undergo mitosis to increase cell mass and replace tissue volume. Epithelialization continues to achieve complete resurfacing of the wound. Finally, the cells in the reepithelialized wound commit to terminal differentiation, undergoing a transient hypertrophy, and eventually reestablish the normal epidermal structure and barrier function.

The wound crust or scab, composed of remnants of the fibrinous clot, dead cells, and debris, remains adherent to the newly formed epithelium until re-formation of the stratum corneum, after which it detaches as part of normal epidermal desquamation. Premature loss or removal of this protective covering can result in reinjury of the healing epidermis. Coordination of degradative and regenerative processes requires a delicate balance of biochemical signaling and cellular responsiveness, which is mediated by local release of growth factors, cytokines, and chemokines, which may act in an autocrine or paracrine manner.[9]

Dermal Wound Healing

Acute Inflammatory Response

When an injury crosses the basement membrane into the dermis, there is usually damage to blood vessels that initiates a cascade of events (Figure 6):

1. Platelet-induced hemostasis is the stopping of blood flow by platelet release and aggregation followed by fibrin clot formation. The fibrin clot is the first provisional matrix for wound healing. Factors released from platelets and mast cells and fibrin-split products produce inflammation and edema.[24,35]

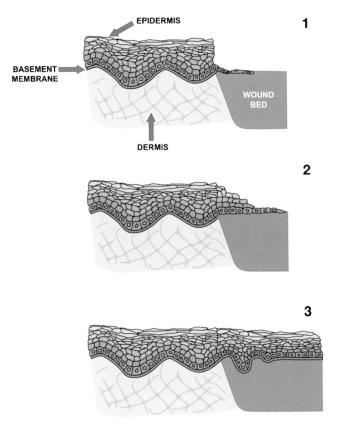

Figure 5. Epidermal wound healing. Injury to the epidermal layer induces epidermal keratinocytes to undergo a process of migration, mitosis, and maturation to reconstitute the epidermis and restore barrier function. See also Table 1 for the key events of each stage.

Table 1. PROCESS OF EPIDERMAL WOUND HEALING*	
Migration events	A. Decrease in desmosomes (cell–cell adhesion junctions)
	B. Increase in gap junctions (for cell–cell communication and coordination)
	C. Reorganization of actin cytoskeleton to form lamellipodia
	D. Altered expression of cell surface integrins Increased integrins for collagen type I and fibronectin Decreased integrin for laminin
	E. Increased secretion of proteases
	F. Temporary inhibition of mitosis in migrating cells
Mitosis events	A. Increased expression of growth factors and growth factor receptors
	B. Removal of mitosis inhibition
	C. Stratification of new epithelium (several cell layers)
	D. Increase in desmosomes
	E. Synthesis of basement membrane proteins— bullous pemphigoid antigen and collagen type IV
Maturation events	A. Stratification and differentiation of new epidermis
	B. Restored barrier function
	C. Re-formed basement membrane with hemidesmosomes
	D. Synthesis of basement membrane laminin, increased integrin for laminin
	E. Restoration of rete ridges, normal architecture with transient hypertrophy

*See Figure 5.

2. Circulating neutrophils are attracted to the site by chemokines. They adhere to endothelial cells and extravasate into the tissue. They rapidly phagocytose and destroy bacteria.
3. Monocytes are similarly attracted to the wound. They enter the tissue, are rapidly activated to become macrophages, and continue where the neutrophils left off. They phagocytose any remaining bacteria, as well as effete neutrophils and tissue debris. They release growth factors that serve as important signals for and mediators of wound healing. In macrophage-deficient animals, the wound healing process is delayed.[36]
4. Granulation tissue formation is induced by the inflammatory response. Granulation tissue is

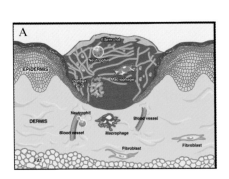
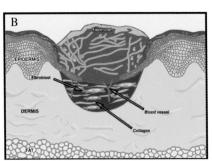
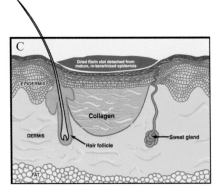

Figure 6. Overview of the wound healing response. The panels show progressive phases of wound healing. *A*, The early wound (day 2) exhibits many migratory responses. *B*, As healing progresses (day 4), there is evidence of mitosis in the several compartments. *C*, In the later stages of healing (day 14), the wound is maturing to establish a new homeostasis. Adapted from Singer AJ and Clark RAF.[24]

the second provisional matrix for wound healing, named for its granular appearance owing to abundant, newly formed blood vessels, which are a major component. Granulation tissue is a loose connective tissue containing blood vessels, macrophages, and fibroblasts but little Collagen. Granulation tissue forms beneath the dried, compacted fibrin clot (also called scab or crust) and under new epidermis. It serves as a scaffold for deposition of new collagen, the third and final matrix of dermal repair.[24]

Connective Tissue Repair

Granulation tissue formation is a provisional matrix formed of cells and blood vessels in a loose connective tissue with relatively little collagen. Blood cells extravasate from postcapillary venules into the tissue. Fibroblasts are recruited into this region by chemoattractants. Granulation tissue serves as a scaffold for fibroblast-mediated deposition of new collagenous connective tissue (Figure 7 and Table 2). A loose connective tissue that facilitates cell migration, granulation tissue provides a nutrient-rich environment for fibro-

Table 2. PROCESS OF DERMAL WOUND HEALING*	
1. Migration Events	A. Chemokines released in the wound diffuse into the surrounding tissue and recruit fibroblasts to migrate toward the wound bed
	B. Fibroblasts stimulated by growth factor and cytokine signals increase their expression of cell surface integrins
	C. Fibroblasts migrate along a path of extracellular matrix components guided by selective integrin expression
2. Mitosis Events	A. In the wound granulation tissue fibroblasts respond to growth factors and undergo mitosis
	B. Fibroblasts upregulate growth factor secretion for autoinduction
	C. Increased fibroblast density (fibroplasia) in the wound contributes to increased wound metabolism
3. Maturation Events	A. Active synthesis of extracellular matrix components, proteases and growth factors
	B. Increased actin microfilaments along membrane, formation of specialized cell-cell attachments (myofibroblasts) for coordinated wound contraction
	C. Decrease in fibroblast density, presumably by apoptosis, leads to decreased wound metabolism with maturation
	D. Extended remodeling of scar tissue over several months to a year, or longer

*See Figure 7

blast proliferation and production of new collagen. Granulation tissue is gradually replaced with a collagenous matrix, which becomes the mature connective tissue matrix of the healed wound. This new matrix, although functionally adequate, imperfectly restores the original tissue structural organization and function (Figure 8). Collagen production is the most prominent aspect of dermal repair—the apparent "default" program for connective tissue healing—but despite upregulation of collagen synthesis by fibroblasts and increased activity of matrix metalloproteinases (MMPs) for collagen remodeling, the functional outcome of collagen production, regain of tensile strength, is incomplete. Normally, full thickness dermal wounds heal with a maximal tensile strength of about 70% of that of uninjured skin.[37] Therefore, the healing process is reparative rather than regenerative, and the end result is fibrotic tissue or scar.

Dermal fibroblasts normally in a resting state become activated by early signals of injury. They migrate into the wound under the direction of chemotactic signals and contact guidance along

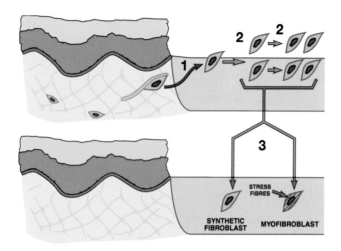

1. FIBROBLASTS INTO THE WOUND
2. SYNTHESIZING COLLAGENS AND OTHER ECM MOLECULES
3. FIBROBLASTS BECOME TWO DISTINCT TYPES

Figure 7. Dermal wound healing. Injury to the dermis induces an inflammatory response that triggers fibroblasts in the adjacent tissues to undergo a process of migration, mitosis, and maturation to repair the dermal connective tissue and restore structural integrity. See also Table 2 for the key events of each stage.

DERMAL WOUND HEALING

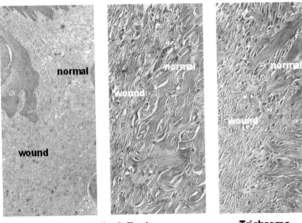

Hematoxylin & Eosin　　　　**Trichrome**

Figure 8. Dermal wound healing. The wound healing response of dermal connective tissue produces imperfect reconstruction of the extracellular matrix architecture, with the end result of collagenous scar tissue, as depicted in the microscopic images of wound margins above showing normal collagen fibril organization and wound tissue with smaller, more densely packed collagen fibrils (stained pink with hematoxylin and eosin and stained blue with trichrome stain) (×20 original magnification).

the ECM, attaching to binding sites on collagen and fibronectin in the tissue and wound.[35] Once in the wound bed, they proliferate in the granulation tissue, a transient process called fibroplasia, which generally occurs simultaneously with angiogenesis (see below). Then some of the fibroblasts recommit to the synthesis of collagen and other ECM molecules, whereas others undergo a morphologic transition to become myofibroblasts, a smooth muscle–like cell with prominent actin stress fibers.[38] These cells are associated with contraction and remodeling of the healing wound as it matures.[27,39] Fibroblasts also secrete MMPs, which degrade some of the newly formed collagen as part of the remodeling process. This elevated synthetic and digestive activity continues over a period of several weeks to months as new collagen fibers are integrated into the surrounding dermal matrix to increase tensile strength and improve structural integrity.[24,27,35]

Angiogenesis

The viability and metabolism of all tissues, including skin, depend on an adequate blood supply, which is disrupted by injury and must be restored as part of the healing process. Wound granulation tissue contains a rich blood supply to support the elevated tissue metabolic activity involved with wound healing. As healing proceeds and metabolic activity decreases, there is regression of angiogenesis through apoptosis to return to essentially normal blood vessel densities.[35]

Endothelial cells, like fibroblasts, become activated shortly after wounding. The disruption of blood supply and the higher metabolic activity in the wound contribute to a hypoxic environment that triggers an angiogenic response, so more vessels are formed from existing vessels in the wound margins.[23,35]

The process of angiogenesis is driven by the endothelial cells, which respond to changes in the wound environment and undergo first migration through areas in the blood vessel walls weakened by locally secreted proteases, and then mitosis of cells following the leading migratory edge into the wound tissue, producing numerous capillary buds that fuse to form capillary loops, thereby bringing a blood supply to the activated fibroblasts in the granulation tissue and to the keratinocytes undergoing reepithelialization. Third, the blood vessels mature and undergo regression, in coordination with the decreasing demands of the wound as it matures (Figure 9 and Table 3).

Wound Healing Process

It is important to bear in mind that the events described above, although discussed individually, occur in simultaneous or overlapping time frames. Wound healing is a complex, dynamic process dependent on the coordinated activities of multiple cell types in the epithelium, connective tissue, and vasculature (see Figure 4). Although still incompletely understood, there clearly is intercommunication among the cells in different tissue compartments that helps regulate the normal healing process and that involves the production of both "start" and "stop" signaling mediators.

One example of a stop signal mechanism is the laminin of the epidermal basement mem-

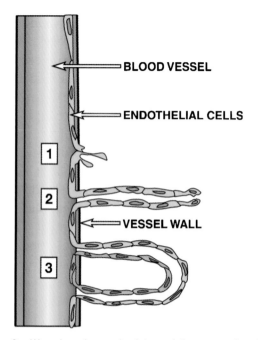

Figure 9. Wound angiogenesis. Injury of the connective tissue includes damage of the vascular supply. The resulting inflammatory response and relative tissue hypoxia induce endothelial cells in vessels in the adjacent tissue (wound margins) to undergo a process of migration, mitosis, and maturation to bring vessels and a blood supply into the wound bed. As wound healing progresses and metabolic demand decreases, there is regression of new vessels toward a more normal density. See also Table 3 for the key events of each stage.

brane. It is one of the last components to be resynthesized and has the effect of inhibiting epidermal cell migration,[40] whereas collagen and

fibronectin in the wound bed strongly stimulate migration.[41] Another example, occurring later in the healing process, is the production of chemokines by maturing endothelial cells and keratinocytes (Interferon-gamma-inducible proteins (IP)-10 and IP-9, respectively) that block growth factor–induced deadhesion of motile fibroblasts.[42,43] This causes the fibroblasts to rechannel intracellular contractility from locomotion to matrix remodeling,[44] which contributes to the dermal maturation process.

Limits of Wound Repair

Destroyed connective tissue is replaced by scar tissue. This imperfect wound repair process results in loss of the normal complement of elastin, PGs, epidermal appendages, subcutaneous fat, muscle, and nerve. Repeated tissue injury and certain chronic diseases cause a continuation of tissue repair that can lead to pathologic fibrosis, as in the case of keloids in the skin.[27] This can also occur in other organs; tissue fibrosis is the general condition in which specialized tissue components (parenchyma) are gradually replaced by collagenous connective tissue (stroma). Eventually, there is loss of specialized function and, ultimately, organ failure.

Table 3. PROCESS OF DERMAL WOUND ANGIOGENESIS*	
1. Migration Events	A. Tissue injury causes plasma leak from vessel, amplified by fibronectin fragments, fibroblast growth factor, heparin.
	B. Plasminogen activator and plasminogen leak into the tissue, plasminogen is converted to plasmin (active protease).
	C. Plasmin converts latent collagenase to active collagenase.
	D. Collagenase attacks the basement membrane surrounding capillaries.
	E. Endothelial cells release proteases that help break down the adjacent basement membrane.
	F. Endothelial cells migrate through weak spots in the basement membrane in response to chemotactic agents including fibronectin fragments, fibroblast growth factor (FGF) and vascular endothelial cell growth factor (VEGF).
2. Mitosis Events	A. At the vessel margins endothelial cells proliferate in response to VEGF, FGF, insulin-like growth factors (IGFs) and other growth factors in the wound bed.
	B. Endothelial cells release growth factors for autoinduction.
	C. Capillary buds are abundant in granulation tissue (hypertrophy).
3. Maturation Events	A. Capillary buds join to form capillary loops, re-establishing circulatory pathways.
	B. Remodeling results in a net decrease and regression of blood vessels toward a normal density. The mechanism by which this process occurs is not fully understood, but is believed to be triggered by increased levels of oxygen in the tissue and to occur by means of apoptosis.
	C. Metabolic demands of the tissue are coordinately decreased.

*See Figure 9

The kidney, liver, and lungs are especially vulnerable to functional loss by fibrosis.[45]

Interestingly, many fibrotic diseases have been linked to abnormalities in the expression or activity of transforming growth factor β (TGF-β). TGF-β is a key cytokine for the initiation and termination of normal wound healing.[45] It is sometimes called the master growth factor because it modulates the effects of other growth factors and cytokines. The sustained production of TGF-β leads to tissue fibrosis.[45,46] Neutralizing antibodies to TGF-β_1 reduce scarring, whereas TGF-β_1-deficient mice show severely impaired late-stage healing (the remodeling or maturation phase).[47,48]

Yet TGF-β is only part of the story. Regulation of the inflammatory response with respect to fibrosis has also been examined. Interleukin-10 (IL-10) is thought to play a major role in limiting and terminating the inflammatory response. The temporal restriction of inflammation is critical for normal wound healing because many inflammatory mediators and products that help remove bacteria and dead cells and tissues are detrimental to tissue reconstruction.[49] Recent studies have found that the addition of IL-10 neutralizing antibodies to experimental wounds in animals increases infiltration of neutrophils and macrophages, effectively prolonging inflammation.[50]

FETAL WOUND HEALING

The early-gestation mammalian fetus has the capacity to heal full-thickness skin wounds scarlessly and regeneratively.[51] This observation has triggered an extensive exploration of this phenomenon to understand the underlying mechanism(s) with the hope of finding new therapeutic solutions for scarring.[27] Scarless fetal healing has been studied from several angles, focusing on the fetal environment and the fetal cells and tissues. It is now fairly well accepted that the fetal environment alone is not the driving force and that fetal cells are crucial to the process and are poised in a unique environment. When fetal skin is injured, the cascade of events is markedly different from postnatal wound repair. One key difference is the minimal inflammatory response.[52] In addition, there are differences in the complement of soluble mediators and in the cellular response to these signals. Taken together, the outcome is regenerative healing.

Absence of Fibrosis

Among growth factors, TGF-β has been the most extensively studied in fetal wound healing. There are three TGF-β isoforms in humans: TGF-β1, -β_2, and –β_3. TGF-β_1 is the most abundant form and is responsible for increased collagen synthesis by fibroblasts and decreased collagen degradation by MMPs.[24,45,46] Relative to adult wounds, fetal wounds have little messenger ribonucleic acid and protein levels of TGF-β_1.[27] Exogenous TGF-β_1 added to fetal wounds produces fibrotic healing (scarring); therefore, it has been proposed that the absence of TGF-β_1 in fetal wounds is important for the scarless fetal wound healing.[53]

More recently, fetal skin has been found to have higher levels of TGF-β_3. In experimental studies, a high ratio of TGF-β_3 to TGF-β_1 was found to be associated with scarless healing, suggesting that relative proportions of these two isoforms may be a determining factor; furthermore, it was reported that treating wounds with TGF-β_3 have shown increased rates of healing and reduced wound fibrosis.[54] However, this antifibrotic effect of TGF-β_3 was not reproduced by another group using a different animal wound healing model.[55]

TGF-β receptor expression also changes during both development and wound repair. In fetal rat skin, of the three TGF-β receptors, R-I and R-II expression decreases and R-III expression remains unchanged during the gestational transition from fetal to adult healing phenotype.[27] During fetal wound healing, R-I decreased in scarless wound healing but not after the transition to adult-type healing, whereas R-II showed little change in scarless fetal wounds but a large increase following the transition to adult-type healing. One suggested interpretation is that less efficient signal transduction may occur in the scarless fetal wound.

Furthermore, fibromodulin and decorin, two ECM molecules that modulate TGF-β activity in situ, each undergo changes in tissue levels during the transition from fetal to adult-type healing.[56,57] Therefore, it seems that differential expression of TGF-β isoforms, receptors, and activity modulators, rather than the mere presence or absence of TGF-β, may determine the scarless fetal wound healing phenotype.

Reduced Inflammation

In studies with IL-10 knockout mice, fetal skin wound healing was found to be altered in the absence of IL-10, with significantly higher amounts of inflammatory cells, increased collagen deposition, and abnormal, scar-like organization, resembling the pattern of adult wound healing.[58] These results suggest an important role for IL-10 in the control of inflammation and the significance of suppressed inflammation for the regenerative wound healing phenotype.

Recently, prostaglandin E_2 (PGE$_2$) was studied for its contribution to healing. Differential expression of the receptors for PGE$_2$ was reported in fetal rabbit wounds compared with postnatal wounds, suggesting a mechanism for divergent responses to this key inflammatory signal.[59] Fetal dermal fibroblasts were also found to be partially refractory to the effects of PGE$_2$.[60] Taken together, these findings may have significant and specific relevance to the scarless fetal wound healing phenotype.

STEM CELLS FOR CUTANEOUS WOUND HEALING

Our understanding of wound repair and tissue regeneration has been radically changed by recent discoveries of stem cell plasticity and of dedifferentiation of supposedly determined cells in both animals and humans.[61,62] Stem cells, exhibiting the capacity for self-renewal over the lifetime of the organism, have been found in various tissues throughout the body, and some have been isolated

for further study. Epidermal stem cells have been shown to have a regenerative capacity for the healing of minor or simple injury, as in pure epidermal wounds, the most prominent clinical use being the culture of confluent epithelial sheets that can be gently removed from the culture dish and applied to reconstitute the epithelial portion of burns, chronic wounds, and ulcers.[11] However, this technology falls short of the mark in more extensive or complex wounds; in full-thickness wounds covered with epidermal autografts, the pattern of epidermal differentiation is abnormal and the neodermis that forms beneath the epidermal sheet is lacking in structural elements that contribute to tissue integrity.[63] Nonetheless, this regenerative capacity of stem cells, present even in the tissues of adults, is a promising area for further exploration and clinical applications.[11,61,62]

Exploration of the potential use of stem cells for true regenerative healing is ongoing. Several sources of stem cells have been identified. These include cells from the early embryo or embryonic stem cells that have the potential for development along multiple differentiation pathways. In addition, there are fetal stem cells (isolated from fetal membranes, umbilical cord, cord blood) and adult stem cells (from several different tissue compartments, including bone marrow, muscle, epidermis, and others).[61] Adult stem cells have received the greatest attention in wound healing research, with the potential for autologous donor cell applications.[64]

Seemingly, these mechanisms should provide our bodies with intrinsic regenerative healing powers. Yet failure to achieve just that is among the most pressing problems of modern medicine. Apparently, counterbalancing forces have evolved that prevent the orderly replacement of lost cells. Moreover, the basic mechanisms of stem cell differentiation that lead to the formation of solid organ tissue are still not completely understood. The present challenge for regenerative medicine is to unravel those barriers and find ways to overcome them. One approach that may hold future promise is the combining of stem cells with bioengineered scaffolds implanted for tissue engineering in situ.[65]

COMMON WOUND HEALING PROBLEMS AND CONDITIONS

Inflammation and the inflammatory response can be considered to be a double-edged sword in the wound environment. It plays an important role in protection against microorganisms and the removal of tissue debris. Growth factors, enzymes, and other regulatory mediators released by inflammatory cells help advance the healing process. However, prolonged inflammation can be detrimental, producing mediators, such as proteases, at the wrong time and place that can disrupt healing and lead to either fibrotic or impaired healing.

As already discussed, scarring and fibrosis are the normal outcome in postnatal wounds, with collagen type I being the predominant component of the scar, taking the place of less readily produced components, such as elastic fibers, minor collagens, PGs, and adipose tissue. In addition, hyper- and hypopigmentation may result from the angiogenetic process.

Keloids and hypertrophic scars (earlobe keloids, burn hypertrophic scars, acne keloids) are infrequent but concerning healing outcomes in susceptible individuals. These result in marked and potentially progressive fibrosis of the wound and surrounding tissue in the case of keloids. Management of these types of wounds is difficult as there are no ideal antifibrotic therapies.

Wound contracture is a result of late-stage remodeling and can be particularly problematic on the face if it causes distortion of the facial features. For surgical procedures that involve full-thickness wounding, the facial anatomy must be taken into account for optimal cosmesis.[66]

Chronic wounds may result from a variety of etiologies. In the head and neck region, these may arise following breakdown of surgical incisions in tissues that have received radiation to reduce the size of tumors.

Aging skin should be considered as potentially having two components that contribute to its healing properties, chronologic aging and actinic or photoaging caused by ultraviolet irradiation damage. It is clear that there are differences in wound healing that come with aging, including a diminished inflammatory response and subsequently reduced activities in migratory, mitotic, and maturation responses, all of which contribute to slower healing,[67] and all of which can be compounded by various pathologic conditions, such as diabetes. A slower regain of tensile strength has been reported in older individuals, documented by a markedly higher rate of wound dehiscence.[68] It seems that there is also a decreased fibrosis owing to this overall attenuated response, so once the wound heals, there is less fibrosis. At the other extreme, young skin in the pediatric patient heals quickly and exuberantly under normal conditions.

FACTORS THAT INFLUENCE WOUND HEALING

A multitude of biologic signals help regulate the delicate balance of the wound healing response. They may induce migration by chemotaxis or pathway guidance, or they may stop migration. They may be on or off signals for mitosis. They may also suppress or induce differentiation of the target cell. The response or set of responses that they invoke depends on the target cell, its state of receptivity, and the local tissue environment, including other factors. Additionally, their effects depend on their spatial and temporal expression in the wound; being in the right place at the right time is critically important in determining outcome.

Approaches to good wound care should include the following considerations: supporting the normal healing process, supplementing healing, reducing scar formation, and promoting regeneration to restore function. The culmination of wound healing research and evidence-based clinical practice has identified exogenous factors and interventions that can affect the rate of healing, outcome of healing, or both. These approaches are addressed in other chapters of this book.

REFERENCES

1. Streilein JW. Skin-associated lymphoid tissue (SALT): origins and functions. J Invest Dermatol 1983;80:12s–6s.

2. Bentsianov B, Blitzer A. Facial anatomy. Clin Dermatol 2004;22:3–13.

3. Grove GL, Kligman AM. Age-associated changes in human epidermal cell renewal. J Gerontol 1983;38:137–42.

4. Odland GF. Structure of the skin. In: Goldsmith LA, editor. Physiology, biochemistry, and molecular biology of the skin. 2nd ed. New York: Oxford University Press; 1991. p. 3–62.

5. Allison JP, Havran WL. The immunobiology of T cells with invariant gamma delta antigen receptors. Annu Rev Immunol 1991;9:679–705.

6. Jameson J, Ugarte K, Chen N, et al. A role for skin γδT cells in wound repair. Science 2002;296:747–9.

7. Born WK, O'Brien RL. The healing touch of epidermal T cells. Nat Med 2002;8:560–1.

8. Mackool RJ, Gittes GK, Longaker MT. Scarless healing. The fetal wound. Clin Plast Surg 1998;25:357–65.

9. Hebda PA, Sandulache VC. The biochemistry of epidermal healing. In: Rovee DT, Maibach HI, editors. The epidermis in wound healing. Boca Raton (FL): CRC Press; 2004. p. 59–86.

10. Cummings CW, Flint PW, Harker LA, et al. Cummings Otolaryngology: Head & Neck Surgery, 4th ed. Elsevier Mosby, Philadelphia 2004. ISBN: 0323019854.

11. Alonso L, Fuchs E. Stem cells of the skin epithelium. Proc Natl Acad Sci U S A 2003;100 Suppl 1:11830–5.

12. Winter GD. Epidermal regeneration studied in the domestic pig. In: Maibach HI, Rovee DT, editors. Epidermal wound healing. Chicago: Year Book Medical Publishers; 1971. p. 71–112.

13. Stenn KS, Malhotra R. Epithelialization. In: Cohen IK, Diegelmann RF, Lindblad WJ, editors. Wound healing. Biochemical and clinical aspects., Philadelphia: W.B. Saunders; 1992. p. 115–27.

14. Uitto J, Pulkkinen L. Molecular complexity of the cutaneous basement membrane zone. Mol Biol Rep 1996;23:35–46.

15. Woodley DT, Briggaman RA. Re-formation of the epidermal-dermal junction during wound healing. In: Clark RAF, Henson PM, editors. The molecular and cellular biology of wound repair. New York: Plenum Press; 1988. p. 559–86.

16. Demarchez M, Hartmann DJ, Herbage D, et al. Wound healing of human skin transplanted onto the nude mouse. II. An immunohistological and ultrastructural study of the epidermal basement membrane zone reconstruction and connective tissue reorganization. Dev Biol 1987;121:119–29.

17. Chetty BV, Boissy RE, Warden GD, Nordlund JJ. Basement membrane and fibroblast aberration in blisters at the donor, graft, and spontaneously healed sites in patients with burns. Arch Dermatol 1992;128:181–6.

18. Uitto J, Olsen DR, Fazio MJ. Extracellular matrix of the skin: 50 years of progress. J Invest Dermatol 1989;92:61S–77S.

19. Keene DR, Marinkovich MP, Sakai LY. Immunodissection of the connective tissue matrix in human skin. Microsc Res Tech 1997;38:394–406.

20. Kielty CM, Shuttleworth A. Microfibrillar elements of the dermal matrix. Microsc Res Tech 1997;38:413–27.

21. Singh S, Swerlick RA. Structure and function of the cutaneous vasculature. In: Freinkel RK, Woodley DT, editors. The biology of the skin. New York: Parthenon; 2001. p. 177–89.

22. Metze D, Luger T. Nervous system in the skin. In: Freinkel RK, Woodley DT, editors. The biology of the skin. New York: Parthenon; 2001. p. 153–76.

23. Hunt TK, Knighton DR, Thakral KK, et al. Cellular control of repair. In: Hunt TK, Heppenstall RB, Pines E, Rovee D, editors. Soft and hard tissue repair: biological and clinical aspects. New York: Praeger; 1984. p. 3–19.

24. Singer AJ, Clark RAF. Cutaneous wound healing. N Engl J Med 1999;341:738–46.

25. Diegelmann RF. Collagen metabolism. Wounds 2001;13:177–82.

26. Uitto J, Paul JL, Brockley K, et al. Elastic fibers in human skin. Quantitation of elastic fibers by computerized digital image analyses and determination of elastin by radioimmunoassay of desmosine. Lab Invest 1983;49:499–505.

27. Lorenz HP, Longaker MT. Wound healing: repair biology and wound and scar treatment. In: Mathes SJ, editor. Plastic surgery. 2nd ed. Vol 1. Philadephia: Saunders Elsevier; 2006. p. 209–34.

28. El-Domyati M, Attia S, Saleh F, et al. Intrinsic aging vs. photoaging: a comparative histopathological, immuno-histochemical, and ultrastructural study of skin. Exp Dermatol 2002;11:398–405.

29. Olszewski WL, Grzelak I, Ziolkowska A, Engeset A. Immune cell traffic from blood through the normal human skin to lymphatics. Clin Dermatol 1995;13:473–83.

30. Kanzler MH, Gorsulowsky DC, Swanson NA. Basic mechanisms in the healing cutaneous wound. J Dermatol Surg Oncol 1986;12:1156–64.

31. Bucala R, Spiegel LA, Chesney J, et al. Circulating fibrocytes define a new leukocyte subpopulation that mediates tissue repair. Mol Med 1994;1:71–81.

32. Abe R, Donnelly SC, Peng T, et al. Peripheral blood fibrocytes: differentiation pathway and migration to wound sites. J Immunol 2001;166:7556–62.

33. Hamann W. Mammalian cutaneous mechanoreceptors. Prog Biophys Mol Biol 1995;64:81–104.

34. De Ugarte DA, Morizono K, Elbarbary A, et al. Comparison of multi-lineage cells from human adipose tissue and bone marrow. Cells Tissues Organs 2003;174:101–9.

35. Clark RAF. Overview and general considerations of wound repair. In: Clark RAF, Henson PM, editors. The molecular and cellular biology of wound repair. New York: Plenum Press; 1988. p. 3–33.

36. Leibovich SJ, Ross R. The role of the macrophage in wound repair. A study with hydrocortisone and antimacrophage serum. Am J Pathol 1975;78:71–100.

37. Levenson SM, Geever EF, Crowley LV, et al. The healing of rat skin wounds. Ann Surg 1965;161:293–308.

38. Gabbiani G, Lelous M, Bailkey AJ, Delauney A. Collagen and myofibroblasts of granulation tissue. A chemical, ultrastructural and immunologic study. Virchows Arch 1976;21:133–45.

39. Darby I, Skalli O, Gabbiani G. Alpha-smooth muscle actin is transiently expressed by myofibroblasts during experimental wound healing. Lab Invest 1990;63:21–9.

40. Woodley DT, Bachmann PM, O'Keefe EJ. Laminin inhibits human keratinocyte migration. J Cell Physiol 1988;136:140–6.

41. Guo M, Toda K, Grinnell F. Activation of human keratinocyte migration on type I collagen and fibronectin. J Cell Sci 1990;96(Pt 2):197–205.

42. Shiraha H, Glading A, Gupta K, Wells A. IP-10 inhibits epidermal growth factor-induced motility by decreasing epidermal growth factor receptor-mediated calpain activity. J Cell Biol 1999;146:243–53.

43. Satish L, Yager D, Wells A. Glu-Leu-Arg-negative CXC chemokine interferon gamma inducible protein-9 as a mediator of epidermal-dermal communication during wound repair. J Invest Dermatol 2003;120:1110–7.

44. Allen FD, Asnes CF, Chang P, et al. Epidermal growth factor induces acute matrix contraction and subsequent calpain-modulated relaxation. Wound Repair Regen 2002;10:67–76.

45. Border WA, Noble NA. Transforming growth factor beta in tissue fibrosis. N Engl J Med 1994;331:1286–92.

46. Blobe GC, Schiemann WP, Lodish HF. Role of transforming growth factor beta in human disease. N Engl J Med 2000;342:1350–8.

47. Shah M, Foreman DM, Ferguson MW. Neutralising antibody to TGF-β 1, 2 reduces cutaneous scarring in adult rodents. J Cell Sci 1994;107:1137–57.

48. Crowe MJ, Doetschman T, Greenhalgh DG. Delayed wound healing in immunodeficient TGF-beta 1 knockout mice. J Invest Dermatol 2000;115:3–11.

49. Haslett C, Henson PM. Resolution of inflammation. In: Clark RAF, Henson PM, editors. The molecular and cellular biology of wound repair. New York: Plenum Press; 1988. p. 185–211.

50. Sato Y, Ohshima T, Kondo T. Regulatory role of endogenous interleukin-10 in cutaneous inflammatory response of murine wound healing. Biochem Biophys Res Commun 1999;265:194–9.

51. Lorenz HP, Longaker MT, Perkocha LA, et al. Scarless wound repair: a human fetal skin model. Development 1992;114:253–9.

52. Cowin AJ, Brosnan MP, Holmes TM, Ferguson MW. Endogenous inflammatory response to dermal wound healing in the fetal and adult mouse. Dev Dyn 1998;212:385–93.

53. Sullivan KM, Lorenz HP, Meuli M, et al. A model of scarless human fetal wound repair is deficient in transforming growth factor beta. J Pediatr Surg 1995;30:198–203.

54. Shah M, Foreman DM, Ferguson MWJ. Neutralisation of TGF-b1 and TGF-b2 or exogenous addition of TGF-b3 to cutaneous rat wounds reduces scarring. J Cell Sci 1995;108:985–1002.

55. Wu L, Siddiqui A, Morris DE, et al. Transforming growth factor β3 (TGFβ3) accelerates wound healing without alteration of scar prominence: histologic and competitive reverse-transcription-polymerase chain reaction studies. Arch Surg 1997;132:753–60.

56. Soo C, Hu FY, Zhang X, et al. Differential expression of fibromodulin, a transforming growth factor-beta modulator, in fetal skin development and scarless repair. Am J Pathol 2000;157:423–33.

57. Beanes SR, Dang C, Soo C, et al. Down-regulation of decorin, a transforming growth factor-beta modulator, is associated with scarless fetal wound healing. J Pediatr Surg 2001;36:1666–71.

58. Liechty KW, Kim HB, Adzick NS, Crombleholme TM. Fetal wound repair results in scar formation in interleukin-10-deficient mice in a syngeneic murine model of scarless fetal wound repair. J Pediatr Surg 2000;35:866–72; discussion 872–3.

59. Li HS, Hebda PA, Kelly LA, et al. Upregulation of prostaglandin EP4 receptor messenger RNA in fetal rabbit skin wound. Arch Otolaryngol Head Neck Surg 2000;126:1337–43.

60. Sandulache VC, Parekh A, Li-Korotky HS, et al. Prostaglandin E2 differentially modulates human fetal and adult dermal fibroblast migration and contraction: implication for wound healing. Wound Repair Regen 2006;14:633–43.

61. Körbling M, Estrov Z. Adult stem cells for tissue repair—a new therapeutic concept? N Engl J Med 2003;349:570–82.

62. van Bekkum DW. Phylogenetic aspects of tissue regeneration: role of stem cells: a concise overview. Blood Cells Mol Dis 2004;32:11–6.

63. Petersen MJ, Lessane B, Woodley DT. Characterization of cellular elements in healed cultured keratinocyte autografts used to cover burn wounds. Arch Dermatol 1990;126:175–80.

64. Harty M, Neff AW, King MW, Mescher AL. Regeneration or scarring: an immunologic perspective. Dev Dyn 2003;226:268–79.

65. Caplan AI. In vivo remodeling. Ann N Y Acad Sci 2002;961:307–8.

66. Zitelli JA. Wounds healing by secondary intention. J Am Acad Dermatol 1983;9:407–15.

67. Eaglstein WH. Wound healing and aging. Dermatol Clin 1986;4:481–4.

68. Mendoza CB, Postlethwait RW, Johnson WD. Incidence of wound disruption following operation. Arch Surg 1970;101:396–8.

2

Facial Bones

Jack Yu, MD; Robert Dinsmore, MD

ANATOMY

Craniofacial anatomy is traditionally divided into three regions: the upper third, consisting of the frontal bone; the middle third, consisting of the orbits, zygoma, maxilla, and nasal bones; and the lower third, consisting of the mandible. However, when treating facial fractures, it is often more useful to think in terms of function rather than location. The two approaches result in the same divisions, but the conceptual framework of form following function allows for a fuller appreciation of the interrelationships between regions and consequently results in a more comprehensive and refined treatment plan. For this reason, we first discuss facial anatomy from a functional aspect and then discuss each region in detail.

The skull can be thought of as two functional territories, the cranium and the facial skeleton. The cranium consists of those bones that house and protect the brain, that is, the frontal, occipital, sphenoid, ethmoid, and paired temporal and parietal bones. The facial skeleton can, in turn, be broken down into several functional subcomponents. The mandible functions as a class III lever to apply the crushing and grinding forces of mastication. The maxilla functions as an anvil to oppose these forces. The remaining bones of the midface have three functions: (1) to position the maxilla in apposition to the mandible and to distribute the masticatory forces to the base of the skull, (2) to position and protect the eye, and (3) to allow for inhalation and humidification of the air when the mouth is closed.

These three functions are achieved by a system of buttresses, which also determine facial height, width, and projection. Midface height is determined by three vertical buttresses: the central buttress projecting around the piriform aperture to the frontomaxillary suture and two lateral buttresses projecting from the lateral maxilla through the zygoma to the zygomatico-frontal suture. The vertical buttresses serve to position the maxilla and to distribute the masticatory forces across the base of the skull. Lower facial height is determined by the mandibular rami, which is of pivotal importance to proper dental occlusion. Facial width is determined by the frontal bar superiorly and the width of the mandible inferiorly. In the midface, facial width is determined by the maxillary width and the horizontal buttress extending laterally from the maxilla through the zygoma to the zygomatic process of the temporal bone (Figures 1 and 2). Midface projection is determined by the anterior-posterior positioning of the maxilla. Maxillary positioning is established by the horizontal buttress of the zygomatic arch, the vertical buttresses, and the interface of the maxilla with the base of the skull through the palatine and sphenoid bones.

Frontal Anatomy

The frontal bone extends anteriorly from its interface with the parietal bones at the coronal suture and comprises the upper third of the face. Inferiorly, it turns inward to form the roof of the orbit. The vertical buttresses of the face intercept

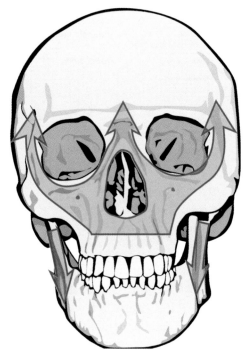

Figure 1. Vertical facial buttresses.

the base of the frontal bone at the maxillofrontal and zygomaticofrontal sutures. Within the orbit, the inferior portion of the frontal bone interfaces medially with the superior portion of the lacrimal bone and the cribriform plate of the ethmoid

bone and posteriorly with both the greater and lesser wings of the sphenoid bone.

Along the inferior aspect, before turning in to form the orbital roof, the frontal bone forms the supraorbital ridge. This ridge defines the facial width in the upper third of the face. Laterally, it is rigid and quite resistant to fracture. When it is fractured, the injury pattern tends toward large fragments, which can be precisely reduced. Once reduced, fragments tend to be stable as there are no significant muscular forces on them. Centrally, beginning between ages 3 and 7 years, the frontal sinuses develop. Although still quite resistant to fracture, the frontal sinuses when fractured have a more comminuted pattern than the lateral portions of the supraorbital ridge. The frontal sinus is drained on each side by the frontonasal duct. The frontonasal duct extends from the inferomedial portion of the sinus into the middle meatus, behind the middle concha of the nose. Injury to this outflow tract results in frontal sinusitis, mucocele, and/or mucopyocele and can progress to meningitis and frontal abscess owing to its close proximity to the frontal lobe.

Orbital Anatomy

The orbit is a four-sided pyramidal structure with the optical canal at its apex. The orbital rim is quadrangular in shape. The frontal bone comprises the superior third, the maxillary bone the medial-inferior third, and the zygoma the lateral-inferior third. The orbital rim does not form a plane but rather an inward spiral. Beginning at the inferomedial rim, the maxilla continues laterally with the zygoma and superiorly to the frontal bone. The superior orbital rim continues medially and ends with the medial portion of the frontal bone in continuity with the posterior crest of the lacrimal bone, which lies just posterior to the maxillary start point. The fossa of the lacrimal sac rests between these two crests. The orbit at the rim is approximately 35 mm in height and 40 mm in width. The orbital depth varies from 45 to 55 mm, as measured to the orbital

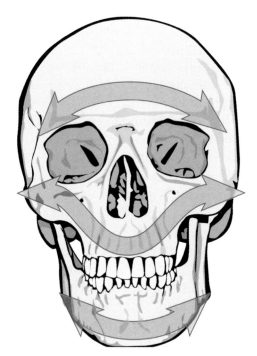

Figure 2. Horizontal facial buttresses.

strut located between the optic foramen and the superior orbital fissure.

Working from the orbital rim toward the apex, the maximal safe depth of dissection varies. For dissection along the medial wall, this distance is approximately 30 mm, as measured from the maxillary rim. The same distance applies for the roof of the orbit. Laterally and inferiorly, however, this distance is limited to 25 mm.[1] Along the superomedial wall, there are two landmarks that aid in determining the depth of safe dissection: the anterior and posterior ethmoidal foramina. The anterior ethmoidal foramen is located approximately 17 to 20 mm from the orbital rim, and the posterior ethmoidal foramen is located just 5 to 7 mm anterior to the optic foramen, approximately 30 mm from the orbital rim.

The roof of the orbit is formed by the orbital plate of the frontal bone. The floor of the orbit is formed by the orbital plate of the maxilla, with a small contribution by the zygoma. Within the orbital plate of the maxilla lies the infraorbital groove, which leads from the inferior orbital fissure to the infraorbital foramen and is the path of the infraorbital nerve (cranial nerve V2). The strong lateral wall is formed by the frontal process of the zygoma and, near the apex, by the greater wing of the sphenoid bone.

The medial wall is formed most superficially by the maxilla, where it is quite strong. However, the medial wall quickly becomes paper thin as it continues deeper into the orbit. Starting at the orbital rim and moving toward the apex of the orbit, the maxilla is located most superficially and is followed by the lacrimal bone, which is, in turn, followed by the orbital plate of the ethmoid bone, also known as the "lamina papyracea." Just beyond the ethmoid is found the diminutive orbital process of the palatine bone. The apex of the orbit is formed by the lesser wing of the sphenoid bone. The lesser wing of the sphenoid houses the optic canal and is separated from the greater wing by the superior orbital fissure (Figure 3). The superior orbital fissure conducts cranial nerves III, IV, V1, and VI and the ophthalmic vein. Injury to these structures results in superior orbital fissure syndrome, a constella-

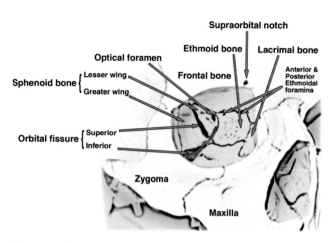

Figure 3. Orbital anatomy.

tion of symptoms consisting of ptosis of the eyelid, proptosis of the globe, and paralysis of cranial nerves III, IV, and VI with anesthesia in the first division of the trigeminal nerve. When these symptoms are accompanied by blindness in the affected eye, the condition is termed *orbital apex syndrome.*

Midface Anatomy

The zygoma is a major "connector" of the facial skeleton in all three major planes, uniting the frontal bone anterior-superiorly, the maxilla medically and inferiorly, and the temporal bone posteriorly. In the sagittal plane, it contributes to the anterior projection. In the coronal plane, it contributes to the facial height. In the axial plane, it defines the midfacial width, also known as bizygomatic width. Structurally, it is very strong as such fractures commonly involve the sutural connections. Horizontally, it extends from the zygomatic process of the temporal bone and forms the lateral and inferior thirds of the orbital rim before interfacing with the zygomatic process of the frontal bone superiorly and with the maxilla inferiorly and medially. Sometimes incorrectly referred to as a tripod, the zygoma is actually a tetrapod. The zygomaticotemporal suture and zygomaticofrontal suture legs are obvious. The zygomaticomaxillary suture, however, is not one leg but two. The inferior orbital rim is formed by dense bone, as is the inferior margin of the zygoma. Between these regions is the maxillary sinus, and the bone overlying it is quite thin. The zygoma has two foramina, conducting the zygomaticotemporal and zygomaticofacial branches of the second division of cranial nerve V. It is important to emphasize that the zygoma is the primary determinant of facial width and projection. In general, proper reduction requires reestablishment of its anatomic alignment and secure fixation in three of the four legs.

The maxilla comprises the major portion of the midface. This bone is essentially hollow, with a honeycombed structure designed to withstand and distribute the compressive forces of mastication without excessive weight. It forms the medial and inferior portions of the orbital floor, where it conducts the infraorbital branch of the second division of cranial nerve V via the infraorbital foramen. From the middle portion of the orbital rim, it extends obliquely outward and inferiorly to a point almost directly inferior to the lateral orbital rim. Medially, it surrounds the piriform aperture, and inferiorly, it forms the maxillary plate. The maxillary plate at its periphery is thickened to form the alveolar process containing the 16 dental alveoli that correspond to those of the mandible, housing 16 teeth: 2 incisors, 1 canine, 2 premolars, and 3 molars on each side, in the unaltered adult. Anteriorly, masticatory forces are directed superiorly, around the piriform aperture to the maxillofrontal suture, dissipating into the cranium. Laterally, they are directed via the zygoma to the zygomaticofrontal suture, again ending at the cranium.

In the central midline of the face is the pear-shaped opening, the piriform aperture. At the apex of the piriform aperture, medial to the frontal process of the maxilla, are the paired nasal bones. Owing to their anteriorly projecting position, these two small bones are the most frequently injured of all facial bones. In the midline within the piriform aperture, the ethmoid gives off a perpendicular plate, the ethmoidal plate, which is contiguous with the septal cartilage anteriorly and the perpendicular plate of the vomer inferiorly. The vomer, a plowshare-shaped bone, extends from the sphenoid bone to the maxillary crest of the maxillary plate ante-

riorly and the palatine bone posteriorly. A large portion of the vomer and ethmoid is thin and complex; these bones are frequently fractured and almost never amenable to open reduction and screw/plate fixation. Along the medial orbital wall, from external to deep, lie the nasal and maxillary processes of the frontal bone, the frontal process of the maxilla, the lacrimal bone, and the ethmoid bone. Severe nasal fractures involving these structures are termed naso-orbital-ethmoid fractures. Without careful reduction and fixation, the distance between the medial canthi, the medial intercanthal distance, will be wider than normal, a condition known as post-traumatic telecanthus.

Mandibular Anatomy

The mandible provides a U-shaped platform for the lower dentition and brings them into apposition with the maxilla with a force of 650 to 1,300 N. As viewed laterally, the mandible is a class III lever bent at the gonial angle to approximately 45°. The pivot point is formed by the mandibular condyle articulating with the glenoid fossa. Upward force is applied to the coronoid process by the temporalis and to the outer body by the masseter. The pterygomassetric sling is formed by the medial pterygoid, which inserts on the inner body of the mandible, and the masseter, which inserts on the external surface of the mandible. The medial pterygoid muscles contribute to the elevation and side-to-side motion (lateral excursion) of the mandible, whereas the masseter provides compressive forces. The lateral pterygoids insert on the mandibular condyle and fine-tune this motion by protruding the mandible and producing grinding side-to-side motions.

The upper surface of the mandible provides 16 alveoli for the dentition—8 on each side with the same dental formula as the maxillary arch, $I_2C_1P_2M_3$. The blood and nerve supply comes from the inferior alveolar artery and nerve. The inferior alveolar nerve is the terminal trunk of the third division of the trigeminal nerve, which exits the middle cranial fossa vertically through the foramen ovale and enters into the mandibular foramen in the upper portion of the inner surface of the ramus just posterior to the lingula. From there, it travels within the body of the mandible until it exits anteriorly at the mental foramen near the mandibular second premolar. It is accompanied by the inferior alveolar artery, a branch of the internal maxillary artery.

Facial Bone Strength

There is wonderful optimization in the facial skeleton: reinforcement is by thickening or rounding the junctions of beams, and the columns are precisely where they are needed and only to the extent that is required. Since the principal direction of masticatory force is vertical, the maxilla does very well with dissipating vertically oriented forces. The anterior to posterior or lateral forces typically encountered with trauma are not as well tolerated. Numerous studies have been performed to determine the relative strengths of the facial bones. From these studies, several generalizations can be made. Male skeletons are significantly stronger than those of female skeletons. Age does not significantly affect skeletal strength, once mature, until the eighth decade. Lastly, the duration of the force impulse is at least as important as the magnitude of force applied.[2] Facial bones are poroviscoelastic; as such, the load rate is an important element. Facial bone is able to withstand very high forces for short periods, with the critical force required for fracture decreasing rapidly as the duration of force is increased. The frontal bone is most resistant to fracture, followed by the maxilla, mandible, and zygoma. The nasal bones are most susceptible to fracture (Table 2-1).

HISTOLOGY

The mechanisms by which bone first develops and then is subsequently remodeled are the root causes of its eventual histologic structure. Likewise, the steps of bone healing are based on these same fundamental processes. For this reason, rather than merely describing normal bone histology in its mature state, we first discuss its development, growth, and physiology. This basic understanding of bone development and remodeling will then serve as a foundation for understanding both normal bone histology and the process of bone healing.

Cell Types

There are three primary types of cells found within bone: osteoblasts, osteocytes, and osteoclasts. Osteoblasts are derived from specialized mesenchymal cells called osteoprogenitor cells

Table 1. FACIAL BONE TOLERANCES				
Bone	Force Tolerance (N)	Reference	Pressure Tolerance (N/mm^2)	Reference
Frontal	1,000–6,494	Allsop et al (1988) Nyquist et al (1986) Gadd et al (1968)	7.58	Gadd et al (1968)
Maxilla	668–1,801	Allsop et al (1988) Hodgson (1967)	1.03–2.07	Nahum (1976) Schneider and Nahum (1974) Gadd et al (1968)
Mandible	685–1,779	Nyquist et al (1986) Gadd et al (1968)	2.76–6.2	Schneider and Nahum (1974)
Zygoma	489–2,401	Allsop et al (1988) Nyquist et al (1986) Gadd et al (1968) Hodgson (1967)	1.38–4.17	Nahum (1976) Gadd et al (1968)
Zygomatic arch	890–1,779	Nahum (1976) Schneider and Nahum (1974)	1.38–2.76	Nahum (1976) Hodgson (1967)
Nose	342–450	Nyquist et al (1986) Swearingen (1965)	0.13–0.34	Nahum (1976)

Adapted from Hampson D.[2]

and are responsible for bone deposition. Osteoprogenitor cells are typically found within tissues that are in direct contact with bone, such as periosteum and endosteum, as well as within bone marrow and both the haversian and Volkmann's canal systems. These progenitor cells, which are similar to fibroblasts in appearance, do not directly differentiate into osteoblasts. Instead, they respond to inductive stimuli by proliferation. The daughter cell population of cells subsequently differentiates into osteoblasts.

Mature osteoblasts are cuboidal or ovoid in shape and orient themselves in a line along the bone formation site, similar to epithelium. They then secrete bone matrix, or osteoid. As might be expected of protein-secreting cells, osteoblasts have a well-developed endoplasmic reticulum, Golgi bodies, and abundant mitochondria with an eccentrically located nucleus. Osteoblasts have a high metabolic demand, which requires close association with capillaries to provide an adequate blood supply.

Osteocytes are osteoblasts that become incorporated within the lacunae of solid bone and are responsible for bone maintenance. This occurs when the preosteocyte ceases production of osteoid and is encapsulated in osteoid by its neighboring osteoblasts. Osteoblasts maintain connections to existing osteocytes via cytoplasmic processes within cannaliculi. As it is buried, the new osteocyte establishes and maintains new connections with the secreting osteoblasts around it, eventually covering them. As it is cocooned within osteoid, these connections become canaliculi. The system of canaliculi between the lacunae provides for both passive diffusion from interstitial fluid and active cytoplasmic transport between cells via gap junctions.

Osteoclasts are not derived from mesenchymal cells but are instead multinucleated cells derived from the macrophage-monocyte system.[3] They are multinucleated giant cells with between 3 and 30 nuclei and a diameter ranging from 10 to 100 μm. These specialized cells resorb bone only along the surface with which they are in intimate direct contact. In the region of this tight contact, a ruffled cytoplasmic border is formed that increases the surface area of the cell in the region. From this surface, hydrochloric acid is secreted to dissolve the mineral phase, and exposed collagen is then enzymatically digested. The rate of resorption can be 50 μm or more per day.[4]

Bone Formation

Bone can be formed through intramembranous ossification or endochondral ossification. Direct or intramembranous ossification results in membranous bone. In this type of ossification, mesenchymal cells within the membranous substrate differentiate directly into osteoblasts, which then secrete osteoid directly within the condensations of mesenchymal tissue. This is considered to be the most primitive form of osteogenesis and is restricted to the cranial vault and maxilla. The cranial vault is a good donor site for bone graft because of low donor-site morbidity when taking just the outer table. Although debated, some authors feel membranous bone to be a preferred donor site for bone graft over endochondral bone, claiming that it undergoes more rapid neovascularization and a lower proportion of resorption than endochondral bone.[5,6] However, other authors feel that these properties can be attributed to the cortical-to-cancellous ratio of the bone graft donor site and not to its embryologic tissue of origin. The mandible, sphenoid, portions of the temporal and occipital bones, and the clavicle demonstrate dual mechanisms of both membranous and endochondral ossification.[7]

Most bone develops via endochondral, rather than intramembranous, ossification. Endochondral ossification begins with mesenchymal condensation, forming the primitive anlage. When the cellular density has reached the required threshold, these cells begin to secret matrices rich in glucosaminoglycan and chondroitin sulfate, leading eventually to the formation of a cartilaginous template. This template then undergoes mineralization followed by vascular invasion and replacement of the cartilaginous template with new bone. Initially, chondrocytes are surrounded by a matrix of cartilage. After several proliferative generations, these chondrocytes begin to hypertrophy. Secretion shifts from proteoglycans and collagen to production of matrix vesicles. These matrix vesicles migrate into the surrounding cartilaginous matrix, where they participate in the mineralization of this matrix. This process is not yet fully elucidated. However, it has been shown that these vesicles transport calcium and contain enzymes for proteolytic degradation of the extracellular matrix. Phosphatases are also present, which degrade matrix phosphodiesters, allowing precipitation of the transported calcium and newly released phosphate ions.[8] Calcification of the cartilage triggers vascular invasion in association with macrophage degradation of the noncalcified extracellular matrix, thus exposing the calcified cartilage. Chondroclasts absorb approximately half to two-thirds of the calcified septa, thus widening the space between the trabeculae and preparing the way for osteoblastic replacement of the calcified framework. Osteoblasts then line up along the surfaces of exposed calcified septae and begin the process of osteoid secretion. The structure thus formed is called primary spongiosa.

This process is prototypically demonstrated at the growth plates. However, the midshaft portions of long bones undergo ossification through a slightly different process. Following midshaft chondrocyte hypertrophy and calcification of the intercellular matrix, perichondral ossification begins. The osteoprogenitor cells within the periosteum (the former perichondrium) multiply and then differentiate into osteoblasts, which begin bone deposition in the form of a bony collar on the surface of the calcified cartilage. This bony collar has a structure that resembles the spongiosa. This transformation continues proximally and distally along the surfaces of the growing bone and results in stabilization of the midshaft. Blood vessels and accompanying osteoclasts invade the calcified cartilage in this region and begin deeper bony substitution in the endochondral ossification pattern.[3] The surface spongiosum is transformed by further bone deposition into a compact layer of cortical bone. This layer of cortical bone is further thickened by appositional bone formation along periosteal and endosteal bone surfaces.

Bone can be deposited in one of two primary forms: lamellar bone and woven bone. Lamellar bone is the primary form found within the adult skeleton; it is characterized by organized type I collagen bundles, which are closely associated with apatite crystals. It is secreted at a rate of approximately 1 μm per day. It undergoes mineralization after approximately 10 days of maturation; thus, the mineral front is found at a relatively constant distance of 10 μm from the actively secreting osteoblasts. Woven bone is formed in response to the need for rapid growth. Woven bone is deposited at a rate that is two to four times the rate of lamellar bone. It is characterized by disorganized type I cartilage and a very short delay before mineralization and is typically present only in very young growing skeletons. In adults, woven bone is present in response to trauma or disease.

Functional Histology

In adults, there are two primary histologic types of bone: compact bone and cancellous bone, sometimes referred to as trabecular bone. The outer compact bone can be further subdivided into osteonal compact bone and cortical compact bone. Although sometimes the term *cortical bone* is used to refer to the entire outer layer of compact bone, this is an imprecise use of terminology as the two have differing histologic structures. Osteonal compact bone is organized along the functional unit of bone from which it derives its name, the osteon. Cortical compact bone consists of the layered rim of compact bone surrounding the osteonal bone, which is deposited by the osteoblasts of the periosteum.

Each osteon is created by the serial deposition of concentric rings of lamellar bone around a central haversian canal. The layered nature is reflective of the method of deposition. Initially, the central canal is wide, but as bone is deposited at the periphery, there is a gradual narrowing of the central canal until it is between 50 and 90 μm in diameter. Within this canal is found a neurovascular bundle and a lining of modified osteoblasts called bone-lining cells. Each of the concentric layers, or lamellae, is approximately 7 µm thick. Under polarized light, these structures evidence birefringence. This is due to the parallel fibers of collagen of each layer lying at an angle to that of the preceding layer, similar to the grain of wood found within the individual layers of plywood.[9] Osteocytes cannot survive more than a limited distance from their blood supply. This results in a maximal wall thickness that rarely exceeds 100 µm in humans. The central haversian canals of the osteon are intercepted by Volkmann's canals at right angles and communicate with the endosteum and periosteum.

The inner surface of compact bone is covered with a thin endosteum, which is another source of osteoprogenitor cells. Here the lamellar structure changes and merges with the trabecular structure of cancellous bone. Cancellous bone is characterized by open spaces bridged by trabeculae. These trabeculae have a lamellar structure and contain lacunae, but the osteocytes within these lacunae receive their blood supply from the sinusoids within the open spaces of the bone. As a result of the same diffusion limitations that apply to compact bone, the maximal trabecular diameter is approximately 200 µm. The trabeculae are lined by a thin layer of endosteum that contains mesenchymal osteoprogenitor cells, osteoblasts, and osteoclasts (Figure 4).

Bone remodeling results in the same morphologic structure as that found in primary bone.[10] The process begins with the formation of a cutting cone by osteoclasts. Osteoclasts begin resorbing bone at a rate of approximately 50 µm per day, with a diameter of approximately 200 µm. Osteoblasts then line the margins over a distance of 100 to 200 µm and begin osteoid secretion. Given the 1 µm per day rate of osteoid deposition, it takes 3 to 4 months to complete a new osteon.

BONE HEALING AFTER INJURY

Bone healing is strongly influenced, if not determined, by the degree of immobilization

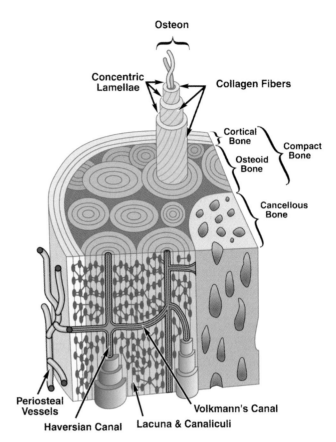

Figure 4. Bone histology.

and vascularity. Fracture healing will often occur in the face of little or no external immobilization. Rigid fixation can facilitate direct bone healing across the fracture site, without callus formation. The process of bone healing without callus formation is sometimes referred to as primary or direct bone healing. Between these two histologic bone healing processes can be found the bone healing continuum, which occurs in response to less than rigid fixation and has characteristics of both primary or direct and secondary bone healing. The objective of fracture management is to promote bone healing by decreasing interfragmentary strains with the fragments in the proper anatomic alignments.

Secondary Bone Healing

Secondary bone healing is healing that occurs using either biologic immobilization alone or medical reduction and incomplete fixation. Secondary bone healing is characterized by the formation of callus. The sequence of bone healing can be summarized as (1) inflammation and hematoma formation; (2) interfragmentary stabilization by periosteal and endosteal callus formation; (3) restoration of continuity by membranous and endochondral ossification; and (4) haversian remodeling and functional adaptation.

The initial inflammation and hematoma formation take place during the first week of fracture healing. It is thought that the hematoma is a source of signaling molecules involved in both the initiation and regulation of fracture healing.[11] Cytokines are known to be important to the process of angiogenesis and to both bone and cartilage metabolism. The expression of interleukins 1 and 6 has been shown to be present throughout the inflammatory phase of bone healing.[12] Transforming growth factor β and platelet-derived growth factor are thought to affect both fracture repair and intramembranous bone formation during callus formation and have been shown to be released by platelets during hematoma formation.[13]

Biologic stabilization of the fracture begins during the inflammatory phase through swelling, hematoma formation, and cessation of motion owing to pain at the fracture site. But it is not until 3 to 4 days later that the hematoma begins to be replaced with granulation tissue, which subsequently differentiates into connective tissue and fibrocartilage. This process continues until by 2 weeks, an abundance of cartilage overlies the fracture site, stabilizing the bone sufficiently to allow for the start of ossification.

Ossification occurs through both intramembranous ossification (hard callus) and endochondral ossification (soft callus). The process of endochondral ossification is very similar to that which takes place at the growth plate. By approximately day 9, the chondrocytes are proliferating. By day 14, the proliferating population is in decline and there is a preponderance of hypertrophic chondrocytes, which begin forming matrix vesicles and initiate the process of mineralization.[6] Once mineralization is complete, bony substitution occurs through the process of

matrix resorption, vascular invasion, and bone formation, similar to that of endochondral ossification. Appositional bone formation occurs along the pattern of intramembranous bone formation. This process is limited to areas that are well vascularized and where there is minimal or no mechanical motion to the substrate. Finally, the healing process enters a more quiescent state in which haversian and functional remodeling occurs in response to mechanical stress encountered, just as it does within non-injured bone.

Direct Bone Healing

The advent of rigid fixation resulted in the clinical appreciation of a different mode of bone healing characterized by the absence of callus formation and the gradual disappearance of fracture lines. The terms *primary bone healing* and *direct bone healing* have been used to describe this phenomenon. However, since the terms *healing by primary intention* and *healing by secondary intention* have come to be used to describe the healing encountered with and without immediate approximation of tissues, and this type of healing does not always follow all forms of reduction, direct healing seems to be the preferable term. This allows the use of the term *indirect healing* to refer to healing in which reduction and fixation have been performed, but direct healing does not occur.

It is clear that bone is capable of healing small defects without callus formation under certain conditions. For example, standardized cortical defects created with a drill of up to 200 μm (0.2 mm) demonstrate osteoblast activation in 1 to 3 days and osteoid deposition within 1 week. Such defects are filled concentrically with lamellar bone, with the end result resembling a transverse osteon. Larger defects up to 0.5 mm are bridged directly with a scaffolding of woven bone, which is subsequently filled in with lamellar bone. The result is that these larger defects are healed at the same rate as the smaller 0.2 mm holes but subsequently must undergo remodeling before their structure again matches osteonal bone. The ability to span a defect with woven bone is limited to 1 mm.[4]

Direct bone healing at a fracture site can be accomplished by recreating the conditions under which bone is able to heal without callus. These conditions are (1) stable fixation, (2) a maximal gap distance of 1 mm or less, and (3) adequate blood supply. In practice, this requires precise reduction and compressive rigid fixation, as well as careful handling of both bone and soft tissue to preserve vascularity. The compressive forces build up enough preload to ensure that interfragmentary contact is maintained under any deforming forces that may be encountered during healing.

Direct contact healing occurs only in those isolated regions where bone fragments are both in direct contact and where no motion occurs. In these areas, cutter cones are able to directly cross the interface from one bone fragment to the next. Osteoid deposition then follows with the establishment of a new osteon directly spanning the fracture site. This type of healing plays a far less important role in direct healing than gap healing for two reasons. First, areas of direct contact are far less extensive than those in which there is a slight gap. Second, the process is much slower. Resorption occurs at a maximal rate of 50 μm per day and osteoid deposition at a rate of 1 μm per day.

Gap healing is a much more rapid process. If a gap has no microinstability, it is said to be "quiet" or stable. In stable gaps of less than 1 mm, angiogenesis and mesenchymal migration begin shortly after injury. Within 3 to 4 days, osteoblast differentiation occurs, and osteoid deposition begins without the need for osteoclastic resorption. For gaps under 200 μm, the deposition is similar to appositional bone formation, and the gap is filled with lamellar bone. Larger gaps, up to 1 mm, are bridged with woven bone. This first phase of healing is usually completed within 4 to 6 weeks. However, the resulting structure differs from uninjured bone both in structure and mechanical strength. The second phase of healing consists of haversian remodeling through the formation of osteoclastic

cutting cones, vascular ingrowth, and osteoblastic deposition within the new haversian canal. These haversian units are about 300 μm in diameter. The remodeling phase overlaps the initial healing but lags the initial fracture by 2 to 3 weeks. It has peak activity lasting for approximately 3 weeks before gradually returning to baseline approximately 6 months after healing.

Indirect Bone Healing

Indirect bone healing occurs under conditions in which the requirements for direct bone healing were not achieved. The most obvious example is when rigid fixation with plates and screws were intended but not fully achieved. Bone regeneration can tolerate only up to 2 to 4% strain. Beyond this limit, no bone will form. Strain is the ratio of the amount of change to the original dimension, $\Delta L/L_0$. If rigid fixation cannot be achieved, there will be microinstability within the gap and the resulting interfragmentary strain will be greater than 2 to 4%. Simply stated, small displacements between the fragments destroy all healing attempts at bridging the gap. The physiologic response to such instability is resorption. The gap is widened, increasing L_0, which reduces the strain experienced within the gap, thus creating conditions under which the healing tissues can survive. Biologic immobilization then occurs using the same mechanisms found in secondary healing, through endosteal and periosteal callus formation. If interfragmentary strain remains high, nonunion will result.

Nonunion and Sequestrum

Nonunion can result from several causes, the most common being insufficient stabilization. They are characterized by abundant callus, a widened fracture cap, and a lack of interfragmentary bony substitution. Persistent instability results in a cessation of mineralization of the fibrocartilage between the fragments. Failure of mineralization prevents the progressive reduction in interfragmentary strain and the next phase of healing, which is vascular invasion and bony substitution. The transition from delayed union to nonunion occurs between the fourth and fifth months after injury. Beyond this point, experimental studies have shown that bony union will not occur even as late as 40 weeks. However, if rigid fixation is established, bony healing will resume, even in well-established nonunions, and union occurs within 5 to 6 weeks.[4] The pattern of healing is the same as that discussed with secondary bone healing.

An adequate blood supply is essential for bony healing. During the remodeling phase, devitalized bone can be revascularized through the process of haversian remodeling. However, it is possible for devitalized bone to persist beyond this phase. After several months, the devascularized bone segment is no longer able to activate remodeling or substitution, even if the surrounding blood supply is adequate. No live osteocytes occupy the lacunae within such bone fragments, or it is fully necrotic and is called a sequestrum. This transition from merely devitalized to necrotic is gradual and is thought to take place 6 to 12 months after insult. Such necrotic fragments are brittle and serve as stress risers, predisposing the bone to refracture.

UNIQUE PHYSIOLOGIC HEALING ASPECTS

The anatomy of the craniofacial skeleton is unique for no other region has such complex surface anatomy. From a mechanical standpoint, the face is not subject to either the magnitude or the multidirectional nature of the mechanical stresses found within other portions of the axial skeleton. The most significant deformational forces to which the craniofacial skeleton is routinely exposed originate from the compressive forces of the muscle of mastication. This is reflected in the structure of the craniofacial skeleton. Since bone remodels in response to the stress, the buttress systems hypertrophy in response to these forces, whereas the regions between the buttresses are thin and easily fragmented. The resultant structural weaknesses are reflected in the unique fracture patterns initially described by René Le Fort in 1901.

The face is resistant to fracture along this vertical plane but susceptible to fracture from forces applied in the anterior-posterior or lateral direction. The honeycomb nature of the midface is of particular significance when it comes to a reduction in fractures. Regions along the vertical and horizontal buttresses are thick enough to allow plate and screw fixation, but within the orbit and overlying the maxillary sinuses, the bone is often too thin.

The craniofacial skeleton has unique structural and functional characteristics: it houses and protects the brain and the three paired distant sensors critical in detecting prey and avoiding predation by registering photonic, acoustic, and olfactory disturbances; related to this is the fact that the apertures for both trophic apparatus and respiratory systems are also present. The major disruption of either of these two functions can be life-threatening without medical intervention. It is frequently necessary to provide temporary mechanisms to fulfill these functions, such as a tracheostomy, a gastrostomy, and/or jejunostomy feeding tubes, while healing of the facial skeleton proceeds.

Lastly, the craniofacial skeleton is unique in its location and importance in social interactions. All other areas of skeletal fixation can accommodate a certain degree of inaccuracy in fixation. Repair of the facial skeleton is unforgiving to such inaccuracies. Owing to its superficial nature and to the sensitivity of the human eye to alterations in the face, minor inaccuracies are rapidly detected. The requirement for precise reduction extends even to areas where inaccuracy would not be immediately visible, such as the jaw. Small discrepancies of occlusion may not be visible to others but will be immediately noticed by the patient.

COMMON WOUND HEALING PROBLEMS

Complication of Trauma and Surgery

A complication is defined as an undesirable occurrence that results in additional damage, delay in recovery, and/or reduction in the final extent or quality of eventual recovery.

Complications occur, on average, in about 5% of the craniofacial surgical cases and have a positive correlation to both injury severity and the length of surgery. Often complications are directly related to factors that are not within the surgeon's control, such as injury severity, patient age, and underlying systemic diseases. Even under the best circumstances, unexpected events may occur during a surgical procedure; it is thus imperative that the surgeon both anticipates such events and has contingency plans in place before they happen. Although this is true of any surgical procedure, this is particularly true with complicated craniofacial operations.

Preoperatively, attention must be directed toward preservation of life and minimizing damages to the brain and ocular globe. Airway complications are the most dreaded and least well tolerated in severe facial trauma and are responsible for the majority of preventable deaths in these patients. The most secure airway is provided by a tracheostomy. Tracheostomy should be performed often and early in patients with panfacial fractures, those requiring postoperative maxillomandibular fixation, and patients with decreased mental status.

The next most important consideration is control of hemorrhage. The face is extremely well vascularized and, as such, can bleed profusely. Without timely control, life-threatening exsanguination is a distinct possibility in patients with significant craniofacial trauma. Any hemorrhage related to the scalp can be controlled with direct pressure. Within the face, the application of such pressure can be problematic. Severe hemorrhage associated with facial fractures is most frequently from the nasal or oral cavities. It can usually be controlled by fracture reduction combined with packing, a Foley catheter balloon, and the application of a Barton dressing for external pressure. Any hemorrhage not controlled by such measures is suspicious for laceration to maxillary arteries or basilar skull fracture with internal carotid involvement. In such cases, angiographic evaluation and embolization are generally preferable to operative attempts at selective ligation.[14]

Complications Related to Anatomic Regions and Misalignment

Successful surgical intervention requires a solid understanding of the underlying anatomy and physiology of involved structures and a practical approach to restoring them. This is particularly true within the craniofacial region as the proximity of key structures, such as the dura mater, cerebrospinal fluid, brain, eye, lacrimal systems, and paranasal sinuses, with their complex geometry and mucosa, makes this an even more challenging problem. The drainage of these glands and sinuses must be reestablished, or their complete ablation should be carried out. Failure to do so will result in chronic dacryocystitis, mucocele, or mucopyocele. The craniofacial region houses the apparatus for nominal nutrient intake and the initial processing. For that, the masticatory system is under cyclic loadings of significant magnitude. Failure to account for this will result in fatigue failure of the fixation hardware (Figure 5). Another requirement, which, if overlooked, can result in significant morbidity, is precise restoration of occlusion. The position of maximum intercuspation and the highly proprioceptive periodontal ligaments require that the reduction and fixation be highly accurate. Precise plate bending is critical to achieving this goal as bone fragments will adapt to the plates. A small angular error of 1:198" at mandibular symphysis will result in about 8 mm displacement at the condyles. The introduction of locking plates has somewhat lessened this stringent requirement but has not eliminated it completely.

Technical Considerations

Intraoperatively, complications can be caused or exacerbated by inappropriate surgical techniques. One of the primary principles that must always be kept in mind is that living tissues must remain viable for healing to occur. Any technique that compromises tissue viability in favor of any other consideration must be avoided. For example, excessive tension can impair blood flow to the region, resulting in cellular death. Failure

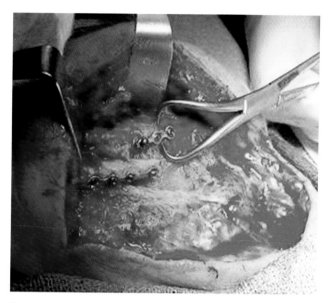

Figure 5. This was found at reexploration; the plate has failed owing to fatigue damage. The cyclic movement of the mandible, although edentulous, eventually broke the titanium plate before the fracture had a chance to heal. A stronger plate or an additional plate would have been better.

to irrigate while drilling can result in excessive heat production during drilling, resulting in focal necrosis of the bone. This can result in loosening of the screw fixation and significantly increase the probability of hardware infection. Overtightening of the screws will cause the bone immediately adjacent to the screw to undergo ischemia or fracture and should be avoided. An additional technical consideration is the precision of alignment and fixation. The prerequisites for osseous healing are stability, blood supply, and restoration of anatomic alignment prior to fixation. Herein resides the dilemma: good reduction requires exposure, but exposure necessarily decreases blood supply. The only possible answer is to expose only that which is absolutely necessary to achieve an accurate reduction in the fractured bone fragments.

FUTURE INNOVATIONS IN CRANIOFACIAL HEALING

Several key areas hold tremendous promise in significantly advancing our ability to care for patients in general, including those with craniofacial deformities. "Significantly" in this case is defined qualitatively as achieving an outcome or

outcomes not previously possible and quantitatively as achieving the same results more efficiently with regard to cost and outcome. By 2010, more than 2.5 trillion dollars will be spent on health care in this country, representing 17% of the projected gross domestic product. How to do what we do better, faster, and cheaper is of critical importance and depends to a large degree on innovations and advances in biotechnology. Such advances will be more dependent on collaboration between physicians, molecular or cellular biologists, and bioengineers. The last section of this chapter approximately parallels the format of the Bioengineering Consortium, BECON, established by the National Institutes of Health (NIH) in 1997 and focuses on the following four major categories:

1. Bioimaging and biosensing
2. Regenerative medicine, biomaterials, stem cell technology, bioreactors
3. Mechanobiology
4. Genomics and modeling

Advances in these areas will not only aid in the diagnosis and treatment of acquired and congenital craniofacial disorders, they will also allow for better understanding of why these disorders occur and how healing can be enhanced. Owing to space limitations, the following categories are not discussed: surgical robotics, micro electromechanical systems, nanotechnology, surgical simulation and surgical simulators, bioinformatics, operational control, and optimization. The Web site <www.becon.nih.gov> contains much pertinent and frequently updated information that is very useful.

Bioimaging and Biosensing

The ability to heal, to self-restore to an intact, preinjured functional state, is a hallmark of biotic processes. Without this ability, an organism will not survive very long. This process has been repeatedly refined and improved over billions of years of evolution to arrive at its current, orchestrated, complex, and complicated state. Many cell types and biochemicals come into play during healing and transition from one stage seamlessly into the next. Each stage has key intermediaries that alter and are altered by the local mechanical environment leading to the ensuing stages, until the remodeling process asymptotically approaches the "normal" basal state metabolically and functionally. Bone, in particular, can regenerate itself almost completely. There are two fundamentally different processes involved in this process: stem cell proliferation and stem cell differentiation. Proliferation permits the increase in cell number, and differentiation drives these uncommitted cells to express the necessary proteins to rebuild the injured tissue.

New imaging methods will allow us to understand better how this complex, hierarchical process is controlled. One such method is by transfection with fluorescent genes such as *EGFP*, coding for a green fluorescent protein, driven by a constitutively active promoter so that all transfected cells can be followed by this green fluorescence as they journey throughout the body. For example, the plRES2 promoter, which is frequently coupled to the *EGFP* gene, allows the tracking of cells such as bone marrow–derived Sca-1 +/CD 34+/CD 105+ mesenchymal stem cells. By coupling *EGFP* to osteoblast-specific promoters such as the RUNX-2 promoter, one can investigate nondestructively cell differentiation in vivo. Because the mechanical environment is very important in shaping cellular responses, biosensors that can report the local stress states will provide the data necessary in constructing the laws governing tissue dynamics. Such sensors will, no doubt, employ nanofabrication technology. The changes in optical property owing to mechanical strain permit the noninvasive measurements of deformation at the tissue levels. Other no-touch modalities or instruments for strain measurements are laser-speckled interferometry, linear variable displacement transducers, and differential acoustic impedance. Levels of various ions, organic compounds, cytokines, and growth factors can be monitored by refinement in technologies such as Fourier transformed infrared spectroscopy,

Raman scattering microscopy, force-amplified biosensors, and the e-tongue type devices developed by NASA to monitor pH.

Regenerative Medicine, Biomaterials, Stem Cell Technology, and Bioreactors

Over a relatively short period of two to three decades, tissue engineering and, more recently, regenerative medicine have grown exponentially in volume and complexity. Using *Google*, a common search engine, more than 460,000 Web sites on regenerative medicine and an amazing 5.5 million sites for tissue engineering were identified as of mid-2005. Regenerative medicine is a new branch of medicine that uses methods and products, including those of tissue engineering, to "synchronize" the life span of the major organs or systems of the human body. The objective is to delay the premature failure of any individual parts so that useful life span of the whole organism can be maximized. As stated by the famous theoretical physicist Erwin Schrödinger, life is avoiding death.

Because the biotic process is fractal in structure and function, often one of the subsystems wears out, whereas all of the others are still in good functional condition. Tissue engineering allows the fabrication of replacement parts to delay the failure of that subsystem until all or most subsystems can wear out at the same time. The principal components in "building" tissue parts, like the native tissue they are to replace, are cells and matrices. In the craniofacial skeleton, matrices perform the macrostructural function of load bearing and shape maintenance. The matrices are synthesized by cells, which, by themselves, are too weak to tolerate the mechanical stress. The cellular elastic modulus is in the range of 5 to 100 kPa, whereas the loading of the skeleton is in the range of 10 to 100 MPa, or a thousand times larger. The loading of the skeleton is cyclic, with variable frequency, load rate, and magnitude. As such, fatigue damage and wear are extremely difficult to overcome if self-renewal cannot occur. This self-renewal requires cells. Cells differ from the extracellular matrices in that they are thermodynamically open and require a continuous supply of nutrients (high enthalpy and low entropy) and elimination of waste products (high entropy and lower enthalpy). This has severely constrained the field of tissue engineering: the requirement of a mass transport system, the vasculature, to move these materials in bulk rather than by diffusion alone.

From the cell's source standpoint, many advances have been made, and more are on the way. Stem cells are the pluripotent, if not totipotent, cells that can self-renew for 15 to 50 doublings, depending on the age and the source of the donor (this maximum number of potential mitoses before senescence is known as the Hayflick constant). Stem cells are either embryonic or adult in origin. It is generally accepted that embryonic stem cells are "better" than adult stem cells. They are derived from blastocysts and are frequently 46XX in karyotype. At least six lines have been established and are available commercially with NIH codes of ES01 to ES06, with a price tag of about $5,000. Adult stem cells can be found in bone marrow, skin, dermis, muscle, and fat. Adipose-derived adult stem cells have enjoyed great popularity in recent years owing to their ease of harvest and abundance.

Stem cells are seeded onto a scaffold polymer construct and placed in a controlled culture environment provided by special culture devices known collectively as tissue reactors. The variables that need to be controlled include temperature, pH, partial pressures of oxygen and carbon dioxide, principal and shear stresses, glucose and amino acid concentrations, growth factors, and ionic contents, to name just a few. Each of these must be kept within a narrow range by servomechanisms with absolute sterility as the constructs may take up to weeks or months to "grow." The scaffolds are typically porous, with an average pore diameter of 100 to 200 μm and high connectivity, which can be achieved by modified salt-leaching methods or selective laser sintering. The three popular polymers approved by the US Food and Drug Administration are poly-L-lactide, polyglycolic acid, and polycaprilactone.

The requirements for scaffolds for bone tissue engineering are to allow cell attachment and proliferation, degrade at the desired rate, be nontoxic, and have sufficient strength in tension, compression, and shear. The compressive strength should be at least 2 MPa, and the tensile modulus should be at least 50 MPa. The scaffold biomaterials affect cell behavior at all scales, from the nano level through the micro and meso levels to the macro levels.

Mechanobiology

How cells respond to external mechanical stresses affects the what, when, where, and how of extracellular matrix production, maintenance, and degradation. The study of these cell-force interactions combines mechanics and cell biology and is known collectively as mechanobiology. The bulk of these interactions are grouped under mechanotransduction, which is the conversion of mechanical perturbation into biochemical events. Cells such as osteocytes and osteoblasts are linked to their external microenvironment by three principal methods: soluble signals, hard-wired connections, and electromagnetic alterations. Of these, the electromagnetic aspects are the least well studied and thus least well understood. Through transmembrane complexes such as the integrins and other cell adhesion molecules, the structural elements within the cells, the cytoskeleton, are firmly attached to the structural elements of the extracellular matrix. Strains at the tissue level are transmitted to individual cells to cause cellular strains.

Only recently, measurements of cellular modulus have become possible through the use of optical tweezers, atomic force microscopy, and micropipeting. Constitutive equations are now being formulated based on these detailed measurements to predict cell mechanical behavior. A major difficulty is that cells are living entities and respond to the changes in their environment; as such, their mechanical properties vary both temporally and spatially. A simplistic, but nonetheless accurate, model of tissue as a smart material views cells as a system of strain gauges, monitoring and adjusting the total stress state at the tissue level. Where stress increases beyond certain threshold level, cells undergo strain and an increase in plasma membrane permeability occurs. Calcium ions move from the extracellular space into the cytosol at a very rapid rate, driven by the concentration gradient. This causes many calcium-dependent processes to proceed, including phosphorylation of members of key pathways, such as the ERK and MAP kinase pathways, which initiate cascades of downstream events, leading to nuclear translocation of factors, which alters the transcriptome and eventually the amount and type of peptides synthesized. The end outcome is reinforcing tissue precisely where reinforcement is needed.

The degradation of the collagenous matrix by matrix metalloproteases (MMPs) is also linked to the strain-inducible genes. There is increasing evidence that shear stress can activate transcription mechanisms, which results in matrix breakdown. Recent data from wound healing research indicate a $\times 30$ increase in MMPs in chronic wounds experiencing high shear stress. A long-recognized characteristic of the living skeletal tissue is the fine-tuning of the trabeculae to better tolerate principal stress and minimize shear stress. If the above two "rules" are repeatedly iterated, such optimization becomes inevitable. Mechanobiology is the foundation on which real practical biomaterials of the next generation can be developed.

Genomics and Modeling

The completion of the Human Genome Project in 2003 brings forward an awesome realization that we, as a species, coded by 3 billion base pairs, have now sequenced this genetic information that has coded ourselves. High-throughput technologies, such as deoxyribonucleic acid (DNA) microarray, protein chips, quantitative trait loci mapping, and expressed sequence tag analysis, have permitted the rapid acquisition of a vast amount of genetic data. This has resulted in a mismatch in meaningful data analysis and data collection. Simply stated, we have more descriptive information than

we know what to do with. Mathematics such as fractal analysis, iterative simulation, and stochastic modeling will help make sense of this massive amount of data. To describe what the genes are is only the first step. How, when, and where these genes are transcribed are equally, if not more, important than the genes themselves. It now appears that the tools used by different animals to achieve their morphology are very well conserved; the theme is repetition, which results in metamerism, and metamerism allows for functional duplication and redundancy. This redundancy, in turn, permits modification without jeopardizing existing systems. Small inhibitory ribonucleic acid is one of the latest therapeutic applications of genomics; functional redundancy in this case is translated to resistance and incomplete responses. New methods in mathematics are required to allow the construction of testable hypotheses and repeated refinements of the theoretical models of the biologic systems. These theoretical frameworks, guided by observations based on real experiments, will lead to a deeper, more complete understanding of these wonderful biologic processes, such as craniofacial wound healing, and from that will come new therapeutics and treatment modalities.

REFERENCES

1. Zide BM, Jelks GW, Craig L. Surgical anatomy of the orbit. New York: Raven Press; 1985.
2. Hampson D. Facial injury: a review of biomechanical studies and test procedures for facial injury assessment. J Biomechan 1995;28:1–7.
3. Wheater PR, Burkitt HG, Daniels VG. Functional histology: a text and colour atlas. New York: Churchill Livingstone; 1987.
4. Schenk RK. Biology of fracture repair; skeletal trauma: fractures, dislocations, ligamentous injuries. Philadelphia: WB Saunders; 1992.
5. Szachowicz EH. Facial bone wound healing. Otolaryngol Clin North Am 1995;28:865–80.
6. Kusaik JF, Zins JE, Whitaker LA. The early revascularization of membranous bone. Plast Reconstr Surg 1985; 76:510–4.
7. Manson PN. Facial bone healing and bone grafts: a review of clinical physiology. Clin Plast Surg 1994;21:331–48.
8. Einhorn TA. The cell and molecular biology of fracture healing. Clin Orthopaed Relat Res 1998;355 Suppl:S7–21.

9. Weiner S, Traub W, Wagner HD. Lamellar bone: structure-function relations. J Struct Biol 1990;126: 241–55.

10. Wornom IL, Buchman SR. Bone and cartilagenous tissue; wound healing biochemical and clinical aspects. Philadelphia: WB Saunders, 1992.

11. Reddi AH, Anderson WA. Collagenous bone matrix-induced endochondral ossification and hematopoiesis. J Cell Biol 1976;69:557–72.

12. Einhorn TA, Majeska RJ, Rush EB, et al. The expression of cytokine activity by fracture callus. J Bone Miner Res 1995;10:1272–81.

13. Bolander ME. Regulation of fracture repair by growth factors. Proc Soc Exp Biol Med 1992;200:165–70.

14. Jurkovich GJ, Carrico CJ. Trauma, management of the acutely injured patient. Sabiston's textbook of surgery. Philadelphia: WB Saunders; 1997.

3

Craniofacial Cartilage Wound Healing: Implications for Facial Surgeons

Craig D. Friedman, MD, FACS; Melissa Kurtis Micou, PhD

Cartilage structures of the face and neck are unique in that they are critical elements in defining an individual's characteristic appearance and also serve important functional roles. Cartilage structures represent a broad array of anatomies within the face and neck. Surgeons routinely perform procedures involving these structures; thus, a thorough knowledge of the tissue and its healing is mandated. This chapter reviews basic anatomy and clinical wound healing of cartilage with a specific focus on facial and neck regions. We also review tissue engineering and regenerative strategies that will impact future clinical practice. This chapter does not serve as an all-inclusive source for facial cartilage anatomy, histology, and physiology but highlights the unique and salient aspects that affect the healing of these tissues and serves as a helpful guideline for surgical decision making.

ANATOMY AND PHYSIOLOGY

Cartilage is a specialized skeletal tissue that is present at anatomic sites where flexible solid structure is required to provide shape and form, with attendant strength and durability. Cartilage provides protection and support of related nonskeletal tissues and organs, the interface of skeletal articulations, and an intermediate scaffold in bone growth and repair. All vertebrate cartilages[1,2] consist of some combination of skeletal or connective tissue cells (chondrocytes), extracellular matrix (ECM) (consisting of fibrous matrix and biopolymers), and water. The structure, composition, and organization of cartilage are intimately related to the physiologic turnover or metabolism of its ECM, which is regulated by chondrocytes under the control of growth factors, cytokines, and mechanical stimuli.

There is a broad distribution of cartilage structures in the face and neck region (Figure 1).

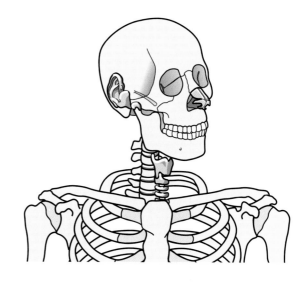

Figure 1. Distribution of cartilage structures in the face and neck, highlighted in *red*.

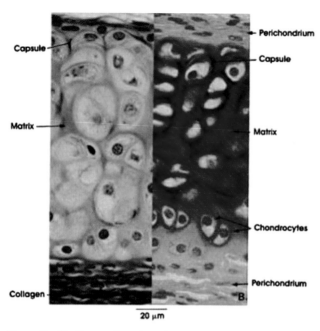

Figure 2. Hyaline cartilage from the trachea (Mallory and toluidine blue stains; ×612 original magnification). http://www.anatomyatlases. org/MicroscopicAnatomy/MicroscopicAnatomy.shtml.

Histologically, cartilage is classically characterized as being hyaline, elastic, or fibrocartilage, defined by the ECM composition and organization. Hyaline cartilage (Figure 2) is seen in various forms of articular surfaces (ie, temporomandibular joint), nasal septum, and larynx or trachea. Elastic cartilage has the significant presence of elastic fibers (Figure 3) within the ECM and is best demonstrated in the external auricle (pinna) and the epiglottis. Fibrocartilage of the head and neck is best demonstrated in the

cranial sutures at birth and the intervertebral disks of the spinal column.

Embryology and Chondrogenesis

Cartilage develops from mesenchyme and mesenchymal chondroprogenitor cells and first appears in embryos of about 5 weeks.[3] In areas in which cartilage forms, the avascular mesenchyme condenses and the cells become rounded. These cells are characterized by high expression of fibronectin and laminin, receptors for these molecules, and the chondroblast or chondrocyte transcription factors homeoprotein 1 and Sox9.[4,5] The latter is required for type II collagen expression and is essential for chondrogenesis. Type II collagen expression is regulated during chondrocyte development to preferentially express IIB collagen as the earlier expressed IIA aminopropeptide binds transforming growth factor (TGF)-β_1 and bone morphogenetic protein (BMP)-2, both growth and differentiation factors for cartilage.[6] Type II collagen and aggrecan (the large cartilage proteoglycan) increase in content and biochemically define cartilage formation. The condensing mesenchyme gives rise to the perichondrium, the main source of chondroblasts during development; it retains chondrogenic potential in the adult, along with periosteum.

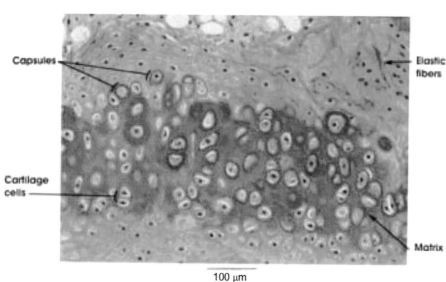

Figure 3. Elastic cartilage from the epiglottis (hematoxylin-eosin stain; ×162 original magnification). http://www.anatomyatlases.org/ MicroscopicAnatomy/Microscopic-Anatomy.shtml.

The differentiation of mesenchyme into chondrocytes involves the superfamily of regulatory molecules called BMPs, which include TGF-β and various BMPs. It is known that mutation of BMP-5 in the short-ear mouse results in a loss of chondrocyte condensations, the overexpression of BMP-2 and Growth Development Factor (GDF)-5 results in overgrowth of cartilage, and null mutations of BMP-7 in mice result in abnormal skeletal development. BMP signaling can be antagonized by noggin or chordin (developmental proteins), each of which can directly bind to their receptors. Retinoic acid or receptor activation can inhibit mesenchymal chondroblast differentiation, whereas inhibition of retinoid signaling induces Sox9 expression, the key transcription factor for chondroblast development. Fibroblast growth factors play a significant role in mesenchyme differentiation, as demonstrated by their presence in limb bud formation and proliferating mesenchyme. Many molecular defects of chondrocytes result in abnormal human skeletal development; therefore, as the complex developmental molecular biology of cartilage becomes better understood, this further elucidation will undoubtedly impact clinical therapies.

Facial and neck cartilage structures form from mesenchyme within the well-known embryologic structures of the branchial apparatus. The cartilage of the ear develops from the first branchial arch derivative mesenchyme; it is distinguished by the elastic fibers present in its ECM. The temporomandibular joint (a diarthrodial joint), which contains the articular (hyaline) cartilage of the condylar head and glenoid fossa and the fibrocartilage of the intra-articular disk, is formed from the first arch, commonly referred to as Meckel's cartilage.

The nasal structures are first noted at 4 weeks with the formation of the bilateral nasal placodes on each side of the lower part of the frontonasal prominence. Over the course of development to the tenth week, the mesenchyme proliferates at the margins of the placodes, forming the nasal pits. The frontonasal prominence forms the nasal dorsum, the lateral nasal prominences form the alar structures, and the nasal septum forms from the fusion of the medial nasal prominences.

The epiglottis develops from the caudal portion of the hypobranchial eminence derived from the third and fourth branchial arches.[3] The laryngotracheal structures begin to develop at 26 days, as indicated by the formation of a groove in the caudal end of the ventral wall of the pharynx. The larynx develops within and about the endodermal lining of the mesenchyme of the fourth and sixth branchial arches. The mesenchyme proliferates and produces paired arytenoids swellings; the laryngeal cartilages develop within the swellings and the condensating cartilage bars of the branchial arch. The tracheal cartilages similarly form from the splanchnic mesenchyme of the pulmonary buds.

Structural Organization of Cartilage

The structural organization of cartilage reflects the biomechanical forces that act on the tissue. This organization has been studied in detail with regard to articular (hyaline) cartilage but maintains relevance for nonarticular cartilage as well. Figure 4 shows the typical regional organization with superficial zone cells, which are exposed to the maximal biomechanical forces (tension, shear, compression). The collagen fibers are oriented to maximize strength, and the most plentiful are mainly type II and, to a lesser extent, type IX and type XI collagens, whereas the large proteoglycan aggrecan shows an inverse concentration gradient. Roberts and colleagues studied the ultrastructure of tracheal cartilage and confirmed how the organizational relationships of the collagen fibrils to other matrix components varied based on the anatomic zone and maximized the biomechanical performance.[7]

Cartilage matrix can have distinct regions with different populations of proteoglycan and other matrix molecules. Chondrocytes are surrounded by a thin pericellular matrix that contains few collagen fibrils but instead has a fibrillar material of a different biochemical composition. The ECM contains 65 to 80% water content, collagens up to 25% of wet weight,

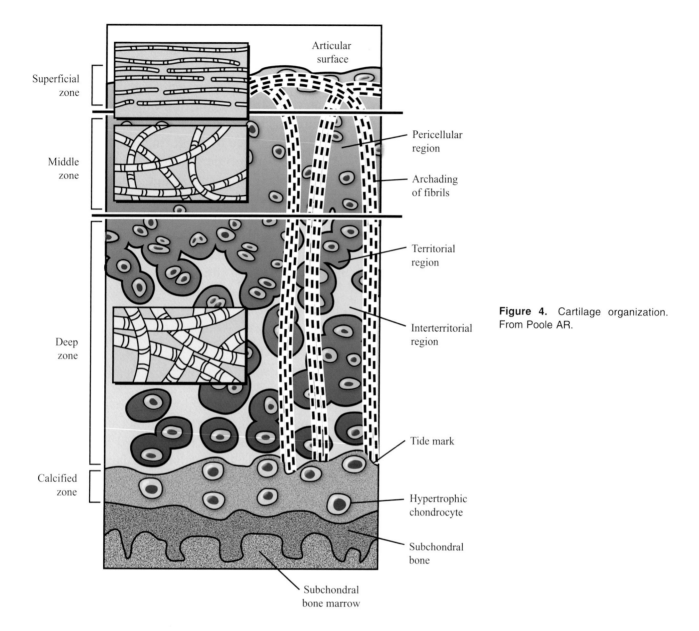

Figure 4. Cartilage organization. From Poole AR.

and proteoglycan up to 10% of wet weight. Figure 5 shows the structural relationships of the proteoglycan glycosaminoglycan.[8] The primary proteoglycan of cartilage matrix, aggrecan, binds, orients, and aggregates hyaluronic acid to the collagen fibrils. Aggrecan binds keratin sulfate and chondroitin sulfate directly within its structure. This unique structure allows for the proteoglycan to maintain the significant water content of cartilage and the resultant biomechanical properties. The proteoglycan glycosaminoglycan structure can bind up to 50 times its weight in water. The negative electrical charge clouds generated by the structure help orient the positive dipole of the oxygen dipole within the water molecule. The swelling (hydrostatic) pressure generated from this unique physical structure is manifested biomechanically in compressive stiffness and resistance to deformation (elastic modulus). Beyond these major components, numerous other matrix proteins and biopolymers play critical roles in the general metabolism and response to injury of cartilage. Certain ones, for example, matrilin 1 (cartilage matrix protein 1), are present in nasal and laryngeal cartilages. Matrilin 1 is absent in

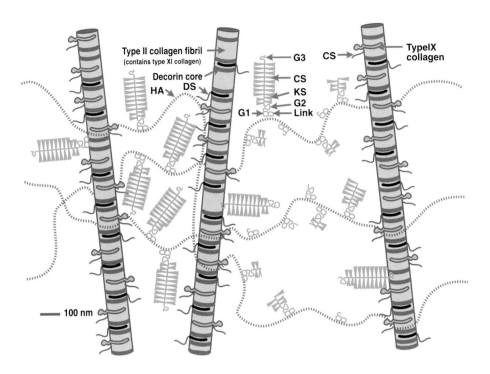

Figure 5. Cartilage structural organization of matrix. From Poole.

healthy articular cartilage but is present when chronic injury occurs.[8] Degradation of cartilage matrix is a highly complex process controlled by the expression of various proteinases acting on aggrecan and collagen and regulated by the TGF-β superfamily. Much of the work studying the healing response of cartilage following injury has been focused on noncraniofacial sites at appendicular skeletal joint surfaces. However, more knowledge specifically related to the face and neck cartilage has been increasing. Most clinically observed wound healing at these sites is commonly the result of trauma, chronic degeneration, and congenital anomalies.

Aging has very specific effects on cartilage, ranging from the change in matrix composition to gross morphologic changes. With age, chondrocytes progressively decrease their response to growth factors and their mitotic potential.[9] The matrix changes show an overall decrease in proteoglycan synthesis and accumulation of related glycation products, such as pentosidine, which can cross-link collagen and make fibrils stiffer biomechanically. Also, proteoglycan content and structure change by the shortening of aggrecan complexes and increase in the keratin sulfate–rich domains. Within the head and neck,

human auricular cartilage increases in size after adulthood maturity. Ito and colleagues performed a morphologic study that confirmed the change in matrix organization, noting an increase in elastic fiber heterogeneity and collagen fibril orientation.[10] Age-related composition and mechanical properties of human nasal septal cartilage parallel those seen in articular cartilage, suggesting that the matrix changes of senescence are independent of specific anatomic site mechanical loading.[11] Age-related gross morphologic changes of cartilage include the presence of calcifications in the nasal septum and laryngeal cartilages and a color change from white to yellow-brown owing to matrix deposition of pigments.[12]

Gross Anatomy of Facial Cartilage

The auricle, nose, larynx, and temporomandibular joint constitute the major cartilaginous anatomic structures of the face and neck. All of these structures have a well-defined perichondrium, which serves as the primary vascular supply to the gross structure. The perichondrium consists of two general zones: an outer fibrous zone and an inner cellular zone. The outer zone is a dense structure that interfaces with surrounding connective tissues and maintains the capillary vascular network. The inner zone is cellular, with chondroblastic stem cells, and merges seamlessly with the cartilage matrix. The outer perichondrium houses the well-organized capillary network, serving as the primary vascular supply for nutrition. The use and preservation of perichondrium are an important technical consideration during surgical procedures as they enable the necessary vascularization for wound healing to proceed.

The auricle is a highly shaped structure with many significant anatomic contours. The cartilages of the external ear (Figure 6) are framed by the helix and antihelical ridges, which define the scaphoid fossa and cavum conchae. These extend into the acoustic meatus canal cartilage. The tragal cartilage extends to define the anterior limit of the auricle. The increased elastic fiber content of the matrix in the auricular cartilage explains the very deformable mechanical nature of the structure. Similarly, the nasal cartilage structures, which support the distal airway, have significant deformable memory. The gross anatomy is well understood and consists mainly of the upper lateral cartilages and alar cartilages and the central nasal septum with the anterior portion consisting of the quadrangular cartilage and the interfacing posterior osseous components of the ethmoid and vomer (Figure 7).

The laryngeal cartilages include the epiglottis, thyroid cartilage, cricoid cartilage, and arytenoid cartilage (Figure 8). The complex ligamentous attachments of all of the cartilages within the organ allow for the performance of physiologic activities. Significant age-related changes within the thyroid and cricoid cartilages are manifested by calcification and ossification within the structures.

The temporomandibular joint consists of three main components: the condylar head, with its articular cartilage surface, the intra-articular disk of fibrocartilage and ligamentous attachments, and the glenoid fossa of the temporal bone, with its cartilaginous articulating surface and proximity to the external ear canal. The entire joint is intimately surrounded by controlling muscles of mastication. The reader is referred to standard anatomic texts for detailed anatomy of the facial cartilages and the relationships to other structures.

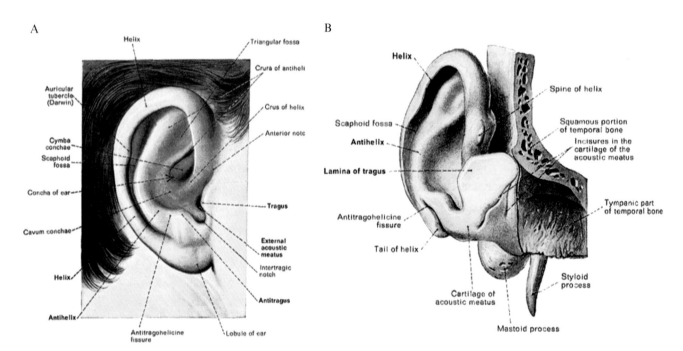

Figure 6. *A*, Auricular external surface anatomy; *B*, auricular cartilages.

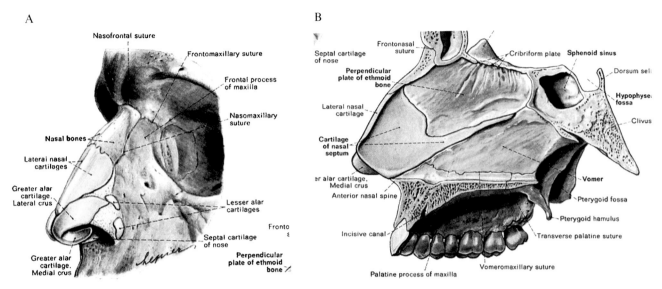

Figure 7. *A*, Nasal cartilages; *B*, nasal septal cartilage and bone articulations.

FACIAL CARTILAGE WOUND HEALING PROCESSES

Normal Wound Healing

Wound healing is a dynamic process requiring cells to express a variety of substances to interact with the ECM. There is inherent structural and functional redundancy, so the process of tissue healing and scarring is not usually a clinically significant problem. Given the skeletal nature of facial cartilage, most wound healing studies have used clinical observation and surrogate animal models. With respect to facial cartilages, primary healing would be reconstitution of the ECM, reconstitution or continued viability of the

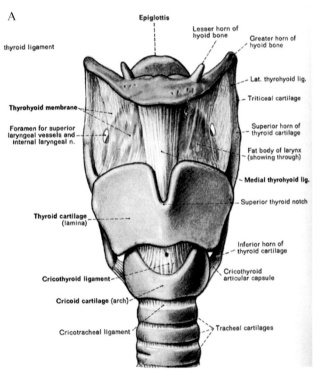

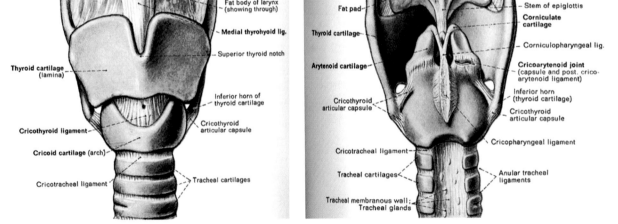

Figure 8. *A*, Laryngotracheal cartilages; *B*, posterior view.

chondrocyte population, and reestablishment of an intact perichondrium. Secondary healing would be the incorporation of fibrous unions between the cartilage fragments and discontinuity of the matrix and its highly oriented structure.

The most simple facial cartilage wound, laceration or full-thickness incision, is most often repaired with a simple suturing technique for achieving apposition and enabling the local vascular supply to support the metabolic demands of healing. Over the last 50 years, it has become well accepted that limiting movement with fixation aids in the reestablishment of the microvascular supply. Given that cartilage derives its vascular supply from the perichondrium, the incorporation of a viable perichondrium or periosteum into the repair is essential. Early investigation into primary facial cartilage healing by Peer[13,14] led to concepts that influenced the repair of facial cartilage but also contributed to the use of facial cartilage to reconstruct other facial cartilage defects. These observational and experimental findings have been modified subsequently but still offer fundamental insight into facial cartilage wound healing. Cartilage cells do not routinely regenerate tissue defects; however, given the chondrogenic potential of the perichondrium, it has been noted that cartilage can heal primarily and can support cartilage graft incorporation into augmentation and defect models. Thus, primary laceration cartilage wounds with adequate perichondrium coverage will heal with remodeling of the matrix and a preservation of viable chondrocyte populations. Verwoerd-Verhoef and colleagues studied various wound scenarios in young and old hyaline cartilage, confirming the ability of young cartilage to heal primarily and mature cartilage to heal via fibrous union.[15] The introduction of immature cartilage tissue into mature cartilage wounds can contribute to viable cartilage healing, with the injury orientation determining the degree of necrosis and viability.

Given the deformable nature of cartilage, much attention has been given to understanding the intrinsic shape behavior and how to modify surgical techniques to enhance its final shape.

Cartilage deforms under applied force, and less force is required over time to maintain its deformation. This property of being able to conformally shape cartilage is important and is reflective of matrix remodeling and the resultant change in the elastic modulus. We are now beginning to understand the changes in cartilage matrix organization that are the result of biomechanical load and/or injury. Fry described "interlocked stresses" of the nasal septal cartilage to explain the memory behavior of cartilage.[16,17] These stresses can predict the deviation of the cartilage when the outer layers are incrementally disrupted via incision (with the cartilage tending to bend away from the relaxing incision). Murray disputed the findings of Fry[18]; however, these arguments do not integrate the variable factors, such as perichondrium and other soft tissue attachments, as well as the matrix remodeling that can change shape over time. What is critically important is that the organization of the most superficial portions of the matrix contain highly oriented collagen fibrils, which, in turn, affect the three-dimensional shape behavior of cartilage. The intrinsic memory of cartilage (with perichondrium removed) and the effect of sharp incision contouring were noted by Gibson and Davis to produce random changes, which can, over time, be manifested by shape distortion.[19] These studies confirmed the importance of surgical technique when modifying cartilage shape, especially when cartilage is used as a graft.

Site-Specific Facial Cartilage Healing

Auricle

The auricle requires an integrated approach to enhance its cartilaginous healing to achieve a favorable and predictable outcome. Auricular trauma can result from a direct laceration or blunt injury and present as an auricular hematoma. Recently, Calhoun and Chase reviewed most of the standard techniques for defect repair.[20] Blunt trauma resulting in auricular hematoma can lead to cartilage necrosis and secondary deformity, commonly referred to as "cauliflower" ear. Ghanem and colleagues outlined the current therapeutic rationale for incision, drainage, and bolster dressings versus needle aspiration for treating this type of injury.[21]

Perhaps the best example of altering the shape and memory modulus or stress forces within auricular cartilage in a predictable fashion is in the neonate with an auricular deformation. Tan et al and Ullamnn reviewed their institutions' experience with using molding of neonatal auricular deformities, including prominent, lop, and Stahl's ear and inverted concha.[22,23] Overall, the outcomes with mold stents in cartilage reshaping were excellent and long-lasting, thus precluding the need for direct surgical intervention. Beyond molding therapy for neonatal deformity, many patients are deferred for correction at a later age. Hoehn and Ashruf and Gosain and colleagues detailed the issues of timing and sequence as well as the spectrum of techniques that are essential for the surgeon to employ.[24,25] Surgical correction involves sutural modeling, wedge excision, reshaping and reversing cartilage segments, and morselization. The mainstay techniques were popularized by Mustarde and Furnas with sutural modeling via mattress sutures.[26,27] Otoplasty has become a common facial cartilage procedure, and most facial surgeons employ a combination of techniques with aesthetic judgment to achieve routinely positive outcomes.

Nasal Cartilages

The cartilage of the nasal septum and alar or dorsum has been extensively studied and reviewed by generations of facial surgeons. Many lessons have been renewed and reinforced with a greater depth of understanding and more refined technical approaches. In 1884, Mackenzie published an early work on the most commonly encountered cartilage pathologic condition, the deviated septum.[28] Pirsig studied the effect of early trauma on nasal septal development and concluded that although nasal septal cartilage does heal and maintains a viable cartilage cell population, gross structural deformities persist, such as deviation away from the injured surface.[29] Traumatic injuries to the face and nasal region can give rise to nasal septal injuries, which, when not completely evaluated, can lead to cartilage loss from a hematoma or an abscess or a major structural deformity.[30,31]

Historically, nasal septal surgery evolved from "submucous" cartilage resection to more conservative cartilage resection procedures.[33–36] The role of perichondrium and the use of "morselization" crush techniques have been studied in recent experimental models by Verwoerd-Verhoef and colleagues and Verwoerd and colleagues.[37,38] They showed the plasticity of young naive cartilage tissues, confirming the earlier work of Peer on graft survival when placed as interposition grafts. Morselized grafts do survive better in younger animals; however, they often result in poorly oriented gross structure secondary to the matrix damage and remodeling. The perichondrium, under the regulatory expression of the TGF-β superfamily, influences cartilage survival and remodeling but also permits the formation of intervening fibrous tissue between graft and recipient site that does not contribute to organized growth of the entire cartilage structure.[39,40]

Recent experimental and clinical studies used an internal polydioxane membrane as a guiding splint to direct growth of the graft and avoid recurrent deviations in the healed state.[41,42] This is an obvious extension of knowledge to enhance predictable morphologic healing. Clinically, the use of sutural modeling has been a mainstay of nasal cartilage surgical technique. Recent reports confirmed the continued valid use of this for various nasal plastic surgical procedures.[43–46]

Further studies have shown the usefulness of adjunctive wound healing agents to enhance results in nasal surgery. The use of fibrin glue adhesives has been studied in nasal septal surgery alone and in combination with auricular cartilage grafts for the prevention and treatment of septal perforations. Daneshrad and colleagues, in a series of 100 patients undergoing nasal septal surgery, used fibrin glue alone as the sole closure technique for reopposing of the nasal flaps, with excellent outcomes.[47] Lee and colleagues used auricular cartilage grafts and fibrin glue in nasal septal repair and had better outcomes in the group with fibrin glue.[48] Another area of great interest that is discussed in detail in this chapter is the use of autologous tissue-engineered implants for healing. Yanaga and colleagues used autologous auricular conchal cartilage cultured into a gel form for dorsal nasal implants.[49] Patients were followed for up to 24 months with maintenance of augmentation. This exciting technology surely represents the vanguard of new tissue-engineered products and technologies for wound healing of facial cartilage defects. This topic is discussed further at the end of this chapter.

Temporomandibular Joint

The temporomandibular joint is most commonly afflicted with conditions that affect function and result in joint disk degeneration and secondary ankylosis. The facial surgeon is often challenged to address disk replacement versus condylar head or glenoid fossa reconstruction as many congenital deformities and adult pathologic entities have been the focus of detailed study and controversial arguments over the years.[50] In the pediatric congenital form of joint ankylosis, the mainstay of therapy has been the use of costal chondral rib grafts.[51] Some authors advocate the use of partial sternoclavicular grafts with better histologic outcome of the repair, but it is clear that in this young patient group, healing with autogenous grafts is positive overall.[52] Costal chondral grafts can be the source of overgrowth, with resultant malocclusion and dysmorphia, but do have predictable healing.[53,54]

Many joint arthroplasties have focused on the disk and disk replacement strategies. Experimental observations have confirmed the use of spacer material as being beneficial to healing.[55] In reviewing alloplastic versus autogenous disk arthroplasties, it remains to be determined whether either approach offers an advantage. The use of local flaps, particularly vascularized temporalis muscle flaps, has been advocated recently, with good early experimental and clinical results.[56,57] Healing of experimental osteochondral joint defects with BMP is currently under study and should have a direct impact on condylar head wound healing in the future.[58–60]

Laryngeal Cartilages

The majority of surgery on the laryngeal cartilages has been focused on ablative procedures, with a focus on survival and patent airway outcomes. Similarly, the treatment of laryngeal fractures focused on the reconstitution of a patent airway. Methods traditionally employed were those of closed reduction with the use of airway stents and, when necessary, suture fixation.[61–63] Little attention was focused on actual cartilage wound healing. Concurrently, the development of laryngeal framework surgery renewed interest in surgical techniques.[64] Application of rigid fixation[65] to the laryngeal cartilages has been followed by studies that document the ease and superior wound healing of internal rigid fixation.[66,67] Dray, Coltrera, and Pinczower performed experimental laryngeal fractures and showed the superiority of rigid fixation in permitting cartilaginous healing, with evidence of matrix reconstitution and cell viability with an intact perichondrial layer, in contrast to semi-rigid wire fixation repairs, which showed fibrous unions and poorly aligned interfaces (see Figure 9).[68] Recently, Tcacencu and colleagues studied the use of BMP-2 in laryngeal wound healing, with encouraging results.[69,70] They confirmed the ability to heal experimental defects with cartilage and bone and that the healing response appeared to be under the control of proliferating perichondrium, with a more robust response in younger animals. Growth factors such as BMP, along with other known positive inducers of cartilage proliferation, hold promise for new therapies in locally delivered laryngeal therapy.

Cartilage Grafts

Beginning with the work of Peer,[14] cartilage grafts have been extensively studied and employed in facial surgery. Autogenous grafts

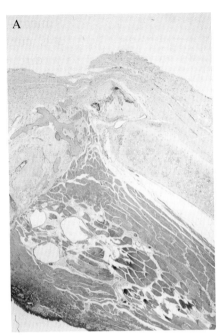 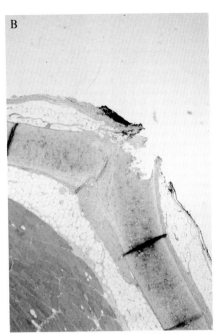 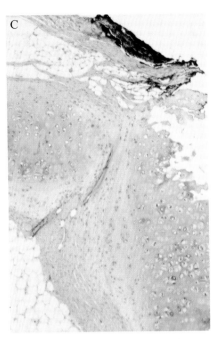

Figure 9. Experimental laryngeal fracture healing. (*A*, Fibrous union in laryngeal fracture. *B*, Cartilaginous union healing. *C*, Cartilaginous union healing with viable chondrocytes and martrix reconstitution. Courtesy of Marc Coltrera, MD, and Eric Pinczower, MD, Seattle, WA.

have always been the preferred source for reconstructive procedures (Figure 10).[43,71] Most studies use purely gross clinical estimates of morphology to determine the success of such grafting, with defect reformation being evidence of graft resorption. It is expected that in younger patients with viable perichondrial coverage, cartilage grafts will be integrated into the donor site,[72,73] yet with onlay grafting, one would expect a fibrous interface at best. Brent detailed his experience with autologous cartilage grafting in auricular reconstruction; the outcomes suggest that long-term survival with volume maintenance is quite predictable in the younger patient.[74]

Often there is limitation on autogenous cartilage for grafting, and alternative sources have been described.[75] Sailer reported the use of lyophilized allograft cartilage for facial augmentation procedures.[76] Irradiated costal cartilage has been extensively used in facial surgery.[77,78] Two common issues with the use of irradiated (costal) cartilage grafts are warping and long-term survival with volume maintenance. A common outcome when using irradiated costal cartilage for facial reconstruction is significant warping of the graft with deformity (Figure 11). Recent studies have shown that there is little difference in the potential for warping of costal cartilage that has been irradiated as opposed to nonirradiated.[79] Clinically, the caveats of removing the perichondrium of irradiated grafts and internal reinforcement[80,81] and using the central portion of the costal graft help minimize such deformation and are consistent with our understanding of the structural organization of cartilage. The long-term survival of irradiated grafts for facial augmentation has been quite controversial. Many authors have reported reasonable results, whereas others have reported volume loss with most irradiated cartilage graft implants.[82] Yet because the volume loss is replaced by fibrous tissue, the contour correction can still be maintained.

Special Situation Cartilage Wound Healing

The widespread introduction of the carbon dioxide laser to clinical surgery in the 1980s opened potential new approaches to cartilage surgery and its impact on wound healing. Smoot and colleagues demonstrated that the region of laser cartilage incision results in chondrocyte loss and a tissue necrosis zone that is significant.[83] Zuger and colleagues examined the use of

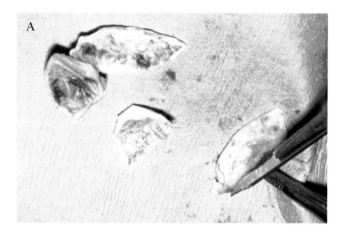
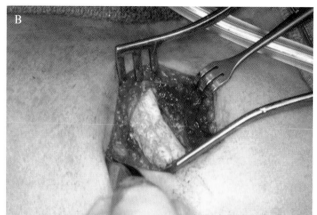
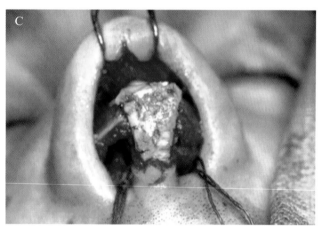
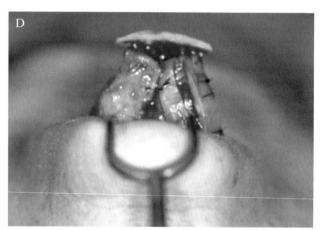

Figure 10. Autogenous cartilage graft harvest from costal and auricular sources and grafting to the nose.

albumin solder and found effective welding of cartilage, but significant chondrocyte loss related to local heat effects still occurred.[84] Interest in the use of laser irradiation to effect changes in the shape and shape-memory biome-

chanical properties was examined in great detail by Wong and colleagues (Figure 12).[85] The basic approach is accomplished with a feedback-controlled laser device (a neodymium:yttrium-aluminum-garnet [YAG] laser) to induce localized temperature-dependent stress relaxation of the cartilage matrix, which permits rapid thermal equilibrium recovery and allows the creation of stable shape changes.[85] These

Figure 11. Warping of nasal irradiated cartilage graft. Courtesy of Fred J. Bressler, MD, Houston, TX.

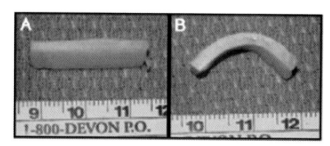

Figure 12. Laser-shaped cartilage by Youn and Milner. http://www.ece.utexas.edu/bell/xprojects/cartilage/main.htm) posted March 27 2000.

investigators have found that the addition of a localized cooling mechanism can enhance the efficiency of the technique and improve chondrocyte viability.[86]

Clinically, nasal septal reshaping using a holmium:YAG laser was studied in 110 patients with good results, accomplishing a truly minimally invasive approach.[87] Although this specialized approach to cartilage wound healing appears to have unique clinical utility, much more basic understanding of the long-term effects on cartilage and its biomechanical properties remains to be explored.[88]

CARTILAGE TISSUE ENGINEERING

Tissue engineering is a new paradigm that integrates the principles and methods of engineering and biomedical technology toward the development of biologic substitutes to restore, maintain, or improve function.[30] By providing an alternate source of graft material for facial reconstruction, tissue engineering of cartilage may help overcome the limitations associated with conventional procedures, such as limited supply, donor-site morbidity, complex three-dimensional morphology, graft resorption, and poor biocompatibility. Tissue engineering methods can be generally categorized as either the implantation of cells alone, a scaffold alone, or a combination of cells within a scaffold.

Cells are intimately involved in the synthesis and organization of ECM components into a functional tissue before and/or after implantation. Accordingly, cells used for tissue engineering generally have a phenotype that is the same or similar to those residing in the target tissue. Ideally, cells for tissue engineering would be easily obtained in large numbers, express the desired phenotype, not transmit disease, and be nonimmunogenic. Scaffolds function by providing mechanical integrity to the engineered tissue and by positively modulating cell behavior. Scaffolds can be composed of synthetic materials, biologic materials, or a combination of both. Ideally, a scaffold for tissue engineering would

support cell attachment and growth, impart the desired anatomic shape on a tissue construct, withstand loads encountered following implantation, and degrade into nontoxic products at a controllable rate. Although tissue engineering is not routinely used for face or neck cartilage reconstruction clinically, experimental investigations have been under way for over a decade to determine the right combination of components and growth conditions to produce functional engineered cartilage.[31]

Cells for Cartilage Tissue Engineering

The vast majority of tissue engineering therapies for cartilage repair and reconstruction incorporate cells are derived from autogenic, allogeneic, or xenogenic sources as therapeutic agents. Mature chondrocytes are most commonly used and have been isolated from a number of sources, including auricular,[2,5,Hutmacher,2003#898,14,16,21,23,29,34] articular,[4,15,23,24] septal,[7,10,12,14,17,21,28] and tracheal cartilage.[17,35] Although these cells share similar characteristics, chondrocytes obtained from different types of cartilage (eg, elastic vs hyaline) have been shown to produce tissue-engineered constructs with different morphologic and biochemical compositions.[21,23] In addition, chondrocytes obtained from similar types of cartilage performing distinctly different functions at different anatomic sites (eg, hyaline cartilage from nasal septum vs articular surface) exhibit inherent dissimilarities.[10,17] Therefore, selection of the type and anatomic location of cartilage to be used as a source of chondrocytes for tissue engineering is an important determinant of the outcome.

As an alternative to chondrocytes, a precursor cell population may be isolated and coerced to undergo differentiation into the desired mature phenotype prior to or following implantation. Mesenchymal stem cells capable of differentiating into chondrocytes have been identified in a number of tissues, including bone marrow, periosteum, and adipose tissue.[26,Nakahara,1990#966,36] Use of mesenchymal stem cells for engineering cartilage for the face and neck was recently investigated.[18,22] A primary benefit of mesenchymal stem cells is their enormous proliferative capacity, meaning that a large number of cells can be obtained from a small biopsy. Furthermore, autologous mesenchymal stem cells can be procured with limited donor-site morbidity.

Most cartilage tissue engineering methods currently under investigation require cell densities equal to or higher than that of native tissue. As a result, amounts on the order of tens of millions of cells are needed per cubic centimeter of tissue. Since chondrocyte availability is limited, particularly for autologous procedures, isolated cells must be expanded over time in culture. Expansion is typically achieved by serially passaging cells cultured in media supplemented with serum and a combination of growth factors, including TGF-β_1, fibroblast growth factor 2, and platelet-derived growth factor.[8,13] It is well established that passaged chondrocytes dedifferentiate to a fibroblast-like phenotype, characterized by a switch from production of collagen type II to collagen type I and by decreased glycosaminoglycan production.[1] Such phenotypic changes have been shown to alter the composition of tissue-engineered cartilage.[12] Attempts to redifferentiate nonarticular chondrocytes in three-dimensional culture systems for tissue engineering applications have produced mixed results.[6,10,21,27] In contrast to chondrocytes, mesenchymal stem cells can be vastly expanded in culture and then induced to differentiate down a desired pathway.[19,25] A recent study suggested that on the order of 1×10^{12} chondrogenic cells can be generated in about a month from 1 mL of human bone marrow.[22] Although mesenchymal stem cells are a promising option, their use also poses a number of obstacles, including how to routinely obtain a pure population, achieve expansion, and control differentiation.

Recently, the approach of using chondrocytes in the absence of a scaffold to engineer cartilage for facial reconstruction was explored.[7,21] Using a macroaggregate system, human septal or auricular chondrocytes were expanded in mono-layer culture and then seeded via centrifugation onto a membrane.[21] Over the course of several weeks in culture, the densely packed cells formed cohesive constructs, with a matrix composition resembling native cartilage in some respects but with significantly lower glycosaminoglycan content and a lack of elastin fibers in the auricular constructs.[21] Using the alginate-recovered chondrocyte method, originally developed using articular chondrocytes, human septal chondrocytes were expanded in monolayer culture and then transferred to a three-dimensional alginate bead culture system, where they accumulated a glycosaminoglycan-rich cell-associated matrix.[7,20] Next, the chondrocytes and their associated matrix were seeded onto a membrane that allowed the cells to integrate and form a cohesive, cartilage-like construct. Direct comparison of scaffold-less constructs formed from monolayer and alginate cultured cells showed that alginate cultured cells produced tissue with greater structural stability and a biochemical composition more like that of native tissue.[7] Although scaffold-less systems may circumvent problems specifically associated with the use of biomaterials, achieving other design criteria, such as an anatomic shape and sufficient mechanical strength, may be more challenging in scaffold-less systems.

Scaffolds for Cartilage Tissue Engineering

Scaffolds are used to impart various macroscopic and microscopic properties on tissue-engineered cartilage constructs and may be used to deliver biologically active substances, such as growth factors, to the implantation site. Important biomaterial characteristics include biocompatibility, biodegradation rate, geometry, surface characteristics, and mechanical integrity. Biocompatibility of a material for the desired function is a foremost necessity. Most scaffold materials are biodegradable and are intended to be replaced by tissue synthesized by implanted or the surrounding native cells. Consequently, the rate of biodegradation should ideally be matched to the rate of matrix synthesis and deposition.

Moldable materials have been extensively used to control the initial construct geometry, a feature particularly relevant for craniofacial reconstruction.[2,4,5,16,34] Over time, postimplantation in animal models, these constructs tend to lose their structural integrity and complex geometries.[2,16,34] This may be due in part to a mismatch in degradation and matrix deposition rates. The pore size and the degree of porosity of scaffold materials should be optimized for a particular application to effectively promote ECM deposition, to facilitate cell seeding, to allow cell migration throughout the construct, and to ensure nutrient delivery and gas exchange for indwelling cells. Surface properties of the material are also an important consideration for cell attachment and growth. For long-term success, materials should be selected to suit the in vivo mechanical environment. Materials used as scaffolds for tissue engineering can be synthetic or biologic in origin.

The most commonly used synthetic materials for cartilage tissue engineering are polylactic acid,[28] polyglycolic acid (PGA),[12,16,17,31,32] and their copolymers.[2,14,27,28] In static culture, chondrocytes attach to these scaffolds, proliferate to varying degrees, and deposit ECM.[10,12,14?,27] The extent to which the newly deposited matrix resembles native cartilage depends on many factors, including cell phenotype prior to seeding onto the scaffold and the duration of culture.[12,Rodriguez,1999#294] A number of in vivo models have demonstrated limitations, including an inflammatory response to PGA in immunocompetent animals,[16] the persistence of inferior mechanical properties compared with native tissue,[2,17] the importance of controlling degradation rates,[28] and difficulty with shape retention.[2] Synthetic hydrogels are currently under investigation, with promising initial results. For example, Pluronic F-127 has been shown to support the formation of cartilaginous tissue in vivo, with no evidence of inflammation.[3,16,29] Nevertheless, in consideration of the complexity of the problem, additional in vitro experimentation is needed to elucidate the complex interactions of cells with various synthetic scaffolds.

Biologic scaffolds that have been used for tissue engineering of cartilages of the face and neck include collagen,[33] fibrin,[34] and alginate.[4,5] Cells can be seeded onto preformed collagen sponges or mixed with soluble collagen prior to polymerization into a gel. When thyroid cartilage chondrocytes were seeded onto collagen sponges, minimal cartilaginous matrix deposition was observed after 8 weeks in culture.[33] In contrast, collagen has produced favorable in vitro and in vivo results when used as a scaffold for articular cartilage engineering, indicating that further research is necessary to elucidate such biphasic responses. Another gelling substance used as a carrier for chondrocytes is fibrin. Auricular chondrocytes embedded in a fibrin gel and subcutaneously implanted in mice formed a cartilaginous tissue after 12 weeks; however, no quantitative biochemical or biomechanical data were presented.[34] Alginate is a natural polymer capable of reversible gel formation. Encapsulation of chondrocytes within alginate allows for prolonged maintenance of the chondrocyte phenotype and accumulation of cartilaginous matrix.[9] Autologous chondrocytes embedded in alginate, molded into anatomic shapes, and implanted for 30 weeks in immunocompetent animals yielded tissue with approximately 60% glycosaminoglycan, 82% collagen, and 85% deoxyribonucleic acid (DNA) content of native tissue. Mechanical properties, specifically the modulus and hydraulic permeability, were also comparable to those of native tissue.[5]

Cartilage tissue engineering is the exciting next phase of medical therapeutics in which targeted therapy benefits from understanding and controlling the cellular molecular biology in various pathologic states. The impact of these developing technologies is vast, and they have potential for significant benefits in facial and neck cartilage surgery.

CONCLUSION

Cartilage wound healing of the face and neck is governed by a complex interrelated set of biologic and biomechanical domains. The fundamental structural organization of cartilage and the various regulatory factors that govern repair and regeneration are beginning to be better understood and correlated with surgical experience and knowledge. Facial cartilage healing can be approached with a sound basis for therapy and predictable outcomes. Future advances, particularly in cellular and tissue regeneration, will continue to enhance the ability of the surgeon to successfully treat the challenging clinical case.

REFERENCES

1. Moss ML, Moss-Saientijn L. Vertebrate cartilages. In: Hall BK, editor. Cartilage. Vol 1. Structure, function, and biochemistry Academic Press, New York, 1983.
2. Caplan AI. Cartilage. Sci Am 1984;251:84.
3. Moore KL, editor. The developing human. 2nd ed. WB Saunders, Philadephia; 1977.
4. Zhao GQ, Zhou X, Eberspaecher H, et al. Cartilage homeoprotein 1, a homeoprotein selectively expressed in chondrocytes. Proc Natl Acad Sci U S A 1993;90: 8633–7.
5. Lefebvre V, de Crombrugghe B. Toward understanding SOX9 function in chondrocyte differentiation. Matrix Biol 1998;16:529–40.
6. Bi W, Deng JM, Zhang Z, et al. Sox9 is required for cartilage formation. Nat Genet 1999;22:85–9.
7. Roberts CR, Rains JK, Pare PD, et al. Ultrastructure and tensile properties of human tracheal cartilage. J Biomech 1998;31:81–6.
8. Poole AR. Cartilage in health and disease. In: Koopman WJ, Moreland LW, editors. Arthritis and allied conditions: textbook of rheumatology Lippincott Williams and Wilkins, Philadephia; 2005.
9. Martin JA, Buckwalter JA. Telomere erosion and senescence in human articular cartilage chondrocytes. J Gerontol A Biol Sci Med Sci 2001;56:B172–9.
10. Ito I, Imada M, Ikeda M, et al. A morphological study of age changes in adult human auricular cartilage with special emphasis on elastic fibers. Laryngoscope 2001; 111:881–6.
11. Rotter N, Tobias G, Lebl M, et al. Age-related changes in the composition and mechanical properties of human nasal cartilage. Arch Biochem Biophys 2002;403:132–40.
12. Sokoloff L. Aging and degenerative diseases affecting cartilages. In: Hall BK, editor. Cartilage. Vol 3. Biomedical aspects, Academic Press, New York; 1983.
13. Peer LA. The fate of living and dead cartilage transplanted in humans. Surg Gynecol Obstet 1939; 68:603.
14. Peer LA. Fate autogenous septal cartilages after transplantation in human tissues. Arch Otolaryngol 1941; 34:696.
15. Verwoerd-Verhoef HL, ten Koppel PG, van Osch GJ, et al. Wound healing of cartilage structures in the head and neck region. Int J Pediatr Otorhinolaryngol 1998;43:241–51.
16. Fry H. Nasal skeletal trauma and the interlocked stresses of the nasal septal cartilage. Br J Plast Surg 1967;20: 146–58.
17. Fry HJH. The healing of cartilage. In: Kernahan DA, Vistnes LM, editors. Biological aspects of reconstructive surgery. Boston: Little Brown; 1977. p. 351, .
18. Murray JA. The behaviour of nasal septal cartilage in response to trauma. Rhinology 1987;25:23–7.
19. Gibson T, Davis WB. The distortion of autogenous cartilage grafts: its cause and prevention. Br J Plast Surg 1958;10:257.
20. Calhoun KH, Chase SP. Reconstruction of the auricle. Facial Plast Surg Clin North Am 2005;13:231.
21. Ghanem T, Rasamny JK, Park SS. Rethinking auricular trauma. Laryngoscope 2005;115:1251–5.
22. Tan ST, Abramson DL, MacDonald DM, Mulliken JB. Molding therapy for infants with deformational auricular anomalies. Ann Plast Surg 1997;38:263–8.
23. Ullmann Y, Blazer S, Ramon Y, et al. Early nonsurgical correction of congenital auricular deformities. Plast Reconstr Surg 2002;109:907–13.
24. Hoehn JG, Ashruf S. Otoplasty: sequencing the operation for improved results. Plast Reconstr Surg 2005;115: 5e–16e.
25. Gosain AK, Kumar A, Huang G. Prominent ears in children younger than 4 years of age: what is the appropriate timing for otoplasty? Plast Reconstr Surg 2004;114:1042–54.
26. Mustarde JC. The treatment of prominent ears by buried mattress sutures: a ten-year survey. Plast Reconstr Surg 1967;39:382–6.
27. Furnas DW. Correction of prominent ears with multiple sutures. Clin Plast Surg 1978;5:491–5.
28. Mackenzie M. Deviation of the nasal septum. 2nd ed London: J & A Churchill; 1884.
29. Pirsig W. Morphologic aspects of the injured nasal septum in children. Rhinology 1979;17:65–75.
30. Olsen KD, Carpenter RJ III, Kern EB. Nasal septal injury in children. Diagnosis and management. Arch Otolaryngol 1980;106:317–20.
31. Holt GR. Related biomechanics of nasal septal trauma. Otolaryngol Clin North Am 1999;32:615–9.
32. Daniel M, Raghavan U. Relation between epistaxis, external nasal deformity, and septal deviation following nasal trauma. Emerg Med J 2005;22(11):778–9.
33. Metzenbaum M. Replacement of the lower and of the dislocated septal cartilage. Arch Otolaryngol 1929;9: 282.
34. Peer L. An operation to repair lateral displacement of the lower border of the septal cartilage. Arch Otolaryngol 1937;25:475.
35. Fomon S, Gilbert J, Syracuse V. Plastic repair of obstruction septum. Arch Otolaryngol 1948;47:7.
36. Harrison DH. Related nasal injuries: their pathogenesis and treatment. Br J Plast Surg 1979;32:57–64.

37. Verwoerd-Verhoef HL, Meeuwis CA, van der Heul RO, Verwoerd CD. Histologic evaluation of crushed cartilage grafts in the growing nasal septum of young rabbits. ORL J Otorhinolaryngol Relat Spec 1991;53: 305–9.

38. Verwoerd CD, Verwoerd-Verhoef HL, Meeuwis CA, van der Heul RO. Wound healing of the nasal septal perichondrium in young rabbits. ORL J Otorhinolaryngol Relat Spec 1990;52:180–6.

39. Duynstee ML, Verwoerd-Verhoef HL, Verwoerd CD, van Osch GJ. The dual role of perichondrium in cartilage wound healing. Plast Reconstr Surg 2002;110:1073–9.

40. Kuettner KE, Pauli BU. Vascularity of cartilage. In: Hall BK, editor. Cartilage. Vol 1. Structure, function, and biochemistry, Academic Press, New York; 1983.

41. Boenisch M, Tamas H, Nolst Trenite GJ. Influence of polydioxanone foil on growing septal cartilage after surgery in an animal model: new aspects of cartilage healing and regeneration (preliminary results). Arch Facial Plast Surg 2003;5:316–9.

42. Boenisch M, Mink A. Clinical and histological results of septoplasty with a resorbable implant. Arch Otolaryngol Head Neck Surg 2000;126:1373–7.

43. Johnson CM Jr, Toriumi DM, editors. Open structure rhinoplasty. WB Saunders, Philadelphia; 1990.

44. Baker SR. Suture contouring of the nasal tip. Arch Facial Plast Surg 2000;2:34–42.

45. Gruber RP, Nahai F, Bogdan MA, Friedman GD. Changing the convexity and concavity of nasal cartilages and cartilage grafts with horizontal mattress sutures: part II. Clinical results. Plast Reconstr Surg 2005;115:595–606.

46. Dyer WK, Kang J. Correction of severe caudal deflections with a cartilage "plating" rigid fixation graft. Arch Otolaryngol Head Neck Surg 2000;126:973–8.

47. Daneshrad P, Chin GY, Rice DH. Fibrin glue prevents complications of septal surgery: findings in a series of 100 patients. Ear Nose Throat J 2003;82: 196–7.

48. Lee JY, Lee SH, Kim SC, et al. Usefulness of autologous cartilage and fibrin glue for the prevention of septal perforation during septal surgery: a preliminary report. Laryngoscope 2006;116:934–7.

49. Yanaga H, Yanaga K, Imai K, et al. Clinical application of cultured autologous human auricular chondrocytes with autologous serum for craniofacial or nasal augmentation and repair. Plast Reconstr Surg 2006; 117:2019–30.

50. Chossegros C, Guyot L, Cheynet F, et al. Comparison of different materials for interposition arthroplasty in treatment of temporomandibular joint ankylosis surgery: long-term follow-up in 25 cases. Br J Oral Maxillofac Surg 1997;35:157–60.

51. Kaban LB, Perrott DH, Fisher K. A protocol for management of temporomandibular joint ankylosis. J Oral Maxillofac Surg 1990;48:1145–51.

52. Daniels S, Ellis E III, Carlson DS. Histologic analysis of costochondral and sternoclavicular grafts in the TMJ

of the juvenile monkey. J Oral Maxillofac Surg 1987; 45:675–83.

53. Matsuura H, Miyamoto H, Ishimaru JI, et al. Costochondral grafts in reconstruction of the temporomandibular joint after condylectomy: an experimental study in sheep. Br J Oral Maxillofac Surg 2001;39: 189–95.

54. Guyuron B, Lasa CI Jr. Unpredictable growth pattern of costochondral graft. Plast Reconstr Surg 1992;90:880– 6.

55. Tucker MR, Watzke IM. Autogenous auricular cartilage graft for temporomandibular joint repair. A comparison of technique with and without temporary Silastic implantation. J Craniomaxillofac Surg 1991;19:108– 12.

56. Feinberg SE, Larsen PE. The use of a pedicled temporalis muscle-pericranial flap for replacement of the TMJ disc: preliminary report. J Oral Maxillofac Surg 1989; 47:142–6.

57. Umeda H, Kaban LB, Pogrel MA, Stern M. Long-term viability of the temporalis muscle/fascia flap used for temporomandibular joint reconstruction. J Oral Maxillofac Surg 1993;51:530–3.

58. Cook SD, Patron LP, Salkeld SL, Rueger DC. Repair of articular cartilage defects with osteogenic protein-1 (BMP-7) in dogs. J Bone Joint Surg Am 2003;85A Suppl 3::116–23.

59. Suzuki T, Bessho K, Fujimura K, et al. Regeneration of defects in the articular cartilage in rabbit temporomandibular joints by bone morphogenetic protein-2. Br J Oral Maxillofac Surg 2002;40:201–6.

60. Ueki K, Takazakura D, Marukawa K, et al. The use of polylactic acid/polyglycolic acid copolymer and gelatin sponge complex containing human recombinant bone morphogenetic protein-2 following condylectomy in rabbits. J Craniomaxillofac Surg 2003;31:107– 14.

61. Olson NR, Miles WK. Treatment of acute blunt laryngeal injuries. Ann Otol Rhinol Laryngol 1971;80:704–9.

62. Olson NR. Surgical treatment of acute blunt laryngeal injuries. Ann Otol Rhinol Laryngol 1978;87(5 Pt 1): 716–21.

63. Schaefer SD, Close LG. Acute management of laryngeal trauma. Ann Otol Rhinol Laryngol 1989;98:98–104.

64. Isshiki N. Progress in laryngeal framework surgery. Acta Otolaryngol (Stockh) 2000;120:120–7.

65. Woo P. Laryngeal framework reconstruction with miniplates. Ann Otol Rhinol Laryngol 1990;99(10 Pt 1): 772–7.

66. Lykins CL, Pinczower EF. The comparative strength of laryngeal fracture fixation. Am J Otolaryngol 1998;19: 158–62.

67. Sasaki CT, Marotta JC, Lowlicht RA, et al. Efficacy of resorbable plates for reduction and stabilization of laryngeal fractures. Ann Otol Rhinol Laryngol 2003; 112(9 Pt 1):745–50.

68. Dray TG, Coltrera MD, Pinczower EF. Thyroid cartilage fracture repair in rabbits: comparing healing with wire

and miniplate fixation. Laryngoscope 1999;109:118–22.

69. Tcacencu I, Carlsoo B, Stierna P. Effect of recombinant human BMP-2 on the repair of cricoid cartilage defects in young and adult rabbits: a comparative study. Int J Pediatr Otorhinolaryngol 2005;69:1239–46.

70. Tcacencu I, Carlsoo B, Stierna P. Cell origin in experimental repair of cricoid cartilage defects treated with recombinant human bone morphogenetic protein-2. Wound Repair Regen 2005;13:341–9.

71. de Jong AL, Park AH, Raveh E, et al. Comparison of thyroid, auricular, and costal cartilage donor sites for laryngotracheal reconstruction in an animal model. Arch Otolaryngol Head Neck Surg 2000;126:49–53.

72. Cheney M. Reconstructive grafting by the open nasal approach. Facial Plast Surg Clin North Am 1993;1:99–109.

73. Pirsig W, Bean JK, Lenders H, et al. Cartilage transformation in a composite graft of demineralized bovine bone matrix and ear perichondrium used in a child for the reconstruction of the nasal septum. Int J Pediatr Otorhinolaryngol 1995;32:171–81.

74. Brent B. Auricular repair with autogenous rib cartilage grafts: two decades of experience with 600 cases. Plast Reconstr Surg 1992;90:355–74; discussion 375–6.

75. Allcroft RA, Friedman CD, Quatela VC. Cartilage grafts for head and neck augmentation and reconstruction autografts and homografts. Otolaryngol Clin North Am 1994;27:69–80.

76. Sailer HF. Experiences with the use of lyophilized bank cartilage for facial contour correction. J Maxillofac Surg 1976;4:149–57.

77. Kridel RW, Konior RJ. Irradiated cartilage grafts in the nose. A preliminary report. Arch Otolaryngol Head Neck Surg 1993;119:24–30; discussion 30–1.

78. Burke AJ, Wang TD, Cook TA. Irradiated homograft rib cartilage in facial reconstruction. Arch Facial Plast Surg 2004;6:334–4.

79. Adams WP Jr, Rohrich RJ, Gunter JP, et al. The rate of warping in irradiated and nonirradiated homograft rib cartilage: a controlled comparison and clinical implications. Plast Reconstr Surg 1999;103:265–70.

80. Gunter JP, Clark CP, Friedman RM. Internal stabilization of autogenous rib cartilage grafts in rhinoplasty: a barrier to cartilage warping. Plast Reconstr Surg 1997;100:161–9.

81. Kim DW, Shah AR, Toriumi DM. Concentric and eccentric carved costal cartilage: a comparison of warping. Arch Facial Plast Surg 2006;8:42–6.

82. Welling DB, Maves MD, Schuller DE, Bardach J. Irradiated homologous cartilage grafts. Long-term results. Arch Otolaryngol Head Neck Surg 1988;114:291–5.

83. Smoot EC III, Bergman B, Lyons S. Effect of the carbon dioxide laser on viability of ear cartilage in a rabbit model. J Craniofac Surg 1995;6:147–50.

84. Zuger BJ, Ott B, Mainil-Varlet P, et al. Laser solder welding of articular cartilage: tensile strength and chondrocyte viability. Lasers Surg Med 2001;28:427–34.

85. Wong BJ, Milner TE, Harrington A, et al. Feedback-controlled laser-mediated cartilage reshaping. Arch Facial Plast Surg 1999;1:282–7.

86. Karamzadeh AM, Rasouli A, Tanenbaum BS, et al. Laser-mediated cartilage reshaping with feedback-controlled cryogen spray cooling: biophysical properties and viability. Lasers Surg Med 2001;28:1–10.

87. Ovchinnikov Y, Sobol E, Svistushkin V, et al. Laser septochondrocorrection. Arch Facial Plast Surg 2002;4:180–5.

88. Karam AM, Protsenko DE, Li C, et al. Long-term viability and mechanical behavior following laser cartilage reshaping. Arch Facial Plast Surg 2006;8:105–16.

89. Benya PD, Shaffer JD. Dedifferentiated chondrocytes reexpress the differentiated collagen phenotype when cultured in agarose gels. Cell 1982;30:215–24.

90. Britt JC, Park SS. Autogenous tissue-engineered cartilage: evaluation as an implant material. Arch Otolaryngol Head Neck Surg 1998;124:671–7.

91. Cao Y, Rodriguez A, Vacanti M, et al. Comparative study of the use of poly(glycolic acid), calcium alginate and pluronics in the engineering of autologous porcine cartilage. J Biomater Sci Polym Ed 1998;9:475–87.

92. Chang SC, Rowley JA, Tobias G, et al. Injection molding of chondrocyte/alginate constructs in the shape of facial implants. J Biomed Mater Res 2001;55:503–11.

93. Chang SC, Tobias G, Roy AK, et al. Tissue engineering of autologous cartilage for craniofacial reconstruction by injection molding. Plast Reconstr Surg 2003;112:793–9; discussion 800–1.

94. Chia SH, Homicz MR, Schumacher BL, et al. Characterization of human nasal septal chondrocytes cultured in alginate. J Am Coll Surg 2005;200:691–704.

95. Chia SH, Schumacher BL, Klein TJ, et al. Tissue-engineered human nasal septal cartilage using the alginate-recovered-chondrocyte method. Laryngoscope 2004;114:38–45.

96. Hardingham T, Tew S, Murdoch A. Tissue engineering: chondrocytes and cartilage. Arthritis Res 2002;4 Suppl 3:S63–8.

97. Hauselmann HJ, Fernandes RJ, Mok SS, et al. Phenotypic stability of bovine articular chondrocytes after long-term culture in alginate beads. J Cell Sci 1994;107:17–27.

98. Homicz MR, Chia SH, Schumacher BL, et al. Human septal chondrocyte redifferentiation in alginate, polyglycolic acid scaffold, and monolayer culture. Laryngoscope 2003;113:25–32.

99. Homicz MR, McGowan KB, Lottman LM, et al. A compositional analysis of human nasal septal cartilage. Arch Facial Plast Surg 2003;5:53–8.

100. Homicz MR, Schumacher BL, Sah RL, Watson D. Effects of serial expansion of septal chondrocytes on tissue-engineered neocartilage composition. Otolaryngol Head Neck Surg 2002;127:398–408.

101. Jakob M, Demarteau O, Schafer D, et al. Specific growth factors during the expansion and redifferentiation of adult human articular chondrocytes enhance chondrogenesis and cartilaginous tissue formation in vitro. J Cell Biochem 2001;81:368–77.

102. Kamil SH, Eavey RD, Vacanti MP, et al. Tissue-engineered cartilage as a graft source for laryngotracheal reconstruction: a pig model. Arch Otolaryngol Head Neck Surg 2004;130:1048–51.

103. Kamil SH, Kojima K, Vacanti MP, et al. In vitro tissue engineering to generate a human-sized auricle and nasal tip. Laryngoscope 2003;113:90–4.

104. Kamil SH, Vacanti MP, Aminuddin BS, et al. Tissue engineering of a human sized and shaped auricle using a mold. Laryngoscope 2004;114:867–70.

105. Kojima K, Bonassar LJ, Ignotz RA, et al. Comparison of tracheal and nasal chondrocytes for tissue engineering of the trachea. Ann Thorac Surg 2003;76:1884–8.

106. Kojima K, Ignotz RA, Kushibiki T, et al. Tissue-engineered trachea from sheep marrow stromal cells with transforming growth factor beta2 released from biodegradable microspheres in a nude rat recipient. J Thorac Cardiovasc Surg 2004;128:147–53.

107. Mackay AM, Beck SC, Murphy JM, et al. Chondrogenic differentiation of cultured human mesenchymal stem cells from marrow. Tissue Eng 1998;4:415–28.

108. Masuda K, Sah RL, Hejna MJ, Thonar EJ. A novel two-step method for the formation of tissue-engineered cartilage by mature bovine chondrocytes: the alginate-recovered-chondrocyte (ARC) method. J Orthop Res 2003;21:139–48.

109. Naumann A, Dennis JE, Aigner J, et al. Tissue engineering of autologous cartilage grafts in three-dimensional in vitro macroaggregate culture system. Tissue Eng 2004;10:1695–706.

110. Pang Y, Cui P, Chen W, et al. Quantitative study of tissue-engineered cartilage with human bone marrow mesenchymal stem cells. Arch Facial Plast Surg 2005;7:7–11.

111. Panossian A, Ashiku S, Kirchhoff CH, et al. Effects of cell concentration and growth period on articular and ear chondrocyte transplants for tissue engineering. Plast Reconstr Surg 2001;108:392–402.

112. Peretti GM, Randolph MA, Zaporojan V, et al. A biomechanical analysis of an engineered cell-scaffold implant for cartilage repair. Ann Plast Surg 2001;46:533–7.

113. Pittenger MF, Mackay AM, Beck SC, et al. Multilineage potential of adult human mesenchymal stem cells. Science 1999;284:143–7.

114. Prockop DJ. Marrow stromal cells as stem cells for nonhematopoietic tissues. Science 1997;276:71–4.

115. Rodriguez A, Cao YL, Ibarra C, et al. Characteristics of cartilage engineered from human pediatric auricular cartilage. Plast Reconstr Surg 1999;103:1111–9.

116. Rotter N, Aigner J, Naumann A, et al. Cartilage reconstruction in head and neck surgery: comparison of resorbable polymer scaffolds for tissue engineering of human septal cartilage. J Biomed Mater Res 1998;42:347–56.

117. Saim AB, Cao Y, Weng Y, et al. Engineering autogenous cartilage in the shape of a helix using an injectable hydrogel scaffold. Laryngoscope 2000;110:1694–7.

118. Skalak RC, Fox F, editors. Tissue engineering. New York: Liss; 1988.

119. Vacanti CA, Langer R, Schloo B, Vacanti JP. Synthetic polymers seeded with chondrocytes provide a template for new cartilage formation. Plast Reconstr Surg 1991;88:753–9.

120. Vacanti CA, Paige KT, Kim WS, et al. Experimental tracheal replacement using tissue-engineered cartilage. J Pediatr Surg 1994;29:201–4; discussion 204–5.

121. Wambach BA, Cheung H, Josephson GD. Cartilage tissue engineering using thyroid chondrocytes on a type I collagen matrix. Laryngoscope 2000;110:2008–11.

122. Xu JW, Johnson TS, Motarjem PM, et al. Tissue-engineered flexible ear-shaped cartilage. Plast Reconstr Surg 2005;115:1633–41.

123. Yang L, Korom S, Welti M, et al. Tissue engineered cartilage generated from human trachea using DegraPol scaffold. Eur J Cardiothorac Surg 2003;24:201–7.

124. Zuk PA, Zhu M, Mizuno H, et al. Multilineage cells from human adipose tissue: implications for cell-based therapies. Tissue Eng 2001;7:211–28.

125. Nakahara H, Bruder SP, Haynesworth SE, et al. Bone and cartilage formation in diffusion chambers by subcultured cells derived from the periosteum. Bone 1990;11:181–8.

4

Peripheral Nerve

David J. Rowe, MD; Hani Matloub, MD

The response to peripheral nerve injury in the face involves a complex milieu of substances that leads to regeneration. The process of nerve regeneration is unique in that the damaged nerve must not only undergo growth and maturation but also, in spanning the nerve gap, must reach its target in a site-specific manner to achieve a positive functional outcome. The process of nerve regeneration involves creation of the appropriate environment for growth and site-specific targeting of the end-organ. This chapter describes the unique regenerative qualities of peripheral nerves of the face and provides an overview of anatomy and possible future technologies to improve nerve regeneration after injury.

UNIQUE HISTOLOGY AND HEALING PHYSIOLOGY

Nerves may be injured from ischemic insult, radiation, traction, infection, inflammation, and pressure from oncologic sources. Degeneration affects the neuron both proximally and distally, as well as producing changes in the Schwann cells surrounding the affected nerve. Proximal to the site of injury, the cell body undergoes retrograde degeneration, chromatolysis, retraction of dendrites, swelling of the cell body, and displacement of the nucleus to the periphery of the cell. The proximal axon may exhibit atrophy within 2 days.

Macrophage proliferation is paramount for both the clearance of cellular debris, namely myelin and extruded axoplasm, and stimulation of the Schwann cells. Following injury, the process of regeneration is multifactorial, involving the proximal and distal stumps of the injured nerve, Schwann cells, glial cells, and macrophages, as well as neurotrophic, molecular, and paracrine factors.

MAJOR STEPS IN HEALING OVER TIME

Following axotomy, there is a resultant gap between the proximal and distal stumps. A fibrin clot resulting from blood products and clotting factors initially fills the gap. Macrophages and ultimately fibroblasts enter this space. Axonal sprouting begins from the proximal stump, and sprouts are accompanied by Schwann cells. Phagocytosis of neuronal debris by macrophages and Schwann cells begins to occur within the first 7 days after axonotmesis. The Schwann cells appear by 1 to 2 days and have peak mitosis by 2 to 3 days postinjury.

Growth of the regenerating axon continues until the distal stump is encountered. Reinnervation of target tissues after axotomy has shown remarkable specificity. The specificity by which the axon is regenerated (neurotropism) and the growth and survival of the axon itself (neurotrophism) are thought to be highly contingent on humoral factors. Neurotrop(h)ic factors are endogenous soluble proteins that are capable of neurotrophism and/or neurotropism. Nerve growth factor (NGF), the first neurotrophic factor to be identified, is postulated to be associated with establishing the basic network of the nervous system during embryologic and fetal development, as well as its regenerative properties in the peripheral nervous system.

Many other factors have been investigated and are reviewed in this chapter.

FUTURE PROMISE FOR HEALING IMPROVEMENT

The use of exogenous neurotropic factors has been investigated. NGF has demonstrated improved quality of the regenerated nerve when NGF was placed in silicone tubes, along with the proximal and distal stumps of the injured nerve. Other factors, such as ciliary neurotrophic factor (CNTF) and insulin-like growth factor (IGF)-1 and IGF-2, have had initial positive results in promotion of regeneration. Neural tubes have been investigated extensively in bridging nerve gaps following injury. The advantages posed by using an allogeneic nerve conduit over a traditional interpositional nerve graft are that of donor nerve harvest and morbidity. Nerve conduits have been demonstrated to have an efficacy similar to that of the nerve graft in instances in which nerve deficits are less than 3 cm; however, at distances greater than 3 cm, nerve conduits have been largely unsuccessful at initiating regeneration across the gap. Multiple neurotrophic and neurotropic factors have been evaluated in the context of neural tubes in the hope of overcoming the critical 3 cm gap, with equivocal results. There is much future promise for the use of nerve conduits and exogenous neurotrophic and neurotropic factors in effectively bridging nerve gaps.

ANATOMY

Many peripheral nerves exist within the face and neck; therefore, a detailed description of the anatomy of this region is beyond the scope of this chapter. However, several key anatomic interests are discussed.

Facial Nerve

The facial nerve (cranial nerve [CN] VII) is the sole motor supply controlling the muscles of facial expression but is not involved in mastication or oculomotor activity. Of the CNs, it is the most susceptible to injury.[1] It also has sensory function for a small area surrounding the external acoustic meatus. The facial nerve is also the parent nerve for secretomotor fibers to the submandibular and salivary glands.[2] The causes of facial nerve injury are multiple and include maxillofacial trauma and neoplastic, idiopathic (Bell's palsy), and iatrogenic (surgical manipulation) causes. Impairment of facial nerve function affects not only facial animation but also cosmesis, communication skills, and the psychology of the patient. Determination of the level of injury is paramount in the ultimate treatment of facial nerve paralysis; thus, the anatomy of the facial nerve is crucial for those operating on the face. A brief overview of the facial nerve anatomy is described below. The interested reader is referred to more comprehensive discussions of facial nerve anatomy.[3]

Pretemporal and Intratemporal Facial Nerves

The origin of the motor nucleus of the facial nerve is deep within the ventrolateral portion of the pons. The facial nerve emerges from the brainstem at the junction of the pons and medulla at the cerebellopontine angle. At this time, two branches exist: the motor root (facial expression) and the intermediate nerve, which contains taste, parasympathetic, and sensory fibers.[2] Once the facial nerve enters the temporal bone, three major branches are formed before exiting the stylomastoid foramen. These are the greater petrosal nerve, the nerve to the stapedius, and the chorda tympani. The greater petrosal nerve traverses through the petrous portion of the temporal bone, middle cranial fossa, pterygoid canal, and pterygopalatine fossa to ultimately supply secretory function to the lacrimal gland. Defects of the greater petrosal nerve may be tested with Schirmer's test for secretory function of the lacrimal gland. The second intratemporal branch is the nerve to the stapedius, which is responsible for sound dampening. Injury to this nerve results in hyperacusia. The third branch, the chorda tympani, joins the lingual nerve to supply taste sensation to the anterior two-thirds of the tongue and soft palate.

The intratemporal facial nerve is particularly succeptable to compression forces within the labyrinthine portion and shearing forces as it enters the tympanic segment.[4]

Post-temporal Facial Nerve

The facial nerve exits the skull through the stylomastoid foramen. The foramen is located posterolateral to the styloid process and anteromedial to the mastoid process. At this location, the facial nerve is approximately 2 cm deep to the skin. After exiting the stylomastoid foramen, the posterior auricular branch, which supplies the auricularis posterior and the occipital belly of the occipitofrontalis muscle, is formed. The facial nerve enters the parotid gland and bifurcates into temporofacial and cervicofacial branches. The two branches then divide into five separate terminal branches leaving the parotid gland: the frontal, zygomatic, buccal, mandibular (marginal mandibular), and cervical branches (Figure 1).

The terminal branches of the facial nerve may have multiple interconnections, as evidenced by Baker and Conley's analysis and that of others.[5-7] Although up to 90% of patients have multiple interconnections within the five terminal branches of the facial nerve, the frontal and mandibular branches have interconnections in only 10 to 15% of cases.[5] Thus, injury to the frontal and mandibular branches may not be compensated for and may lead to disruption of kinetic movement.

Trigeminal Nerve (CN V)

The trigeminal nerve provides sensation to the face, scalp, auricle, external auditory meatus, nose, paranasal sinuses, mouth, parts of the nasopharynx, auditory canal, and cranial dura mater. Also, the trigeminal nerve provides motor function to the muscles of mastication, mylohyoid, anterior belly of the digastric muscle, tensor veli palitini, and tensor tympani (Figure 2). The trigeminal nerve emerges from the pons as a motor root and a sensory root, which enter the trigeminal ganglion in the petrous portion of the temporal bone. From the trigeminal ganglion, the neurons divide into three separate nerves: the ophthalmic nerve (CN V1), the maxillary nerve (CN V2), and the mandibular nerve (CN V3).

The ophthalmic nerve (CN V1) traverses the lateral wall of the cavernous sinus and enters the orbit through the superior orbital fissure. The frontal division of the ophthalmic nerve branches along the orbital roof to ultimately form the supraorbital and supratrochlear nerves, which supply sensation to the forehead and scalp. The supraorbital nerve is commonly injured as a result of trauma to the forehead region. The maxillary nerve (CN V2) enters the lateral wall of the cavernous sinus and passes through the foramen rotundum to supply sensation to the midface, palate, paranasal sinuses, and maxillary teeth. The maxillary nerve divides into the zygomaticotem-

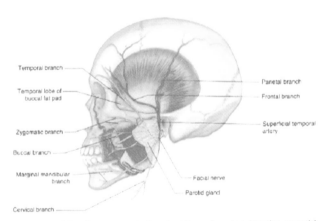

Figure 1. The five separate terminal branches leaving the parotid gland.

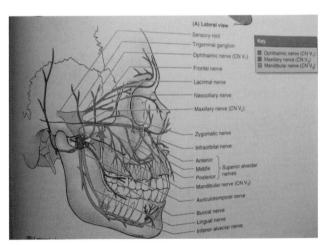

Figure 2. The trigeminal nerve provides motor function to the muscles of mastication, mylohyoid, anterior belly of the digastric muscle, tensor veli palitini, and tensor tympani.

poral, zygomaticofacial, posterior superior middle and anterior alveolar nerves, and infraorbital nerve. Of note, the infraorbital nerve is most commonly injured during orbital floor fractures owing to the disruption of the infraorbital groove or foramen. The mandibular nerve (CN V3) is a mixed motor and sensory nerve, providing motor function for the trigeminal nerve and sensation for the lower third of the face. The mandibular nerve passes through the foramen ovale and terminates in three main sensory branches and motor fibers to the muscles of mastication: the auriculotemporal, the buccal, and inferior alveolar nerves. The mental nerve branches from the inferior alveolar nerve and enters the mandible posteromedially. It traverses the mandible within the inferior alveolar canal and exits the mental foramen anteromedially as the mental nerve to provide sensation to the chin, lower lip, and gingiva.

Great Auricular Nerve

The great auricular nerve is formed from C2 and C3 dorsal sensory roots and supplies the lower two-thirds of the ear, as well as the pre- and postauricular skin. Transient numbness in the great auricular distribution is a relatively common complication following face-lift surgery. The great auricular nerve crosses the sternocleidomastoid muscle 6.5 cm inferior to the inferior border of the external auditory canal.

HISTOLOGY

Anatomy of a Nerve

Peripheral nerves are composed of three distinct types of nerve fibers, motor (efferent), sensory (afferent), and sympathetic, each of which differs in structure and function. The ventral roots of the spinal cord contain the efferent fibers that transmit signal output from the spinal cord to the muscle, including motor and sympathetic information. The cell body of the motor nerve lies within the ventral root itself, whereas the axon of the motor nerve travels to the neuromuscular junction at the muscle terminus.[8] The fibers leaving the spinal cord from the ventral root contain α motoneurons, γ motoneurons, and preganglionic autonomic neurons. The dorsal roots of the spinal cord consist of sensory fibers transmitting information from the periphery to the spinal cord. The cell bodies of these afferent nerves are located in the dorsal root ganglia. The size, type, and description of sensory and motor nerves are listed in Table 1.

Myelinated and unmyelinated nerve fibers leave the spinal cord and are covered by the endoneurium, a thin collagen-containing layer (Figure 3). Ultimately, groupings of nerve fibers are surrounded by the perineurium, a multilayered connective tissue sheath that provides a barrier to diffusion.[8] This concentration of nerve fibers and perineurium is denoted as a fascicle. Multiple fascicles may then be surrounded by

Table 1. CLASSIFICATION OF NERVE FIBERS			
Fibers	Diameter (μm)	Conduction Velocity (m/sec)	Function
Sensory			
Ia (A-α)	12–20	70–120	Primary afferents of muscle spindle
Ib (A-α)	12–20	70–120	Golgi tendon organ
			Touch and pressure receptors
II (A-β)	5–14	30–70	Touch, pressure, and vibratory sense receptors
III (A-δ)	2–7	12–30	Touch, pressure, pain, and temperature receptors
IV (C)	0.5–1	0.5–2	Pain and temperature receptors (unmyelinated)
Motor			
Alpha (A-α)	12–20	15–120	Innervate extrafusal muscle fibers
Gamma (A-γ)	2–10	10–45	Intrafusal muscle fibers
Preganglionic autonomic fibers (B)	< 3	3–15	Myelinated preganglionic autonomic fibers
Postganglionic autonomic fibers (C)	1	2	Unmyelinated postganglionic autonomic fibers

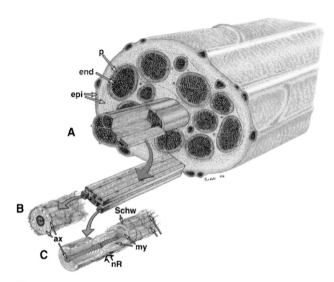

Figure 3. Myelinated and unmyelinated nerve fibers leave the spinal cord and are covered by the endoneurium, a thin collagen-containing layer.

another connective tissue layer called the epineurium. The epineurium is essentially the prolongation of the dural sleeve of the nerve roots.[9] The blood supply to the peripheral nerve is via an intrinsic system located within the endoneurium, perineurium, and epineurium, as well as segmental external blood supplies contingent on nerve location.

Axoplasmic Transport

All cells must have a system to distribute intracellular proteins, energy, and cytoskeletal elements. The neuron is distinct in that its individual cell may stretch from one end of the body to the other. A complex system of anterograde and retrograde transport exists for the maintenance of cellular elements within the neuron. Organelles and neurotransmitter precursors are transported throughout the neuron via fast anterograde transport. Fast transport is typically mediated by microtubules and has a rate of distribution of 200 to 400 mm/d. Other cytoskeletal and cytoplasmic material is transported via slow anterograde transport (1–5 mm/d) mediated by microtubules. Materials are returned to the cell body from the axon terminal primarily via fast retrograde transport. The rate of retrograde transport is 100 to 200 mm/d and is mediated by microtubules and dynein. This

intricate process must function for the peripheral nervous system to maintain optimal function. If significant defects of the system occur, there will likely be cessation of nerve conduction and therefore degeneration of the cell.

Nerve Histology

Sunderland originally mapped the arrangement of nerve bundles along the course of peripheral nerves, showing multiple points of branching, fusion, and changes in the number of fascicles.[10,11]

Histochemical Evaluation

Following transection of mixed motor and sensory nerves, reanastomosis of the nerve fascicles may be performed. However, selectivity of the nerve stumps to reanastomose is problematic with conventional histology and electron microscopy. When transection occurs proximally, the motor and sensory neurons may be quite mixed, whereas further distally, they are organized into distinct fascicles.[12] Mapping of the peripheral nerve may aid the surgeon in distal fascicular repair and thus may lead to improved outcomes. Several techniques have been investigated for intraoperative fascicular mapping of peripheral nerves.

Acetylcholinesterase. Acetylcholinesterase was first used by Karnovsky and Roots to evaluate sectioned nerves.[13] When acetylcholine, copper sulfate, and potassium ferricyanide are combined, a dark brown precipitate visible by light microscopy is produced. This technique was further refined for differentiation of motor and sensory neurons, whereby motor nerves were preferentially stained.[14] Acetylcholinesterase has been used as an intraoperative histochemical aid; however, accurate staining of the nerve may take from 4 to 36 hours.[15,16]

Choline Acetyltransferase. Choline acetyltransferase activity has also been investigated as a method for intraoperative histochemical analysis. Choline acetyltransferase is an enzyme that is found in cholinergic axons and is in more abundance in motor nerves when compared with sensory nerves.[17,18] The test, as described by Lang and colleagues and Engel and colleagues,[19,20] uses a radioimmunoassay technique to evaluate the enzyme activity in the nerve stumps. According to these authors, the analysis takes between 2 and 4 hours to perform.

Carbonic Anhydrase. Unlike acetylcholinesterase and choline acetyltransferase, carbonic anhydrase is more sensitive to sensory axons. It is a ubiquitous enzyme that has multiple functions, including carbon dioxide metabolism and bicarbonate transport. Riley and colleagues demonstrated differentiation of motor and sensory neurons in a rat model and postulated that carbonic anhydrase may be clinically applicable.[21,22]

Histochemical analysis via the aforementioned techniques has been proven to aid in the reanastomosis of fascicles in the peripheral nerves. However, these techniques have not been used routinely by the microsurgeon owing to the prohibitively long duration of the tests. Future investigations will likely focus on decreasing intraoperative time while maintaining high sensitivity. Long-term studies are needed to evaluate the return of function in patients who have had histochemical-aided reanastomoses compared with those who have not.

HEALING STEPS AFTER INJURY

Degeneration

Nerves may be injured in a variety of ways, including ischemic insult, radiation, traction, infection, inflammation, and pressure from oncologic sources (pressure, direct invasion). Nerve injury is also likely to be associated with concomitant damage to other important local or distant structures, such as muscle, bone, or blood vessels. The types of nerve injuries can be broadly subdivided into nondegenerative and degenerative injuries. Nondegenerative lesions are described as those lesions that do not cause interruption of the axon itself. External pressure via tumor, hematoma, bony prominence, or transient ischemia may produce local demyelination and thus a conduction block.[23,24] Once the nidus for the local insult is removed, function or sensation may be restored.[25] Once disruption of the axon occurs and there is damage to the neuron itself, the lesion is categorized as degenerative.

In 1951, Sunderland introduced a five-tiered classification system for neuronal injury based on histologic findings (Table 2).[26,27] The first degree of injury was classified as a conduction block or nondegenerative lesion. Second-degree severity occurs when the axon is disrupted but the Schwann cell layer is maintained. The following three degrees range from disruption of the endoneurium to complete loss of nerve continuity. Recently, more simplified classification systems have begun to reclassify injuries as conduction block versus axonal degeneration, a basic return to earlier nondegeneration versus degeneration terms.[28] The remainder of this section concentrates on the reactions of the neuron to degenerative (axonal degeneration) lesions.

Degeneration caused by damage to the neuron was first described by Waller in 1850

Table 2. SUNDERLAND CLASSIFICATION OF NERVE INJURY			
Degree of Injury	Histology	Findings	Rate/Type of Recovery
First	Nerve in continuity, possible demyelination, no axonal disruption	Partial conduction block, no advancing Tinel's sign (no axonal injury)	Days–3 mo, complete
Second	Axonal disruption, intact endoneurium, perineurium	Advancing Tinel's sign with recovery	1 inch/mo, complete
Third	Disruption of endoneurium, fascicular disorganization	Advancing Tinel's sign	1 inch/mo, incomplete
Fourth	Disruption of endoneurium, severe scarring restricting regeneration	Nonadvancing Tinel's sign at level of injury	Surgical intervention needed owing to scar
Fifth	Transection of nerve	Nonadvancing Tinel's sign at level of injury	Surgical intervention needed

Adapted from Sunderland S.[27]

and thus was coined "wallerian degeneration."[29] Following injury to the neuron, wallerian degeneration affects the neuron both proximally and distally, as well as producing changes in the Schwann cells. Proximal to the site of injury, the cell body undergoes retrograde degeneration, with changes in the axon and the cell body itself. Within the cell body, there is disappearance of Nissl-staining substances (chromatolysis), retraction of dendrites, swelling of the cell body, and displacement of the nucleus to the periphery of the cell. The proximal axon may exhibit atrophy within 2 days.

Changes are quite profound in the distal stump following axotomy (Table 3). The distal axon and myelin sheath undergo degradation and phagocytosis. Degradation of the myelin sheath leads to local macrophage infiltration and removal of the injured distal axon, usually within 4 to 6 weeks.[30] This macrophage proliferation is paramount for both the clearance of cellular debris, namely myelin and extruded axoplasm, and stimulation of the Schwann cells. Following injury, Schwann cells undergo proliferation and demyelation. The phenotype of the Schwann cell is altered, transforming from a relatively quiescent myelinating cell to a highly mitotically active, nonmyelinating cell.[31] The proliferating Schwann cells migrate to form organized columns (Büngner's bands).[32] If Schwann cell migration does not occur, axonal regeneration does not occur.[33]

Regeneration

Following injury, the process of regeneration is multifactorial, involving the proximal and distal stumps of the injured nerve, Schwann cells, glial cells, and macrophages, as well as neurotrophic, molecular, paracrine, and perhaps gene regulatory factors. A detailed description of all of the cellular constituents thought to be involved in neuronal regeneration is beyond the scope of this chapter. For the interested reader, Choi and Dunn, Stoll and Müller, and Moran and Graeber provide good reviews of the topic.[34–36] Several of the more important humoral factors involved in nerve regeneration are discussed in the following section.

Following axotomy, there is a resultant gap between the proximal and distal stumps, as described in the previous section. A fibrin clot resulting from blood products and clotting factors initially fills the gap. Macrophages and ultimately fibroblasts enter this space. Axonal sprouting begins from the proximal stump, and sprouts are accompanied by Schwann cells. Growth of the regenerating axon continues until the distal stump is encountered. The specificity by which the axon is regenerated and the survival of the axon itself are thought to be highly contingent on humoral factors, as discussed in the following section.

Schwann Cells

Phagocytosis of neuronal debris by macrophages and Schwann cells begins to occur within the first 7 days after axonotmesis. The Schwann cells appear by 1 to 2 days and have peak mitosis by 2 to 3 days postinjury. Activation occurs by a myriad of growth factors, including NGF, transforming growth factor β, platelet-derived growth factor, and interleukin-1. By 4 days postinjury, L1, neural cell adhesion molecule, and ninjurin, all cell surface adhesion molecules involved in neurite extension, are expressed on the Schwann cell surface.[37–39] Schwann cells also secrete extracellular matrix constituents, including laminin, collagen, and fibronectin, which are essential for neuronal extension.[40] Growth factors secreted by the Schwann cells include NGF.

UNIQUE PHYSIOLOGIC HEALING ASPECTS

Bridging the Gap: Neurotrophism, Neurotropism, and Contact Guidance

The process of nerve regeneration is unique in that the damaged nerve must not only undergo growth and maturation but also, in spanning the nerve gap, must reach its target in a site-specific manner to achieve a positive functional outcome. In 1898, Forssman reported that regeneration could occur across nerve gaps.[41] Cajal, the father of modern neuroscience, postulated that endogenous soluble proteins secreted from the distal injury site were responsible for the attraction of nerve sprouts from the proximal site of injury.[42] The mechanisms and factors now believed to sustain axonal sprouts and lead to the conduction of the neuron to the distal stump are referred to as neurotrophism, neurotropism, and contact guidance.

Neurotrophism refers to a process controlled by a particular substance that leads to the maturation and survival of the nerve cells, whereas neurotropism describes a process that influences the directionality of nerve growth.[43] The combination of these, neurotrop(h)ism, has been used to describe factors that influence both maturation and directionality of growth.[44]

Reinnervation of target tissues after axotomy has shown remarkable specificity. Bruschart and Seiler demonstrated that motor axons preferentially reinnervate distal motor branches.[45] Furthermore, there is evidence that specificity exists for reinnervation of sensory axons.[46] The effects of neurotrophism were further defined by Mackinnon and colleagues with the use of a siliconY-shaped chamber.[47] The regenerating axonal stump was placed in one section of the Y, and two targets were placed equidistant from the stump in the other two respective ends. After 6 weeks, axons uniformly reinnervated the Y end with the distal nerve as opposed to the ends containing either tendon, muscle, or granulation tissue. Axonal direction was further elucidated by Kuffler in the frog cutaneous pectoris nerve.[48] Regenerating axons from the proximal stump were seen to sprout randomly when no distal stump was present. When the distal stump was present, the proximal axon stump exhibited directionality toward the distal stump. Research has since focused on the identification of neurotrophic and neurotropic substances involved in nerve regeneration. Several of the major factors described are discussed below (Table 3).

Factors Involved in Neurotrophism and Neurotropisn

Nerve Growth Factor

Neurotrophic factors, as first postulated by Cajal (above), are endogenous soluble proteins that are

Table 3. SUMMARY OF EVENTS AFTER AXOTOMY
Intrinsic neuronal events
Anterograde degeneration
Wallerian degeneration (1–14 d)
Distal myelin swells, retracts, and fragments
Retrograde signaling
Activation of phospholipases, increase in nitric oxide, and free radical production
Increase in cytokine production
Loss of trophic signals
Retrograde degeneration
Swelling of neuron cell body, chromatolysis, eccentric location of nucleus
Seeping of axoplasm from cut end sealed by 24 h
Disassembly of damaged microtubules and neurofilaments (3–10 d)
Axonal bulb formation at cut end
Regrowth of proximal axon (1–2 mm/d)
Gene expression
Increase in bax and bac correlates with apoptosis
c-fos, c-jun, and jun-B expressed (5 h–8 d)
Increase in GAP 43 mRNA and CGRP
Extrinsic events
Schwann cells (appear at 1–2 d)
Mitosis peaks at 2–3 d
Schwann cells activated by NGF, TGF-β, PDGF, IL-1, and macrophage factors
Production of cytokines, growth factors, extracellular matrix, and surface adhesion molecules
Macrophages (appear at 2–3 d)
Phagocytosis of debris
Production of cytokines
Activation of Schwann cells and fibroblasts

Adapted from Choi D and Dunn L.[34]
CGRP = calcitonin gene–related peptide; IL = interleukin; mRNA = messenger ribonucleic acid; NGF = nerve growth factor; PDGF = platelet-derived growth factor; TGF = transforming growth factor.

capable of neurotrophism and/or neurotropism.[42,49] NGF, the first neurotrophic factor to be identified, was first described in the 1950s by Levi-Montalcini and colleagues and Cohen and Levi-Montalcini.[50–53] They found that this substance, first isolated in mouse sarcoma models, profoundly affected nerve growth. Ultimately, the role of NGF in the regeneration of peripheral nerves was elucidated.[54–56] Also, within this class of neurotrophic factors are brain-derived neurotrophic factor and neurotrophins NT-3 through NT-7. NGF is postulated to be associated with establishing the basic network of the nervous system during embryologic and fetal development, as well as its regenerative properties in the peripheral nervous system.

Two receptor types for NGF have been identified: a low-affinity rapidly binding receptor (p75) and a high-affinity slowly binding receptor.[57] Debate exists as to whether these two receptor types act separately or in conjunction with each other to affect the binding of NGF.[58] Once bound, the NGF receptor complex, through both the phospholipase C pathway and the tyrosine kinase pathway, acts to produce protein syntheses and production of additional neurotransmitters. After transection of the nerve, Schwann cells and macrophages are instrumental in the paracrine-like increase in NGF and NGF receptor levels at the site of injury.[59] Following axotomy, the NGF receptor is found on the surface of denervated Schwann cells; however, following regeneration and axonal contact, these levels are decreased.[60] Thus, the Schwann cells may be instrumental in providing trophic support for the injured nerve.

Ciliary Neurotrophic Factor

Ciliary neurotrophic factor (CNTF) has been found to support the survival of primarily motor neurons in cell culture.[61] CNTF is predominantly located in the cytoplasm of myelinating Schwann cells and the axoplasm of neurons.[62,63] Its function in nerve regeneration may largely be a factor involved in general somatic support rather than a neurotrophic factor as it is present after injury predominantly in the extracellular environment and not intracellularly or on the cell surface.[64] Thus, the addition of endogenous CNTF may benefit axonal regeneration as a neurotropic factor.

IGF-1 and IGF-2

Both IGF-1 and IGF-2 stimulate neuronal growth in tissue culture.[65] IGF-1 messenger ribonucleic acid levels have been found to increase in the injured neurons after axotomy, whereas IGF-2 levels increase primarily in the muscle. This may signify the importance of IGF-I to axonal regeneration and of IGF-2 to neuromuscular regeneration.[66]

Many other factors have been investigated for their neuroregenerative roles. These include fibroblast growth factors (acidic, and basic), transforming growth factor β, platelet-derived growth factor, and erythropoietin. As with

CNTF, described above, these molecules have been found to have a role in neuroregeneration and neurotropism; however, their neurotrophic value remains unknown (Table 4).

Contact Guidance

Contact guidance, or pathway specificity, is the concept of use of contact of the peripheral nerve fragment with the surrounding structures, thereby allowing orientation toward the distal nerve stump via "feel." In this scenario, multiple collaterals sprout from the proximal stump. Those that contact an inappropriate substance (eg, muscle, sensory nerve) may be terminated, whereas those going toward the distal stump continue to grow until contact is made.

Martini and colleagues postulated that L2/HNK-1 carbohydrate epitopes were instrumental in reinnervating the motor axons of the femoral nerve in the rat model.[67] The L2-HNK-1 carbohydrate moiety is preferentially expressed on Schwann cells present in motor axons and the ventral nerve roots, although not present on sensory nerves. During regeneration of the neuron across the nerve gap, the Schwann cells associated with the distal motor nerve express L2/HNK-1, whereas the sensory branches do not. Contact by the proximal regenerating motor neuron to the distal stump expressing L2 may therefore lead to preferential regeneration of the motor pathway.

As more research on neurotropism, neurotrophism, and contact guidance is reported, it may become evident that the three processes are not mutually exclusive and that, in fact, all are necessary in the complex milieu surrounding the regenerating stump.

FUTURE PROMISE FOR HEALING

Neurotrop(h)ic Factors

The use of exogenous NGF has been studied extensively in the context of peripheral nerve regeneration. The facial nerve of the rabbit has been investigated for this purpose. Chen and colleagues demonstrated improved quality of the regenerated nerve when NGF was placed in

Table 4. EXPRESSION OF GENES/PROTEINS FOLLOWING FACIAL NERVE AXOTOMY

Category	Gene Expressed	Cell Type
Up-regulated substances		
Cell adhesion molecules	ICAM-1	Glia
	CD44	Neurons
	$\alpha_7\beta^1$ integrin	Neurons
	Integrin subunit β_1	Neurons
Cell death inhibitors	Nitric oxide synthase	Neurons
Chemoattractants	MCP-1 receptor	Glia
Chemokines	Fractalkine receptor (CX3CR1)	Glia
	Phospholipase Cα	Facial nucleus
Cytokines	IL-6	Neurons, glia
	IL-1β	Facial nucleus
	IFN-γ	Neurons
	TGF-β_1	Facial nucleus
	TNF-α	Facial nucleus
Cytoskeleton	GFAP	Glia
	Vimentin	Glia
	Actin, tubulin	Facial nucleus
Growth-associated proteins	GAP-43	Neurons
Neuropeptides	Galanin	Neurons
	Cholecystokinin	Neurons
	FasL	Neurons
Neurotransmission	Glutamate receptor (GLT-1)	Glia
	NOS	Neurons
	NADPH-d	Neurons, Glia
Neurokines	PGDF A chain	Neurons, Glia
	PGDF B chain	Neurons
	PGDF α receptor	Glia
	BNDF	Neurons
Protein translation	Ribosomal proteins S3, S6, S7	Glia
Receptors	PGDF α receptor	Glia
	Transferrin receptors	Neurons
Structural proteins	Connexin 43	Glia
Transcription factors	c-jun	Neurons
	Jun-B	Neurons
	JAK2, JAK3, STAT1, STAT3, STAT5	Neurons
	c-maf	Neurons
Down-regulated substances		
Cotransporters	K-Cl (KCC2)	Neurons
Metalloprotein	MT-III	Neurons
Neurokines	CNTF receptor α	Neurons
Neuropeptides	β-Calcitonin gene–related protein	Neurons
Neurotransmission	Acetylcholine esterase	Neurons
	M2 muscarinic receptors	Facial nucleus
	Neurodap1	Neurons
Transcription factors	Cytochrome oxidase	Facial nucleus
	Protease-activated/thrombin receptor 1	Neurons

Adapted from Moran L and Graeber M.[36]
BNDF = brand derived neurotrophic factor; CNTF = ciliary neurotrophic factor; GFAP = glial fibrillary acidic protein; ICAM = intercellular adhesion molecule; IFN = interferon; IL = interleukin; MCP = monocyte chemotactic protein; NADPH = reduced nicotinamide adenine dinucleotide phosphate; NOS = nitric oxide synthase; PGDF = ; TGF = transforming growth factor; TNF = tumor necrosis factor.

silicone tubes along with the proximal and distal stumps of the rabbit facial nerve.[68] In particular, at the end of 5 weeks, the nerve cable itself was significantly larger than those nerves placed in the silicone tube without NGF. Successful regeneration, however, was the same for both groups. Other studies on exogenous NGF in the rat sciatic nerve have shown improved initial outgrowth of the axon stump when compared with controls, but the final regeneration with both 10 and 15 mm gap models is similar with and without NGF.[69,70]

CNTF may be useful after axotomy as an injury factor, as described above. Its extracellular presence after injury intimates that it may support axonal regeneration rather than help direct regeneration. Both systemic application and local application of CNTF have been shown to increase the number of myelinated axons following nerve repair.[71] Both IGF-1 and IGF-2 have also been found to increase the regeneration of motor nerves after injury.[72,73] IGF-1 has been shown to increase nerve sprouting and regeneration following axotomy in the mouse hypoglossal nerve.[74]

Pharmacologic Agents

Several pharmacologic agents have been investigated in nerve regeneration. Administration of the calcium channel blocker nimodipine after transection of the rat facial nerve has resulted in improved axonal sprouting.[75] Polyamine and aminoguanidine treatment after facial nerve injury in rats has also led to improved nerve regrowth.[76]

Conduits

Neural tubes have been investigated extensively in bridging nerve gaps following injury. The advantages posed by using an allogeneic nerve conduit over a traditional interpositional nerve graft are those of donor nerve harvest and morbidity. Several different materials have been used, including synthetic (silicone, polyglycolic acid, and polyglactin) and autogenous (vein, artery, muscle, bone) materials.[77] Nerve conduits have been demonstrated to have an efficacy similar to that of the nerve graft in instances in which nerve deficits are less than 3 cm.[78] However, at distances greater than 3 cm, nerve conduits have been largely unsuccessful at initiating regeneration across the gap.[35,79]

Multiple neurotrophic and neurotropic factors have been evaluated in the context of neural tubes in the hope of overcoming the critical 3 cm gap. Spector and colleagues evaluated silicone tube grafts containing NGF.[80] In the NGF tube grafts, the quality of the regenerating nerve was more histologically organized than was that of the autologous interpositional nerve graft control. However, there were a smaller total number of regenerating myelinated nerve fibers in the NGF-silicone tube graft group. Neural tubes seeded with cultured Schwann cells have shown promise in overcoming the 3 cm gap. Neural tubes seeded with cultured Schwann cells are more successful in bridging gaps when compared with plain neural tubes.[81,82]

Allograft

Reconstruction of large nerve deficits is limited by the availability of expendable donor nerves for interposition. As discussed above, synthetic nerve conduits have been clinically successful in bridging gaps only of 3 cm or less. The concept of allograft use was first introduced by Albert in 1885; however, the results were poor.[83] To be effective as a conduit, nerve allografts must have intact basal laminae and functional Schwann cells, as well as a reduction in the expression of major histocompatibility complex antigens.[77]

Suppression of the host immune system must be performed temporarily for the nerve allograft to be effective.[84,85] Immunosuppression must continue until that time in which the recipient Schwann cells have replaced the donor cells and the recipient axons have traversed the gap. Once this process is complete, the neural elements within the conduit are of host origin only and immunosuppression may cease.[86] Recent clinical trials using this methodology have shown the ability to bridge long peripheral nerve gaps with restoration of motor or sensory function.[87] In this study by Mackinnon and colleagues, patients were maintained on immunosuppression therapy for 6 months following neurologic evidence of regeneration. Six of seven patients had motor and/or sensory return to the affected area. Although further investigation is necessary, the use of a nerve allograft in bridging long nerve gaps may become clinically applicable in the near future.

REFERENCES

1. Dai CF, Kanoh N, Li KY, et al. Study on facial motorneuronal death after proximal or distal facial nerve transection. Am Otolaryngol 2000;21:115–8.

2. Moore K, Dalley A. Cranial nerves. In: Clinically oriented anatomy, Philadelphia: Lippincott Williams & Wilkins; 1999. p. 1083–12.
3. May M. Anatomy for the clinician. In: May M, Schaitkin B, editors. The facial nerve. New York: Thieme; 2000. p. 19–56.
4. Myckatyn T, Mackinnon S. The surgical management of facial nerve injury. Clin Plast Surg 2003;30:307–18.
5. Baker DC, Conley J. Avoiding facial nerve injuries in rhytidectomy: anatomical variations and pitfalls. Plast Reconstr Surg 1979;64:781.
6. McCormack LJ, Cauldwell EW, Anson BJ. The surgical anatomy of the facial nerve with special reference to the parotid gland. Surg Gynecol Obstet 1945;80:620.
7. Davis RA, Anson BJ, Budinger JM, et al. Surgical anatomy of the facial nerve and parotid gland based upon a study of 350 cervicofacial halves. Surg Gynecol Obstet 1956;102:385.
8. Thomas P. The connective tissue of peripheral nerve; an electron microscope study. J Anat 1963;97:35–42.
9. Gamble H, Eames R. An electron microscope study of the connective tissues of the human peripheral nerve. J Anat 1964;98:655–62.
10. Sunderland S. Nerves and nerve injuries. Edinburgh: E&S Livingstone; 1968.
11. Sunderland S, Bradley K. The cross sectional area of peripheral nerve trunks devoted to nerve fibers. Brain 1949;72:428–49.
12. Sunderland S. The anatomic basis of nerve repair. In: Jewett D, McCarroll H, editors. Nerve repair and regeneration. St. Louis: CV Mosby; 1980. p. 35–50.
13. Karnovsky M, CARoots. A "direct coloring" thiocholine method for cholinesterases. J Histochem Cytochem 1964;12:219–21.
14. Grueber H, Zenksa W. Acetylcholinesterase: histochemical differentiation between motor and sensory fibers. Brain Res 1973;51:207–14.
15. Grueber H, Freilinger G, Houe J. Identification of motor and sensory funiculi in cut nerves and their selective reunion. Br J Plast Surg 1976;29:70.
16. Deutinger M, Girsch W, Burgasser G. Clinical and electroneurographic evaluation of sensory/motor-differentiated nerve repair in the hand. J Neurosurg 1993;78:709–13.
17. Ganel A, Engel J, Luboshitz S. Choline acetyltransferase nerve identification method in early and late nerve repair. Ann Plast Surg 1980;4:228–30.
18. Ganel A, Farine I, Aharowson Z. Intraoperative nerve fascicle identification using choline acetyltransferase: a preliminary report. Clin Orthop 1982;165:228–32.
19. Lang D, Lister G, Jevans AW. Histochemical and biochemical aids to nerve repair. In: Gelberman R, editor. Operative nerve repair and reconstruction. Philadelphia, JB: Lippincott; 1991. p. 259–70.
20. Engel J, Ganel A, Melamed S. Choline acetyltransferase for differentiation between motor and sensory nerve fibers. Ann Plast Surg 1980;4:5.
21. Riley D, Ellis S, Bain J. Carbonic anhydrase histochemistry reveals subpopulations of myelinated axons in the dorsal and ventral roots of rat spinal nerves [abstract]. Soc Neurosci Abst 1981;7:257.
22. Riley D, Lang D. Carbonic anhydrase activity of human peripheral nerves: a possible histochemical aid to nerve repair. J Hand Surg [Am] 1984;9A:112–20.
23. Gilliatt R. Physical injury to peripheral nerves. Mayo Clin Proc 1981;56:361–70.
24. Fowler T, Dunta G, Gilliatt R. Recovery of nerve conduction after a pneumatic tourniquet: observations in the hind limb of a baboon. J Neurol Neurosurg Psychiatry 1972;35:638–47.
25. Birch R, St Clair Strange F. A new type of peripheral nerve lesion. J Bone Joint Surg Br 1990;72B:312–3.
26. Sunderland S. A classification of peripheral nerve injuries producing loss of function. Brain 1951;74:491–516.
27. Sunderland S. Some anatomical and pathophysiological data relevant to the facial nerve injury and repair. In: Fisch U, editor. Facial nerve surgery. Amstelveen: Kugler; 1977. p. 47–61.
28. Thomas P, Holdorff B. Neuropathy due to physical agents. In: Dyck P, et al, editor. Peripheral neuropathy. Philadelphia: WB Saunders; 1993. p. 990–1013.
29. Waller A. Experiments on the section of the glossopharyngeal and hypoglossal nerves of the frog, and observations of the alterations produced thereby in the structure of their primitive fibres. Philos Trans R Soc Lond 1850;140:423–9.
30. Griffin J, Hoffman P. Degeneration and regeneration in the peripheral nervous system. In Dyck P, et al, editors. Peripheral neuropathy. 3rd ed. Philadelphia: WB Saunders; 1993. p. 361–76.
31. Curtis R, Stawart H, Hall S. GAP-43 is expressed by nonmyelin-forming Schwann cells of the peripheral nervous system. J Cell Biol 1992;116:1455–64.
32. Fawcett J, Keynes R. Peripheral nerve regeneration. Annu Rev Neurosci 1990;13:43–60.
33. Bruschart T, Gerber J, Kessens P. Contributions of pathway and neuron to preferential motor reinnervation. J Neurosci 1998;18:8674–81.
34. Choi D, Dunn L. Facial nerve repair and regeneration: an overview of basic principles for neurosurgeons. Acta Neurochir (Wien) 2001;143:107–14.
35. Stoll G, Müller HW. Nerve injury, axonal degeneration and neural regeneration: basic insights. Brain Pathol 1999;9:313–25.
36. Moran L, Graeber M. The facial nerve axotomy model. Brain Res Rev 2004;44:154–78.
37. Martini R, Schachner M. Immunoelectron microscopic localization of neural cell adhesion molecules (L-1, N-CAM, and myelin-associated glycoprotein) in regenerating adult mouse sciatic nerve. J Cell Biol 1988;106:1735–46.
38. Seilheimer B, Schachner M. Studies of adhesion molecules mediating interactions between cells of peripheral nervous system indicate a major role for L1 in mediating sensory neuron growth on Schwann cells in culture. J Cell Biol 1988;107:341–51.

39. Arai T, Milbrandt J. Ninjurin, a novel adhesion molecule, is induced by nerve injury and promotes axonal growth. Neuron 1996;17:353–61.

40. Martini R. Expression and functional roles of neural surface molecules and extracellular matrix components during development and regeneration of peripheral nerves. J Neurocytol 1994;23:1–28.

41. Forssman J. Ueber die Ursachen, welche die Wachstumsrichtungg der peripheren Nervenfasern bei der Regeneration bestimmen. Beitr Z Pathol Anat 1898; 24:56.

42. Cajal Ry. Mechanismo de la degeneracion y regeneration de nervos. Madrid: Trab Lab Inbest Biol 1905;4:119–210.

43. Lundborg G. Neurotrophism, frozen muscle grafts and other conduits. J Hand Surg [Br] 1991;16B:473–6.

44. Mackinnon SE, Dellon AL. Future directions in peripheral nerve surgery. In: Mackinnon SE, Dellon AL, editors. Surgery of the peripheral nerve., New York: Thieme Medical Publishers; 1988. p. 551–74.

45. Bruschart T, Seiler W. Selective reinnervation of distal motor stumps by peripheral motor axons. Exp Neurol 1987;97:289–300.

46. Madison R, Archibald S, Bruschart T. Reinnervation accuracy of the rat femoral nerve by motor and sensory neurons. J Neurosci 1996;16:5698–703.

47. Mackinnon SE, Dellon AL, Lundborg G, et al. A study of neurotrophism in a primate model. J Hand Surg [Am] 1986;11A:888.

48. Kuffler D. Regeneration of muscle axons in the frog is directed by diffusable factors from denervated muscle and nerve fibers. J Exp Neurol 1989;281:416.

49. Cajal Ry. Neurotrophic action of the distal stump. In: May RM, editor. Degeneration and regeneration in the nervous system. London: Oxford University Press; 1928. p. 3–26.

50. Levi-Montalcini R, Hamburger V. Selective growth stimulating effects of mouse sarcoma on the sensory and sympathetic nervous system of the chick embryo. J Exp Zool 1951;116:321–62.

51. Levi-Montalcini R, Meyer H, Hamburger V. In vitro experiments on the effects of mouse sarcomas 180 and 37 on the spinal and sympathetic ganglia of the chick embryo. Cancer Res 1954;14:49–57.

52. Cohen S, Levi-Montalcini R. A nerve growth-stimulating factor isolated from snake-venom. Proc Natl Acad Sci U S A 1956;42:571–4.

53. Cohen S, Levi-Montalcini R, Hamburger V. A nerve growth stimulating factor isolated from sarcomas 37 and 180. Proc Natl Acad Sci U S A 1954;40: 1014–8.

54. Gunderson R, Barrett J. Neuronal chemotaxis: chick dorsal root axons turn towards high concentrations of nerve growth factor. Science 1979;206:1079–80.

55. Martini R, Schatner M. Immunoelectron microscopic localization of neural cell adhesion molecules (l1, N-cam and MAG) and their shared carbohydrate epitope and myelin basic protein in developing sciatic nerve. J Cell Biol 1986;103:2439–48.

56. Rich KM, Alexander TD, Pryor JC, et al. Nerve growth factor enhances regeneration through silicone chambers. Exp Neurol 1989;105:162–70.

57. Johnson D, Lanahan A, Buck C, et al. Expression and structure of human NGF receptor. Cell 1986;47:545.

58. Bothwell M. Keeping track of neurotrophin receptors. Cell 1991;65:915.

59. Lindholm D, Heumann R, Meyer M, et al. Interleukin-1 regulates synthesis of nerve growth factor in non-neuronal cells of rat sciatic nerve. Nature 1987;330: 658.

60. Taniuchi M, Clark H, Schweitzer J, et al. Expression of nerve growth factor receptors by Schwann cells of axotomized peripheral nerves: ultrastructural location, suppression by axonal contact, and binding properties. J Neurosci 1988;8:664.

61. Oppenheim R, Prevette D, Qin-Wei Y, et al. Control of embryonic motoneuron survival in vivo by ciliary neurotrophic factor. Science 1991;251:1616.

62. Rende M, Muir D, Ruoslahti E, et al. Immunolocalization of ciliary neuronotrophic factor in adult rat sciatic nerve. Glia 1992;5:25.

63. Friedman B, Scherer SS, Rodge JS, et al. Regulation of ciliary neurotrophic factor expression in myelin-related Schwann cells in vivo. Neuron 1992;9:295.

64. Sendtner M, Stockli K, Thoenen H. Ciliary neuronotrophic factor prevents the degeneration of motor neurons after axotomy. Nature 1992;345:440.

65. Caroni P, Grandes P. Nerve sprouting in innervated adult skeletal muscle induced by exposure to elevated levels on insulin-like growth factors. J Cell Biol 1990;110: 1307.

66. Glazner G, Wright W, Ishii D. Kinetics of insulin-like growth factor (IGF) mRNA changes in rat nerve and muscle during IGF-dependent nerve regeneration [abstract]. Soc Neurosci Abstr 1993;19:253.

67. Martini R, Schachner M, Brushart T. The L2/HNK-1 carbohydrate is preferentially expressed by previously motor axon-associated Schwann cells in reinnervated peripheral nerves. J Neurosci 1994;14:7180–91.

68. Chen Y, Wang-Bennett L, Coker N. Facial nerve regeneration in the silicon chamber: the influence of nerve growth factor. Exp Neurol 1989;103:52.

69. Hollowell J, Villadiego A, Rich K. Sciatic nerve regeneration across gaps with silicon chambers: long term effects of NGF and consideration of axonal branching. Exp Neurol 1990;110:45.

70. Derby A, Engelman W, Frierdich G, et al. Nerve growth factor facilitates regeneration across nerve gaps: morphological and behavioral studies in rat sciatic nerve. Exp Neurol 1993;119:76.

71. Sahenk Z, Seharaseyon J, Mendell J. CNTF potentiates peripheral nerve regeneration. Brain Res 1994;655:246.

72. Sjoberg J, Kanje M. Insulin-like growth factor (IGF-I) as a stimulator of regeneration in the freeze-injured rat sciatic nerve. Brain Res 1989;485:102.

73. Near S, Whalen R, Miller JA, et al. Insulin-like growth factor II stimulates motor nerve regeneration. Proc Natl Acad Sci U S A 1992;89:11716.

74. Gruner J, Wagner L, Chiu D, et al. RhIGF-I protects against motorneuron loss following nerve transecton in adult mice [abstract]. Soc Neurosci Abst 1996;22: 1961.

75. Angelov D, Meiss WF, Streppel M, et al. Nimodipine accelerates axonal sprouting after surgical repair of the rat facial nerve. J Neurosci 1996;16:1041–8.

76. Gilad V, Tetzlaff WG, Rebey JM, et al. Accelerated recovery following polyamines and animoguanidine treatment after facial nerve injury in rats. Brain Res 1996;724:141–4.

77. Dvali L, Mackinnon S. Nerve repair, grafting, and nerve transfers. Clin Plast Surg 2003;30:203–21.

78. Chiu D, Janecka I, Krizek T. Autogenous vein graft as a conduit for nerve regeneration. Surgery 1982;91: 226–33.

79. Chiu D, Strauch B. A prospective clinical evaluation of autogenous vein grafts used as a nerve conduit for sensory nerve deficits of 3 cm or less. Plast Reconstr Surg 1990;86:928–34.

80. Spector J, Lee P, Derby A, et al. Rabbit facial nerve regeneration in NGF-containing Silastic tubes. Laryngoscope 1993;103:548–58.

81. Francel P, Francel TJ, Machinnon SE, et al. Enhancing nerve regeneration across a silicone tube conduit by using interposed short-segment nerve grafts. J Neurosurg 1997;87:887–92.

82. Bryan D, Wank K, Summerhayes C. Migration of Schwann cells in peripheral nerve regeneration. J Reconstr Microsurg 1999;15:591–6.

83. Albert T. Einige Operationen an Nerven. Wien Med Presse 1885;26:1285.

84. Bain J, Mackinnon S, Hudson A. The nerve allograft response in the rat immunosuppressed with cyclosporin A. Plast Reconstr Surg 1988;82:1052–66.

85. Mackinnon S, Midha R, Bain J. An assessment of regeneration across peripheral nerve allografts in rats receiving short courses of cyclosporin A immunosuppression. Neuroscience 1992;46:585–93.

86. Atchabahian A, Mackinnon S, Doolabh V. Indefinite survival of peripheral nerve allografts after temporary cyclosporin A immunosuppression. Restor Neurol Neurosci 1998;13:129.

87. Mackinnon SE, Doolabh VB, Novak CB, et al. Clinical outcome following nerve allograft transplantation. Plast Reconstr Surg 2001;107:1419–29.

Salient Healing Features of Muscles of the Face and Neck

Loree K. Kalliainen, MD, FACS

The purpose of skeletal muscle is to generate force and allow voluntary motion by way of coordinated contractions. Muscle in the head and neck has an identical histology to muscle in the trunk and limbs, but differences in contractile protein composition and innervation of ocular and jaw muscles have been described. There is a fair amount of anatomic diversity with respect to the presence or absence of muscles of facial expression, and they have the distinguishing features of inserting into the skin and not crossing joints.

The muscle cell, the myofiber, is almost completely filled by longitudinally arrayed contractile proteins. Muscle contraction has been explained by the sliding filament theory of Huxley and Niedergerke[1] and has been well accepted for decades. Contraction occurs when a nerve impulse depolarizes a muscle fiber and myofibrils slide past one another by a calcium-dependent process. Muscle injuries are very common in trauma of the head and neck, but until recent times, it was thought that muscle was incapable of healing because the nuclei are postmitotic. What was not initially realized was that the satellite cells present at the perimeter of the myofiber are capable of up-regulation and regeneration of new fibers. As is true with other tissues, muscle healing passes through the phases of inflammation, proliferation, and remodeling, and healing can be delayed if inflammation is prolonged or extensive fibrosis develops. Recommendations to optimize healing include restoration of muscle continuity, obtaining hemostasis, and removing muscles from fractures. Early protected motion has been shown to limit fibrosis. Future interventions have the goals of preservation of function and limiting fibrosis and are focusing on growth factors, gene therapy, and stem cell therapy.

ANATOMY AND PHYSIOLOGY OF SKELETAL MUSCLE

The role of skeletal muscle is to generate force, allowing voluntary movement by means of coordinated contractions. Muscle structure has been well described, and its mechanism of action has been accepted since Huxley and Niedergerke described the sliding filament theory in 1954.[1] Histologically, skeletal muscle of the head and neck is identical to that elsewhere in the body; but myosin isoform and morphologic differences have been described, and these are reviewed below.[2]

Skeletal muscle architecture has been described as parallel, pennate, sphincteric, and convergent. The distinction is determined by the direction of the fibers relative to the line of pull. Parallel or fusiform muscles are rectangular and are not especially strong. The sternohyoid and thyrohyoid muscles are parallel-fibered. Pennate or pinnate muscle fibers insert into the tendon or aponeurosis at an angle. They can be unipennate, bipennate, or multipennate. The masseter is a multipennate muscle. Sphincteric muscles, such as the orbicularis oris and orbicularis oculi, surround body orifices and have less distinct origins, insertions, and tendons. Convergent muscles, of which the pectoralis is an example, are very strong as the forces created by the fibers converge on a tendon.[3,4] Muscles in the head and neck can be difficult to classify because their anatomy can be complex, with extensive admixing of adjacent muscles.[5] Little has been written about muscle architecture in the craniofacial region.

Skeletal muscle can be distinguished from other muscle types by striation, multinucleated cells, and voluntary action. Smooth and cardiac muscle cells have individual nuclei and are involuntary. Smooth muscle has no discrete neuromuscular junctions, is activated via gap junctions, and can have an intrinsic rhythm.[4] Cardiac cells are striated and involuntary and are joined end to end via intercalated disks, on which myofilaments are attached and through which contractions are transmitted.[4]

Each skeletal muscle is enveloped in epimysium and is composed of bundles of fascicles. Fascicles are groups of muscle cells encased within perimysium. The cells, called myofibers, are wrapped in a basal lamina surrounded by an extracellular matrix called the endomysium and are filled with myofibrils and sarcoplasm (Figure 1). Myofibrils are 1 to 2 μm in diameter and are made of repeating contractile units called sarcomeres (see Figure 1, B and C). They make up about two-thirds of the dry weight of the myofiber; the sarcoplasm makes up about one-third.[6] The endomysium is the site of vascular and ion exchange.[4] Beneath the endomysium lies the outer layer of the myofiber, which is called the sarcolemma or plasma membrane. The basal lamina borders the outer layer of the sarcolemma, and this encloses both satellite cells and muscle fibers. The size of a myofiber varies between muscles and can range from millimeters to centimeters long and from 10 to 100 μm in diameter.[4,7,8]

Cellular Anatomy of the Myofiber

The muscle cell membrane, the sarcolemma, has features unique to muscle. At the myotendinous

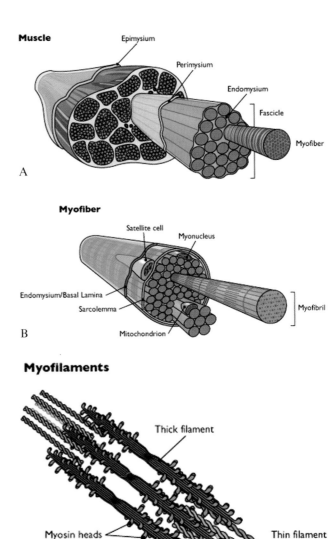

Figure 1. Diagram illustrating skeletal muscle organization. *A* shows the three-dimensional organization of the various components of the muscle cell, or myocyte. Adapted from Salmons S.[4] *B* shows a diagram of the organization of the components forming the sarcomere, the functional contractile unit. *C* shows the regions of the sarcomere that form the striations of skeletal muscle.

junctions, the outer layer is composed of fibrils that attach to tendon, and the sarcolemma is folded to increase the surface area of attachment of the myofiber to the tendon.[9] The epimysium, perimysium, and endomysium all coalesce to strengthen the attachment of muscle to tendon. In tendons, integrins and dystrophin-glycoprotein complexes connect sarcomeres to extracellular matrix elements and act to transmit force and transduce signals from the muscle across the tendons.[7,10] Whereas integrins are more common at the ends of myofibers, dystrophin-glycoprotein complexes are found along the entire myofiber membrane.[7] In the extremities, the muscles cross joints, and the myotendinous junctions need greater force stress and shear tolerance than in the face, where muscles insert directly into skin.[4]

Sarcoplasm, or myofiber cytoplasm, contains adenosine triphosphate (ATP), enzymes, metabolic by-products, and organelles necessary for cellular function. Mitochondria are found between the myofibrils or in the I band. The concentration of mitochondria varies between muscles with different metabolic demands and can change to meet new demands.[4]

Transverse, or T, tubules are invaginations of the sarcolemma lying between myofibrils at the level of the A to I band junction (Figure 2). The function is to spread membrane potential changes caused by nerve impulses between the fibers. The interior of the tubules is contiguous with the extracellular space.[4] Sarcoplasmic reticulum (SR) sacs, called terminal cisternae, surround the T tubules, and the function of the SR is to regulate storage and reuptake of calcium. Calcium, necessary for muscle contraction, is stored in the terminal cisternae bound to calsequestrin.[11] The excitation-contraction coupling mechanism is discussed below.

Sarcomeres are the functional units of contraction in the muscle and have a half-life of 5 to 7 days.[12] They are arranged in series; each one is about 2.5 μm long in the resting muscle, and sarcomeres in adjacent myofibers are aligned such that their internal structure creates transverse banding appreciated in longitudinal section with light microscopy (see Figures 1B and 2). Sarcomeres are composed of thick myosin filaments and thin actin filaments. Dark A bands (anisotropic) alternate with lighter I bands (isotropic). The sarcomere extends from the center of one I band to the next, and in the center of each I band is the Z line, also known as the Z disk or Z band (see Figure 1, B and C). The

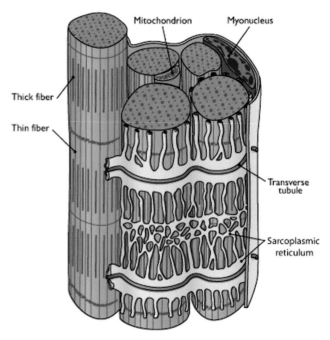

Figure 2. Diagram illustrating a muscle fiber showing the organization of the transverse (T) tubules and sarcoplasmic reticulum relative to the myofibrils. Note the T tubules aligned along the A to I junctions of the sarcomeres. Adapted from Salmons S.[4])

A band spans the length of the thick myosin filaments and includes the areas of overlap between thick and thin filaments. The A-band length remains constant in muscle contraction. The central area of the A band, the H zone, is paler than the borders and is the site in which there is no overlap of thick and thin fiber. The M line lies at the center of the A band and consists of connections between adjacent myosin filaments. I bands contain thin but no thick filaments and narrow with muscle contraction.[4,6]

The primary protein filaments in the sarcomere are actin, myosin, and titin (ie, connectin). Additional proteins serving important functional roles in muscle contraction are tropomyosin, troponin, nebulin, α-actinin, and the intermediate filaments nestin, vimentin, and desmin.[2,4,6,13] Thin filaments are primarily composed of actin, which is associated with troponin and tropomyosin.

Actin is highly conserved phylogenetically and, for all practical purposes, can be considered to have a common structure within and between organisms. Actin filaments are 9 nm in diameter and 1.0 μm long and make up 20% of the fibrillar protein in muscles. Actin takes two forms: F-actin (filamentous actin) and G-actin (globular actin). G-actin molecules polymerize to form a double-chain helix of F-actin. Each globular molecule is associated with a calcium ion and a molecule of ATP. Actin has polarity, and filaments in serial sarcomeres point away from the Z line, thereby ensuring that activation of actin-myosin cross-bridges will shorten the sarcomere. Troponin and tropomyosin molecules are arranged along the thin filament: at every seventh G-actin lies one of each of the proteins. Tropomyosin and troponin are required for calcium-mediated contractile activity. Tropomyosin lies in the groove of the actin helix and adds stiffness to it. Troponin is a complex of three subunits: T, I, and C. T binds tropomyosin, I inhibits binding between actin and myosin, and C binds calcium ions.

Myosin (thick) filaments are 15 nm in diameter and 1.6 μm long. Myosin comprises 60% of myofibrillar protein and is composed of two heavy and four light chains (Figure 3). The heavy chain has a tail and two globular heads. The tail consists of two heavy α helical chains wound around each other. The four light chains are associated with the two globular heads. The globular heads of the heavy myosin chains are mobile and are the sites of binding with actin and of hydrolysis of ATP. Each head can bind to a different actin molecule. Myosin isoforms vary depending on age, the location within the body, and injury states. Heavy-chain isoforms are thought to play a large role in determining fiber type (fast twitch or slow twitch), muscle force, velocity, and power.[14,15]

Titin is a large filament (> 1.0 μm long) that connects the ends of thick filaments to the Z disk and helps prevent injury to muscle by acting as an internal spring.[13,16] Six titin molecules surround each end of a myosin fiber and extend from the M band in the center of the A band to the Z band. Within the A band, titin is stiffer and binds myosin and C protein, and in the I band, the titin filament is more elastic and serves to modulate passive sarcomeric tension.[13,17] Titin filament termini overlap in both the M and Z

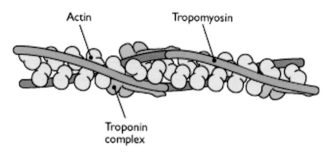

Figure 3. Diagram of skeletal muscle thin filaments illustrating the relative positions of the tropomyosin and troponin along the actin double helix and thick filaments showing assembly of light and heavy myosin chains and polymerization to form the thick filament. Note the position of myosin heads in close proximity to binding sites along the actin filaments, which facilitates the opposed sliding movements of actin and myosin during muscle contraction.

bands.[8] Nebulin travels along the length of the actin filament and may play a role in signal transduction, force generation, and maintenance of actin. α-Actinin connects actin fibers to each other at the Z disk.[8,18,19] The intermediate filaments are expressed at different times in the life of the organism, but all are up-regulated to various degrees with denervation. The intermediate filaments are thought to play roles in maintaining the structure of the myofiber. Nestin is found where there are acetylcholine receptors, vimentin is associated with fibroblasts in the muscle connective tissue, and desmin is more diffusely located within the myocyte near the sarcolemma.[20]

Excitation-Contraction Coupling and the "Sliding Filament" Model of Muscle Contraction

Huxley and Niedergerke described the sliding filament model of muscle contraction in 1954.[1] They found, via x-ray diffraction and electron microscopy, that although muscle fiber length shortens, individual actin and myosin filaments do not change in length. In shortening contractions, I-band width decreases, but the A-band width does not change (Figure 4). This supports the hypothesis that muscle fiber shortening occurs when filaments slide past one another. Muscle contraction occurs proportionally in all

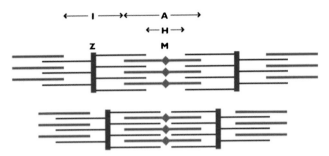

Figure 4. Diagrams of the relaxed (*top*) and contracting (*bottom*) sarcomere. The Z disk is in *blue*, the actin filaments are in *black*, and the myosin is in *red*. The *red diamonds* represent the cross connections between the myosin strands that help maintain the orientation and stability of the sarcomere in space. This is the location of the M line. Note that the A band does not change in width with contraction, whereas the I and H bands shrink. Adapted from Salmons S.[4]

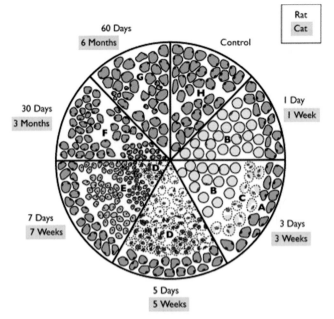

Figure 5. Schematic of muscle that has been excised and grafted showing histologic changes over time. Cross sections of muscles from normal controls to devascularized and necrotic fibers to fully healed muscle are presented in a clockwise direction. In this paradigm, the superficial muscle fibers survived, whereas the deeper ones died and were the last to regenerate. *A*, Surviving muscle fibers. *B*, Original muscle fibers in a state of ischemic necrosis. *C*, Muscle fibers invaded by macrophages that are phagocytizing the necrotic cytoplasm. *D*, Myoblasts and early myotubes within the basal laminae of the original muscle fibers. *E*, Early cross-striated muscle fibers. *F*, Maturing regenerating muscle fibers. *G*, Mature regenerated muscle fibers. *H*, Normal control muscle fibers. (**Permission pending** from Carlson.)

sarcomeres in series along the length of the fiber, and muscle tension is related to the overlap of thick and thin filaments, but the fibers within a muscle are arranged such that they do not all reach maximum tension simultaneously. Fiber bundles activate in different orders and to differing degrees depending on the local load requirements.

The excitation-contraction coupling mechanism provides the energy for muscle contraction.[21] Muscle contraction is initiated by a depolarizing nerve impulse. When a muscle fiber is at rest, the rod-like tropomyosin prevents actin from interacting with myosin by blocking one of the contact sites for the cross-bridges (see Figure 5-3). An action potential travels from the neuromuscular junction across the sarcolemma, through the T tubules, and releases calcium from the cisternae of the SR through an inrush of sodium ions into the cell.[21] The increase in free cytosolic calcium ions changes the shape of troponin. The shape change moves tropomyosin away from the cross-bridge binding site, allowing actin and myosin to interact.[22]

Except in the H zone, myosin fibers have multiple "heads" along their length (see Figure 3). Bound to each head is an adenosine diphosphate (ADP) and an inorganic phosphate. When tropomyosin moves away from the actin binding site, the myosin head cross-bridge contacts actin, ADP and phosphate are released, the head tilts,

and myosin slides 5 to 10 nm along actin. Cross-bridges are bound at about 45°. Multiple cycles are involved in each muscle contraction, and the myosin heads do not contract and release in unison. At the end of each stroke, ATP binds to the myosin head and causes it to be released from actin. The ATP hydrolyzes to ADP and phosphate, and the next cycle can begin. The ratcheting action of cross-bridges pulls the Z lines closer to the H zone.[4,6]

Muscles generate maximum tension when there is an intermediate degree of overlap between the filaments and the sarcomere length is about 2.3 μm. When sarcomeres are stretched past 3.5 μm, there is not enough overlap between thick and thin filaments to generate significant tension; and when muscle fibers are shortened excessively, the actin filaments from half of the sarcomere run into those on the far side of the H zone (see Figure 4). The sarcomere length-tension relationship was first defined by Blix in the late 1800s and expanded on by Gordon and Huxley in the 1960s.[3]

Contractions can be isometric (no length change), eccentric (lengthening or pliometric), or concentric (shortening).[23] Two general principles apply to muscle contractions, which generate variable amounts of force at varying rates. Force is proportional to the physiologic cross-sectional area of the muscle (summation of all areas of all fibers), but muscle contractile speed is proportional to fiber length and fiber type.[3,21] As the shortening velocity increases, the force decreases.[24] Concentric contractions are less likely to cause damage to the muscle fibers, and eccentric contractions allow high tension to persist and cause more damage. The magnitude of strain determines the degree of injury, although the noncontractile elements bear some of the tension.[25]

Fiber-Type Distinction

Muscle fibers can be distinguished in several ways: tonic and twitch; red, white, and intermediate; and types 1, 2A, and 2B (Table 1).[4] Tonic muscle fibers are rare in humans: they are slow to contract and do not propagate action potentials. Extraocular muscles (EOMs) and the stapedius muscle are tonic. Other human skeletal muscle fibers are of the twitch type, and action potentials travel along their surfaces. The tonic-twitch distinction is too broad for human muscles as twitch-type muscle fibers vary significantly. A more common classification for human muscles is that of the red, white, and intermediate fibers, which are distinguished by histochemistry. Fibers can also be divided functionally by staining for adenosine triphosphatase (ATPase) activity. Groups are noted as types 1, 2A, and 2B. Type 1 fibers are also known as slow-twitch muscle fibers, and type 2 are fast twitch. Human muscles have fiber-type heterogeneity, and the proportion of each type within a muscle varies with the demands placed on it. Postural muscles, for example, are more likely to have a greater proportion of red (high mitochondrial and vascular content) and type 1 (fatigue resistant) fibers than are muscles used for delicate activity.

Unique Features of Muscles in the Head and Neck

The muscles of facial expression are unique in that their attachment is frequently to skin, not to bone, and they do not cross joints. Many of the head and neck muscles lack the discrete, well-formed tendons found in the extremities, and there is wide variability in the size and presence of muscles (Table 2).[26] In a series of cadaver hemiface dissections, the most common pattern of facial musculature was present only in 44% of hemifaces dissected, and not all expected muscles existed in those faces.[27] There has been limited investigation of the functional significance of structural variances in facial muscle.

Neck muscles have complex architecture.[5] Multiple insertions, complex internal geometry, and the potential to cross multiple joints put them at increased risk of eccentric strain injuries.[28]

Table 1. CHARACTERISTICS OF MAJOR SKELETAL MUSCLE FIBER TYPES						
Color	Metabolism	Contraction Speed	Mitochondrial Count	Vascularity	Function	Fatigue Resistance
Type 1: red	Oxidative (aerobic)	Slow	High	High	Postural support	Resistant
Type 2A: intermediate	Oxidative-glycolytic	Intermediate	Intermediate	Intermediate	Rapid activity	Resistant
Type 2B: white	Glycolytic (anaerobic)	Fast	Low	Low	Rapid activity	Susceptible

Extraocular Muscles

In the craniofacial skeleton, extraocular, jaw, and laryngeal muscles display anatomic and physiologic characteristics that make them significantly different from skeletal muscle in the trunk and limbs. EOMs differ in several ways.[29–31] They must maintain activity over a dynamic range that requires greater contraction speed and resistance to fatigue than displayed by regular skeletal muscles. They do not act across joints. Because forces on the eye are relatively small and constant, 70% of EOM motor units are constantly active. The load on the eye does not change, and sensory feedback is neural, not based on forces acting on the globe.[30] Myonuclei of skeletal muscles are postmitotic unless injured, but those of EOMs display continuous remodeling.[32] Skeletal muscles usually have one neuromuscular junction, but EOMs have singly innervated fibers, as well as multiply innervated fibers (MIFs). MIFs in the EOM are similar to those seen in amphibians and may play a role in proprioception.[33] EOM MIFs display myosin heterogeneity and include developmental and α-cardiac isoforms.

Grossly, EOMs are compartmentalized into two layers: orbital and global. The layers contain different myosin isoforms between and within layers depending on the position within the muscle.[34] The functional implications of this pattern are unknown. Interestingly, EOMs may be selected or spared in certain disease conditions.[35] One hypothesis is that satellite cells in the EOM are continuously dividing. In most muscles, injury with loss of basal lamina integrity is required for satellite cell proliferation. Their activity may cause differing responses to acquired disease states.[31,36] Myasthenia gravis causes weakness of the EOMs and of the levator palpebrae. Because of the high firing rates of ocular motor nerves, these muscles may be at increased risk of fatigue. Botulism, but not nerve laceration, causes atrophy in EOMs but not in truncal skeletal muscles.[33,37] In Graves' disease, EOMs are enlarged by increased extracellular matrix and connective tissues owing to inflammation, but the degree of intrinsic destruction of the muscle is variable. EOMs are not affected in Duchenne muscular dystrophy or motoneuron disease.[30]

Jaw Muscles

Jaw muscles are phylogenetically diverse and contain four main families of myosins: limb, developmental, α-cardiac, and masticatory.[38] Limb myosin can be further distinguished as fast or slow. Slow fibers have a large blood supply, high concentrations of mitochondria, low ATPase activity, and conservative energy production. They are most frequently seen in low-speed muscles and muscles of posture. Fast fibers are divided into three subtypes (IIa, IIx, and IIB). They are used for rapid development of speed and power and lack endurance. The ATPase activity is high. In the human, muscles of the jaw contain developmental, α-cardiac, fast IIa and IIx, and slow fibers.[38] Among mammals, the speed of jaw closing is more variable than that of jaw opening. Carnivores, monkeys, and chimps have a high percentage of superfast type II fibers; humans have none.[2,38] In the limb, fast type II fibers are larger than slow type I, but in human jaw-closing muscles, the type II fibers are smaller than type I fibers. The differences seen in human jaw-closing muscles may be due to altered oral requirements, embryologic derivation, innervation, and delays in maturation.[2]

From a biomechanical standpoint, the muscles of the jaw are complex. Creating models to better understand function and dysfunction has been challenging as the muscle architecture is not straightforward, it is difficult to estimate cross-sectional areas (and thus predict forces), passive and active forces act on the muscles and joints, and muscle recruitment patterns are poorly understood.[39]

Laryngeal Muscles

Laryngeal muscles of the rat and rabbit also display myosin heterogeneity. The myosin isoforms differ between muscles within the larynx and are changeable with denervation and reinnervation.[40,41] The human laryngeal musculature has been shown to have fast and slow myosin

Table 2. KEY ANATOMIC FEATURES OF THE MUSCLES OF THE HEAD AND NECK				
Muscle	Origin	Insertion	Cranial Nerve	Action
Epicranial				
Occipitalis	Occipital and temporal bones	Epicranial aponeurosis (aka galea aponeurotica)	VII (temporal branch)	Occipitalis and frontalis act together to move scalp back and forth and elevate brows
Frontalis	Superficial fascia of scalp	Epicranial aponeurosis	VII (posterior auricular branch)	Tightens scalp, moves skin over temples, raises auricle
Temporoparietalis	Temporal fascia above auricle	Skin and temporal fascia near superior temporal line	VII (temporal branch)	
Circumorbital and palpebral				
Orbicularis oculi	Frontal bone, maxilla, medial palpebral ligament	Skin of brow, lateral palpebral raphe, tarsi of eyelids	VII (temporal and zygomatic branches)	Closes eyelids
Corrugator supercilii	Superciliary arch of frontal bone	Skin over supraorbital rim	VII (temporal branch)	Draws eyebrow inferomedially
Levator palpebrae superioris	Lesser wing of sphenoid	Upper eyelid, tarsus	III	Elevates the upper eyelid
Extraocular				
Superior rectus	Common annular tendon	Sclera	III	Elevates globe (with inferior oblique)
Inferior rectus	Common annular tendon	Sclera	III	Downward gaze (with superior oblique)
Lateral rectus	Common annular tendon	Sclera	VI	Abduction of globe
Medial rectus	Common annular tendon	Sclera	III	Adduction of globe
Superior oblique	Sphenoid superomedial to optic canal	Sclera between superior and lateral rectus	IV	Rotates globe down and lateral
Inferior oblique	Orbital surface of maxilla	Sclera between inferior and lateral rectus	III	Rotates globe up and lateral
Nasal				
Procerus	Fascia over lower nasal bone and upper lateral nasal cartilage	Skin between eyebrows	VII (buccal branch)	Draws down medial eyebrow and creates transverse wrinkles
Nasalis (transverse and alar parts)	Maxilla	Procerus (transverse) and nasal alar cartilage (alar)	VII (buccal branch)	Transverse compresses nasal aperture Alar widens alar aperture
Depressor septi	Maxilla	Mobile nasal septum	VII (buccal branch)	Widens alar aperture
Buccolabial				
Levator labii superioris alaeque nasi	Frontal process of maxilla	Alar cartilage, overlying skin, lateral upper lip	VII (buccal branch)	Raises, everts upper lip; deepens nasolabial crease
Levator labii superioris	Inferior orbital margin	Upper lip muscles	VII (buccal branch)	Raises, everts upper lip; deepens nasolabial crease
Levator anguli oris	Canine fossa of maxilla below infraorbital foramen	Modiolus at lateral oral commissure	VII (buccal branch)	Raises corners of mouth; deepens nasolabial crease
Zygomaticus major	Zygoma	Modiolus	VII (buccal branch)	Raises corners of mouth and draws posteriorly
Zygomaticus minor	Zygoma	Upper lip muscles	VII (buccal branch)	Raises upper lip; deepens nasolabial crease
Risorius	Zygomatic arch, facial fascia	Modiolus	VII (buccal branch)	Draws angle of mouth laterally
Mentalis	Incisive fossa of mandible	Skin of lower chin	VII (marginal mandibular branch)	Raises and everts lower lip
Depressor labii inferioris	Oblique line of mandible	Skin and mucosa of lower lip	VII (marginal mandibular branch)	Depresses lower lip and pulls it slightly laterally

Table 2. CONTINUED				
Muscle	Origin	Insertion	Cranial Nerve	Action
Depressor anguli oris	Mental tubercle and oblique line of mandible	Modiolus and levator anguli oris	VII (marginal mandibular branch)	Depresses lower lip and pulls it laterally
Buccinator	Alveolar processes of maxilla and mandible; anterior border of pterygomandibular raphe	Orbicularis oris, lips, oral mucosa	VII (inferior buccal branches)	Compresses the cheeks toward the teeth
Orbicularis oris	Buccinator, levator labii superioris, zygomaticus major, depressor labii inferioris	Skin, mucosa of lips	VII (inferior buccal and marginal mandibular)	Closes lips; alters the shape of the mouth in speaking, eating, and drinking
Incisivus labii superioris	Incisive fossa of maxilla	Modiolus, levator anguli oris	VII (buccal branches)	Alters shape of mouth
Incisivus labii inferioris	Incisive fossa of mandible	Modiolus	VII (buccal branches)	Alters shape of mouth
Masticatory				
Masseter	Superficial: maxillary process of zygoma Middle: anterior zygomatic arch Deep: deep surface of zygomatic arch	Superficial: angle and lateral mandibular ramus Middle: central mandibular ramus Deep: upper mandibular ramus and coronoid	V3 (mandibular)	Elevates the mandible
Temporalis	Temporal fossa and deep surface of temporal fascia	Coronoid and anterior border of mandibular ramus	V3 (mandibular)	Elevates and retracts the mandible
Lateral pterygoid	Upper head: greater wing of sphenoid Lower head: lateral surface lateral pterygoid plate	Anterior neck of mandible and capsule and disk of TMJ	V3 (mandibular)	Opens mouth, protrudes mandible, grinds teeth
Medial pterygoid	Deep head: medial surface of lateral pterygoid plate, palatine bone Superficial head: lateral palatine and maxillary tuberosity	Inferior and posterior medial surface of ramus and angle of mandible	V3 (mandibular)	Elevates and protrudes mandible, grinds teeth
Anterolateral neck				
Platysma	Fascia over pectoralis major and deltoid	Lower mandible, lower lateral lip, lower face	VII (cervical branch)	Depresses mandible and lower lip
Sternocleidomastoid	Medial head: manubrium Lateral head: medial clavicle	Medial head: occiput Lateral head: mastoid process	XI, C2, C3, C4	Bends head laterally, rotates head
Suprahyoid				
Digastric	Posterior belly: mastoid process Anterior belly: digastric fossa	Intermediate tendon (attached to hyoid)	Posterior belly: VII Anterior belly: V3	Depresses mandible, elevates hyoid
Stylohyoid	Styloid process	Hyoid	VII	Elevates and retracts hyoid
Mylohyoid	Mandible	Hyoid and median raphe	V3	Elevates floor of mouth
Geniohyoid	Symphysis menti	Hyoid	C1 traveling with XII	Elevates and protrudes hyoid
Infrahyoid				
Sternohyoid	Medial clavicle, posterior sternoclavicular ligament, manubrium	Hyoid	C1, C2, C3 (ansa cervicalis)	Depresses hyoid
Sternothyroid	Manubrium, first rib	Thyroid cartilage	C1, C2, C3 (ansa cervicalis)	Depresses larynx
Thyrohyoid	Thyroid cartilage	Hyoid	C1 traveling with XII	Depresses hyoid

Table 2. CONTINUED				
Muscle	Origin	Insertion	Cranial Nerve	Action
Omohyoid	Inferior belly: scapula	Inferior belly: intermediate tendon	Inferior belly: C2, C3	Depresses hyoid
	Superior belly: intermediate tendon	Superior belly: hyoid	Superior belly: C1	

TMJ = temporomandibular joint.

fibers, but there is no evidence of cardiac or developmental fiber types.[42]

STEPS IN HEALING

Muscle contusions and lacerations are extremely common in facial trauma. Strains caused by excessive stretch of the muscle are less a significant consideration for the muscles intrinsic to the face but may be clinically significant in the muscles of the neck. Muscles can also be injured when subject to ischemia and denervation. The redundancy of blood supply to the face makes the former a less clinically significant problem.

Until fairly recently, it was believed that muscle could not regenerate because myofibers were thought to be postmitotic and, therefore, incapable of regeneration. The recognition that satellite cells were capable of up-regulation and induction of the formation of new myofibers changed the way in which muscle injury and recovery were viewed.[7,43] Muscle damage, through processes as varied as vigorous exercise and trauma, up-regulates the activity of satellite cells. Muscle has a high rate of metabolic activity, and although damage progresses rapidly, it regresses in much the same way (Figure 5).[43,44] As is true with injuries to other soft tissues, muscles heal by a three-phase process: inflammation, proliferation, and remodeling. The phases overlap, and wound healing problems can prolong the duration of a phase. The most common obstruction to complete muscle healing is fibrosis, but relatively little work has been done on the nature of fibrosis in skeletal muscle.[21]

Inflammation

Inflammation is a complex balance of injury and repair that begins shortly after the injury and persists for about 5 days.[45,46] When the sarcoplasm is torn, myofibrils retract, extracellular calcium flows in, and injury is exacerbated via proteases.[21,47] A novel process called contraction banding limits the longitudinal extent of myofiber damage by quickly sealing the open sarcomere.[47,48] Transection of blood vessels and the subsequent collection of a hematoma initiate the inflammatory cascade.[7] Platelets are released, fibrin clots are formed, phagocytosis begins, and satellite cells are up-regulated.[49]

Polymorphonuclear leukocytes (PMNs) and macrophages are the primary cells in the inflammatory response following muscle injury.[45] PMNs appear in the wound within 1 hour, peak at 1 day postinjury, and are present for up to 5 days. Although an intrinsic part of the inflammatory response, PMNs may exacerbate local tissue damage and impair recovery of muscle fibers.[45,50] The PMN has no known reparative role. Ridding the muscle of PMNs preinjury has been shown to limit muscle damage, and administration of an antibody that blocks the respiratory burst and degranulation of PMNs decreases visible muscle damage.[45] PMNs lyse cell membranes via superoxide, hydrogen peroxide, and myeloperoxidase (MPO)-dependent paths (Figure 6). The more clinically relevant of the three are likely to be hydrogen peroxide and MPO. MPO is produced by PMNs and is increased in muscle injury or exercise. Both superoxide and hydrogen peroxide can react with MPO to generate agents that are capable of lysing cell membranes, and the redox environment in the muscle determines the extent of PMN-mediated damage.[45]

The PMNs are soon joined by monocytes, which metamorphose into macrophages, which both phagocytose cellular debris and aid in

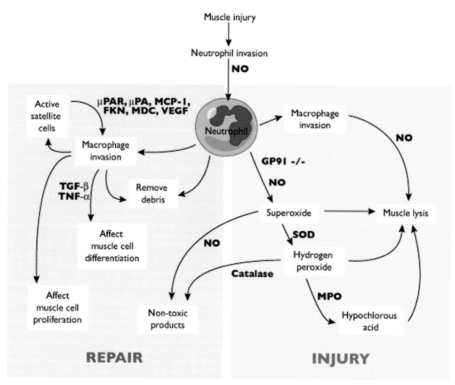

Figure 6. Schematic of potential mediators of inflammatory cell interactions with injured muscle. Experimental observations that support the potential interactions between neutrophils, macrophages, and muscle are discussed in the text. Neutrophils are shown as having a potential role in promoting injury or repair, although their role in promoting repair in injured muscle is speculative. FKN = fractalkine; MCP-1 = monocyte chemoattractant protein 1; MDC = macrophage-derived chemokine; MPO = myeloperoxidase; NO = nitric oxide; SOD = superoxide dismutase; uPA = urokinase-type plasminogen activator; uPAR = urokinase-type plasminogen-activator receptor; VEGF = vascular endothelial growth factor. Reproduced with permission from Tidball JG.[45]

reconstruction.[51] Macrophages, aided by PMNs, lyse myofibers through a nitric oxide–dependent and superoxide-independent mechanism.[45] Reconstructive roles of the macrophage have been elucidated, and macrophage-depleted cells show impaired muscle regeneration. Macrophage-derived growth factors include transforming growth factor β (TGF-β), heparin-binding epidermal growth factor–like growth factor (HB-EGF), and nitric oxide. TGF-β inhibits differentiation of myogenic cells, HB-EGF may increase muscle survival during oxidative stress, and nitric oxide regulates inflammation and damage caused by invading cells by scavenging radicals or inhibiting molecules that allow PMNs to adhere to the vascular endothelium.

Fibroblasts attach to the early fibrin clot and secrete proteins needed for reconstruction of the muscle's supportive matrix.[52] Adjacent to the site of injury, the inflammatory cells rid the myo-

tubes of necrotic cellular material yet leave the endomysium intact. Common cytokines and growth factors playing roles in stages of muscle regeneration are tumor necrosis factor α, TGF-β, fibroblast growth factor (FGF), insulin-like growth factor (IGF), vascular endothelial growth factor, leukemia inhibitory factor (LIF), platelet-derived growth factor, and interleukins 1β, 6, and 8.[7,53–56] Cytokines control the inflammatory response and local vascularity; growth factors control satellite cell up-regulation and myofiber development. Thrombospondin is an "adhesive glycoprotein" produced by a variety of cells involved in the inflammatory cascade. It may mediate interactions between the extracellular matrix and the myofibrils.[49]

Given that injury is necessary for activation of satellite cells, it has been hypothesized that muscle injury is a necessary evil for optimal function, growth, and adaptation.[45,49] Satellite cells are located between the sarcolemma and basal lamina, and two cell populations of satellite cells are present in adult muscle cells: mature and stem satellite cells.[7,21] Mature satellite cells are ready to differentiate; stem cells proliferate, restock the supply of stem cells, and differentiate.[7] Myofiber damage caused by resistance training, exercise-induced trauma, and direct (external) trauma promotes the influx of macrophages. The macrophage secretes numerous growth factors, including IGF-I, IGF-II, hepatocyte growth factor (HGF), and FGF, and these stimulate satellite cell proliferation within hours of the injury. Satellite cell proliferation is maximal during the first few days after the injury.[36] Activated satellite cells also release factors that attract macrophages: monocyte chemoattractant protein 1 and urokinase-type plasminogen-activator receptor.[45,57] The activated satellite cells crawl along tissue bridges to get to the site of injury, proliferate, differentiate into myotubes, mature, and fuse with each other or with preexisting muscle fibers. Once the myofibers are healed, the satellite cell again becomes quiescent.[36] Age-related impairment of muscle healing is due not so much to the presence of fewer satellite cells but to suboptimal factors in the local environment: new myofibers are more delicate, the immune response is less robust, the capillary concentration is decreased, and reinnervation is less successful.[36] Despite the simultaneous destructive activity of macrophages, satellite cells are able to use macrophages to begin the regenerative process shortly after injury.[57,58] Inhibition of satellite cell proliferation with irradiation has been found to inhibit force recovery following contraction-induced injury.[59] Ultimately, the capacity of satellite cells to replicate is not infinite, and the ability of muscles to regenerate can be exhausted.[52]

Proliferation and Remodeling

The proliferative phase is characterized by phagocytosis of necrotic tissue by macrophages, continued satellite cell proliferation, neovascularization, reinnervation, and regeneration of muscle fibers and of connective tissue. The proliferative phase peaks at 2 weeks and lasts up to 6 weeks. Mature myofibers appear by 10 days postinjury.[46] Remodeling can last months and is the time of reorganization of regenerating myofibers into fused mature myofibers.[7]

Neovascularization and reinnervation precede maturation and ingrowth of mature muscle fibers. Immature myotubes can use anaerobic metabolism, but mature myofibers require aerobic metabolism, so vascularity must be established before myofibers can mature.[60] A motor nerve branch travels within the endomysium and innervates each myofiber. The transection of the myofiber may occur proximal to, at, or distal to the neuromuscular junction, but nerves are capable of regrowth if cut. Motor units are the muscle fibers innervated by a single nerve branch, and their size is inversely proportional to the degree of control required by the muscle.[21]

Fibroblasts produce tenascin C and fibronectin, which confer elasticity to the healing tissue.[61] Type III and then type I collagen forms within the first week after injury and quickly remodels into a scar mass by 2 to 3 weeks following injury.[5,62,63] Unless immobilization of the muscle is prolonged, the scar mass does not significantly increase the total amount of connective tissue in the muscle, but the persistence of fibrotic tissue limits the ability of muscle to completely heal.[5,62,63] New myofibers begin growing toward the scar and attempt to pierce it, and if the scar is too thick, the myofibers create pseudomyotendinous junctions to the scar. The scar gradually decreases in width, and the myofibers may eventually fuse.[64,65] Between the first and second month postinjury, the myofiber cross-sectional area increases.[44] It has been demonstrated that some mechanical tension is necessary for optimal recreation of the myotendinous junctions.[66]

FUTURE PROMISE FOR HEALING

Currently, optimization of recovery from muscle injury consists of the standard RICE protocol (rest, ice, compression, and elevation) for non-surgical injuries.[67] Recommendations to avoid muscle-associated complications of healing in the head and neck include restoring muscle continuity to limit fibrosis, removing muscles from fractures to optimize osseous union, and obtaining adequate hemostasis to avoid hematoma-related complications of trismus and myositis ossificans.[68,69] Epimysial repair of muscle facilitates early motion, optimizes force generation, and limits fibrosis.[70,71]

A variety of oral and intravenous agents have been proposed to optimize global body protein retention and maintain muscle integrity, with promising yet inconsistent results. Dietary manipulations have included supplementation with arginine, omega-3 fatty acids, protein, vitamins, and amino acids, but they have had contradictory results. It is well supported that trauma-induced malnutrition must be avoided.[72] Glutamine supplementation has been shown to increase muscle protein synthesis in elective surgery patients and has had beneficial physiologic effects in burn and trauma patients.[73] Nonsteroidal anti-inflammatory agents (NSAIDs) have been used widely in the post-injury phase, but there has been concern that NSAIDs can be detrimental to muscle healing. The purported mechanism of this may be via inhibition of cyclooxygenase enzymes and subsequent inhibition of satellite cells, but no harmful effects on force production and muscle size have been demonstrated when NSAIDs are administered at the usual doses.[45,74–76] The anabolic steroid oxandrolone has been shown to attenuate lean body mass loss and promote wound healing in burn patients, but it may be potentially harmful to the ventilator-dependent surgical patient by potentiating pulmonary fibrosis.[77,78] A β2-adrenoreceptor agonist (fenoterol) was shown to increase muscle force, mass, myofiber cross-sectional area, and total muscle protein content in both bupivicaine-injured and control rat limb muscles.[79]

Categories of therapies under intense investigation include growth factors, gene therapy, and stem cell therapy. The ideal therapeutic agent would promote muscle regeneration and limit fibrosis—the enemy of function.[7] Combining agents that stimulate myogenesis with those that inhibit fibrosis may be the best alternative. Parameters requiring standardization in the use of growth factors include timing, volume, and site of application. Unfortunately, the short biologic half-life of growth factors makes administration challenging and limits clinical efficacy.[67]

Growth Factors for Muscle Regeneration

IGF-1 has been found to be mitogenic for myoblasts, and application has increased protein in muscles, has increased tetanic and twitch strength in regenerating muscle, and has been protective against denervation atrophy.[21,80] When administered in viral vectors, IGF-1 can block age-related atrophy. However, IGF is also mitogenic for fibroblasts and can increase collagen production and possibly increase muscle fibrosis.[21]

Several other growth factors have not thus far shown promise for clinical application. Kasemkijwattana and colleagues found FGF to increase muscle force development,[67] but Mitchell and colleagues noted inhibition of myoblast differentiation and regeneration and no enhancement of muscle regeneration.[81] HGF has been shown to stimulate satellite cells and to inhibit myoblast regeneration, but it does not appear to be clinically effective.[21,81] LIF stimulates satellite cells, and although LIF messenger ribonucleic acid increases by a factor of seven after skeletal muscle injury, exogenous administration of LIF does not appear to improve muscle regeneration.[21,56,82] Recombinant human growth hormone has not proven to be useful, and harmful effects have been noted. Takala and colleagues found an increased mortality in critically ill patients treated with growth hormone.[83] Biolo and colleagues saw preservation of muscle bulk but were concerned by the depression of glutamine synthesis and potential inhibition of necessary anabolic cellular functions.[84]

Gene Therapy

Gene therapy is performed by using a viral or nonviral vector to deliver a gene that has a desired action on a muscle or scar into the host.[7,21,67] Because of technical difficulties involved in getting sufficient quantities of growth factors into the injured muscle, using gene therapy could aid healing by providing a mechanism for increased long-term production of growth factors.[21] The gene for IGF-1 has had mixed efficacy when injected into injured murine muscles. Some functional improvement was noted, but deficits remained.[21] Plasmids have been proposed as a means to transfer genes for selected myosin isoforms. As noted above, myosin isoforms determine muscle contractile properties, and gene transfer may allow tailoring of muscle properties.[15]

Stem Cell–Based Therapy

Stem cells are tissue specific or hematopoietic. Both can be recruited into muscle tissue in the face of injury, but it is more likely for stem cells residing in muscle to be activated.[7] Natsu and colleagues found that injection of bone marrow–derived stem cells into an injured muscle improved muscle force generation; but they were unable to determine the mechanism of action (direct incorporation of cells into fibers or release of growth-mediating agents).[85] Abedi and colleagues irradiated mice, injected a limb muscle with cardiotoxin, and performed a bone marrow transplant with fluorescent cells. They demonstrated the presence of chimerism in the area of muscle injury and concluded that bone marrow stem cells fuse with muscle fibers.[86]

Antifibrosis Therapy

A major impediment to muscle healing is fibrosis. Fibrosis tends to begin during the second week after an injury and is progressive.[87] TGF-β has been found to play a significant role in the development of fibrosis by stimulating myofibroblast proliferation and activating the extracellular matrix.[21,88] Neutralization of TGF-β has been performed with decorin, suramin, and interferon-γ.[21,87–89] Decorin is a human proteoglycan that, when injected into lacerated murine muscle, has been shown to decrease the stimulatory effect of TGF-β on myofibroblasts and improve muscle regeneration.[87] Suramin is a naphthylurea compound and, likewise, inhibits the activity of TGF-β and improves twitch and tetanic forces.[90] As a reverse transcriptase inhibitor, it has a wide array of cellular activities and may not be sufficiently selective for correction of fibrosis without induction of unwanted side effects.[91] Interferon-γ is a cytokine that inhibits the induction of fibroblast proliferation by TGF-β.[89]

Bionic Replacement

When an injured muscle cannot be fixed, "bionic" replacements may someday be an alternative. As is true for muscles, electroactive polymers respond to electrical stimulation by changing shape and size.[92] They can be activated by electrical or ionic mechanisms; the electrical mechanism is more likely to be clinically useful. The newest polymers can develop clinically functional amounts of strain, resist fracture, and damp vibrations, giving them "lifelike aesthetics," and the key advantages are resilience, tolerance, and quiet operation. Proposed uses include cardiac valves, eyelid muscles and EOMs, muscles of facial expression, and muscles of the limbs. Despite rapid progress, the current state of the art is that electroactive polymers have low conversion efficiency, are not robust, and develop low torque. In addition, no standard commercial materials are available, and a commercial and research infrastructure must be developed before they can be fully exploited as a treatment alternative.

SUMMARY

It is being increasingly appreciated that muscle is a highly plastic tissue capable of recovery following injury. Research related to muscle tissue in the face and neck has largely centered on extraocular and jaw muscles. A large body of work exists on reinnervation of facial musculature, but relatively few investigations have looked at strategies to optimize healing specifically in the facial and neck muscles. Given the social and functional importance of these muscles, it is an area rich in possibility for future research.

REFERENCES

1. Huxley AF, Niedergerke R. Structural changes in muscle during contraction. Interference microscopy of living muscle fibers. Nature 1954;173:971–3.
2. Sciote JJ, Horton MJ, Rowlerson AM, Link J. Specialized cranial muscles: how different are they from limb and abdominal muscles? Cells Tissues Organs 2003;174:73–86.
3. Lieber RL. Skeletal muscle is a biological example of a linear electro-active actuator. In: Proceedings of SPIE's 6th Annual International Symposium on Smart Structures and Materials, 1–5 March, 1999, San Diego, CA. Paper No.: 3669-03.
4. Salmons S. Muscle. In: Williams PL, Bannister LH, Berry MM, et al, editors. Gray's anatomy. 38th ed. Edinburgh: Churchill Livingstone; 1995. p. 737–900.
5. Kamibayashi LK, Richmond FJR. Morphometry of human neck muscles. Spine 1998;23:1314–23.
6. Alberts B. The cytoskeleton. In: Alberts B, Bray D, Lewis J, et al, editors. Molecular biology of the cell. 1st ed. New York: Garland Publishing; 1983. p. 550–61.
7. Järvinen TAH, Järvinen TLN, Kääriäinen M, et al. Muscle injuries: biology and treatment. Am J Sports Med 2005; 33:745–64.
8. Sanger JW, Chowrashi P, Shaner NC, et al. Myofibrillogenesis in skeletal muscle cells. Clin Orthop Relat Res 2002;403 Suppl:S153–62.
9. Eisenberg BR, Milton RL. Muscle fiber termination at the tendon in the frog's sartorius: a stereological study. Am J Anat 1984;171:273–84.
10. Chargé SBP, Rudnicki MA. Cellular and molecular regulation of muscle regeneration. Physiol Rev 2004; 84:209–38.
11. Jorgensen AO, Kalnins VI, Zubrzyca E, MacLennan DH. Assembly of the sarcoplasmic reticulum proteins in differentiating rat skeletal muscle cell cultures: localization by immunofluorescence of sarcoplasmic reticulum proteins in differentiating rat skeletal muscle cell cultures. J Cell Biol 1977;74:287–98.
12. Zak R, Martin AF, Prior G, Rabinowitz M. Comparison of turnover of several myofibrillar proteins and critical evaluation of double isotope method. J Biol Chem 1977;252:3430–5.
13. Labeit S, Kolmerer B, Linke WA. The giant protein titin. Emerging roles in physiology and pathophysiology. Circ Res 1997;80:290–4.
14. Bárány M. ATPase activity of myosin correlated with speed of muscle shortening. J Gen Physiol 1967;50:197–218.
15. Lutz GJ, Lieber RL. Studies of myosin isoforms in muscle cells: single cell mechanics and gene transfer. Clin Orthop Relat Res 2002;403 Supply:S51–8.
16. Tatsumi R, Maeda K, Hattori A, Takahashi K. Calcium binding to an elastic portion of connectin/titin filaments. J Muscle Res Cell Motil 2001;22:149–62.
17. Lindstedt SL, Reich TE, Keim P, LaStayo PC. Do muscles function as adaptable locomotor springs? J Exp Biol 2002;205:2211–6.
18. McElhinny AS, Kazmierski ST, Labeit S, Gregorio CC. Nebulin: the nebulous, multifunctional giant of striated muscle. Trends Cardiovasc Med 2003;13:195–201.
19. Waterman-Storer CM. The cytoskeleton of skeletal muscle: is it affected by exercise? A brief review. Med Sci Sports Exerc 1991;23:1240–9.
20. Vaittinen S, Lukka R, Sahlgren C, et al. Specific and innervation-regulated expression of the intermediate filament protein nestin at neuromuscular and myotendinous junctions in skeletal muscle. Am J Pathol 1999; 154:591–600.
21. Huard J, Li Y, Fu F. Muscle injuries and repair: current trends in research. J Bone Joint Surg Am 2002;84A: 822–32.
22. Ebashi S, Endo M, Otsuki I. Control of muscle contraction. Q Rev Biophys 1969;2:351–84.
23. Faulkner JA. Terminology for contractions of muscles during shortening, while isometric, and during lengthening. J Appl Physiol 2003;95:455–9.
24. Katz B. The relation between force and speed in muscular contraction. J Physiol (Lond) 1939;96:45–64.
25. Kirkendall DT, Garrett WE. Clinical perspectives regarding eccentric muscle injury. Clin Orthop Relat Res 2002;403 Supply:S81–9.
26. Goodmurphy CW, Ovalle WK. Morphological study of two human facial muscles: orbicularis oculi and corrugator supercilii. Clin Anat 1999;12:1–11.
27. Pessa JE, Zadoo VP, Adrian EK, et al. Variability of the midfacial muscles: analysis of 50 hemifacial cadaver dissections. Plast Reconstr Surg 1998;102:1888–93.
28. Best TM, Hasselman CT, Garrett WE Jr. Muscle strain injuries: biomechanical and structural studies. In: Salmons S, editor. Muscle damage. Oxford: Oxford University Press; 1997. p. 145–67.
29. Porter JD. Extraocular muscle: cellular adaptations for a diverse functional repertoire. Ann N Y Acad Sci 2002; 956:4–16.
30. Ruff RL. More than meets the eye: extraocular muscle is very distinct from extremity skeletal muscle. Muscle Nerve 2002;25:311–3.
31. McLoon LK, Rios L, Wirschafter JD. Complex three-dimensional patterns of myosin isoform expression: differences between and within specific extraocular muscles. J Muscle Res Cell Motil 1999;20:771–83.
32. McLoon LK, Wirtschafter JD. Continuous myonuclear addition to single extraocular myofibers in uninjured adult rabbits. Muscle Nerve 2002;25:348–58.
33. Porter JD, Baker RS, Ragusa RJ, Brueckner JK. Extraocular muscles: basic and clinical aspects of

structure and function. Surv Ophthalmol 1995;39:451–84.

34. Rubinstein NA, Porter JD, Hoh JFY. The development of longitudinal variation of myosin isoforms in the orbital fibers of extraocular muscles of rats. Invest Ophthalmol Vis Sci 2004;45:3067–72.

35. Kaminski HJ. Differential susceptibility of the ocular motor system to disease. Ann N Y Acad Sci 2002;956:42–54.

36. Hawke TJ, Garry DJ. Myogenic satellite cells: physiology to molecular biology. J Appl Physiol 2001;91:534–51.

37. Christiansen SP, Baker RS, Madhat M, Terrell B. Type-specific changes in fiber morphometry following denervation of canine extraocular muscle. Exp Mol Pathol 1992;56:87–95.

38. Hoh JFY. 'Superfast' or masticatory myosin and the evolution of jaw-closing muscles of vertebrates. J Exp Biol 2002;205:2203–10.

39. Koolstra JH. Dynamics of the human masticatory system. Crit Rev Oral Biol Med 2002;13:366–76.

40. Rhee HS, Lucas CA, Hoh JFY. Fiber types in rat laryngeal muscles and their transformations after denervation and reinnervation. J Histochem Cytochem 2004;52:581–90.

41. Hoh JFY. Laryngeal muscle fibre types. Acta Physiol Scand 2005;183:133–49.

42. Li ZB, Lehar M, Nakagawa H, et al. Differential expression of myosin heavy chain isoforms between abductor and adductor muscles in the human larynx. Otolaryngol Head Neck Surg 2004;130:217–22.

43. Dop Bar PR, Reijneveld JC, Wokke JHJ, et al. Muscle damage induced by exercise: nature, prevention and repair. In: Salmons S, editor. Muscle damage. Oxford: Oxford University Press; 1997. p. 1–27.

44. Carlson BM, Faulkner JA. The regeneration of skeletal muscle fibers following injury: a review. Med Sci Sports Exerc 1983;15:187–98.

45. Tidball JG. Inflammatory processes in muscle injury and repair. Am J Physiol Regul Integr Comp Physiol 2005;288:R345–53.

46. Stauber WT, Fritz VK, Dahlmann B. Extracellular matrix changes following blunt trauma to rat skeletal muscles. Exp Mol Pathol 1990;52:69–86.

47. Miyake K, McNeil PL, Suzuki K, et al. An actin barrier to resealing. J Cell Sci 2001;114:3487–94.

48. McNeil PL. Repairing a torn cell surface: make way, lysosomes to the rescue. J Cell Sci 2002;115:873–9.

49. Watkins SC, Lynch GW, Kane LP, Slayter HS. Thrombospondin expression in traumatized skeletal muscle. Correlation of appearance with post-trauma regeneration. Cell Tissue Res 1990;261:73–84.

50. Pizza FX, Peterson JM, Baas JH, Koh TJ. Neutrophils contribute to muscle injury and impair its resolution after lengthening contractions in mice. J Physiol 2005;562:899–913.

51. Best TM, Hunter KD. Muscle injury and repair. Phys Med Rehabil Clin N Am 2000;11:251–66.

52. Goetsch SC, Hawke TJ, Gallardo TD, et al. Transcriptional profiling and regulation of the extra-cellular matrix during muscle regeneration. Physiol Genom 2003;14:261–71.

53. Lefaucheur JP, Gjata B, Lafont H, Sebille A. Angiogenic and inflammatory responses following skeletal muscle injury are altered by immune neutralization of endogenous basic fibroblast growth factor, insulin-like growth factor-1 and transforming growth factor-beta 1. J Neuroimmunol 1996;70:37–44.

54. Ouchi N, Shibata R, Walsh K. AMP-activated protein kinase signaling stimulates VEGF expression and angiogenesis in skeletal muscle. Circ Res 2005;96:838–46.

55. Uutela M, Wirzenius M, Paavonen K, et al. PDGF-D induces macrophage recruitment, increased interstitial pressure, and blood vessel maturation during angiogenesis. Blood 2004;104:3198–204.

56. Reardon KA, Kapsa RM, Davis J, et al. Increased levels of leukemia inhibitory factor mRNA in muscular dystrophy and human muscle trauma. Muscle Nerve 2000;23:962–6.

57. Chazaud B, Sonnet C, Lafuste P, et al. Satellite cells attract monocytes and use macrophages as a support to escape apoptosis and enhance muscle growth. J Cell Biol 2003;163:1133–43.

58. Grounds MD. Towards understanding skeletal muscle regeneration. Pathol Res Pract 1991;187:1–22.

59. Rathbone CR, Wenke JC, Warren GL, Armstrong RB. Importance of satellite cells in the strength recovery after eccentric contraction-induced muscle injury. Am J Physiol Regul Integr Comp Physiol 2003;285:R1490–5.

60. Jarvinen M. Healing of a crush injury in rat striated muscle, 3: a microangiographical study of the effect of early mobilization and immobilization on capillary ingrowth. Acta Pathol Microbiol Scand 1976;84A:85–94.

61. Järvinen TAH, Jozsa L, Kannus P, et al. Mechanical loading regulates the expression of tenascin-C in the myotendinous junction and tendon but does not induce de novo-synthesis in the skeletal muscle. J Cell Sci 2003;116:857–66.

62. Lehto M, Duance VC, Restall D. Collagen and fibronectin in a healing skeletal muscle injury: an immunohistochemical study of the effects of physical activity on the repair of injured gastrocnemius muscle in the rat. J Bone Joint Surg Br 1985;67:820–8.

63. Lehto M, Jarvinen M, Nelimarkka O. Scar formation after skeletal muscle injury: a histological and autoradiographical study in rats. Arch Orthop Trauma Surg 1986;104:366–70.

64. Vaittinen S, Hurme T, Rantanen J, Kalimo H. Transected myofibres may remain permanently divided in two parts. Neuromuscul Disord 2002;12:584–7.

65. Aarimaa V, Kääriäinen M, Vaittinen S, et al. Restoration of myofiber continuity after transection injury in the rat soleus. Neuromuscul Disord 2004;14:421–8.

66. Kääriäinen M, Liljamo T, Pelto-Huikko M, et al. Regulation of α7 integrin by mechanical stress during skeletal muscle regeneration. Neuromuscul Disord 2001;11:360–9.

67. Kasemkijwattana C, Menetrey J, Bosch P, et al. Use of growth factors to improve muscle healing after strain injury. Clin Orthop Relat Res 2000;370:272–85.

68. Leopard PJ. Complications. In: Williams JL, editor. Rowe and Williams' maxillofacial injuries. Vol 2. Edinburgh: Churchill Livingstone; 1994. p. 853–6.

69. Yano H, Yamamoto H, Hirata R, Hirano A. Post-traumatic severe trismus caused by impairment of the masticatory muscle. J Craniofac Surg 2005;16:277–80.

70. Kragh JF Jr. Svoboda SJ, Wenke JC, et al. Epimysium and perimysium in suturing in skeletal muscle lacerations. J Trauma 2005;59:209–12.

71. Menetrey J, Kasemkijwattana C, Fu FH, et al. Suturing versus immobilization of a muscle laceration. A morphological and functional study in a mouse model. Am J Sports Med 1999;27:222–9.

72. Jeschke MG, Herndon DN, Ebener C, et al. Nutritional intervention high in vitamins, protein, amino acids, and ω3 fatty acids improves protein metabolism during the hypermetabolic state after thermal injury. Arch Surg 2001;136:1301–6.

73. Wilmore DW. The effect of glutamine supplementation in patients following elective surgery and accidental injury. J Nutr 2001;131:2543S–9S.

74. Prisk V, Huard J. Muscle injuries and repair: the role of prostaglandins and inflammation. Histol Histopathol 2003;18:1243–56.

75. Mendias CL, Tatsumi R, Allen RE. Role of cyclooxygen-ase-1 and -2 in satellite cell proliferation, differentiation, and fusion. Muscle Nerve 2004;30:497–500.

76. Vignaud A, Cebrian J, Martelly I, et al. Effect of anti-inflammatory and antioxidant drugs on the long-term repair of severely injured mouse skeletal muscle. Exp Physiol 2005;90:487–95.

77. Bulger EM, Jurkovich GJ, Farver CL, et al. Oxandrolone does not improve outcome of ventilator dependent surgical patients. Ann Surg 2004;240:472–8.

78. Demling RH, DeSanti L. Oxandrolone induced lean mass gain during recovery from severe burns is maintained after discontinuation of the anabolic steroid. Burns 2003;29:793–7.

79. Beitzel F, Gregorevic P, Ryall JG, et al. Beta 2-adrenoreceptor agonist fenoterol enhances functional repair of regenerating rat skeletal muscle after injury. J Appl Physiol 2004;96:1385–92.

80. Fang CH, Li BG, Wray CJ, Hasselgren PO. Insulin-like growth factor-I inhibits lysosomal and proteasome-dependent proteolysis in skeletal muscle after burn injury. J Burn Care Rehabil 2002;23:318–25.

81. Mitchell CA, McGeachie JK, Grounds MD. The exogen-ous administration of basic fibroblast growth factor to regenerating skeletal muscle in mice does not enhance the process of regeneration. Growth Factors 1996;13:37–55.

82. Gregorevic P, Hayes A, Lynch GS, Williams DA. Functional properties of regenerating skeletal muscle following LIF administration. Muscle Nerve 2000;23:1586–8.

83. Takala J, Ruokonen E, Webster NR, et al. Increased mortality associated with growth hormone treatment in critically ill patients. N Engl J Med 1999;341:785–92.

84. Biolo G, Iscra F, Bosutti A, et al. Growth hormone decreases muscle glutamine production and stimulates protein synthesis in hypercatabolic patients. Am J Physiol Endocrinol Metab 2000;279:E323–32.

85. Natsu K, Ochi M, Mochizuki Y, et al. Allogeneic bone marrow-derived mesenchymal stromal cells promote the regeneration of injured skeletal muscle without differentiation into myofibers. Tissue Eng 2004;10:1093–112.

86. Abedi M, Greer DA, Colvin GA, et al. Robust conversion of marrow cells to skeletal muscle with formation of marrow-derived muscle cell colonies: a multifactorial process. Exp Hematol 2004;32:426–34.

87. Fukushima K, Badlani N, Usas A, et al. The use of an antifibrosis agent to improve muscle recovery after laceration. Am J Sports Med 2001;29:394–402.

88. Li Y, Foster W, Deasy BM, et al. Transforming growth factor-beta 1 induces the differentiation of myogenic cells into fibrotic cells in injured skeletal muscle: a key event in muscle fibrogenesis. Am J Pathol 2004;164:1007–19.

89. Foster W, Li Y, Usas A, et al. Gamma interferon as an antifibrosis agent in skeletal muscle. J Orthopaed Res 2003;21:798–804.

90. Chan YS, Li Y, Foster W, et al. The use of suramin, an antifibrotic agent, to improve muscle recovery after strain injury. Am J Sports Med 2005;33:43–51.

91. Micromedex[R] healthcare series, Vol 126. Available at: www.micromedex.com (accessed March 28, 2007).

92. Bar-Cohen Y. Bionic humans using EAP as artificial muscles: reality and challenges. Int J Advanced Robotic Systems Robotics J 2004;1(3). Available at: http://ndeaa.jpl.nasa.gov.

6

Salient Features of the Oral Mucosa

Falk Wehrhan, MD, DDS; Stefan Schultze-Mosgau, MD, DDS, PhD;
Henning Schliephake, MD, DDS, PhD

UNIQUE HISTOLOGY AND HEALING PHYSIOLOGY

Intraoral squamous epithelia consist of up to 20 keratinocyte cell layers. Cellular elements of the human oral mucosa are interconnected by desmosomes and adhesion molecules. Healing of oral mucosa wounds results from complex biochemical and cellular interactions and is regulated by cytokines and growth factors, mediating inflammatory reactions and matrix production.

MAJOR STEPS IN HEALING OVER TIME

Oral mucosa wounds heal faster than wounds of extraoral skin. Epithelial-mesenchymal interactions obviously play a pivotal role in the regulation of proliferation and maturation of the newly formed epithelium during wound healing.

COMMON WOUND HEALING PROBLEMS

Common wound healing problems are characterized by delayed epithelialization, aberrant matrix synthesis, and reduced vascularization. Malnutrition, such as ascorbic acid depletion, may result in clinical wound healing problems.

FUTURE PROMISE FOR HEALING IMPROVEMENT

Future promise for healing improvement is held by composite grafts, consisting of oral mucosa keratinocytes and underlying fibroblasts, as well as in vivo strategies for improvement of wound healing in fibrotic conditions by blocking overexpression of transforming growth factor $(TGF)\beta_1$.

ANATOMY AND HISTOLOGY: MORPHOLOGY AND FUNCTION OF THE ORAL MUCOSA

Oral mucosa is composed of a stratified epithelial layer and underlying connective tissue. The structure of the oral mucosa and the connection of the epithelial layer to the underlying connective tissue are highly variable, depending on the intraoral region. The structural features of the different types of intraoral mucosa develop during the fetal period. Human gingival epithelium consists of up to 20 cell layers, measuring 200 to 300 μm in thickness. The epithelial layer is stratified into four layers: stratum basale, stratum spinosum, stratum granulosum, and stratum corneum.[1] The cells of the stratum basale are characterized by high mitotic activity, and they maintain epithelial regeneration. The keratinocytes of the stratum spinosum undergo differentiation. The stratum granulosum contains only a few cells expressing hyaline granules. The keratinized stratum corneum is the outermost layer and is of variable thickness, depending on intraoral location. Nuclei of these keratinocytes show signs of pyknosis. Three types of keratinization are found in human oral epithelia: nonkeratinized buccal mucosa, parakeratinized gingiva, and orthokeratinized hard palate mucosa.[2,3]

All cells of the oral gingival epithelium are interconnected by desmosomes and nexi, or gap junctions. Narrow intercellular spaces contain proteoglycans and glycoproteins.[4,5] The epithelial layers and the underlying connective tissue are separated by the basal lamina, measuring 50 to 100 nm. The basal membrane, consisting of collagen IV, laminin, and heparin-proteoglycan, connects the differentially keratinized epithelial regions with the underlying submucosal connective tissue. Patterns of proteins in skin and oral mucosa share similarities in the expression of basement membrane components but differ in expression of cytokeratins.[6] All stratified oral squamous epithelia express cytokeratins K5 and K14 in their basal layers, but sulcular gingiva also expresses K19, K4, and K13, and marginal gingiva expresses K6 and K19.[6] Moreover, in contrast to extraoral skin, the collagenous network of intraoral submucosa does not contain elastic fibers and directly connects the lamina propria with the periosteum of jaws and hard palate.

FEATURES OF MUCOSA HEALING

Summary

The healing of oral mucosa wounds results from complex biochemical and cellular interactions. Tissue injury activates a cascade of events that lead to tissue healing. The process of wound healing can be divided into a sequence of three partially overlapping phases: (1) inflammation, (2) proliferation, and (3) remodeling. Inflammation is the initial step, characterized by hemostasis, platelet degranulation, and plug formation. Activation of neutrophils and macrophages leads to cell recruitment and further signaling cascades by released early-phase cytokines, such as interleukin (IL)-1, IL-6, tumor necrosis factor α (TNF-α), and platelet-derived growth factor (PDGF). The second stage of wound healing, the phase of proliferation, is characterized by wound contraction, epithelialization, and fibroplasia. A provisional wound coverage is formed by deposition of matrix proteins and vascularization of the fibrin plug. Collagens, mainly types I and III, are synthesized and deposited. Epithelial coverage of the wound surface is accomplished by migrating keratinocytes. During remodeling, the third stage of wound healing, the final composition of the extracellular matrix (ECM) is defined. This is mediated by both matrix-synthesizing and matrix-degrading enzymes. The quality of the regenerated tissue is determined during this process of remodeling. The common result of postnatal wound healing is scar formation.

Wound healing is regulated by cytokines and growth factors, mediating inflammatory reactions and matrix production. Cytokines coordinate inflammation and cell recruitment (IL-1, IL-6, TNF-α, TGF-β), vascularization (fibroblast growth factor [FGF]-1, FGF-2, vascular endothelial growth factor), tissue homeostasis, and matrix synthesis (keratinocyte growth factor [KGF], PDGF, TGF-β). They are synthesized and secreted by several types of cells and have pleiotropic effects depending on local tissue conditions. Cytokines mediate their cellular actions through specific receptors and intracellular downstream effector proteins. TGF-β in particular plays a fundamental role in regulating all phases of wound healing. It stimulates matrix deposition and collagen cross-linking. TGF-β is a major player in determining the definitive ECM composition and tissue architecture. Depletion and overexpression of TGF-β lead to wound healing disorders.

Morphology of Mucosal Healing

The healing of the oral mucosa is a complex biologic process of carefully orchestrated cellular and biochemical events. Initiated by tissue injury, wound healing leads to the restoration of the biologic matrix and results in the reestablishment of tissue integrity. All biologic tissues, except bone, heal by scarring through formation of fibrotic connective tissue of reduced biologic functionality. The quality of this tissue is affected by wound healing conditions. Given that surgical procedures in oral and maxillofacial surgery induce injury, a thorough understanding of the events of oral mucosa healing is of fundamental importance for surgical practice. More detailed knowledge about the repair processes and their regulation has led to improvements in wound care and improved functional and esthetic results of oral surgery procedures. Wound healing can be separated into three phases: inflammation, proliferation, and remodeling (Figure 1). These partially overlap in their temporal sequence and their biologic characteristics.[7–9] In the inflammation phase, hemostasis and acute inflammatory infiltrate ensue. Proliferation is mainly characterized by formation of granulation tissue, wound contraction, and epithelialization. The final remodeling phase is described as maturation of scar tissue.

Inflammation, the first stage of wound healing, starts with constriction of lacerated vessels. Subendothelial thromboplastic components are exposed after tissue injury. Permeability of vessels for inflammatory cells is increased. Platelets degranulate, aggregate, and form the initial hemostatic plug. The coagulation system and the complement cascade are initiated. The intrinsic and extrinsic coagulation pathways lead to activation of prothrombin to thrombin,

converting fibrinogen to fibrin. Fibrin is subsequently polymerized into a stable clot.[9–12] Following hemostasis, the aggregated platelets release potent chemoattractant factors for activation of local endothelial cells and fibroblasts. Platelet adhesiveness is mediated by integrins, such as integrin αIIbβ3.[13–15] White blood cells, neutrophils at first, followed by monocytes, migrate into the wound site, stimulated by local release of bradykinin and activated complement factors. Neutrophils infiltrating injured tissue scavenge cellular debris, foreign bodies, and bacteria. Within 2 to 3 days after injury, the inflammatory cell population starts to shift to monocyte predominance.[16] Circulating monocytes migrate into the tissue and differentiate into macrophages. They orchestrate the early wound repair process. Besides phagocytosis, macrophages secrete over 20 different cytokines and growth factors that are involved in wound healing.[17–19] These growth factors activate and attract endothelial cells, fibroblasts, and keratinocytes during tissue repair. Therefore, depletion of monocytes and macrophages leads to severe wound healing disorders, delayed fibroblast proliferation, and inadequate angiogenesis.[20,21]

The second stage of wound repair, the proliferation phase, is characterized by matrix

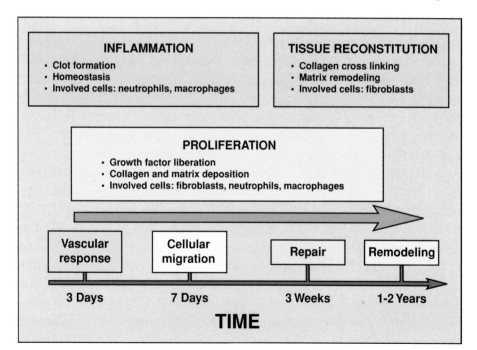

Figure 1. The temporal sequence of repair phases in wound healing.

synthesis, starting with the deposition of fibrin and activation of the fibroblast mitosis (fibroplasia). Fibroblasts proliferate and become the predominant cell type in clean, noninfected oral mucosal wounds by 3 to 5 days following injury. The deposition of ECM components is complex and regulated by growth factors and by interactions between integrins and other cell membrane receptors. Integrins, composed of alpha and beta subunits, are heterodimeric transmembrane proteins that interact to form active protein receptors.[22–24] The initial matrix deposited in the wound is provisional and is composed of fibrin, glycosaminoglycans (GAGs), and hyaluronic acid. Adhesion proteins, including laminin, tenascin, and fibronectin, are present during provisional matrix synthesis and facilitate cell attachment and migration. Integrins are of particular importance for the interaction of matrix synthesis, tissue regeneration, and vascularization because integrin $\alpha_5\beta_6$ has been shown to be involved in vascular sprouting during wound healing.[25,26] Fibroblasts use hyaluronidase step by step and digest the provisional matrix. Larger sulfated GAGs are subsequently deposited, followed by collagens and fibronectin.

Collagens I and III are the major fibrillar components in human oral mucosa.[27] Their ratio is 4:1 in both subcutaneous tissue and scar tissue.[28] Collagens are secreted mainly by fibroblasts into the extracellular fiber network. Intra- and extracellular post-translational modifications during collagen maturation have been described.[7,9,29,30] Messenger ribonucleic acid splicing variants occur after transcription. Signal peptides are added in the rough endoplasmic reticulum to form the triple helix. After translation, the signal peptide is cleaved, followed by hydroxylation of selected proline and lysine residues. Right-handed triple-helical procollagens are formed. Most collagens have three identical chains (eg: collagens II, III, VII, and X), whereas others have two different chains (eg: collagens I and IV), coded by different genes.[28,31–34]

Besides fibroplasia, epithelialization is the major process during the proliferation phase of wound healing. Morphologic changes in keratinocytes adjacent to the wound margins occur within hours after wounding.[35,36] In skin and oral mucosa wounds, the epidermis thickens and basal cells enlarge and start to migrate across the epithelial defect of the wound. The necrotic parts of the superficial mucosa are sequestrated by newly formed epithelial layers. Interestingly, epithelial cells do not divide until epithelial continuity is restored. Epithelial tissue near the wound margins provides a source of keratinocytes needed for superficial wound closure. Migration over the wound matrix is mediated by cell adhesion glycoproteins, such as fibronectin and tenascin. Following reconstitution of the continuity of the epithelial layer, keratinocytes start to secrete laminin and type IV collagen, reforming a basement membrane.

Reestablishment of the epidermis is completed by columnar shaping of the keratinocytes at the basal membrane, forming a barrier against further contamination and loss of moisture.[37–39] Fibroplasia and epithelialization would halt if neovascularization failed to accompany the newly synthesized oral keratinocyte-connective tissue matrix. Endothelial cell division and migration can be observed in granulation tissue beginning on days 1 to 2 after wounding.[7,30,40,41] This tissue, characterized by a dense capillary network and representing strong vascular potency, serves as a source for migrating microvascular endothelial cells, forming microvessels to interconnect the wound margins with a rich vascular network.[42] Contraction of the wound occurs after trauma or open oral mucosa wounds and is not present in closed surgical incisions. Wound contraction decreases the size of the wound. The underlying mechanisms are not completely understood. Contractile forces are likely to be generated by activated myofibroblasts, containing small muscle actin and tenascin C.[43,44]

During wound healing, the ECM is subject to a constantly changing balance of synthesis and degradation. The regulation of tissue remodeling is yet poorly understood. Collagen cross-linking, mediated by cytokines and integrins, modifies the connective tissue architecture and improves mechanical breaking strength. Matrix metalloproteinases (MMPs) degrade collagens and ECM and regulate the final ECM deposition.[45] Ultimately, the result of mammalian wound healing is scar formation. Morphologically, scars are characterized by a loss of tissue organization compared with the normal surrounding tissue. Scars show aberrant and disorganized collagen deposition.[46,47] The ratio of collagen types is altered compared with the normal tissue, and this is accompanied by a lack of functionality. Collagen fibers in scars are more densely packed than in normal connective tissue. The reticular pattern of collagen bundles, found in normal oral mucosa connective tissue, is lost in scar tissue. Newly formed scar tissue remodels slowly over months to years into mature scar. The early scar is densely capillarized, regressing over time and resulting in fibrotic, hypopigmented, and poorly vascularized tissue. During remodeling, tissue breaking strength increases rapidly until the eighth week after wounding. Thereafter, the breaking strength increases slowly, reaching its maximum approximately 1 year after injury. However, the final breaking strength reaches only 80% of the strength of normal, unwounded skin or oral mucosa.[46,47] Furthermore, scar tissue usually lacks epithelial appendages, such as ducts and glands, which do not regenerate after injury.

Regulation of Wound Healing

Regulation of oral mucosa wound healing is mediated by growth factors and cytokines (see Chapter 30, "Growth Factors: Modulators of Wound Healing"). These are polypeptides, released by a variety of activated cells at the wound site. Cytokines can act in either an autocrine or a paracrine fashion. Cytokine-mediated stimulation or inhibition of protein synthesis or signal transduction processes is realized by highly specific cell surface receptors.[10] Growth factors and cytokines additionally chemoattract cells to the wound area. The biologic functions of cytokines are pleiotropic and depend on local concentration, the state of activation, the presence of cofactors, and expression patterns of their signal transducing receptors (Table 1).[7,48,49]

Depending on the biologic activity in different stages of wound healing, different cytokines play a role in the regulation of tissue repair and homeostasis. During inflammation in early wound healing, activation and recruitment of neutrophils and macrophages are mediated by IL-1, IL-6, TNF-α, insulin-like growth factor 1, and TGF-β.[9,50] PDGF, released from degranulating platelets immediately after injury, attracts neutrophils, macrophages, and fibroblasts to the

Table 1. CYTOKINES INVOLVED IN ORAL MUCOSA HEALING, THEIR CELLULAR SOURCES, AND THEIR TARGETS

Cytokine	Cellular Source	Cellular Target	Biologic Activity
TGF-β₁, TGF-β₂	Macrophages, platelets, fibroblasts	Keratinocytes, fibroblasts, macrophages	Chemotaxis, proliferation collagen synthesis
TGF-β₃	Macrophages	Fibroblasts	Remodeling
TGF-α	Macrophages, platelets	Keratinocytes, fibroblasts, endothelial cells	Proliferation
TNF-α	Neutrophils	Macrophages, keratinocytes, fibroblasts	Activation of cytokines
PDGF	Macrophages, platelets, firoblasts, endothelial cells	Neutrophils, macrophages, fibroblasts, endothelial cells	Chemotaxis, proliferation
FGF-1, FGF-2, FGF-4	Macrophages, fibroblasts, endothelial cells	Keratinocytes, fibroblasts, endothelial cells	Angiogenesis, proliferation, chemotaxis
FGF-7 (KGF)	Fibroblasts	Keratinocytes	Proliferation, chemotaxis
EGF	Platelets, macrophages, keratinocytes	Keratinocytes, fibroblasts, endothelial cells	Proliferation, chemotaxis
IGF-1	Fibroblasts, macrophages	Fibroblasts, endothelial cells	Proliferation, collagen synthesis
IL-1α, IL-1β	Macrophages, neutrophls	Macrophages, fibroblasts, keratinocytes	Proliferation, chemotaxis
VEGF	Macrophages, keratinocytes	Endothelial cells	Angiogenesis

EGF = epidermal growth factor; FGF = fibroblast growth factor; IGF = insulin-like growth factor; IL = interleukin; KGF = keratinocyte growth factor; PDGF = platelet-derived growth factor; TGF = transforming growth factor; TNF = tumor necrosis factor; VEGF = vascular endothelial growth factor.

wound margins and serves as a powerful mitogen. PDGF is also synthesized and secreted by endothelial cells, macrophages, and fibroblasts. PDGF stimulates fibroblasts to express GAG adhesion proteins. During tissue remodeling, PDGF increases the secretion of MMPs, indicating a role in tissue remodeling.[51,52]

Vascular endothelial cell growth factor (VEGF) is a potent angiogenic stimulus. It stimulates microvascular endothelial cells to proliferate and can be secreted from platelets, macrophages, fibroblasts, and keratinocytes. Its expression is strongly induced in hypoxic tissue conditions.[53] Fibroblast growth factors (FGF-1 and FGF-2) also contribute to angiogenesis. Endothelial cells, fibroblasts, and macrophages are able to secrete FGF-1 and FGF-2. FGFs stimulate endothelial cells to divide and form new capillaries.[54] They are bound by heparin and heparin sulfate in the ECM. The basement membrane can serve as a possible storage reservoir for FGF-2.

TGF-β plays a pivotal role in the regulation of the wound healing processes. It stimulates the synthesis and deposition of collagens in all stages of wound repair. TGF-β is of crucial importance for the determination of tissue architecture and quality. Both depletion or elevated levels of TGF-β have been shown to be associated with wound healing disorders. TGF-β is secreted by fibroblasts and epithelial cells and can act in an autocrine and a paracrine fashion. It thus can amplify its own expression. TGF-β has been shown to act as a profibrotic factor. Increased TGF-β expression has been described to be associated with fibrotic tissue conditions in multiorgan systems, such as the lung, heart, liver, kidney, and skin (Figure 2). TGF-β increases integrin expression and therefore stimulates increased collagen cross-linking.

During epithelialization, TGF-β induces induction of specific integrins, which coordinate epithelial cell migration across the wound surface.[55] Particularly, collagen I and III synthesis by fibroblasts is stimulated by TGF-β during proliferation and remodeling.[56–59] Regulation of collagen turnover during remodeling determines the definitive matrix conditions and is TGF-β dependent, as activators and inhibitors of matrix deposition are TGF-β sensitive.[60–62] Therefore, tissue homeostasis is influenced by TGF-β concentration in healing oral mucosa and underlying connective tissue.[56,63]

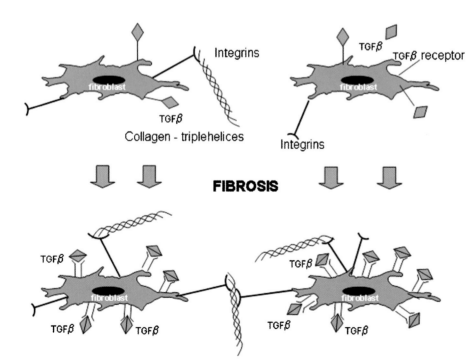

Figure 2. Transforming growth factor β stimulates matrix deposition and collagen cross-linking by receptor complexes and integrins.

The role of TGF-β in vascularization and angiogenesis during wound healing is subject to controversy. Several authors describe the stimulation of angiogenesis by TGF-β depending on the total dose and time during wound healing.[64-67] Other groups have reported inhibition of angiogenesis by TGF-β.[68]

Several other cytokines are involved in oral mucosa regeneration, such as FGF-7, also named KGF. FGF-7/KGF is stored and secreted by fibroblasts of subepithelial connective tissue, thus stimulating reconstitution of the basal lamina and keratinocyte proliferation, migration, and differentiation.[69,70] Insulin-like growth factor 1 (IGF-1) is also involved in the stimulation of matrix synthesis synergistically and facilitates fibroblast proliferation.[71]

Wound healing has been shown to be enhanced by exogenous modulation of growth factors in pathologic conditions. This indicates that profound knowledge of cytokine interactions and their biologic impact on tissue healing is required for the future to advance the care and management of oral mucosal wounds. For example, TGF-β is involved in regulation of all wound healing phases, but its own regulation and signal transduction depend on the local microenvironment and on the ECM conditions. The ECM serves as a storage reservoir of latent, biologically inactive forms of cytokines. Following injury or surgical procedures, these factors are activated by proteolysis. TGF-β signal transduction may serve as an example to study the interaction of systemic and local growth factors or cytokines with wound healing mechanisms. Latent, biologically inactive TGF-β is bound to the proteoglycan decorin. After wounding, these complexes are released from the ECM. TGF-β, bone morphogenetic proteins, and activins belong to the TGF-β superfamily, representing cytokines of similar biologic structure. Three TGF-β isoforms (TGF-β_1, TGF-β_2, TGF-β_3) have been identified in mammals. TGF-β represents a highly conserved cytokine.[72,73] TGF-β isoforms are synthesized as biologically inactive homodimeric precursor proteins and intracellularly cleaved (Figure 3).[74] C-terminal TGF-β_1 remains noncovalently bound to the N-terminal latency-associated peptide (LAP). TGF-β and LAP occur as disulfide-linked homodimers.[75] LAP itself is linked to latent TGF-β binding protein, mediating cell and matrix interaction.[76,77]

Activation of TGF-β is enhanced under acidic conditions due to hypoxia in traumatized tissue. LAP dissociates, and active TGF-β complexes are formed.[74,78,79] Active TGF-β binds to three different forms of serine-threonine-kinase receptors (TGF-βR-I, TGF-βR-II, and TGF-βR-III), presented on fibroblasts, macrophages, and endothelial cells (Figure 4).[80-82]

Following binding of TGF-β, TGF-βR-I and TGF-βR-II form heterodimeric complexes and initiate TGF-β-mediated intracellular receptor

precursor-protein   **biologically active TGFβ**

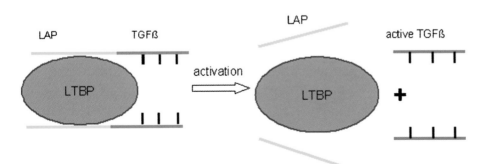

Figure 3. Activation of transforming growth factor β is realized by proteolytic cleaving of the precursor protein.

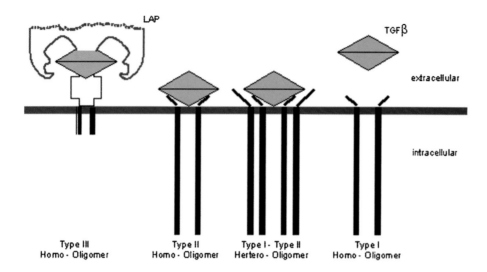

Figure 4. Structure of transforming growth factor β binding receptors.

downstream signaling.[83,84] To date, the role of TGF-βR-III in TGF-β-related signal transduction remains unclear.[85]

Intracellular receptor–associated kinases activate intracellular TGF-β signal transducing proteins (so-called Smad proteins) (Figure 5).[84] Smad proteins represent a class of highly conserved intracellular transcription factors, mediating signals from activated receptor complexes to the nucleus. They can be classified into three groups: receptor-regulated Smads (R-Smads), common mediator Smads (co-Smads) and inhibitory Smads (I-Smads).[86] Activated TGF-βR-I and TGF-βR-II complexes specifi-

cally phosphorylate Smad 2 and 3 complexes. Following binding to Smad 4, these activated transcription complexes translocate into the nucleus.[87]

UNIQUE PHYSIOLOGIC HEALING ASPECTS

Summary

Fetal healing in early gestation is characterized by tissue repair without scar formation. Scarless repair appears to be inherent to fetuses and not dependent on exogenous factors. An important difference to postnatal wound healing is that TGF-β is not expressed during fetal skin wound healing. Likewise, inflammation, a fundamental step of postnatal tissue healing, is not observed in fetal healing.

Oral mucosa wounds heal faster than wounds of extraoral skin. The proliferation and turnover rate of oral mucosa cells are faster than in normal skin. Cell adhesion proteins, influencing motility and velocity of migrating keratinocytes, appear to be differentially expressed between skin and oral mucosa. Epithelial-mesenchymal interactions obviously play a pivotal role in the regulation of proliferation and maturation of the newly formed epithelium during wound healing. The desquamation rate of oral mucosa keratinocytes is increased compared with skin, contributing to a lower bacterial colonization of oral mucosa epithelium.

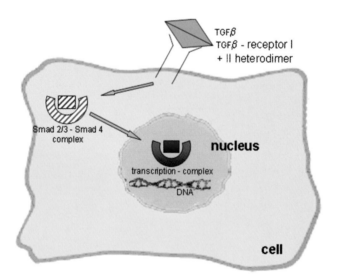

Figure 5. Intracellular transforming growth factor β–related receptor downstream signaling is mediated by Smad proteins.

Scarless Wound Repair

Compared with adult tissue, the early-gestation fetus can heal skin wounds without scar formation (see Chapter 1). Both epidermis and dermis are restored to normal tissue without visible sequelae of wound healing. The resulting skin architecture is normal and unchanged from unwounded dermis. Hair follicles and sweat glands are reexpressed regularly.[88,89] Scarless repair appears to be independent from exogenic factors, such as amniotic fluid or an intrauterine environment.[63] Moreover, inflammation is not observed in fetal tissue healing, although it is of fundamental importance in postnatal tissue repair. The expression of certain cytokines, such as TGF-β, has been found to be significantly reduced during fetal wound healing as well.[88] To date, numerous approaches have been made to analyze the paradigm of fetal scarless wound healing; however, understanding of the major regulating factors is poor.[88–90]

Unique Oral Mucosa Healing Aspects

The process of oral mucosa wound healing highly coordinates inflammation, proliferation, tissue remodeling, and regeneration. Compared with cutaneous wound healing, oral mucosal healing occurs more rapidly.[91] The dynamic nature of gene expression in oral mucosal healing, especially in the early phase, is not completely understood. In contrast to skin epithelium and dermal connective tissue, the oral mucosa is composed of a rapidly proliferating and continually renewing sheet of epithelial cells. In intact oral mucosa, a variety of genes involved in oral tissue regeneration and wound healing regulation are constitutively expressed, indicating a primed mucosa, ready to respond to a variety of noxious tissue influences.[92] Recent studies suggest a transient down-regulation of corneodesmosin during early oral mucosa healing. Corneodesmosin is involved in intercellular adhesion between keratinocytes and contributes to epithelial integrity.[93,94] Reduced expression of corneodesmosin in oral mucosa healing may

contribute to increased cellular migration and acceleration of wound closure.

Epithelial-mesenchymal interactions have been described to be essential for oral epithelial morphogenesis, homeostasis, and repair.[95,96] Connective tissue underlying the oral epithelium has been reported to essentially modulate restoration of oral mucosa. FGF-7/KGF, secreted by fibroblasts, has been found to modulate the proliferation and differentiation of oral mucosal keratinocytes in particular.[97,98] FGF-7/KGF is a typical paracrine growth factor that is synthesized and secreted by underlying stromal fibroblasts. The effects of fibroblasts on oral epithelial regeneration appear to be biphasic in that proliferation is stimulated initially, whereas differentiation is promoted at later stages of healing.[99] It has been shown that oral fibroblasts produce more FGF-7/KGF than their dermal counterparts.[100] The cell desquamation rate, removing material adherent to the superficial epithelium, is higher in oral mucosa compared with dermal tissue. This might contribute to the lower rate of bacterial colonization of oral epithelium compared with dermal epithelium.[101] The presence of fibroblasts induces an inhibition of spontaneous cell death in the basal epithelial compartment, accompanied by increased terminal differentiation of the cells, which are shed from the superficial cell layer.[102,103]

COMMON WOUND HEALING PROBLEMS

Summary

Common wound healing problems are characterized by delayed epithelialization, aberrant matrix synthesis, and reduced vascularization. Bacterial infections in oral mucosa healing are rare and depend on the bacterial load of the affected tissue. Well-vascularized wounds and transplanted tissue heal more successfully even despite sometimes high bacterial contamination. Malnutrition, such as ascorbic acid depletion, may result in clinical wound healing problems. Ascorbic acid is required to synthesize the collagenous matrix during proliferation and remodeling. Absence of vitamin C leads to impaired collagen deposition and impaired tissue quality. Diabetes and obesity affect wound healing by decreased KGF and PDGF expression, which are important mediators for epithelial cell migration. Therefore, diabetic wounds are associated with delayed wound closure. Corticosteroid treatment affects wound healing, particularly during the early stages. Depleting KGF and PDGF levels by corticosteroid treatment results in delayed wound closure. Radiation-impaired wound healing is characterized by structural changes in irradiated vessels and by a reduced capillary area. Radiation of oral mucosa results in altered TGF-β_1 expression, leading to matrix accumulation and fibrosis.

Wound healing can be affected by several clinical factors, which may affect epithelialization and matrix synthesis, as well as matrix degradation and vascularization. Wound infection occurs owing to an imbalance between host resistance and bacterial invasion.[104–106] In oral mucosa wound healing, the rate of wound infection is low compared with that of skin wounds owing to the unique features of the oral mucosa. Acute and chronic inflammatory infiltrates retard fibroblast proliferation at the wound margins and thereby delay ECM synthesis and remodeling. A threshold of bacterial load determines whether a clinical infection occurs. It has been shown that bacterial loads at or above 10^5 organisms per gram of tissue lead to infection and delayed healing. Well-vascularized muscle flaps can heal open wounds successfully when the bacterial load is less than 10^5 organisms per gram tissue (see Chapter 26, "Controlling Infection").[107,108]

Wound healing disorders can occur owing to malnutrition, which results in depletion of essential factors required for undisturbed wound healing. For example, an increased risk of wound dehiscence is associated with protein depletion after wounding. Vitamin C (ascorbic acid) deficiency results in arrest of wound healing in the stage of fibroplasia. Inadequate amounts of collagen are synthesized, and hydroxylation of proline and lysine fails in the absence of vitamin C, which is an essential cofactor for prolyl and lysyl hydroxylases. Secretion of collagen fibrils

into the extracellular space is suppressed, and the degree of cross-linking of collagen fibrils is reduced (see Chapter 25, "Nutrition and Wound Healing").[109,110]

Ischemia leads to poor wound healing and increases the risk of infection. Ischemia can be caused by excessive suture tension, trauma, vascular diseases, vasoconstriction, and hypovolemia. Wound healing can be improved by increased oxygen delivery. Collagen synthesis by fibroblasts is enhanced by an increase in oxygen supply (see Chapter 28, "Hyperbaric Oxygen and Wound Healing in the Head and Neck").[111]

Diabetes mellitus and obesity also impair wound healing. It has been shown that a lack of KGF and PDGF in diabetic wounds results in delayed reepithelialization. Microangiopathy, associated with diabetes mellitus, additionally impairs perfusion and oxygen delivery to the wound sites. Poor wound perfusion and necrotic adipose tissue in obese patients contribute to further impairment in healing.[112,113]

Topically and systemically applied corticosteroids impair wound healing, especially when given early, between days 1 and 3 after wounding.[114] Inflammation, as well as wound contraction and collagen synthesis, is reduced following steroid treatment.[47] Glucocorticoids have been shown to decrease PDGF and KGF expression, resulting in delayed wound closure.[115,116] As lysosomal membranes are stabilized by steroids, the release of lysosomes at the wound site is inhibited. As a result of a reduced inflammatory reaction, steroid use increases the risk of bacterial infection.[116]

Radiation therapy impairs wound healing in a dose-dependent manner. Mitosis of fibroblasts, keratinocytes, and endothelial cells is impaired; therefore, wound closure is retarded. Blood vessels in the preirradiated surgical sites undergo structural changes, such as degeneration of tunica intima, tunica media fibrosis, and loss of a relative capillary area.[117,118] It has been shown that VEGF, the major stimulatory cytokine for vascularization, is depleted by radiotherapy.[119] TGF-β_1, implicated in the development of tissue fibrosis, has been reported to be strongly up-regulated following irradiation.[120] This results in fibrocontractive wound healing disorders and scarring.[121–125] As TGF-β_1 mainly stimulates expression of collagen I and suppresses matrix-degrading enzymes, such as MMP-1 and MMP-3, overwhelming ECM deposition associated with poor angiogenesis characterizes radiation-impaired wound healing.[126–129] TGF-βR-II-mediating TGF-β-related cell-cycle arrest is not expressed on migrating keratinocytes during nonimpaired wound closure. In preirradiated epithelium, TGF-βR-II is reexpressed on keratinocytes at the wound margins, contributing to delayed and insufficient epithelial integrity (see Chapter 15, "Irradiated Skin and Its Postsurgical Management").[130,131]

FUTURE PROMISE FOR HEALING

Summary

Surgical repair of mucosal wounds in the oral cavity is accomplished by nonvascularized grafts of oral mucosa or split-thickness skin grafts from extraoral skin. The disadvantages of split-thickness skin are donor-site morbidity and simultaneous transfer of dermal adnexes. Numerous attempts have been made to overcome the problem of limited availability of oral mucosa by tissue engineering procedures. Dermal replacement products, based on collagen and other biodegradable matrices, have been developed and clinically used. However, no acellular graft has been able to sufficiently reduce wound shrinkage and scarring. Mucosa-like equivalents have been created by culturing oral mucosa keratinocytes on biodegradable membranes. Maturation and differentiation of epithelium remained crucial because epithelial-mesenchymal interaction could not be realized without fibroblast coculture. Composite grafts, consisting of oral mucosa keratinocytes and underlying fibroblasts, showed improved stratification and maturation of synthesized epithelium. In vivo strategies for improvement in wound healing under fibrotic conditions have been able to reduce collagen

deposition during wound healing by blocking overexpression of TGF-β_1. Following radiotherapy of the head and neck region, anti-TGF-β_1 therapy has been shown to be capable of reducing scarring and improving angiogenesis.

Many procedures in preprosthetic and reconstructive surgery in oral and maxillofacial surgery require surgical repair and/or replacement of oral mucosa. Nonvascularized mucosal grafts from the oral cavity are a common means and well established in practice to prevent microbial infection, excessive fluid loss, and excessive wound contraction. Use of intraoral mucosa grafting, however, is limited as the supply of donor tissue is restricted to the oral region. Alternatively, split-thickness skin grafts are available almost from the whole body surface. However, use of donor skin grafts in the oral cavity may be problematic. Besides donor-site morbidity, skin adnexal structures are transferred into the oral cavity with split-thickness skin grafts, which may prove to be difficult in terms of patient acceptance and untoward effects, such as hair growth and scar contraction.[132] Therefore, numerous approaches have been tried to establish artificial mucosal substitutes.[132] Biodegradable polymers have been used as templates for dermal ECM. In one of the earliest tissue engineering approaches, a collagen-GAG sponge served as a scaffold for dermal regeneration.[133,134] The goal was to promote fibroblast repopulation in a controlled way. Several variations of collagen sponges have been tested. Enhanced fibroblast penetration and improved resistance of the collagen lattice to proteolytic attack have been achieved by the use collagen cross-linked matrices. Modifications of the matrix by inclusion of additional matrix proteins and hyaluronic acid have been performed.[133,134] The microporosity of scaffolds was modified to improve adherence of cells. Although these matrix scaffolds showed some improvement in scar morphology, no acellular matrix has led to true oral mucosa regeneration. Therefore, mucosal substitutes containing oral mucosa keratinocytes have been tested.[135,136] Multilayered keratinocyte collagen sheets have

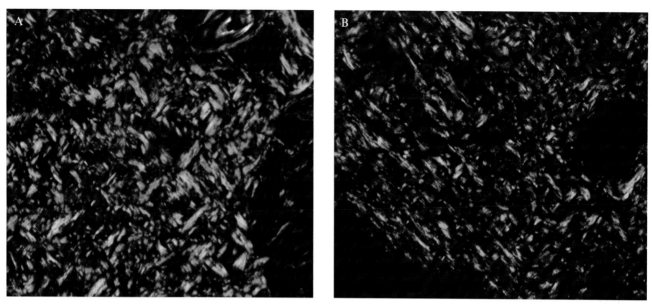

Figure 6. Fibrotic, scarring skin from the preirradiated wound healing area (*A*) compared with healing skin following anti–transforming growth factor β₁ treatment (*B*). The observation time point is postoperative day 28. The method of sirius red staining and observation between crossed polarized filters enables quantitative assessment of expressed collagen (×400 original magnification).

been cultured in vitro since the method of keratinocyte isolation and amplification was established.[137] However, oral mucosa–like differentiation of cultured keratinocytes[138] and formation of a true basal membrane and stratified epithelial layers, which is crucial to achieve biologic and mechanical tissue-like properties, have not yet been reached. Skin-derived biologic

matrices showed better in vitro results for oral mucosa reconstitution compared with artificial collagen–based scaffolds, suggesting that inherent skin factors regulating differentiation and maturation are important yet still unknown.[135,136] Composite grafts, consisting of living fibroblasts and keratinocytes, may improve the biologic quality and hence the

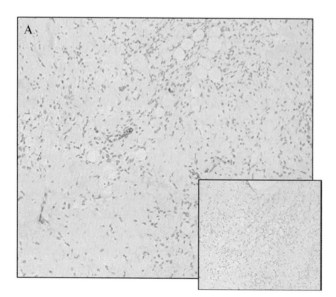
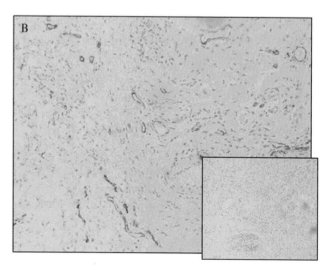

Figure 7. Vascularization (transforming growth factor βR-III [TGF-βR-III] labeling) in fibrotic, scarring skin from the preirradiated wound healing area (*A*) compared with healing skin following anti-TGF-β₁ treatment (*B*). The observation time point is postoperative day 28. The method of immunohistochemical labeling of TGF-βR-III-associated capillaries enables quantitative assessment of newly formed blood vessels; negative control checks at *right bottom* (×400 original magnification).

clinical success of oral mucosa substitutes formed ex vivo.[138] KGF, which is secreted by underlying fibroblasts, is necessary for the proliferation and maturation of keratinocytes. Thus, a composite graft can provide advantages in reestablishment of oral epithelium.

Other experimental and clinical approaches that address improvement in wound healing disorders in vivo have modified cytokine expression.[90,119,139,140] Fibrocontractive wound healing disorders, which may occur in scleroderma or submucosal fibrosis following radiotherapy of the head and neck, are caused by altered and sustained expression of profibrotic TGF-β_1. Neutralization of overexpressed TGF-β_1 with anti-TGF-β_1 treatment during wound healing has been shown to reduce scarring.[88] In an animal model of radiation-impaired head and neck skin and oral mucosa healing, topically administered anti-TGF-β_1 successfully diminished collagen deposition and was able to reduce scarring (Figure 6).[119,139,141] Additionally, anti-TGF-β_1 treatment in vivo was associated with increased neovascularization, as shown in an immunohistochemical study measuring the relative capillary area in the head and neck region of rats during wound healing in preirradiated skin (Figure 7).

In conclusion, future strategies to improve oral mucosa wound healing should include both cell-based devices of improved biologic quality and the modification of growth factor and cytokine activity involved in mucosal regeneration.

REFERENCES

1. Bernimoulin JP, Schroeder HE. Quantitative electron microscopic analysis of the epithelium of normal human alveolar mucosa. Cell Tissue Res 1977;180: 383–401.
2. Phillips TJ, Gilchrest BA. Clinical applications of cultured epithelium. Epithelial Cell Biol 1992;1:39–46.
3. Tsai CY, Ueda M, Hata K, et al. Clinical results of cultured epithelial cell grafting in the oral and maxillofacial region. J Craniomaxillofac Surg 1997; 25:4–8.
4. Sisca RF, Langkamp HH, Thonard JC. Histochemical demonstration of acid mucopolysaccharide production by tissue cultured epithelial-like cells. Histochemie 1971;27:173–81.
5. Thonard JC, Migliore SA, Blustein R. Isolation of hyaluronic acid from broth cultures of streptococci. J Biol Chem 1964;239:726–8.
6. Dale BA, Salonen J, Jones AH. New approaches and concepts in the study of differentiation of oral epithelia. Crit Rev Oral Biol Med 1990;1:167–90.
7. Gailit J, Clark RA. Wound repair in the context of extracellular matrix. Curr Opin Cell Biol 1994;6:717–25.
8. Samuels P, Tan AK. Fetal scarless wound healing. J Otolaryngol 1999;28:296–302.
9. Witte MB, Barbul A. General principles of wound healing. Surg Clin North Am 1997;77:509–28.
10. Ono I, Gunji H, Zhang JZ, et al. Studies on cytokines related to wound healing in donor site wound fluid. J Dermatol Sci 1995;10:241–5.
11. Vegesna V, McBride WH, Taylor JM, Withers HR. The effect of interleukin-1 beta or transforming growth factor-beta on radiation-impaired murine skin wound healing. J Surg Res 1995;59:699–704.
12. Vogt PM, Lehnhardt M, Wagner D, et al. Determination of endogenous growth factors in human wound fluid: temporal presence and profiles of secretion. Plast Reconstr Surg 1998;102:117–23.
13. Penick GD, Roberts HR. Intravascular clotting: focal and systemic. Int Rev Exp Pathol 1964;3:269–328.
14. Penick GD, Roberts HR, Dejanov II. Covert intravascular clotting. Fed Proc 1965;24:835–9.
15. Webster WP, Roberts HR, Penick GD. Dental care of patients with hereditary disorders of blood coagulation. Mod Treat 1968;5:93–110.
16. Smith PD, Suffredini AF, Allen JB, et al. Endotoxin administration to humans primes alveolar macrophages for increased production of inflammatory mediators. J Clin Immunol 1994;14:141–8.
17. DiPietro LA. Wound healing: the role of the macrophage and other immune cells. Shock 1995;4:233–40.
18. Kovacs EJ, DiPietro LA. Fibrogenic cytokines and connective tissue production. FASEB J 1994;8:854–61.
19. Nissen NN, Gamelli RL, Polverini PJ, DiPietro LA. Differential angiogenic and proliferative activity of surgical and burn wound fluids. J Trauma 2003;54: 1205–10.
20. Leibovich SJ, Wiseman DM. Macrophages, wound repair and angiogenesis. Prog Clin Biol Res 1988;266:131–45.
21. Leibovich SJ, Chen JF, Pinhal-Enfield G, et al. Synergistic up-regulation of vascular endothelial growth factor expression in murine macrophages by adenosine A(2A) receptor agonists and endotoxin. Am J Pathol 2002;160:2231–44.
22. Chen CC, Mo FE, Lau LF. The angiogenic factor Cyr61 activates a genetic program for wound healing in human skin fibroblasts. J Biol Chem 2001;276:47329–37.
23. Eckes B, Zigrino P, Kessler D, et al. Fibroblast-matrix interactions in wound healing and fibrosis. Matrix Biol 2000;19:325–32.

24. Haapasalmi K, Zhang K, Tonnesen M, et al. Keratinocytes in human wounds express alpha v beta 6 integrin. J Invest Dermatol 1996;106:42–8.

25. Lim JM, Kim JA, Lee JH, Joo CK. Downregulated expression of integrin alpha6 by transforming growth factor-beta(1) on lens epithelial cells in vitro. Biochem Biophys Res Commun 2001;284:33–41.

26. Xu J, Clark RA. Extracellular matrix alters PDGF regulation of fibroblast integrins. J Cell Biol 1996; 132:239–49.

27. Becker J, Schuppan D, Hahn EG, et al. The immunohistochemical distribution of collagens type IV, V, VI and of laminin in the human oral mucosa. Arch Oral Biol 1986;31:179–86.

28. Moore JC, Matukas VJ, Deatherage JR, Miller EJ. Craniofacial osseous restoration with osteoinductive proteins in a collagenous delivery system. Int J Oral Maxillofac Surg 1990;19:172–6.

29. Ruoslahti E, Noble NA, Kagami S, Border WA. Integrins. Kidney Int Suppl 1994;44:S17–22.

30. Slavin J. The role of cytokines in wound healing. J Pathol 1996;178:5–10.

31. Miller EJ, Gay S. Collagen: an overview. Methods Enzymol 1982;82(Pt A):3–32.

32. Miller EJ, Gay S. The collagens: an overview and update. Methods Enzymol 1987;144:3–41.

33. Berthod F, Germain L, Guignard R, et al. Differential expression of collagens XII and XIV in human skin and in reconstructed skin. J Invest Dermatol 1997; 108:737–42.

34. Berthod F, Germain L, Li H, et al. Collagen fibril network and elastic system remodelling in a reconstructed skin transplanted on nude mice. Matrix Biol 2001;20:463–73.

35. Woodley DT, Bachmann PM, O'Keefe EJ. The role of matrix components in human keratinocyte re-epithelialization. Prog Clin Biol Res 1991;365:129–40.

36. Woodley DT, Chen JD, Kim JP, et al. Re-epithelialization. Human keratinocyte locomotion. Dermatol Clin 1993;11:641–6.

37. Woodley DT, O'Keefe EJ, Prunieras M. Cutaneous wound healing: a model for cell-matrix interactions. J Am Acad Dermatol 1985;12:420–33.

38. Woodley DT, Kalebec T, Banes AJ, et al. Adult human keratinocytes migrating over nonviable dermal collagen produce collagenolytic enzymes that degrade type I and type IV collagen. J Invest Dermatol 1986; 86:418–23.

39. Woodley DT, Briggaman RA, Herzog SR, et al. Characterization of "neo-dermis" formation beneath cultured human epidermal autografts transplanted on muscle fascia. J Invest Dermatol 1990;95:20–6.

40. Mann A, Breuhahn K, Schirmacher P, Blessing M. Keratinocyte-derived granulocyte-macrophage colony stimulating factor accelerates wound healing: stimulation of keratinocyte proliferation, granulation tissue formation, and vascularization. J Invest Dermatol 2001;117:1382–90.

41. Matsumoto K, Robb E, Warden G, Nordlund J. The expression of cytokines, growth factors and ICAM-1 in the healing of human cutaneous xenografts on nude mice. Exp Dermatol 1997;6:13–21.

42. de FC, Latini G, Parrini S, et al. Oral mucosal microvascular abnormalities: an early marker of bronchopulmonary dysplasia. Pediatr Res 2004;56: 927–31.

43. Chiquet-Ehrismann R, Mackie EJ, Pearson CA, Sakakura T. Tenascin: an extracellular matrix protein involved in tissue interactions during fetal development and oncogenesis. Cell 1986;47:131–9.

44. Chiquet-Ehrismann R, Kalla P, Pearson CA, et al. Tenascin interferes with fibronectin action. Cell 1988;53:383–90.

45. Kobayashi H, Ishii M, Chanoki M, et al. Immunohistochemical localization of lysyl oxidase in normal human skin. Br J Dermatol 1994;131:325–30.

46. Geever EF, Levenson SM, Manner G. The role of noncollagenous substances in the breaking strength of experimental wounds. Surgery 1966;60:343–51.

47. Levenson SM, Geever EF, Crowley LV, et al. The healing of rat skin wounds. Ann Surg 1965;161:293–308.

48. Miyazono K. Positive and negative regulation of TGF-beta signaling. J Cell Sci 2000;113(Pt 7):1101–9.

49. Pepper MS, Mandriota SJ, Vassalli JD, et al. Angiogenesis-regulating cytokines: activities and interactions. Curr Top Microbiol Immunol 1996; 213:31–67.

50. Goretsky MJ, Harriger MD, Supp AP, et al. Expression of interleukin-1alpha, interleukin-6, and basic fibroblast growth factor by cultured skin substitutes before and after grafting to full-thickness wounds in athymic mice. J Trauma 1996;40:894–9.

51. Grayson LS, Hansbrough JF, Zapata-Sirvent RL, et al. Quantitation of cytokine levels in skin graft donor site wound fluid. Burns 1993;19:401–5.

52. Kaiura TL, Itoh H, Kubaska SM III, et al. The effect of growth factors, cytokines, and extracellular matrix proteins on fibronectin production in human vascular smooth muscle cells. J Vasc Surg 2000;31:577–84.

53. Brogi E, Wu T, Namiki A, Isner JM. Indirect angiogenic cytokines upregulate VEGF and bFGF gene expression in vascular smooth muscle cells, whereas hypoxia upregulates VEGF expression only. Circulation 1994; 90:649–52.

54. Hakvoort T, Altun V, van Zuijlen PP, et al. Transforming growth factor-beta(1), -beta(2), -beta(3), basic fibroblast growth factor and vascular endothelial growth factor expression in keratinocytes of burn scars. Eur Cytokine Netw 2000;11:233–9.

55. Gailit J, Welch MP, Clark RA. TGF-beta 1 stimulates expression of keratinocyte integrins during re-epithelialization of cutaneous wounds. J Invest Dermatol 1994;103:221–7.

56. Kishi K, Nakajima H, Tajima S. Differential responses of collagen and glycosaminoglycan syntheses and cell proliferation to exogenous transforming growth

factor beta 1 in the developing mouse skin fibroblasts in culture. Br J Plast Surg 1999;52:579–82.

57. Reed MJ, Vernon RB, Abrass IB, Sage EH. TGF-beta 1 induces the expression of type I collagen and SPARC, and enhances contraction of collagen gels, by fibroblasts from young and aged donors. J Cell Physiol 1994;158:169–79.

58. Wang JF, Olson ME, Reno CR, et al. Molecular and cell biology of skin wound healing in a pig model. Connect Tissue Res 2000;41:195–211.

59. Pablos JL, Everett ET, Harley R, et al. Transforming growth factor-beta 1 and collagen gene expression during postnatal skin development and fibrosis in the tight-skin mouse. Lab Invest 1995;72:670–8.

60. Frank R, Adelmann-Grill BC, Herrmann K, et al. Transforming growth factor-beta controls cell-matrix interaction of microvascular dermal endothelial cells by downregulation of integrin expression. J Invest Dermatol 1996;106:36–41.

61. Heino J, Ignotz RA, Hemler ME, et al. Regulation of cell adhesion receptors by transforming growth factor-beta. Concomitant regulation of integrins that share a common beta 1 subunit. J Biol Chem 1989; 264:380–8.

62. Kagami S, Border WA, Ruoslahti E, Noble NA. Coordinated expression of beta 1 integrins and transforming growth factor-beta-induced matrix proteins in glomerulonephritis. Lab Invest 1993;69: 68–76.

63. Lorenz HP, Adzick NS. Scarless skin wound repair in the fetus. West J Med 1993;159:350–5.

64. Border WA, Noble NA. Transforming growth factor beta in tissue fibrosis. N Engl J Med 1994;331:1286–92.

65. Fajardo LF, Prionas SD, Kwan HH, et al. Transforming growth factor beta1 induces angiogenesis in vivo with a threshold pattern. Lab Invest 1996;74:600–8.

66. Yang EY, Moses HL. Transforming growth factor beta 1-induced changes in cell migration, proliferation, and angiogenesis in the chicken chorioallantoic membrane. J Cell Biol 1990;111:731–41.

67. Sankar S, Mahooti-Brooks N, Bensen L, et al. Modulation of transforming growth factor beta receptor levels on microvascular endothelial cells during in vitro angiogenesis. J Clin Invest 1996;97: 1436–46.

68. Roberts AB, Sporn MB, Assoian RK, et al. Transforming growth factor type beta: rapid induction of fibrosis and angiogenesis in vivo and stimulation of collagen formation in vitro. Proc Natl Acad Sci U S A 1986;83: 4167–71.

69. Mustoe TA, Pierce GF, Thomason A, et al. Accelerated healing of incisional wounds in rats induced by transforming growth factor-beta. Science 1987;237: 1333–6.

70. Mustoe TA, Pierce GF, Morishima C, Deuel TF. Growth factor-induced acceleration of tissue repair through direct and inductive activities in a rabbit dermal ulcer model. J Clin Invest 1991;87:694–703.

71. Robertson JG, Pickering KJ, Belford DA. Insulin-like growth factor I (IGF-I) and IGF-binding proteins in rat wound fluid. Endocrinology 1996;137:2774–81.

72. Massague J. TGF-beta signal transduction. Annu Rev Biochem 1998;67:753–91.

73. Roberts AB, Kim SJ, Noma T, et al. Multiple forms of TGF-beta: distinct promoters and differential expression. Ciba Found Symp 1991;157:7–15.

74. Khalil N. TGF-beta: from latent to active. Microbes Infect 1999;1:1255–63.

75. Derynck R, Jarrett JA, Chen EY, et al. Human transforming growth factor-beta complementary DNA sequence and expression in normal and transformed cells. Nature 1985;316:701–5.

76. Olofsson A, Ichijo H, Moren A, et al. Efficient association of an amino-terminally extended form of human latent transforming growth factor-beta binding protein with the extracellular matrix. J Biol Chem 1995; 270:31294–7.

77. Saharinen J, Hyytiainen M, Taipale J, Keski-Oja J. Latent transforming growth factor-beta binding proteins (LTBPs)—structural extracellular matrix proteins for targeting TGF-beta action. Cytokine Growth Factor Rev 1999;10:99–117.

78. Flaumenhaft R, Abe M, Mignatti P, Rifkin DB. Basic fibroblast growth factor-induced activation of latent transforming growth factor beta in endothelial cells: regulation of plasminogen activator activity. J Cell Biol 1992;118:901–9.

79. Brown PD, Wakefield LM, Levinson AD, Sporn MB. Physicochemical activation of recombinant latent transforming growth factor-beta's 1, 2, and 3. Growth Factors 1990;3:35–43.

80. Cheifetz S, Like B, Massague J. Cellular distribution of type I and type II receptors for transforming growth factor-beta. J Biol Chem 1986;261:9972–8.

81. Cheifetz S, Andres JL, Massague J. The transforming growth factor-beta receptor type III is a membrane proteoglycan. Domain structure of the receptor. J Biol Chem 1988;263:16984–991.

82. Cheifetz S, Massague J. Transforming growth factor-beta (TGF-beta) receptor proteoglycan. Cell surface expression and ligand binding in the absence of glycosaminoglycan chains. J Biol Chem 1989;264: 12025–8.

83. Wrana JL, Attisano L, Carcamo J, et al. TGF beta signals through a heteromeric protein kinase receptor complex. Cell 1992;71:1003–14.

84. Zhang Y, Derynck R. Regulation of Smad signalling by protein associations and signalling crosstalk. Trends Cell Biol 1999;9:274–9.

85. Lopez-Casillas F, Wrana JL, Massague J. Betaglycan presents ligand to the TGF beta signaling receptor. Cell 1993;73:1435–44.

86. Miyazono K, ten Dijke P, Heldin CH. TGF-beta signaling by Smad proteins. Adv Immunol 2000;75: 115–57.

87. Liu F, Pouponnot C, Massague J. Dual role of the Smad4/DPC4 tumor suppressor in TGFbeta-induci-

ble transcriptional complexes. Genes Dev 1997;11: 3157–67.

88. Adzick NS, Lorenz HP. Cells, matrix, growth factors, and the surgeon. The biology of scarless fetal wound repair. Ann Surg 1994;220:10–8.

89. Ferguson MW. Skin wound healing: transforming growth factor beta antagonists decrease scarring and improve quality. J Interferon Res 1994;14:303–4.

90. Shah M, Foreman DM, Ferguson MW. Neutralising antibody to TGF-beta 1,2 reduces cutaneous scarring in adult rodents. J Cell Sci 1994;107:1137–57.

91. Angelov N, Moutsopoulos N, Jeong MJ, et al. Aberrant mucosal wound repair in the absence of secretory leukocyte protease inhibitor. Thromb Haemost 2004; 92:288–97.

92. Warburton G, Nares S, Angelov N, et al. Transcriptional events in a clinical model of oral mucosal tissue injury and repair. Wound Repair Regen 2005;13:19–26.

93. Jonca N, Guerrin M, Hadjiolova K, et al. Corneodesmosin, a component of epidermal corneocyte desmosomes, displays homophilic adhesive properties. J Biol Chem 2002;277:5024–9.

94. Simon M, Jonca N, Guerrin M, et al. Refined characterization of corneodesmosin proteolysis during terminal differentiation of human epidermis and its relationship to desquamation. J Biol Chem 2001;276:20292–9.

95. Bohnert A, Hornung J, Mackenzie IC, Fusenig NE. Epithelial-mesenchymal interactions control basement membrane production and differentiation in cultured and transplanted mouse keratinocytes. Cell Tissue Res 1986;244:413–29.

96. Mackenzie IC, Dabelsteen E, Roed-Petersen B. A method for studying epithelial-mesenchymal interactions in human oral mucosal lesions. Scand J Dent Res 1979; 87:234–43.

97. Maas-Szabowski N, Shimotoyodome A, Fusenig NE. Keratinocyte growth regulation in fibroblast cocultures via a double paracrine mechanism. J Cell Sci 1999;112(Pt 12):1843–53.

98. Maas-Szabowski N, Fusenig NE, Stark HJ. Experimental models to analyze differentiation functions of cultured keratinocytes in vitro and in vivo. Methods Mol Biol 2005;289:47–60.

99. Tomakidi P, Breitkreutz D, Fusenig NE, et al. Establishment of oral mucosa phenotype in vitro in correlation to epithelial anchorage. Cell Tissue Res 1998;292:355–66.

100. Okazaki M, Yoshimura K, Suzuki Y, Harii K. Effects of subepithelial fibroblasts on epithelial differentiation in human skin and oral mucosa: heterotypically recombined organotypic culture model. Plast Reconstr Surg 2003;112:784–92.

101. Kvidera A, Mackenzie IC. Rates of clearance of the epithelial surfaces of mouse oral mucosa and skin. Epithelial Cell Biol 1994;3:175–80.

102. Costea DE, Loro LL, Dimba EA, et al. Crucial effects of fibroblasts and keratinocyte growth factor on morphogenesis of reconstituted human oral epithelium. J Invest Dermatol 2003;121:1479–86.

103. Costea DE, Johannessen AC, Vintermyr OK. Fibroblast control on epithelial differentiation is gradually lost during in vitro tumor progression. Differentiation 2005;73:134–41.

104. Robson MC, Heggers JP. Surgical infection. I. Single bacterial species or polymicrobic in origin? Surgery 1969;65:608–10.

105. Robson MC, Heggers JP. Variables in host resistance pertaining to septicemia. I. Blood glucose level. J Am Geriatr Soc 1969;17:991–6.

106. Robson MC, Heggers JP. Delayed wound closure based on bacterial counts. J Surg Oncol 1970;2:379–83.

107. Robson MC, Lea CE, Dalton JB, Heggers JP. Quantitative bacteriology and delayed wound closure. Surg Forum 1968;19:501–2.

108. Robson MC, Krizek TJ, Heggers JP. Biology of surgical infection. Curr Probl Surg 1973. p. 1–62.

109. Levenson SM, Crowley LV, Rosen H, Vinecour HM. Effect of administered ascorbic acid on nitrogen metabolic response to thermal trauma. Proc Soc Exp Biol Med 1955;90:502–4.

110. Levenson SM, Seifter E. Dysnutrition, wound healing, and resistance to infection. Clin Plast Surg 1977;4: 375–88.

111. Allen DB, Maguire JJ, Mahdavian M, et al. Wound hypoxia and acidosis limit neutrophil bacterial killing mechanisms. Arch Surg 1997;132:991–6.

112. Wong AL, Haroon ZA, Werner S, et al. Tie2 expression and phosphorylation in angiogenic and quiescent adult tissues. Circ Res 1997;81:567–74.

113. Frank S, Hubner G, Breier G, et al. Regulation of vascular endothelial growth factor expression in cultured keratinocytes. Implications for normal and impaired wound healing. J Biol Chem 1995;270: 12607–13.

114. Marks JG Jr, Cano C, Leitzel K, Lipton A. Inhibition of wound healing by topical steroids. J Dermatol Surg Oncol 1983;9:819–21.

115. Beer HD, Longaker MT, Werner S. Reduced expression of PDGF and PDGF receptors during impaired wound healing. J Invest Dermatol 1997;109:132–8.

116. Beer HD, Gassmann MG, Munz B, et al. Expression and function of keratinocyte growth factor and activin in skin morphogenesis and cutaneous wound repair. J Investig Dermatol Symp Proc 2000;5:34–9.

117. Schultze-Mosgau S, Rodel F, Keilholz L, et al. Vascularization of free myocutaneous gracilis flaps in replacement transplantation after preoperative radiotherapy. An experimental study. Strahlenther Onkol 2000;176:498–505.

118. Schultze-Mosgau S, Erbe M, Keilholz L, et al. Histomorphometric analysis of irradiated recipient vessels and transplant vessels of free flaps in patients undergoing reconstruction after ablative surgery. Int J Oral Maxillofac Surg 2000;29:112–8.

119. Schultze-Mosgau S, Wehrhan F, Rodel F, et al. Improved free vascular graft survival in an irradiated surgical site following topical application of rVEGF. Int J Radiat Oncol Biol Phys 2003;57:803–12.

120. Schultze-Mosgau S, Wehrhan F, Grabenbauer G, et al. Transforming growth factor beta1 and beta2 (TGFbeta2/TGFbeta2) profile changes in previously irradiated free flap beds. Head Neck 2002;24:33–41.

121. Peat BG, Bell RS, Davis A, et al. Wound-healing complications after soft-tissue sarcoma surgery. Plast Reconstr Surg 1994;93:980–7.

122. Raghow R. Role of transforming growth factor-beta in repair and fibrosis. Chest 1991;99:61–5.

123. Robson H, Spence K, Anderson E, et al. Differential influence of TGFbeta1 and TGFbeta3 isoforms on cell cycle kinetics and postirradiation recovery of normal and malignant colorectal epithelial cells. Int J Radiat Oncol Biol Phys 1997;38:183–90.

124. Rodel F, Schaller U, Schultze-Mosgau S, et al. The induction of TGF-beta(1) and NF-kappaB parallels a biphasic time course of leukocyte/endothelial cell adhesion following low-dose X-irradiation. Strahlenther Onkol 2004;180:194–200.

125. Schwentker A, Evans SM, Partington M, et al. A model of wound healing in chronically radiation-damaged rat skin. Cancer Lett 1998;128:71–8.

126. Langberg CW, Hauer-Jensen M, Sung CC, Kane CJ. Expression of fibrogenic cytokines in rat small intestine after fractionated irradiation. Radiother Oncol 1994;32:29–36.

127. Richter KK, Langberg CW, Sung CC, Hauer-Jensen M. Increased transforming growth factor beta (TGF-beta) immunoreactivity is independently associated with chronic injury in both consequential and primary radiation enteropathy. Int J Radiat Oncol Biol Phys 1997;39:187–95.

128. Geffrotin C, Tricaud Y, Crechet F, et al. Unlike tenascin-X, tenascin-C is highly up-regulated in pig cutaneous and underlying muscle tissue developing fibrosis after necrosis induced by very high-dose gamma radiation. Radiat Res 1998;149:472–81.

129. Schultze-Mosgau S, Grabenbauer GG, Radespiel-Troger M, et al. Vascularization in the transition area between free grafted soft tissues and pre-irradiated graft bed tissues following preoperative radiotherapy in the head and neck region. Head Neck 2002;24:42–51.

130. Gold LI, Sung JJ, Siebert JW, Longaker MT. Type I (RI) and type II (RII) receptors for transforming growth factor-beta isoforms are expressed subsequent to transforming growth factor-beta ligands during excisional wound repair. Am J Pathol 1997;150:209–22.

131. Schultze-Mosgau S, Wehrhan F, Rodel F, et al. Transforming growth factor-beta receptor-II up-regulation during wound healing in previously irradiated graft beds in vivo. Wound Repair Regen 2003; 11:297–305.

132. Boyce ST, Warden GD. Principles and practices for treatment of cutaneous wounds with cultured skin substitutes. Am J Surg 2002;183:445–56.

133. Hafemann B, Ensslen S, Erdmann C, et al. Use of a collagen/elastin-membrane for the tissue engineering of dermis. Burns 1999;25:373–84.

134. Rouabhia M, Germain L, Bergeron J, Auger FA. Allogeneic-syngeneic cultured epithelia. A successful therapeutic option for skin regeneration. Transplantation 1995;59:1229–35.

135. Ophof R, van Rheden RE, Von den HJ, et al. Oral keratinocytes cultured on dermal matrices form a mucosa-like tissue. Biomaterials 2002;23:3741–8.

136. Schultze-Mosgau S, Lee BK, Ries J, et al. In vitro cultured autologous pre-confluent oral keratinocytes for experimental prefabrication of oral mucosa. Int J Oral Maxillofac Surg 2004;33:476–85.

137. Rheinwald JG. Serial cultivation of normal human epidermal keratinocytes. Methods Cell Biol 1980; 21A:229–54.

138. Auger FA, Rouabhia M, Goulet F, et al. Tissue-engineered human skin substitutes developed from collagen-populated hydrated gels: clinical and fundamental applications. Med Biol Eng Comput 1998;36: 801–12.

139. Schultze-Mosgau S, Blaese MA, Grabenbauer G, et al. Smad-3 and Smad-7 expression following anti-transforming growth factor beta 1 (TGFbeta(1))-treatment in irradiated rat tissue. Radiother Oncol 2004;70:249–59.

140. Shah M, Foreman DM, Ferguson MW. Neutralisation of TGF-beta 1 and TGF-beta 2 or exogenous addition of TGF-beta 3 to cutaneous rat wounds reduces scarring. J Cell Sci 1995;108:985–1002.

141. Wehrhan F, Grabenbauer GG, Rodel F, et al. Exogenous modulation of TGF-beta(1) influences TGF-betaR-III-associated vascularization during wound healing in irradiated tissue. Strahlenther Onkol 2004;180:526–33.

7

Wound Healing of the Larynx

Susan L. Thibeault, PhD

The vocal mechanism is an intricate system that is exposed to repetitive biophysical forces. It has been proposed that the unique histologic structure of the vocal folds has evolved to withstand such forces. According to Hirano, the vocal folds' five histologic layers of increasing density break down into two biomechanical layers: the body and the cover.[1,2] The body is composed primarily of muscle, whereas the cover has been described as being composed primarily of extracellular matrix (ECM). The ECM is composed of proteins, glycoproteins, and glycosaminoglycans (GAGs). The fibroblast is the primary cell of the ECM; it is responsible for manufacturing and maintaining the ECM.

When the vocal mechanism undergoes excessive forces, it is not uncommon for injury to occur. Injuries can be acute or chronic in nature. Injuries are typically manifested by a variety of laryngeal lesions and scarring. Histologic and molecular studies have attempted to understand and characterize the pathophysiologic processes of wound healing of the ECM for different lesions. Furthermore, significant strides have been made in understanding the wound healing and repair processes of the ECM involved in vocal fold scarring. It has become evident that the interaction between the ECM in vocal fold lesions and scarring is complicated.

A comprehensive understanding of the biology of vocal fold wound healing will provide a foundation for future research. In addition, there is a clinical need for improved understanding of the pathophysiology of disrupted ECM and the development of advanced biomaterials that appreciate the biomechanical properties of the lamina propria. Development of products would also promote wound repair and induce tissue regeneration. Early tissue engineering approaches demonstrate exciting promise and potential for treatment alternatives that maximize biologic and biomechanical outcomes.

ANATOMY AND HISTOLOGY

The vocal folds, a combination of muscle and mucosa, lie in the laryngeal vestibule. The thyroarytenoid (TA) muscle is situated in an anterior to posterior direction over the lower airway. The origin of the TA muscle is the angle of the thyroid cartilage as it inserts on the vocal process of the arytenoid cartilage, which is mobile in a mediolateral direction. Hirano was the first to provide a detailed description of the morphologic structure of the vocal folds.[1,2] Histologically, the human vocal fold has been divided into three distinct tissue layers: epithelium, lamina propria, and muscle. The epithelium of the vocal fold (medial edge) is composed of stratified squamous epithelium, which is adjacent to ciliated pseudostratified epithelium of the ventricular folds and trachea and stratified columnar epithelium in the epiglottis. The lamina propria has three regions: the superficial (SLP), intermediate (ILP), and deep (DLP) lamina propria. ECM molecules are the major constituent of the SLP and ILP. The innermost vocal fold tissue layer is the TA muscle (Figure 1).

The basement membrane zone (BMZ), a specialized ECM, divides the epithelium and

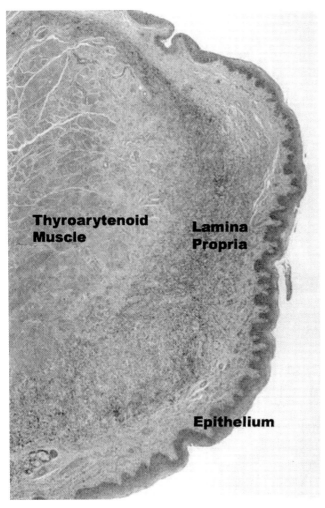

Figure 1. Coronal section of the vocal folds. The vocal folds are a layered entity, covered by epithelium. The lamina propria is made up of extracellular matrix. Moving most medially is the thyroarytenoid muscle. The transition between the lamina propria and the muscle is called the vocal ligament.

SLP. Collagen types IV and VII[3] and fibronectin[4] are found in this zone. The SLP is a pliable, loose region also known as Reinke's space. Generally, the SLP is made up of loose fibrous elements. Hammond and colleagues found relatively small amounts of mature elastin and collagen (types I, II, and III) and hyaluronic acid (HA) in the SLP.[5] They reported that the elastin in the SLP is present in its nonfibrillar forms, elaunin and oxytalan, which are not verified using the common elastic van gieson (EVG) elastin stain. Decorin, keratin sulfate, fibronectin, macrophages, and myofibrils were described by Pawlak and colleagues using immunocytochemical techniques in the SLP.[6]

In this study, the cytoplasm of macrophages and fibroblasts was found to contain heparan sulfate, chondroitin sulfate, and hyaluronate receptor.

The proteoglycans observed in the SLP differ from those seen in the ILP and DLP. The ILP is marked by a distinct elevation in the relative amount of elastin.[2] Fibromodulin and fibronectin are present in the ILP. Additionally, there are fibroblasts and myofibrils. The important GAG HA is present at its highest concentration in the ILP,[7] particularly in the infrafold area of the ILP. Prominent in the DLP are the fibrous proteins collagen and elastin. Fibromodulin, fibronectin, fibroblasts, and myofibrils continue throughout this layer. The ILP and DLP together have been described as the vocal ligament. As observed by several investigators, the presence of fibrous proteins within the lamina propria increases as the TA muscle is approached, accounting for a concomitant increase in stiffness closest to the muscle. It has been postulated that this difference in layer stiffness contributes to vocal quality.

UNIQUE PHYSIOLOGIC HEALING

Because of the inherent difficulties in obtaining human vocal fold tissue of any kind, research investigating wound healing and repair of the vocal folds has been accomplished by studying biologic markers in benign laryngeal lesions. Studies that have measured these markers of wound healing in the vocal mechanism have demonstrated that different traumatic lesions may reflect varied phases of wound repair.[8,9] These varied representations of wound repair most likely have a concomitant varied effect on the mucosal wave and vibratory pattern. The large majority of benign pathologies (edema, nodules, polyps, cysts) demonstrate differences in the cellular composition and ultrastructure of the ECM in the SLP. Traditionally, characterization of lesions has been based on histologic analysis. More recently, lesions have been analyzed using molecular genetic techniques.

Edema of the vocal folds is a generalized swelling of the vocal folds and represents inflammation and capillary leakage. Acute edema is the result of increased vasodilatation and subsequent leakage of plasma into the extravascular compartment.[4] Chronic edema, also known as Reinke's edema and/or polypoid degeneration, represents hemorrhage, fibrin deposition, edematous lakes, thickening of the BMZ, and increased blood vessel wall thickness.[10] Recurrent inflammation may induce a more chronic state of edema and inflammation. The histologic characterization of Reinke's edema represents a recurring injury or repair paradigm, which is not permitted to complete the concluding stages of healing. Decreased gene expression levels measured for fibronectin[11] would support this hypothesis, demonstrating that fibronectin is not able to accumulate as it does in the later stages of repair.

Repetitive vocal trauma, such as that seen in vocal fold nodules, can represent changes in the BMZ, demonstrating a separation of the epithelium from the underlying lamina propria. It has been proposed that this area represents an area of stress when the tissue is put into vibration.[12] Electron microscopy studies have demonstrated thickening of the BMZ and increased fibronectin,[3,4,13] which may represent tearing forces in the subepithelium. Kotby and colleagues described nodular lesions with gaps at the intercellular junctions, disruption and duplication of the BMZ, and collagen fiber.[8,9] The presence of increased fibronectin corresponds to the later stages of wound healing. Gray and colleagues proposed that the disorganized BMZ (particularly injury to the anchoring fibrils) may leave the vocal fold in a predisposed state for repetitious injury and the fibronectin deposition may lead to increased stiffening of that part of the membranous fold.[12]

Polyps have been found to have less fibronectin deposition, less BMZ injury, and more vascular injury[4] compared with normal vocal folds, indicating a primarily acute vascular injury. The vascular injury would correlate to capillary damage and leakage with hemorrhage.

Dikkers and Nikkels described hemorrhage, fibrin and iron deposition, and thrombosis as the "clinical diagnosis" of a polyp.[10] Speculatively, it would appear as if a polyp is in a static state of hemostasis or coagulation, without completing further stages of wound repair. Kotby and colleagues suggested that edematous nodules and polyps may represent a continuum of vocal fold injury.[8,9] The differences depend on chronicity and whether the injury was focal or diffuse.

Recently, Thibeault and colleagues examined the genotypic expression levels of some key ECM proteins in vocal fold polyps.[11] Distinct patterns of ECM regulation for polyps were found, highlighted by up-regulation of the fibronectin gene and down-regulation of the fibromodulin gene. Protein levels, measured by Western blot, corresponded to gene expression levels. Deoxyribonucleic acid (DNA) microarray analysis has been used to analyze transcriptional gene expression for over 4,000 genes. Interesting genes that were found to be significant reflected a tempered wound repair response with increased epithelial manifestations, suggesting that the etiology of polyps may be epithelial in nature. Differentiated vocal fold polyp genes did not include inflammatory, wound healing, or matrix remodeling genes. This is significant in light of the prevailing notion in the literature suggesting that vocal fold polyps are a result of vocal trauma and their histology shows evidence of regeneration and repair.[8–10,14] The down-regulated cluster of membrane receptor genes implies anomalies in normal cellular activity, indicating a system that is in inhibition rather than overexpression of ECM regulating genes. The cluster of epithelial regulated genes highly expressed in vocal fold polyp specifies greater activity in the epithelium compared with normal vocal fold. Differing reports regarding alterations in the epithelium of vocal fold polyp have been described in the literature. Loire and colleagues reported atrophy of the epithelium of vocal fold polyps with a thin BMZ,[14] whereas Kotby and colleagues described an intact BMZ in their histologic samples.[8,9] The overexpressed genes in our epithelial cluster are already known as active participants in altering epithelial structure and the BMZ at the level of the anchoring fibers, suggesting anomalies of the epithelium in vocal fold polyps directly related to gene expression. Taken together, these findings indicate a more chronic injury scenario for polyps rather than an acute trauma, as suggested by Dikkers and Nikkels.[10]

Kotby and colleagues hypothesized that vocal fold benign lesions represent a continuum of vocal fold injury and have essentially identical pathogenesis.[8,9] In contrast, vocal fold polyps and Reinke's edema appear to have very different gene expression and overall gene activity levels, which characterize their individual wound healing paradigms. Vocal fold polyp–expressed genes do not include those one would expect in wound healing or repair. Rather, up-regulation of genes involved in epithelial cell alterations, keratin protein malformations, and altered cell–cell interactions were noted, with down-regulation of membrane receptors. These results indicate two different pathologies. Comparing vocal fold polyps with Reinke's edema, levels of gene activity for selected fibrous and interstitial proteins indicate very different overall gene expression that characterizes their differences. Polyps had up-regulated fibronectin, down-regulated fibromodulin, and higher gene expression levels. In Reinke's edema, lower gene expressions were associated with decreased fibronectin and increased fibromodulin. These results indicate a regulation pattern that is distinctly different from that of the polyp.

Vocal fold cysts are often associated with increased vocal trauma, either as a direct cause or by increasing vocal forces because of their interruption of the glottic vibratory cycle, producing a more forceful vocal closure pattern. Cysts can be lined with columnar or squamous epithelium,[15] with a BMZ thickness that is between that of polyps and nodules.[4]

Another active area in wound healing research of the larynx is vocal fold scarring. Vocal fold scarring can occur after surgery or injury. Scarring represents a region of tissue that has completed wound healing, with resultant tissue repair. Repair

is inadequate, directly causing poor vocal fold vibration, with subsequent poor vocal quality (Figure 2). Various animal models have been used to determine the histologic characterization of the ECM in vocal fold scar. Systematic investigations have attempted to characterize wound healing and scarring in vocal fold lamina propria ECM in a variety of animal models. Discussion of this research is organized based on ECM constituents.

COLLAGEN

Collagen in normal vocal fold tissue is organized into bundles that run parallel to the epithelial mucosa above it. Procollagen 1, a collagen

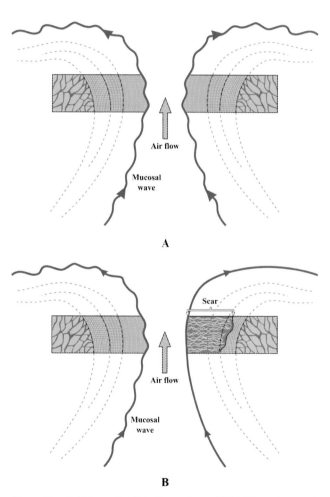

Figure 2. *A*, Schematic of the layered vocal fold. When the vocal folds are normal, airflow passes through the glottis helping to create a mucosal wave that contributes to vocal quality. *B*, Schematic of unilateral vocal fold injury to the lamina propria. When the extracellular matrix of the lamina propria is damaged, muscosal wave is diminished. This is common in vocal fold scarring.

precursor, and elastin are also present in the SLP and DLP of normal vocal folds, respectively. Two months postoperatively, scarred rabbit vocal fold tissue had elevated levels of procollagen in the SLP.[16] Collagen is less dense and without its characteristic organization into parallel bundles.[16] Elastin is also less dense, with fibers that are short and compact.[16] By 6 months, levels of procollagen and elastin have resumed the densities seen in normal vocal folds, although the elastin fibers remain fragmented and disorganized.[17] Collagen densities, however, are significantly higher than in normal vocal folds, with fibers organized into thick bundles.[17] These changes are thought to be indicative of the mature phase of wound remodeling in rabbit vocal folds.

A canine model of vocal fold wound healing showed procollagen, collagen, and elastin levels similar to those of the rabbit model. Procollagen densities were elevated at 2 months, returning to normal levels at 6 months.[18] Elastin fibers were fewer in number at both 2 and 6 months and appeared to be tangled and disorganized. Collagen levels were not significantly different at 2 months, but by 6 months, collagen levels were elevated above that found in normal vocal folds and showed marked disorganization and thick bundling. Here again, vocal fold scarring is characterized by elevated levels of procollagen in the early stage of wound healing, being replaced by thick disorganized collagen bundles and disorganized, fragmented elastin fibers in the later stages of wound healing.

In a pig animal model, collagen deposition in the very early stages of vocal fold wound healing was found to be loose and sparsely organized 3 and 10 days postoperatively in injured and control tissues.[19] On day 15, increased collagen deposition and thick bundling were observed in the scarred vocal folds only.

Finally, in a rat model, collagen types I and III were elevated on day 1, with a more pronounced elevation of collagen type III.[20] Both collagen types were elevated above controls at 2, 4, 8, and 12 weeks.[21] Collagen type I levels declined after the first 8 weeks of wound repair, although still elevated above controls, suggesting that vigorous tissue remodeling in the scarred vocal folds slows after 2 months. Collagen type III levels remained elevated and stable for the duration of the study.

FIBRONECTIN

Fibronectin is an ECM glycoprotein that has been shown to be an important adhesion molecule in the vocal folds. Fibronectin has properties that are chemotactic for inflammatory cells and fibroblasts and contributes to matrix organization.[22] Fibronectin has been found to be overexpressed in hypertrophic[23] and chronic wounds,[24] and its persistence above normal levels in the ECM may contribute to fibrosis at the site of wound repair.[25] Fibronectin in normal vocal fold tissue is found primarily in the BMZ and the SLP.[4,26,27] Levels of fibronectin in scarred vocal fold tissue were studied in rabbit and canine models.[25,26] In 2-month scarred rabbit vocal fold tissue, fibronectin levels were significantly increased over normal vocal fold levels, with more prominent staining patterns seen in the SLP. Similarly, in scarred canine vocal folds, fibronectin was found at significantly higher levels in the SLP at 2 months and continued to be higher 6 months postoperatively. These increased levels imply that even as late as 6 months after injury, matrix reorganization, stimulated at least in part by fibronectin, continues in the SLP, with likely resultant increases in fibrosis and collagen deposition characteristic of scar tissue.

Vocal fold scar in the rat was shown to have increased levels of fibronectin until the fourth week of wound healing, after which levels declined, reaching control levels at 8 and 12 weeks.[21] These fluctuations in levels of fibronectin corresponded roughly to levels of collagen type I found in the same tissues, reinforcing the probable relationship between fibronectin and collagen in wound repair.

DECORIN

Decorin is a small-chain proteoglycan adhesion molecule present in the ECM that attaches to collagen, maintaining collagen fibril organization.[6] Decorin has been previously identified in the SLP and may contribute to the minimal scarring seen when this layer of the lamina propria is disturbed.[6,7] It has been shown in previous studies that decorin regulates collagen assembly in the ECM, influencing its rate of formation and the thickness of fibrils.[6,7] It is possible that if adequate levels of decorin could maintain collagen fibril organization, the thick bundling and disorganized structural regrowth characteristic of scar tissue could be avoided when the DLP is disturbed. Decorin density in scarred rabbit vocal folds 60 days after injury[25] was significantly decreased. As decorin is thought to promote the lateral association of collagen fibrils to form organized collagen bundles, decreased levels of decorin would be expected to lead to regeneration of tissue with an unorganized collagen matrix, and this has been reported for acute vocal fold scar.[16]

FIBROMODULIN

Fibromodulin is an ECM proteoglycan that binds to and potentially inhibits transforming growth factor (TGF)-β; it has been found primarily in the ILP and DLP in association with collagen and elastin fibers of the vocal ligament.[6,7] TGF-β up-regulates collagen synthesis; thus, decreased levels of fibromodulin would be expected to be associated with increased collagen synthesis. It has been shown that procollagen is increased 2 months after scar formation,[16] concomitant with a significantly decreased level of fibromodulin, with distribution of fibromodulin being mainly in the SLP.[25] Decreased fibromodulin in the SLP could lead to increased collagen synthesis in this layer of the vocal fold as the wound heals.

COMBINED EFFECTS OF ECM COMPONENTS

Collectively, decreased levels of decorin and increased fibronectin would be expected with elevated levels of collagen synthesis (owing to decreased fibromodulin), disorganized collagen deposition (owing to decreased decorin), and continued inflammatory cell and fibroblast migration (owing to increased fibronectin). These correlations are supported by recent studies in a rabbit model.[16,27]

The dynamic association between fibronectin and collagen was observed in scarred canine vocal folds by Hirano and colleagues.[27] Fibronectin, but not collagen, was observed at increased levels in 2-month scar tissue. At 6 months, both fibronectin and collagen levels were significantly increased above normal levels. This suggests that replacement of fibronectin by collagen is a prolonged process and is not evident until sometime after the 2-month postoperative period and continuing through the 6-month postoperative period. Although some elevated levels of fibronectin are necessary for the regeneration of vocal fold tissue after injury,[25] manipulation of fibronectin levels may, in turn, affect the deposition of collagen in the later stages of wound healing and reduce the subsequent scarring seen in the vocal folds after injury.

Density and distribution of other adhesion molecules, namely cadherin, syndecan 4, and syndecan 1, were measured in normal versus scarred canine vocal folds.[27] Syndecan 4 was rarely found in normal vocal fold epithelium but was prominently expressed in the basal layer of the mucosal epithelium of scarred vocal folds, 2 months and 6 months postoperatively. Levels of syndecan 1 and cadherin, adhesion molecules found in the epithelial intercellular space, were detectable but unchanged in normal versus scarred vocal fold tissue. From these studies, it seems apparent that the basal layer of the mucosal epithelium continues to experience remodeling in the later stages of wound healing, whereas the intercellular epithelial space undergoes remodeling earlier during the acute stage of wound healing.

INFLAMMATORY MEDIATORS

A new methodology to investigate the mechanisms involved in acute wound healing of the larynx has been proposed by Verdolini and colleagues that measures acute inflammatory mediators in laryngeal secretions.[28] Marked shifts in interleukin (IL)-1β, tumor necrosis factor α, and matrix metalloproteinase 8 levels in secretions collected from the surface of the vocal folds have been reported following an episode of acute phonotrauma.[28] In a rabbit wound model, IL-1β and prostaglandin E2 (PGE$_2$) levels were measured with enzyme-linked immunosorbent assay (ELISA), and their expressed protein levels were consistent with their proposed role in the wound healing cascade noted in other tissues. Maximum expression of IL-1β occurred on day 1 after injury and returned to baseline at day 7. Conversely, PGE$_2$ did not significantly increase immediately following injury. Maximal levels were measured on day 7, and at day 21, PGE$_2$ levels remained elevated above preinjury levels. Branski and colleagues proposed that this methodology may hold scientific and clinical utility for understanding wound healing in the larynx.[29]

FUTURE PROMISE FOR HEALING

State of the art research in the wound healing of the larynx has focused on understanding the roles of HA and growth factors in vocal fold healing. Moreover, tissue engineering approaches have been designed to promote wound repair and induce tissue regeneration. It would be expected that future treatments that improve wound healing and repair in the larynx would resolve the complex interactions among tissue characteristics, biomechanical properties, and surgical requisites necessary to create a suitable clinical outcome.

HA is a nonantigenic GAG found in the ECM throughout the body and is concentrated in the vocal folds and other specialized tissues.[30] Higher concentrations of HA are found in the infrafold region of the vocal fold, which corresponds to the region where the mucosal wave begins its vertical rise.[7] It has been shown that if HA is removed from the vocal folds, there is an increase in viscosity and a reduction in stiffness

of the tissue, creating less than optimal conditions for phonation and vocal fundamental frequency.[31,32] In general, men have a higher concentration of HA in the vocal folds than do women.[33]

The levels of HA in the vocal folds may have an impact on wound healing and scar formation. Exploring the phenomenon of fetal scarless wound healing, Estes and colleagues found that sheep fetal wound fluid contains significantly higher levels of HA than adult wounds, suggesting that HA has a mechanistic role in wound healing.[34] It has been shown that in dermal wound healing, a chemically cross-linked HA hydrogel film and a chondroitin sulfate hydrogel film promoted reepithelialization, vascularization, and dermal collagen organization.[35] GAG films may retain cytokines and other growth factors made by the regenerating tissue, facilitating the assembly of other matrix components and supporting cell migration to the wound site.

Research has been conducted to learn more about the role of HA in the vocal fold healing process. The density and distribution of HA in scarred vocal folds have been compared with those in normal vocal folds in rabbits and canines. Measured levels of HA in injured rabbit vocal folds during the early stages of wound repair were lower than normal during the first 15 days of wound healing.[36] Postoperatively, day 3 injured vocal folds showed expected signs of acute inflammatory response, with infiltration of neutrophils and significantly lower levels of HA than normal vocal folds. Day 5 was the only time during the 15 days that HA levels in scarred tissue were comparable to those of controls. Thus, even in the early stage of wound repair in the mature rabbit, HA levels were never elevated above those found in undisturbed tissue and were actually lower than normal overall during the first 15 days. HA levels in the acute stage of wound healing were studied in a pig model, with similar results being reported: HA levels were reduced in the injured pig vocal folds 3, 10, and 15 days postoperatively compared with controls.[19] In the rat model, it was found that HA levels were lower than controls, although there was evidence of HA in the tissues by day 3 and peaking at day 5. Because collagen and fibronectin levels were found to peak at days 3 and 5 as well,[20] HA may have a role in the regulation or deposition of collagen in the acute phase of wound healing. However, this hypothesis requires further investigation as HA levels were depressed in scarred rat vocal folds when measured at 2, 4, 8, and 12 weeks, even as levels of collagen types I and III were elevated.[21]

It has been shown that the density of HA in the scarred vocal folds at 2 and 6 months postoperatively is not statistically different from normal vocal folds in either the rabbit or the canine model.[16–18] The distribution of HA in normal rabbit vocal folds is predominantly in the DLP, similar to the distribution of HA in normal canine vocal folds. After scarring, rabbit vocal folds show a redistribution of HA to all layers of the lamina propria when viewed 2 and 6 months postoperatively.[16,17] In contrast, scarred canine vocal folds show no redistribution of HA to other layers of the lamina propria after wounding.[18] Because these studies have shown that HA levels in scarred vocal folds 2 and 6 months postoperatively are the same as those in controls, it is thought that the critical time frame for the involvement of HA in wound repair occurs earlier in the wound healing process,[16,17] in the first few days and weeks after injury.

Endogenous HA is rapidly turned over in the body, and its half-life in the vocal fold tissues has been estimated to be between 0.5 and 4 days.[37] The turnover of HA is accomplished by hyaluronidases that enzymatically degrade HA intracellularly after it has been removed from the ECM by receptor-mediated endocytosis.[30] By inhibiting the hyaluronidases, it may be possible to keep HA at normal levels in the early stages of wound healing.[37] Echinacoside, a caffeoyl derivative and known antihyaluronidase from the echinacea plant, was added to human vocal fold fibroblast cell lines, incubated for 24, 48, or 72 hours, which were then analyzed for HA concentrations. Higher levels

of HA were found in the supernatant of the treated cells that had been incubated for 24 hours than were found in controls, presumably because of inhibition of hyaluronidase activity and not owing to stimulation of HA production. No elevated levels of HA were found in samples treated and incubated for 48 or 72 hours, warranting further study.

Because of HA's ubiquitous role in wound healing, maximizing HA levels at the time of injury is a promising line of study. Rousseau and colleagues investigated the use of echinacoside in a pig model.[37] Following injury, treated vocal folds were found to have increased levels of HA over untreated vocal folds, with levels similar to those of uninjured controls on all postoperative days, measured histologically. Collagen accumulation in the scarred vocal folds was reduced compared with untreated vocal folds. Biomechanically, the treated larynges demonstrated lower phonation threshold pressure and improved vocal economy.

The importance of the role of HA in the biomechanics of the vocal folds has led to research that seeks to broaden the understanding of factors that influence HA levels in normal tissue and in the wound healing process. A two-part study was conducted to determine which growth factors influence the production of HA by canine vocal fold fibroblasts in vitro and, second, how maintenance of high levels of HA can be stimulated by repeated administration of growth factors.[27] The growth factors used were hepatocyte growth factor (HGF), epidermal growth factor (EGF), basic fibroblast growth factor (bFGF), and TGF-β. Growth factor was administered to cell cultures according to different predetermined schedules: (a) day 1 only; (b) days 1 and 4; (c) days 1, 3, and 5; or (d) daily for 6 days. The results of the first study showed that all growth factors significantly increased HA synthesis. The second study showed that a single administration of EGF, bFGF, and TGF-β on day 1 was sufficient to increase HA production for at least 7 days. HGF increased HA production in all variations of administration except when given on schedule b, days 1 and 4.

The localization and activity of HGF and its receptor, c-Met, in fibroblasts in the ECM of rat and rabbit vocal folds were studied to substantiate their existence.[38] Normal rat vocal folds were found to express HGF and c-Met in the epithelial and gland cells at significantly detectable levels but not in the lamina propria and muscle. Injured rabbit vocal folds, with a section of epithelium removed, showed no HGF in the lamina propria initially but by day 5 and peaking at day 10 showed the presence of HGF in the regenerating epithelium, lamina propria, and gland cells. The study did not address whether the HGF is produced by fibroblasts in the lamina propria and transported to the epithelium or if the epithelial cells produce HGF in an autocrine fashion. The results of this study suggest that HGF has an antifibrotic role in the healing of vocal fold wounds, similar to its role in other organs. In an in vitro study, HGF was used to stimulate canine vocal fold fibroblasts to increase production of HA and to decrease production of collagen type I.[38] The production of fibronectin was not affected by HGF. Consequently, stimulation of canine fibroblasts with TGF-β_1 not only increased levels of HA, it also increased levels of collagen type I and fibronectin.

The in vitro effects of HGF on human vocal fold fibroblasts from the macula flava (FbMF) and Reinke's space (FbRS) were studied.[39] It was shown that stimulation by HGF up-regulated production of HA by FbRS, down-regulated production of collagen type I in both cell types, and had no effect on fibronectin production by either cell type. HGF also had an effect on cell shape and organelle development in FbRS. More well-developed Golgi apparatus and rough endoplasmic reticulum were observed in FbRS with added HGF, and the shapes of the cells shifted from oval toward spindle and stellate. Organelle development and cell shape showed little change in FbMF when HGF was added. These results suggest that HGF has a greater effect on the FbRS and may have potential for future treatment modalities to control scarring.

Hirano and colleagues studied the effect of HGF at the time of injury in the rabbit and canine models.[40,41] In both studies, treated vocal folds improved biomechanical properties with less collagen deposition and tissue contraction. Unfortunately, HA levels were not measured in either study. The mechanism for improvement can only be speculated.

Three laboratories have published research using tissue engineering approaches specifically to regenerate the vocal folds. Kanemaru and colleagues injected autologous mesenchymal stem cells (MSCs) in an attempt to regenerate injured canine vocal folds.[42] MSCs have the capacity to differentiate into a variety of tissue types. Positive gross morphologic findings (less atrophy, granulation, irregularity of vocal fold surface, and fibrous changes) were observed 2 months after treatment, whereas immature cells thought to originate from the MSCs were present among TA cells. Chhetri and colleagues used a similar canine model to assess the effectiveness of autologous skin fibroblasts injected into scarred vocal folds.[43] Improvements were measured for mucosal wave, jitter, shimmer, and signal to noise ratio. The fibroblast-treated vocal folds stained positive for ECM components. Lastly, Hansen and colleagues used a HA scaffold hydrogel, Carbylan-SX (Sentrex Surgical, Salt Lake City, UT), in a rabbit model in newly scarred vocal folds.[44] The cross-linkable polymer hydrogel was able to adhere to the tissue during gel formation, and the resultant mechanical interlocking arising from surface microroughness was found to strengthen the tissue-hydrogel interface, providing an optimal scaffolding for fibroblast migration. Three weeks after injection, the HA scaffold had degraded as measured by ELISA. Improved viscoelastic properties were measured with the presence of well-organized collagen fibrils. It was hypothesized that the HA scaffolding accelerated wound repair through the improved migration and assembly of matrix components. Each of the above studies is preliminary in nature, with exciting promise and potential for treatment alternatives that maximize biologic and biomechanical outcomes. Substantial further investigation is necessary prior to human trials.

REFERENCES

1. Hirano M. Morphological structure of the vocal cord as a vibrator and its variations. Folia Phoniatr (Basel) 1974; 26:89–94.
2. Hirano M. Structure of the vocal fold in normal and disease states: anatomical and physical studies. ASHA Rep 1981;11:11–30.
3. Gray SD, Pignatari S, Harding P. Morphologic ultrastructure of anchoring fibers in normal vocal fold basement membrane zone. J Voice 1994;8:48–52.
4. Courey M, Shohet J, Scott M, Ossoff R. Immunohistochemical characterization of benign lesions. Ann Otol Rhinol Laryngol 1996;105:525–31.
5. Hammond TH, Zhou R, Hammond EH, et al. The intermediate layer: a morphologic study of the elastin and hyaluronic acid constituents of normal human vocal folds. J Voice 1997;11:59–66.
6. Pawlak AS, Hammond T, Hammond E, Gray SD. Immunocytochemical study of proteoglycans in vocal folds. Ann Otol Rhinol Laryngol 1996;105:6–11.
7. Gray SD, Titze IR, Chan R, Hammond TH. Vocal fold proteoglycans and their influence on biomechanics. Laryngoscope 1999;109:845–54.
8. Kotby MN, Nassar A, Seif EI, et al. Ultrastructural changes of the basement membrane zone in benign lesions of the vocal folds. Acta Otolaryngol (Stockh) 1988;113:98–101.
9. Kotby MN, Nassar A, Seif EI, et al. Ultrastructural features of vocal fold nodules and polyps. Acta Otolaryngol (Stockh) 1988;105:477–82.
10. Dikkers F, Nikkels P. Benign lesions of the vocal folds: histopathology and phonotrauma. Ann Otol Rhinol Laryngol 1995;104:698–703.
11. Thibeault SL, Gray SD, Li W, et al. Genotypic and phenotypic expression of vocal fold polyps and Reinke's edema: a preliminary study. Ann Otol Rhinol Laryngol 2002;111:302–8.
12. Gray SD, Hammond E, Hanson DF. Benign pathologic responses of the larynx. Ann Otol Rhinol Laryngol 1995;104:13–8.
13. Moussallam I, Kotby M, Ghaly A, et al. Histopathological aspects of benign vocal fold lesions associated with dysphonia. In: Kierchner J, editor. Vocal fold histopathology: a symposium. San Diego, CA: College Hill Press; 1986. p. 65–80.
14. Loire R, Bouchayer M, Cornut G, Bastian R. Pathology of benign vocal fold lesions. Ear Nose Throat J 1988;67:357–62.
15. Shvero J, Koren R, Hadar T, et al. Clinicopathologic study and classification of vocal cord cysts. Pathol Res Pract 2000;196:95–8.
16. Thibeault SL, Gray SD, Bless DM, et al. Histologic and rheologic characterization of vocal fold scarring. J Voice 2002;16:96–104.
17. Rousseau B, Hirano S, Chan RW, et al. Characterization of chronic vocal fold scarring in a rabbit model. J Voice 2004;18:116–24.
18. Rousseau B, Hirano S, Scheidt TD, et al. Characterization of vocal fold scarring in a canine model. Laryngoscope 2003;113:620–7.
19. Rousseau B, Sohn J, Montequin DW, et al. Functional outcomes of reduced hyaluronan in acute vocal fold scar. Ann Otol Rhinol Laryngol 2004;113:767–76.
20. Tateya T, Tateya I, Sohn J, Bless DM. Histological study of acute vocal fold injury in a rat model. Ann Otol Rhinol Laryngol 2006;115(3):215–24.
21. Tateya T, Tateya I, Sohn JH, Bless DM. Histological characterization of rat vocal fold scarring. Annals of Otology, Rhinology, Laryngology 2005;114(3):183–191.
22. Grinnell F. Fibronectin and wound healing. J Cell Biochem 1984;26:107–16.
23. Kischer CW, Hendrix MJC. Fibronectin in hypertropic scars and keloids. Cell Tissue Res 1983;231:29–37.
24. Ongenae KC, Phillips TJ, Park HY. Level of fibronection mRNA is markely increased in human chronic wounds. Dermatol Surg 2000;26:447–51.
25. Thibeault SL, Bless DM, Gray SD. Interstitial protein alterations in rabbit vocal fold with scar. J Voice 2003; 17:377–83.
26. Hirano S, Bless DM, Rousseau B, et al. Fibronectin and adhesion molecules on canine scarred vocal folds. Laryngoscope 2003;113:966–72.
27. Hirano S, Bless DM, Heisey D, Ford C. Effect of growth factors on hyaluronan production by canine vocal fold fibroblasts. Ann Otol Rhinol Laryngol 2003;112:617–24.
28. Verdolini K, Rosen CA, Branski RC, Hebda PA. Shifts in biochemical markers associated with wound healing in laryngeal secretions following phonotrauma: a preliminary study. Ann Otol Rhinol Laryngol 2003;112:1021–5.
29. Branski RC, Sandulache VC, Dohar JE, Hebda PA. Mucosal wound healing in a rabbit model of subglottic stenosis: biochemical analysis of secretions. Arch Otolaryngol Head Neck Surg 2005;131:153–7.
30. Ward PD, Thibeault SL, Gray SD. Hyaluronic acid: its role in voice. J Voice 2002;16:303–9.
31. Chan RW, Gray SD, Titze IR. The importance of hyaluronic acid in vocal fold biomechanics. Otolaryngol Head Neck Surg 2001;124:607–14.
32. Thibeault SL. Hyaluronan biology. In: Garg HG, Hales CA, editors. Vocal fold morphology and biomechanics. Chemistry and biology of hyaluronan, New York: Elsevier Press; 2004. p. 339–50.
33. Butler J, Hammond T, Gray SD. Gender-related differences of hyaluronic acid distribution in the human vocal fold. Laryngoscope 2001;111:907–11.
34. Estes JM, Adzick NS, Harrison MR, et al. Hyaluronate metabolism undergoes an ontogenic transition during fetal development: implications for scar-free wound healing. J Pediatr Surg 1993;28:1227–31.
35. Kirker KR, Luo Y, Nielson JH, et al. Glycosaminoglycan hydrogel films as bio-interactive dressings for wound healing. Biomaterials 2002;23:3661–71.

36. Thibeault SL, Rousseau B, Welham NV, et al. Hyaluronan levels in acute vocal fold scar. Laryngoscope 2004;114: 760–4.

37. Rousseau B, Tateya I, Lim X, et al. Investigation of echinacoside on laryngeal hyaluronan production. J Voice 2006;20:443–51.

38. Hirano S, Bless DM, Heisey D, Ford C. Roles of hepatocyte growth factor and transforming growth factor B1 in production of extracellular matrix by canine vocal fold fibroblasts. Laryngoscope 2003;113:144–8.

39. Hirano S, Bless DM, Massey RJ, et al. Morphological and functional changes of human vocal fold fibroblasts with hepatocyte growth factor. Ann Otol Rhinol Laryngol 2003;112:1026–33.

40. Hirano S, Bless DM, Nagai H, et al. Growth factor therapy for vocal fold scarring in a canine model. Ann Otol Rhinol Laryngol 2004;113:777–85.

41. Hirano S, Bless DM, Rousseau B, et al. Prevention of vocal fold scarring by topical injection of hepatocyte growth factor in a rabbit model. Laryngoscope 2004; 114:548–56.

42. Kanemaru S, Nakamura T, Omori K, et al. Regeneration of the vocal fold using autologous mesenchymal stem cells. Ann Otol Rhinol Laryngol 2003;112: 915–20.

43. Chhetri DK, Head C, Revazova E, et al. Lamina propria replacement therapy with cultured autologous fibroblasts for vocal fold scars. Otolaryngol Head Neck Surg 2004;131:864–70.

44. Hansen J, Thibeault SL, Walsh JF, et al. In vivo engineering of the vocal fold ECM with injectable HA hydrogels: early effects on tissue repair and biomechanics in a rabbit model. Ann Otol Rhinol Laryngol 2006; 114(9):662–670.

8

Wound Healing in the Subglottis and Trachea

Vlad C. Sandulache, PhD; Patricia A. Hebda, PhD; Joseph E. Dohar, MD, MS

Wound healing of the upper airway involves multiple cell types, soluble mediators, and extracellular matrix (ECM) components. Complex interactions between these factors, triggered by mucosal injury, result in partial restoration of initial tissue structure and function. The upper airway can be damaged through a variety of mechanisms. Mild mucosal injury resulting in damage to the epithelial layer can be caused by inhaled irritants and repetitive mechanical stress, such as intubation. More severe damage can be caused by trauma or by surgical manipulation of and laser use in the upper airway. Finally, a variety of systemic diseases, including acid reflux and Wegener's granulomatosis (WG), can trigger a wound healing response in the mucosal layer. In a certain subset of cases, such mucosal damage results in an abnormal wound healing response with excessive synthesis of ECM components and may lead to impairment of normal airflow.

The precise cellular and molecular processes comprising mucosal wound healing of the upper airway remain poorly understood. However, studies to date have demonstrated that appropriate repair requires the coordinated activity of epithelial, inflammatory, and endothelial cells, along with fibroblasts and chondrocytes. This coordination is achieved through an array of growth factors and inflammatory mediators, which ensure the timing and extent of wound healing processes such as reepithelialization, restoration of lamina propria ECM, and revascularization. Abnormal cell activity in the mucosal wound bed can result in excessive healing and the development of scarring (stenosis). Although methods exist to exogenously control the degree of mucosal scarring, the ultimate goal remains to create a regenerative wound healing response to injury in upper airway tissues. Fetal wound healing presents us with a useful template of scarless, regenerative mucosal wound healing.

TRACHEAL MUCOSA: WOUND HEALING FEATURES

The subglottis and trachea are complex structures, the major function of which is to maintain airflow to and from the lower airway. A respiratory epithelium lining the upper airway lumen humidifies and sterilizes inspired air. The underlying lamina propria and cartilage layers offer structural and nutrient support to the airway epithelium. Damage to this trilaminar structure can occur by multiple mechanisms, ranging from inhaled irritants to trauma and surgical instrumentation, triggering a wound healing response.

Wound healing of the upper airway is a complex process, involving multiple cell types and soluble mediators. The precise cellular and molecular processes required for appropriate mucosal repair remain only partially understood. Recent work demonstrated a role for inflammatory mediators and growth factors, particularly fibroblast growth factor (FGF) and transforming growth factor (TGF)-β in coordinating the activity of epithelial cells, fibroblasts, and chondrocytes postinjury.

Wound healing is a reparative process that generally fails to completely restore the original structure of the injured tissue, resulting in scar formation. In the upper airway, scarring of the mucosa can cause significant impairment of airflow, whereas damage to the cartilage framework may cause loss of structural rigidity. Current approaches to management of airway stenosis rely primarily on surgical interventions that either expand the cartilaginous framework or resect the injured segment. Such procedures meet with variable success. Understanding the precise cellular and molecular processes that ensue following mucosal damage will be required for the development of improved future clinical approaches. Fetal wound healing, a scarless variant of adult repair, may hold promise as a tool for understanding regenerative healing and highlighting the requirements for minimizing mucosal scarring.

Anatomy, Histology, and Embryology

Tracheal function is the primary determinant of its anatomy. The upper airway is a conduit for air exchange, with its primary function being facilitation of uninterrupted airflow during respiration. As such, it must possess several anatomic traits: (1) a semirigid structure to prevent collapse under pressure from fascia and muscle layers surrounding it, (2) flexibility to allow for distention during breathing, and (3) a smooth internal lumen to allow for undisturbed airflow lined by epithelium, which can maintain a filtering and clearing function for both pathogens and foreign bodies (Figure 1).

The subglottis is defined as the region immediately inferior to the true vocal folds and is continuous with the trachea below. The border between these two structures is demarcated by the cricoid cartilage, which represents the narrowest luminal region of the pediatric airway. In the adult, the narrowest point of the upper airway is generally considered to be the glottis

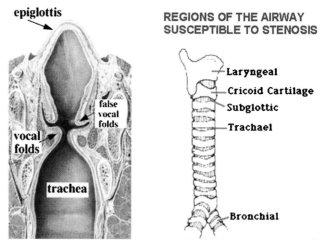

Figure 1. Anatomy of the upper airway. The subglottis lies just inferior to the vocal folds and superior to the rest of the trachea. Several regions of the upper airway are susceptible to the development of stenosis.

(vocal folds). However, some data suggest that the diameter of the glottis is dependent on active functional adduction of the vocal cords. In relaxed adult airways, as in the case of cadaveric airways, the glottic diameter is greater than the subglottic diameter in both male and female airways.[1] In life, however, it is generally accepted that the glottis is the limiting dimension of the adult upper airway. This is in striking contrast to the pediatric upper airway limited by the diameter of the subglottis. The trachea, which ranges between 3 and 5 inches in length in the adult, begins at the cricoid cartilage and divides into the main stem bronchi at the level of the carina. The tracheal lumen is supported by a series of incomplete cartilage rings open posteriorly. These rings are supported by a network of longitudinal and circular muscle fibers, including the trachealis muscle, which controls the size of the lumen. The precise roles of other tracheal muscles remain unclear. The tracheal and subglottic lumina are lined by pseudostratified ciliated columnar (respiratory) epithelium with goblet cells (unicellular secretory glands) underlined by the lamina propria, a thin connective tissue layer, which is separated from the cartilage-muscle layer by an elastic membrane. Seromucous glands are present in the submucosa, primarily interspersed between cartilage rings. The entire structure is supported by a vascular network localized primarily to the surrounding fascia. This network includes the inferior thyroid artery and subepithelial and submucosal venous plexi, which drain into a plexus of thyroid veins.[2] Lymphatic drainage occurs via a complex network of lymph vessels present in the mucosa and submucosa. This network drains into pretracheal, paratracheal, and inferior deep cervical nodes. The tracheal cartilage is a hyaline cartilage containing chondrocytes in evenly spaced lacunae, embedded into a fine matrix of connective tissue composed primarily of cartilage-specific collagen (type II), proteoglycans, and glycosaminoglycans. This dense matrix provides both support and flexibility for the entire upper airway conduit.

External approaches to the subglottis or trachea must take into account the extensive array of structures lying anterior to it, including the brachiocephalic veins, thymus, and thyroid gland, and posterior to it, including the esophagus, recurrent laryngeal nerves, and thoracic duct. Less invasive approaches via laryngoscopy must take into account internal anatomic features. Visualization and manipulation of the subglottis and trachea must occur without damaging the superior vocal cords or the cricoid cartilage. Additional anatomic details that are relevant to specific surgical approaches to the subglottis and trachea are discussed in more detail in subsequent chapters.

The subglottis and trachea are complex tissues organized as multilayer tubular structures. The epithelial layer matures and becomes ciliated by 12 weeks of gestation, with mucosal glands forming and invaginating into the submucosa between 13 and 16 weeks of gestation. The cartilage support structures begin to form around 10 weeks of gestation and are thought to remain relatively stable during subsequent developmental stages.[2] Tracheal cartilage is not a completely static structure, but can eventually ossify.[3] Ossification accompanies aging and is found primarily in the outer tracheal cartilage layer, with hyalinization occurring in the central region. These processes are accompanied by changes in the ECM of the cartilage, with type II collagen within the cartilaginous matrix and type I localized to the perichondrium and ossified areas.

The upper airway epithelium has three main functions: (1) clearing foreign bodies and pathogens, (2) preventing infection, and (3) humidifying inspired air. Ciliation allows for clearance of foreign bodies and pathogens through a continuous, coordinated activity of millions of individual adenosine triphosphate–powered cilia. The distribution of these cilia follows the upper airway anatomy to maximize clearance rates, with retrograde ciliary function occurring in the trachea along the posterior and lateral walls of the lumen.[4]

The protective function of the epithelium is accomplished through multiple mechanisms: (1) a bilayered protective liquid cover containing a fluid and a mucous layer; (2) lectins, immunoglobulin A, transferrin, and lysozyme, all of which have antibacterial activity; and (3) a complex of tight junctions that prevents pathogen invasion of the submucosa. The humidifying function of the epithelium is accomplished through closely controlled secretion of a mucous layer containing a large amount of hydrated glycosaminoglycans. The subglottic region contains multiple submucosal glands with serous tubules that secrete lectins, enzymes, and other bioactive molecules.[5]

The airway epithelium is underlined by connective tissue, the lamina propria, which consists of a collagenous ECM, with interspersed fibroblasts, other connective tissue cells, and prominent blood vessels. The lamina propria provides essential physical support and cushioning to the epithelial layer, along with vascular and lymphatic beds. It also provides an avenue for inflammatory cell infiltration subsequent to mucosal injury. The final support mechanism for the airway epithelium is the cartilage framework, which provides support and maintains the patency of the lumen (Figure 2).

The precise sequence of events involved in tracheal development remains unclear. However, evidence suggests that FGFs and their receptors (FGFRs) play an important role in the appropriate generation of a patent upper airway. Several craniosynostosis syndromes, including Pfeiffer's syndrome, are associated with specific

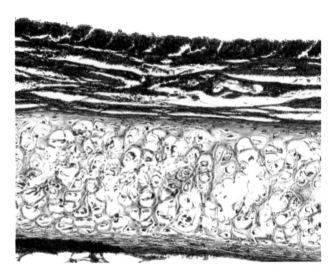

Figure 2. Histology of subglottic mucosa and cartilage framework from a normal adult rabbit airway stained with Masson's trichrome (×100 original magnification). CF = cartilage framework; LP = lamina propria; ME = mucosal epithelium.

mutations in the *FGFR2* gene and have been shown to present with some tracheal anomalies, including the congenital tracheal cartilaginous sleeve.[6,7] Animal modeling has demonstrated that FGF-2 and one of its receptors, FGFR-1, play an important role in the development of the basal membrane that separates the epithelial and lamina propria layers. Improper FGF–FGFR interactions during development have been linked to esophageal atresia and tracheoesophageal fistula formation.[8] Precise regulation of FGF and other signaling pathways during tracheal development is highly dependent on the expression of higher-order genes coding for various transcription factors.[9] Both FGF-2 and FGFR-1 are expressed throughout postnatal production of the basement membrane zone in the basal epithelial cells.[10] FGF-2 has also been implicated in basement membrane zone remodeling subsequent to allergen-induced damage.[11]

Unique Physiologic Healing Aspects and Problems

Wound Healing Overview

The subglottis and trachea are trilaminar structures whose anatomy and physiology dictate that effective wound healing must achieve four key end points: (1) restoration and maintenance of vascu-larity, (2) reepithelialization, (3) control of fibroblast activity, and (4) maintenance of a semirigid cartilaginous structure. To achieve these goals, wound healing of the airway mucosa involves complex interactions between inflammatory cells, epithelial cells, fibroblasts, and chondrocytes, all carefully choreographed by an array of cytokines, chemokines, and growth factors. A consistent component of normal wound healing is the propensity of most connective tissues to heal through a reparative process that only partially approximates the original tissue structure and function and results in a thicker, denser lamina propria, that is, scar formation. Although scarring is never a desirable outcome when wounded tissue heals, the tendency for scar tissue to be excessive can be disastrous when it occurs in the airway. Stenosis of the airway, often caused by what is essentially a type of hypertrophic scarring, reduces the cross section of the lumen through which the body's air supply flows. The seriousness of this narrowing becomes clear in light of Poiseuille's law, which states that the reduction in the laminar flow rate of a fluid or gas through a tube decreases proportionally to the fourth power of the radius. Thus, airway stenosis caused by scarring and cartilage framework deformation can severely impair respiration.

Types of Clinically Relevant Injuries

Wound healing of the upper airway is induced by a variety of mechanisms, ranging from systemic disease and local abnormalities to surgical interventions and attempts at reconstruction. Below is a summary of clinically relevant defects encountered by otolaryngologists.

Congenital Malformations. In neonates, upper airway congenital malformations present with clinically significant correlates. Tracheal atresia or malformation represents the most extreme example, with complete or almost complete impairment of airflow. More commonly, tracheal stenosis occurs and is a result of complete tracheal rings. As stated earlier, the cartilage of the tracheal rings should be incomplete posteriorly. Additional congenital malformations involving the upper airway include subglottic stenosis, tracheomalacia, hemangiomas, and lymphangiomas. Although these congenital conditions do not represent injuries to the upper airway, they do, nevertheless, result in significant mortality and morbidity and as such have been targeted by surgical intervention in recent years. Unfortunately, these same surgical procedures themselves cause injury to airway structures and elicit a wound healing response.

Systemic Disease. Airway stenosis is often a manifestation of larger, systemic diseases, such as sarcoidosis, WG, amyloidosis, and gastroesophageal reflux (GERD). Subglottic stenosis (SGS) resulting from amyloidosis is rare, although clinically significant.[12] Amyloid deposits can give rise to localized tumor-like growths or diffuse pockets undermining the airway mucosa. The precise distribution pattern is important in that it can dictate the type of therapeutic interventions. Tracheal resection[13,14] can be used to remove primary lesions, whereas endoscopic approaches, such as neodymium–yttrium-aluminum-garnet lasers,[15] can manage more diffuse disease. Tracheobronchial manifestations of sarcoidosis are similarly rare, although they have been found to coincide with other known sarcoid entities, such as vena cava syndrome and breast granuloma.[16] WG is a form of vasculitis in which the walls of blood vessels are damaged owing to an inflammatory infiltrate. The most common presentation of WG is localized granulomatous inflammation of the airway mucosa, which may progress to subsequent tissue necrosis. Although the pathophysiology of this disease involves an immune-mediated mechanism, the precise pathophysiology is unknown. SGS is an established symptom of WG, and a diagnosis of SGS in the absence of clear etiology should stimulate further testing for systemic WG.[17]

GERD has been previously linked to the development of otolaryngologic disease.[18] Although the symptoms vary in intensity, ranging from chronic cough to stridor, they may include extensive involvement of the upper airway and larynx, resulting in SGS. In patients requiring intubation for other purposes, GERD-induced airway damage has been shown to be a complicating factor.[19]

Intubation. Endotracheal intubation has become more prevalent in recent years, especially in the neonatal population, and represents an important consideration for the development of upper airway complications. Endotracheal tubes can compress the epithelial and laminar layers against the more rigid cartilage, impairing capillary perfusion and causing ischemia. In addition, continual motion owing to normal breathing can erode the mucosa, resulting in the formation of ulcers. Prolonged intubation is thought to lead to edema and hyperemia, erosion, and necrosis of the mucosa and eventually erosion of the underlying perichondrium. Colonization by pathogenic microorganisms can worsen the mucosal damage resulting from physical injury. The presence of *Neisseria*, *Streptococcus*, *Staphylococcus*, and *Pseudomonas*, along with *Candida* species, has been documented on both the internal and external surfaces of endotracheal tubes.[20] Scanning electron microscopic analysis of endotracheal tube surfaces has indicated the presence of biofilms, an adherent, metabolically less active bacterial phenotype, which may account for the antibiotic resistance of some of these microorganisms.[21] The colonization of injured airway mucosa by active pathogens can continually stimulate the inflammatory or immune response and contribute to excessive fibrosis.

Surgical Wounds. Endotracheal intubation injures the tracheal and subglottic mucosa through an iterative series of small injuries. In contrast, surgical interventions in the upper airway result in acute damage to subglottic and tracheal structures. Incisional damage to the mucosa is an intrinsic component of procedures such as lung transplantation, laryngeal or tracheal reconstruction, tracheostomy, and/or anastomosis. In addition to the immediate risk of restenosis, the long-term outcomes of extensive airway reconstruction leave a lot to be desired with respect to both dysphonia and stridor.[22]

Studies addressing the risk of stenosis following surgical manipulation are largely anecdotal and retrospective. Fortunately, multiple animal models exist that have been used to document the extent of SGS induced by cold steel damage.[23]

In addition to cold steel, the upper airway mucosa is often injured by lasers used for the removal of airway lesions, including amyloid deposits, hemangiomas, or previous fibrotic tissue. In particular, treatment of airway hemangiomas requires the use of CO_2 lasers. Airway hemangiomas display rapid growth during the first few months after birth but regress in the following 2 years, showing a high although variable degree of overall resolution. Management of hemangiomas can be done either by bypassing the obstruction temporarily or by treating or removing the obstruction surgically. The use of lasers results in resolution of hemangiomas but may also induce subsequent, irreversible and possibly morbid stenosis of the trachea and/or subglottis.[24,25] Although laser use causes damage to the airway mucosa, it can also be used to halt the progression of stenosis by stabilizing scar formation through a process that remains unclear. As such, repetitive CO_2 laser treatment has been used for management of intubation-induced stenosis in combination with stenting.[26] Again, the danger in adopting this approach is worsening (ie, deepening) the injury. Although short-term increases in the diameter of the lumen may be achieved, it is often at the expense of long-term compromise of the lumen. Lasers have also been used during laryngotracheoplasty to improve the interlocking of graft and adjacent normal tissue and improve integrity across the margin between graft and normal tissue.[27] This spotty "welding" application is less likely to complicate long-term results.

Spontaneous Injury. Head and neck trauma can result in extensive damage to the upper airway, along with surrounding structures. Although the most prominent symptoms are dyspnea or stridor, subcutaneous emphysema, and pneumothorax, the development of upper airway stenosis has been reported.[28] In extreme cases, combined tracheal and esophageal injuries can result in severe stenosis of both structures with formation of tracheoesophageal fistulae.[29] However, since stenosis can present clinically long after the initial injury, it is difficult to determine whether it resulted from trauma or subsequent iatrogenic interventions, such as surgical manipulation of the damaged airway.[30] In the neonatal population, there have been several reported cases of spontaneous subglottic or trachea rupture following a complicated vaginal delivery.[31] Although these cases are rare, they present with significant mortality and morbidity.

Idiopathic SGS. Idiopathic SGS is seldom encountered and has no clearly identified cause. Although some studies have linked it to a hormonal etiology, owing to its almost exclusive prevalence in female patients, no association with WG or other systemic diseases has been found.[32] Some idiopathic SGS patients have been found to exhibit acidic laryngeal secretions, despite treatment with proton pump inhibitors.[33] The presence of reflux as demonstrated by acidic secretions has been postulated as a possible cause for the idiopathic cases of SGS. The primary challenge associated with idiopathic SGS is that it is often progressive and incurable. Surgical treatment, regardless of the method, often results in recurrence of mucosal fibrosis. Histologically, idiopathic SGS is dominated by subglottic mucosal fibrosis and a continual excessive inflammatory infiltrate, which may account for continuous stimulation of fibrotic processes.[34]

The clinically relevant injury mechanisms discussed in this section are summarized in Table 1, along with the extent of subsequent mucosal injury and relative risk of SGS development.

Extent of Injury Dictates Subsequent Wound Healing

The above-described congenital or acquired mechanisms result in varying degrees of damage to the trachea and subglottis. Chronic conditions with airway involvement generally damage the epithelial and lamina propria layers. Intubation damage involves primarily ulceration of the

Table 1. SUMMARY OF CLINICALLY RELEVANT MUCOSAL INJURIES AND SUBSEQUENT TISSUE DAMAGE

SGS Cause	Extent of Injury	Risk of SGS
Congenital malformation	3	High
Systemic disease	2	Low
Intubation, repetitive injury	2	Medium
Intubation, superficial injury	1	Low
Surgical intervention	3	Medium
Spontaneous injury	3	Medium
Idiopathic SGS	4	Unknown

SGS = subglottic stenosis.
1 = epithelial damage only; 2 = epithelial and lamina propria damage; 3 = full-thickness damage (includes cartilage); 4 = variable damage.

epithelium with secondary damage to the underlying lamina propria and cartilage by both erosion and necrosis secondary to ischemia. Surgical manipulation and laser instrumentation of the upper airway create varying degrees of damage and are sometimes accompanied by manipulation of the overlying muscle and fascia layers, creating a significant risk of impaired blood supply to the airway mucosa.

Anecdotal evidence in various patient populations has been supplemented by multiple animal studies demonstrating that the degree and type of injury dictate the subsequent degree of airway scarring or fibrosis.[35] More specifically, in the case of acquired SGS, the depth of injury is thought to correlate with the extent of long-term stenosis. As such, it is an important indication that any type of surgical injury to the upper airway mucosa, regardless of the extent, will cause a certain degree of stenosis. These data have been further confirmed by recent animal studies, which have demonstrated that the depth of penetrating injury into the underlying cartilage is an important predictor of long-term healing outcome, with complete cartilage resection making regeneration improbable.[36,37]

Wound Healing Response

Epithelium. Epithelial function is often disturbed by damage to the mucosal layer, more so than the other two layers. Even introduction

of allergens in the upper airway has been shown to induce focal sites of epithelial damage and inflammatory infiltrate.[38] Other noxious stimuli, including cigarette smoke, can cause up-regulation of a variety of gene products within the epithelial and lamina propria layers of the trachea, including collagen. Activation of ECM-related genes is thought to occur through multiple mechanisms, such as epidermal growth factor receptor and nuclear factor κB signaling.[39]

Buckling of the overlying cartilaginous layer subsequent to smooth muscle contraction during asthma attacks can exert small but significant forces on the luminal epithelium. Transmembrane pressure changes can then trigger induction of multiple epithelial gene products, including early growth response 1 and TGF-β_1.[40] Following endotracheal intubation, tracheal and subglottic epithelium may be lost within hours, resulting in ulceration and continual damage to the underlying lamina propria. When reepithelialization is not impaired by secondary causes, ulcer repair is rapid and often complete by 30 days' postinjury, indicating that epithelial damage alone does not result in compromising long-term stenosis.[41]

Extensive experience with lung transplantation has revealed that significant epithelial damage can occur in response to endogenous inflammation. Lung transplantation resulting in chronic rejection manifests with obliterative bronchiolitis, primarily represented by epithelial damage.[42] This occurs via complex interactions between inflammatory cells, fibroblasts, and epithelial cells modulated by cytokines and growth factors. Following transplantation, sites of anastomosis are reepithelialized with cells primarily of host origin. Mechanisms of epithelial layer regeneration include migration of the tracheal basal cells from the wound margin followed by proliferation and differentiation into ciliated epithelium.[1] In immunosuppressed hosts, reepithelialization and differentiation occur faster than in their nonimmunosuppressed counterparts, indicating that reepithelialization can be negatively impacted by excessive inflammation. In general, studies of upper airway epithelial repair are difficult and often require extensive animal modeling. Mathematical models may also be highly useful by taking into account multiple variables such as cell spreading, migration, and mitosis in a dynamic model that includes tensile changes on the entire structure, as would be encountered at sites of anastomosis.[44]

Lamina Propria. More extensive mucosal damage often results in disturbance of the lamina propria layer, resulting in fibroblast activation. Excessive fibroblast activity can result in scarring and stenosis, whereas impaired fibroblast activity results in insufficiency of connective tissue repair. Therefore, it must be closely regulated by endogenous factors such as TGF-β_1, a well-characterized master regulator of wound healing in many tissue types. TGF-β_1 has been shown to stimulate conversion of tracheal fibroblasts into myofibroblasts, which are generally associated with wound contraction and increased ECM deposition. The conversion of fibroblasts to myofibroblasts can also be stimulated by the presence of gastric juice, indicating a possible mechanism of GERD-induced SGS formation.[45] Although tracheal fibroblasts share some phenotypic similarities with fibroblasts derived from other tissue types, their precise profile remains poorly characterized. In vitro analysis of expression profiles for multiple ECM component genes in tracheal scar fibroblasts revealed varied expression across isolates and cell passages, although karyotypic stability was high.[46] In vivo, fibroblasts are responsible for both ECM deposition and remodeling activities, which are largely dependent on matrix metalloproteinases (MMPs). During tracheal repair, MMP-2, along with its membrane-bound activator membrane type 1 matrix metalloproteinase (MT1-MMP), is thought to play a major role in ECM reconstruction.[47]

Although fibroblast activation following injury is crucial to mucosal repair, excessive fibroplasia and ECM deposition can result in scar formation, thickening of the lamina propria, and subsequent impairment of airflow. These effects can be contained in both experimental and clinical settings using exogenous antifibrotic or antiproliferative agents. In this group, mitomycin C has been employed to regulate ECM deposition following mucosal injury, with good short-term resolution without restenosis and stridor.[48,49] Additional studies have indicated that such agents can also impair other aspects of mucosal wound healing, such as reepithelialization, wound contraction, and angiogenesis. Other pharmacologic agents, such as rapamycin, have similar effects on tracheal repair.[50,51] In spite of these ostensible therapeutic benefits, safety remains a significant concern and is unproven in children.

Cartilage. Cartilage is the outermost component of the upper airway wall whose function is to provide structural support for the epithelial and lamina propria layers. Cartilage damage is associated with extensive airway injury and results in dramatic alterations in overall airway structure and function. Early studies indicated that extensive cartilage damage is a significant component of persistent SGS, underlying extensive mucosal fibrosis.[52] Damage to the cartilage layer of the trachea compromises its structural properties. This can occur either by direct damage to the perichodrium or indirect damage to the entire cartilage layer following interruption of the vascular supply.

Multiple animal studies have documented the mechanisms of cartilage repair subsequent to injury. Age appears to be an important factor in determining the extent of cartilage repair.[39,40] Early in the repair process, cartilage is replaced by a less differentiated fibrotic tissue following intracartilaginous injury, regardless of age. However, in younger animals, incomplete cartilage damage is completely repaired, although the overall tracheal structure is altered, indicating that young cartilage is constantly being remodeled and that the supracartilaginous structures can alter the structure and function of the cartilage. In adult animals, extensive remodeling of the cartilage does not occur, indicating possible loss of chondrocyte reparative capacity with age progression. Penetration of the perichondrial layer has been shown to be an important component of cartilage damage, leading to significant chronic stenosis. Reactions of the damaged cartilage include thickening by chondroneogenesis on the internal surface, loss of perichondrium and cartilage, conversion to fibrotic tissue, formation of new hyaline cartilage on the exterior surface, and thickening of the entire cartilage layer.[53]

Cartilage healing is largely dependent on synthesis, deposition, and remodeling of ECM components. Analysis of stenotic segments of the upper airway indicates that there is preferential loss of collagen type I and aggrecan in areas of maximal damage, whereas collagen II expression is generally constant. Cartilage regeneration can be observed and identified by relative increased collagen II and aggrecan expression in areas of repair. Cartilage deposition and repair are dependent on chondrocyte activity. This activity is partially intrinsic and partially dictated by soluble mediators and other cell types. The precise phenotypes of tracheal chondrocytes have not been completely defined, but studies of tracheal reconstruction demonstrate that at least part of their secretory activity is similar to that of other chondrocytes. Chondrocytes isolated from both trachea and nasal septum, grown on artificial matrices and implanted subcutaneously, result in structures with hydroxyproline and glycosaminoglycan content similar to that of native trachea.[54] Chondrocyte activity is not completely intrinsic and is partially dictated by the other cell types involved in repair and soluble factors. When chondrocytes are seeded onto polyglycolic acid meshes, covered with a fibroblast-seeded mesh and implanted subcutaneously as bioengineered tracheas, they can grow and mature in vivo, exhibiting morphology similar to that of native cartilage. Appropriate cartilage repair is important to other healing processes that occur following tracheal injury.[55,56] Activated chondrocytes can secrete a variety of factors, including MMP-2 and MMP-9.[57] These enzymes play an important role not only in ECM reconstruction and reorganization but also in regulating the activity of overlying epithelial cells, specifically epithelial cell attachment and proliferation.

Cartilage regeneration subsequent to trauma has been generally considered to be an unlikely possibility. However, it has been demonstrated that application of exogenous growth factors, such as bone morphogenetic protein (BMP)-2, may result in active cartilage remodeling and regrowth. Specifically, exogenous BMP-2 can cause extensive epithelial and cartilage regeneration and integration into the uninjured wound margins.[58,59]

Coordination of Cell Activity via Soluble Mediators

Cell activity in any wound bed is coordinated by interactions with the ECM, cell–cell contacts, and secretion of soluble mediators, including cytokines, chemokines, and growth factors (Table 2). Cytokines and chemokines are an integral part of the inflammatory response that accompanies wound healing and can thus function to provide an insight into the potential course of the healing process. Multiple studies have demonstrated that soluble inflammatory mediators, such as interleukin (IL)-1, IL-6, IL-8, and IL-10, play an important role in dictating the overall outcome of wound healing in other tissue types.[60–62] Although the inflammatory reaction to injury has been well defined in the lower airway, it remains less well characterized in the tracheal mucosa. However, it is relatively clear that inflammatory cell invasion of the airway wound bed occurs through inflammatory mediators released by the endogenous epithelial cells. Alterations in the soluble cytokine or chemokine environment subsequent to mucosal damage have been shown to trigger increases in receptors for adhesive glycoproteins expressed on the surface of neutrophils, specifically intercellular adhesion molecule 1.[63]

Minimally invasive methods for continual upper airway secretion sampling are being developed.[64] These methods can be used to analyze mucosal secretions for the presence of proinflammatory mediators, including IL-1β and prostaglandin E_2 (PGE_2). Data indicate that

Table 2. ROLES OF CELLS, SOLUBLE MEDIATORS, AND EXTRACELLULAR MATRIX COMPONENTS DURING MUCOSAL WOUND HEALING

Component	Component Type	Role during Mucosal Repair
Epithelial cells	1	Restore barrier function
Fibroblasts	1	ECM synthesis/ remodeling
Chondrocytes	1	Repair cartilage
Macrophages	1	Débridement
Neutrophils	1	Débridement
Endothelial cells	1	Restore vascularity
TGF-β1	2	Pro fibrotic; stimulates ECM production
TGF-β_3	2	Antifibrotic; reduces ECM production
VEGF	2	Revascularization
bFGF	2	Revascularization
KGF	2	Regulates epithelial cell activity
BMP-2	2	Cartilage repair; coordinates cell activity
IL-1β	3	Coordinates inflammation
PGE$_2$	3	Coordinates inflammation
iNOS	3	Coordinates inflammation
Collagen	4	Regain of structure
Glycosaminoglycan	4	Tissue rehydration

bFGF = basic fibroblast growth factor; BMP = bone morphogenetic protein; ECM = extracellular matrix; IL = interleukin; iNOS = inducible nitric oxide synthase; KGF = keratinocyte growth factor; TGF = transforming growth factor; PG = prostaglandin; VEGF = vascular endothelial growth factor.
1 = cell; 2 = growth factor; 3 = inflammatory mediator; 4 = ECM component.

both mediators are detectable in mucosal secretions and appear to correlate with the progression and resolution of the mucosal wound healing response. Activation of IL-1β during subglottic mucosal injury is important in that IL-1β has been shown to act as an early master coordinator of inflammation with significant effects on downstream targets, such as PGE$_2$, IL-6, and IL-8. Activation of these pathways can subsequently alter the physiologic parameters of the upper airway. Specifically, IL-1β up-regulation of cyclooxygenase 2 activity and PGE$_2$ secretion can increase mucin gene expression and protein secretion by epithelial cells.[65] Endogenous PGE$_2$ production is also thought to play a role in regulating the effects of

hyperoxic injury to the tracheal epithelium through mechanisms that remain unclear.[66]

Another important inflammatory pathway, revolving around nitric oxide, has also been implicated in upper airway repair. Specifically, inducible nitric oxide synthase has been shown to be an important factor in the inflammatory response to tracheal allograft transplantation and to be responsible for the expression of proinflammatory cytokines and chemokines.[67] Together, these alterations in the inflammatory or immune response to injury can change the degree of airway scarring subsequent to injury.

Growth factors have long been known to coordinate the wound healing process in concert with cytokines and other soluble mediators. Two approaches have been used to more precisely elucidate the role of growth factors in upper airway wound healing: analysis of endogenous growth factor activation following mucosal injury and alterations in the native wound healing response subsequent to administration of exogenous growth factors. In other tissue types, TGF-β_1 has been identified as an early master regulator of mucosal wound healing. Evidence detailed above has demonstrated a role for TGF-β_1 regulation of fibroblast activity following injury of the subglottic mucosa.[48] TGF-β_1 signaling occurs primarily by closely regulated paracrine signaling. In an experimental setting, the presence of tracheal chondrocytes can dramatically alter not only morphologic and functional parameters of airway epithelial cells but also the expression profile of epithelium-derived soluble mediators TGF-α and TGF-β.[68] Whereas TGF-β_1 is generally considered to be a profibrotic factor, another isoform, TGF-β_3, is thought to be antifibrotic. In the airway mucosa, a role for TGF-β_3 has been implicated in the coordination between the epithelial and lamina propria layers. Exogenous TGF-β_3 can accelerate the rate of reepithelialization and connective tissue formation.[69]

The activation of endogenous growth factors following mucosal injury correlates with the type and extent of injury. Keratinocyte growth factor (KGF) has been shown to play an important role during wound healing by regulating the migratory and mitotic rates of epithelial cells. Following upper airway injury, KGF expression is up-regulated in a manner largely dependent on disruption of the basal membrane. Suprabasal exfoliation, unlike complete epithelial denudation, does not trigger KGF up-regulation.[70]

Proper mucosal wound repair necessitates revascularization of the injured tissue. Like other processes, this is growth factor dependent.[71] Treatment of tracheal injury with exogenous vascular endothelial growth factor (VEGF) can increase the mean vascular density early in the repair process and decrease inflammation (lymphocytes and eosinophils), fibrosis, and subsequent airway stenosis. Although the underlying cartilage layer is not affected by exogenous VEGF administration, the rate and degree of reepithelialization subsequent to injury can be increased, improving overall wound healing outcomes.[72] VEGF is not the only growth factor with vasculogenic potential.[73] Basic fibroblast growth factor (bFGF) has also been targeted as a promoter of angiogenesis to enhance the vascularization of tracheal transplantation. Although it was found that allogeneic devascularized tracheal grafts cannot maintain integrity and display graft necrosis, with loss of epithelium and cartilage along with excessive inflammation, administration of exogenous growth factors such as bFGF or surgical vascularization (omental wraps) was shown to significantly improve graft survival and overall quality by increasing vascularity.

Future Promise for Healing

Wound healing is a complex process whose ultimate goal is to restore the original tissue structure and function. As such, it is largely dependent on the functional requirements of the original tissue. In the case of the upper airway, the desirability of mucosal wound healing outcomes can be judged in relation to three overriding functional parameters: (1) maintainance of a patent lumen, which allows for unimpeded airflow; (2) maintenance of a semirigid structure that remains patent under pressure from surrounding muscular and fascial layers; and (3) a high degree of interdigitation of injured tissue and normal margins, resulting in a continuous airway. Damage to the airway, whether resulting from intubation, surgical manipulation, or systemic disease, normally impairs all three functional parameters. Damage to the laminar layer of the mucosa stimulates fibroblast activity, causing fibrosis and thickening of the layer, restricting the diameter of the lumen. Incisions or trauma to the perichondrium or the whole cartilage layer results in replacement of the existing structure with a scar owing to the inability of adult cartilage to regenerate. Finally, natural or surgical anastomosis sites are generally considered to be largely compromised tissue regions at risk of dehiscence and other morbidities.

Multiple approaches are currently under way to serve as adjuncts to the normal wound healing process and provide improved function. Pharmacologic approaches can be used to modulate fibroblast activity in the wound bed. As previously mentioned,[51,52] antiproliferative agents, such as mitomycin C, can control fibroplasia in the context of mucosal repair to varying degrees. The primary function of fibroblasts is to secrete and organize collagen fibers in a replacement ECM. As such, scar formation can be reduced using pharmacologic agents that inhibit ECM deposition. Lathyrogens interfere with the deposition and cross-linking of collagen fibers, which is essential for creating a mature scar.[74] Administration of exogenous TGF-β_1 increases fibroblast ECM deposition during SGS formation. In contrast, antibodies that neutralize endogenous TGF-β_1 activity can dramatically reduce the degree of scarring or stenosis.[75]

Although fibroplasia can be tolerated in the lamina propria, it is extremely compromising in the cartilage layer. Replacement of tracheal cartilage by fibrotic tissue subsequent to injury greatly jeopardizes structural integrity. Therefore, efforts to completely engineer tracheal structures are receiving a lot of attention. Mature chondrocytes can be seeded onto a synthetic mesh and, following subcutaneous implantation, create a tubular structure with a patent lumen, consisting of collagen and glycosaminoglycans in ratios similar to that of endogenous trachea.[57–59] Addition of fibroblasts to the tracheal construct can increase the fidelity of the tissue engineering outcome as it relates to the native tissue with respect to ECM content and organization. Engineering of an intact, functional epithelium has been attempted using tracheal epithelial cells cultured on scaffolds (hyaluronic acid, collagen, and others), which allowed for cell attachment and spreading and differentiation into ciliated secretory epithelium.[76] Survival of these engineered structures once anastomosed to the normal tissue is highly dependent on proper revascularization, which remains a difficult undertaking.[77]

Recent advances in stem cell biology have opened the door for additional tissue engineering constructs that more closely resemble the native tissue. Bone marrow–derived multipotential cells were seeded onto polyglycolic acid meshes and guided in vitro using TGF-β_1 and insulin-like growth factor 1 prior to implantation into hosts; this resulted in constructs resembling native trachea, with mature cartilage containing glycosaminoglycans and collagen fibers.[59]

Fetal Wound Healing: Natural Variant of Mucosal Repair

Mucosal wound healing in the adult upper airway is a reparative process that only approximates by does not recapitulate the initial structure and function. In contrast, fetal mucosal wound healing is a regenerative process in which regeneration of the multilayered structure is flawless and indistinguishable from the uninjured tissue. This phenomenon is species, tissue, and time dependent. The fetal airway mucosal wound healing phenotype has been described in the last few years.[78,79] Whereas adult subglottic wounds heal with scar formation and induction of chronic stenosis, fetal wounds heal in a regenerative manner. Histologic analysis of healed fetal airways reveals complete reconstitution of

the trilaminar structure, with restoration of functional status. These data correlate with long-standing animal studies of fetal dermal wound healing, suggesting that there is a gestational transition from regenerative to reparative wound healing. Additional work is ongoing to correlate the functional requirements of the fetal upper airway with its distinct wound healing phenotype.[80]

SUMMARY

Upper airway wound healing is a complex process that remains incompletely understood. Recent work demonstrated that repair of injured tracheal mucosa requires a carefully coordinated response by epithelial cells, fibroblasts, and chondrocytes, guided by inflammatory mediators and growth factors. Minimizing mucosal scarring subsequent to injury will continue to be a challenge for clinicians and researchers alike. Current approaches that modulate cell and growth factor activity have shown promise in improving healing outcome and decreasing impairment of airflow. Tissue engineering approaches are under development. Detailed studies of fetal mucosal wound healing may provide further clues as to the primary factors responsible for regenerative healing that may be applicable for controlling the degree of mucosal scar formation and stenosis.

REFERENCES

1. Seymour AH, Prakash N. A cadaver study to measure the adult glottis and subglottis: defining a problem associated with the use of double-lumen tubes. J Cardiothorac Vasc Anesth 2002;16:196–8.
2. Seiden AM, Tami TA, Pensak ML, et al. Otolaryngology: the essentials. New York: Thieme; 2002.
3. Kusafuka K, Yamaguchi A, Kayano T, et al. Ossification of tracheal cartilage in aged humans: a histological and immunohistochemical analysis. J Bone Miner Metab 2001;19:168–74.
4. Lee SY, Yeh TH, Lou PJ, et al. Mucociliary transport pathway on laryngotracheal tract and stented glottis in guinea pigs. Ann Otol Rhinol Laryngol 2002;109:210–5.
5. Melgarejo-Moreno P, Hellin-Meseguer D. Different glycoconjugates in the submucosal glands of the supra-

glottis and subglottis. Lectin histochemistry study in the hamster. J Laryngol Otol 1997;111:441–3.

6. Hockstein NG, McDonald-McGinn D, Zackai E, et al. Tracheal anomalis in Pfeiffer syndrome. Arch Otolaryngol Head Neck Surg 2004;130:1298–302.

7. Mathijssen IM, Vaandrager JM, Hoogeboom, et al. Pfeiffer's syndrome resulting from an S351C mutation in the fibroblast growth factor receptor-2 gene. J Craniofac Surg 1998;9:207–9.

8. Spilde TL, Bhatia AM, Marosky JK, et al. Fibroblast growth factor signaling in the developing tracheoesophageal fistula. J Pediatr Surg 2003;38:474–7.

9. Boube M, Llimargas M, Casanova J. Cross- regulatory interactions among tracheal genes support a co-operative model for the induction of tracheal fates in the Drosophila embryo. Mech Dev 2000;91:271–8.

10. Evans MJ, Fanucchie MV, Van Winkle LS, et al. Fibroblast growth factor-2 during postnatal development of the tracheal basement membrane zone. Am J Physiol Lung Cell Mol Physiol 2002;283:L1263–70.

11. Evans MJ, Van Winkle LS, Fanucchi MV, et al. Fibroblast growth factor-2 in remodeling of the developing basement membrane zone in the trachea of infant rhesus monkeys sensitized and challenged with allergen. Lab Invest 2002;82:1747–54.

12. Pena J, Cicero R, Marin J, et al. Laryngotracheal reconstruction in subglottic stenosis: an ancient problem still present. Otolaryngol Head Neck Surg 2001;125:397–400.

13. Grillo HC. Primary reconstruction of airway after resection of subglottic laryngeal and upper tracheal stenosis. Ann Thorac Surg 1982;33:3–18.

14. Naef AP, Savary M, Gruneck JM, et al. Amyloid pseudotumor treated by tracheal resection. Ann Thorac Surg 1977;23:578–81.

15. Fukumura M, Mieno T, Suzuki T, et al. Primary diffuse tracheobronchial amyloidosis treated by bronchoscopic Nd-YAG laser irradiation. Jpn J Med 1990;29:620–2.

16. McPherson JG, Yeoh CB. Rare manifestations of sacroidosis. J Natl Med Assoc 1993;85:869–72.

17. Gluth MB, Shinners PA, Kasperbauer JL. Subglottic stenosis associated with Wegener's granulomatosis. Laryngoscope 2003;113:1304–7.

18. Gilger MA. Pediatric otolaryngologic manifestations of gastroesophageal reflux disease. Curr Gastroenterol Rep 2003;5:247–52.

19. Cantillo J, Cypel D, Schaffer SR, et al. Difficult intubation from gastroesophageal reflux disease in adults. J Clin Anesth 1998;10:235–7.

20. Brown OE, Manning SC. Microbial flora of the subglottis in intubated pediatric patients. Int J Pediatr Otorhinolaryngol 1996;35:97–105.

21. Zur KB, Mandell DL, Gordon RE, et al. Electron microscopic analysis of biofilm on endotracheal tubes removed from intubated neonates. Otolaryngol Head Neck Surg 2004;130:407–14.

22. Monnier P, Savary M, Chapuis G. Partial cricoid resection with primary tracheal anastomosis for subglottic stenosis in infants and children. Laryngoscope 1993;103(11 Pt 1):1273–83.

23. Mitskavich MT, Rimell FL, Shapiro AM. Porcine model of airway mucosal injury. Am J Otolaryngol 1997;18:315–9.

24. Cotton RT, Tewfik TL. Laryngeal stenosis following carbon dioxide laser in subglottic hemangioma. Report of three cases. Ann Otol Rhinol Laryngol 1985;94(5 Pt 1):494–7.

25. Naiman AN, Ayari S, Froehlich P. Controlled risk of stenosis after surgical excision of laryngeal hemangioma. Arch Otolaryngol Head Neck Surg 2003;129:1291–5.

26. Whitehead E, Salam MA. Use of the carbon dioxide laser with the Montgomery T-tube in the management of extensive subglottic stenosis. J Laryngol Otol 1992;106:829–31.

27. Wang Z, Volk MS, Shapshay SM. Endoscopic laryngotracheoplasty and graft soldering with the carbon dioxide laser. An animal study. Ann Otol Rhinol Laryngol 1997;106:989–94.

28. Balci AE, Eren N, Eren S, et al. Surgical treatment of post-traumatic tracheobronchial injuries: 14-year experience. Eur J Cardiothorac Surg 2002;22:984–9.

29. Sokolov VV, Bagirov MM. Reconstructive surgery for combined tracheo-esophageal injuries and their sequelae. Eur J Cardiothorac Surg 2001;20:1025–9.

30. Feat S, Le Clech G, Riffaud L, et al. Complete cervical tracheal rupture in children after closed trauma. J Pediatr Surg 2002;37:E39.

31. Kacmarynski DS, Sidman JD, Rimell FL, et al. Spontaneous tracheal and subglottic tears in neonates. Laryngoscope 2002;112(8 Pt 1):1387–93.

32. Lorenz RR. Adult laryngotracheal stenosis: etiology and surgical management. Curr Opin Otolaryngol Head Neck Surg 2003;11:467–72.

33. Maronian NC, Azadeh H, Waugh P, et al. Association of laryngopharyngeal reflux disease and subglottic stenosis. Ann Otol Rhinol Laryngol 2001;110(7 Pt 1):606–12.

34. Dedo HH, Catten MD. Idiopathic progressive subglottic stenosis: findings and treatment in 52 patients. Ann Otol Rhinol Laryngol 2001;110:305–11.

35. Dohar JE, Klein EC, Betsch JL, et al. Aquired subglottic stenosis-depth and not extent of the insult is key. J Pediatr Otorhinolaryngol 1998;46:159–70.

36. Mankarious LA, Cherukupally SR, Adams AB. Gross and histologic changes in the developing rabbit subglottis in response to a controlled depth of injury. Otolaryngol Head Neck Surg 2002;127:442–7.

37. Mankarious LA, Adams AB, Pires VL. Patterns of cartilage structural protein loss in human tracheal stenosis. Laryngoscope 2002;112:1025–30.

38. Erjefalt JS, Korsgren M, Nilsson MC, et al. Prompt epithelial damage and restitution processes in allergen challenged guinea-pig trachea in vivo. Clin Exp Allergy 1997;27:1458–70.

39. Wang RD, Tai H, Xie C, et al. Cigarette smoke produces airway wall remodelling in rat tracheal explants. Am J Respir Crit Care Med 2003;168:1232–6.

40. Ressler B, Lee RT, Randell SH, et al. Molecular responses of rat tracheal epithelial cells to transmembrane pressure. Am J Physiol Lung Cell Mol Physiol 2000;278:L1264–72.

41. Gould SJ, Young M. Subglottic ulceration and healing following endotracheal intubation in the neonate: a morphometric study. Ann Otol Rhinol Laryngol 1992;101:815–20.

42. Ikonen TS, Brazelton TR, Berry GJ, et al. Epithelial re-growth is associated with inhibition of obliterative airway disease in orthotopic tracheal allografts in non-immunosuppressed rats. Transplantation 2000;70:857–63.

43. Genden EM, Iskander A, Bromberg JS, et al. The kinetics and pattern of tracheal allograft re-epithelialization. Am J Respir Cell Mol Biol 2003;28:673–81.

44. Savla U, Olson LE, Waters CM. Mathematical modeling of airway epithelial wound closure during cyclic mechanical strain. J Appl Physiol 2004;96:566–74.

45. Jarmuz T, Rivera H, Roser S. Transforming growth factor β-1, myofibroblasts, and tissue remodeling in the pathogenesis of tracheal injury: potential role of gastroesophageal reflux. Ann Otol Rhinol Laryngol 2004;113:488–97.

46. Thibeault SL, Li W, Gray SD, et al. Instability of extracellular matrix gene expression in primary cell culture of fibroblasts from human vocal fold lamina propria and tracheal scar. Ann Otol Rhinol Laryngol 2002;111:8–14.

47. Inaki N, Tsunezuka Y, Kawakami K, et al. Increased matrix metalloproteinase-2 and membrane type 1 matrix metalloproteinase activity and expression in heterotopically transplanted murine tracheas. J Heart Lung Transplant 2004;23:218–27.

48. Rahbar R, Valdez TA, Shapshay SM. Preliminary results of intraoperative mitomycin-C in the treatment and prevention of glottic and subglottic stenosis. J Voice 2000;14:282–6.

49. Correa AJ, Reinisch L, Sanders DL, et al. Inhibition of subglottic stenosis with mitomycin-C in the canine model. Ann Otol Rhinol Laryngol 1999;108(11 Pt 1):1053–60.

50. Hardillo J, Vanclooster C, Delaere PR. An investigation of airway wound healing using a novel in vivo model. Laryngoscope 2001;111:1174–82.

51. Dutly AE, Gaspert A, Inci I, et al. The influence of the rapamycin-derivate SDZ RAD on the healing of airway anastomoses. Eur J Cardiothorac Surg 2003;24:154–8, discussion 158.

52. Gould SJ, Graham J. Long term pathological sequelae of neonatal endotracheal intubation. J Laryngol Otol 1989;103:622–5.

53. Bean JK, Verwoerd-Verhoef HL, Verwoerd CD. Injury- and age-linked differences in wound healing and stenosis formation in the subglottis. Acta Otolaryngol (Stockh) 1995;115:317–21.

54. Kojima K, Bonassar LJ, Ignotz RA, et al. Comparison of tracheal and nasal chondrocytes for tissue engineering of the trachea. Ann Thorac Surg 2003;76:1884–8.

55. Kojima K, Bonassar LJ, Roy AK, et al. Autologous tissue-engineered trachea with sheep nasal chondrocytes. J Thorac Cardiovasc Surg 2002;123:1177–84.

56. Kojima K, Ignotz RA, Kushibiki T, et al. Tissue-engineered trachea from sheep marrow stromal cells with transforming growth factor beta2 released from biodegradable microspheres in a nude rat recipient. J Thorac Cardiovasc Surg 2004;128:147–53.

57. Sigurdson L, Sen T, Hall L, et al. Possible impedance of luminal reepithelialization by tracheal cartilage metal-loproteinases. Arch Otolaryngol Head Neck Surg 2003;129:197–200.

58. Tcacencu I, Carlsoo B, Stierna P. Structural characteristics of repair tissue of cricoid cartilage defects treated with recombinant human bone morphogenetic protein-2. Wound Repair Regen 2004;12:346–50.

59. Okamoto T, Yamamoto Y, Gotoh M, et al. Slow release of bone morphogenetic protein 2 from a gelatin sponge to promote regeneration of tracheal cartilage in a canine model. J Thorac Cardiovasc Surg 2004;127:329–34.

60. Liechty KW, Adzick NS, Crombleholme TM. Diminished interleukin-6 (IL-6) production during scarless human fetal wound healing. Cytokine 2000;12:671–6.

61. Liechty KW, Crombleholme TM, Cass DL, et al. Diminished interleukin-8 (IL-8) production in the fetal wound healing response. J Surg Res 1998;77:80–4.

62. Liechty KW, Kim HB, Adzick NS, Crombleholme TM. Fetal wound repair results in scar formation in interleukin-10-deficient mice in a syngeneic murine model of scarless fetal wound repair. J Pediatr Surg 2000;35:866–72.

63. Tosi MF, Stark JM, Smith CW, et al. Induction of ICAM-1 expression on human airways epithelial cells by inflammatory cytokines: effects on neutrophil-epithelial cell adhesion. Am J Respir Cell Mol Biol 1992;7:214–21.

64. Branski RC, Sandulache VC, Dohar JE, Hebda PA. Mucosal wound healing in a rabbit model of subglottic stenosis: biochemical analysis of secretions. Arch Otolaryngol Head Neck Surg 2005;131:153–7.

65. Gray T, Nettesheim P, Loftin C, et al. Interleukin-1b-induced mucin production in human airway epithelium is mediated by cyclooxygenase-2, prostaglandin E2 receptors, and cyclic AMP-protein kinase A signaling. Mol Pharmacol 2004;66:337–46.

66. Dennery PA, Walenga RW, Kramer CM, Alpert SE. Prostaglandin E2 attenuates hyperoxia-induced injury in cultured rabbit tracheal epithelial cells. Pediatr Res 1992;32:87–91.

67. Minamoto K, Pinsky DJ. Recipient iNOS but not eNOS deficiency reduces luminal narrowing in tracheal allografts. J Exp Med 2002;196:1321–33.

68. Hicks W, Sigurdson L, Gabalski E, et al. Does cartilage down-regulate growth factor expression in tracheal epithelium? Arch Otolaryngol Head Neck Surg 1999;125:1239–43.

69. Loewen MS, Walner DL, Caldarelli DD. Improved airway healing using transforming growth factor beta-3 in a rabbit model. Wound Repair Regen 2001;9:44–9.

70. Hicks WL. Increased expression of keratinocyte growth factor represents a stereotypic response to tracheal lumenal insult independent of injury mechanism. Laryngoscope 1999;109:1552–9.

71. Dodge-Khatami A, Backer CL, Holinger LD, et al. Healing of a free tracheal autograft is enhanced by topical vascular endothelial growth factor in an experimental rabbit model. J Thorac Cardiovasc Surg 2001;122:554–61.

72. Govindaraj S, Goron R, Genden EM. Effect of fibrin matrix and vascular endothelial growth factor on reepithelialization of orthotopic murine tracheal transplants. Ann Otol Rhinol Laryngol 2004;113:797–804.

73. Nakanishi R, Hashimoto M, Yasumoto K. Improved airway healing using basic fibroblast growth factor in a canine tracheal autotransplantation model. Ann Surg 1998;227:446–54.

74. Doolin EJ, Tsuno K, Strande LF, et al. Pharmacologic inhibition of collagen in an experimental model of subglottic stenosis. Ann Otol Rhinol Laryngol 1998; 107:275–9.

75. Dillard DG, Gal AA, Roman-Rodriguez J, et al. Transforming growth factor and neutralizing antibodies in subglottic stenosis. Ann Otol Rhinol Laryngol 2001;110(5 Pt 1):393–400.

76. Ziegelaar BW, Aigner J, Staudenmaier R, et al. The characterisation of human respiratory epithelial cells cultured on resorbable scaffolds: first steps towards a tissue engineered tracheal replacement. Biomaterials 2002;23:1425–38.

77. Glatz F, Neumeister M, Suchy H, et al. A tissue-engineering technique for vascularized laryngotracheal reconstruction. Arch Otolaryngol Head Neck Surg 2003;129:201–6.

78. Dohar JE, Klein EC, Betsch JL, et al. Fetal airway wound repair: a new frontier. Arch Otolaryngol Head Neck Surg 1998;124:25–9.

79. Ciprandi G, Nicollas R, Triglia JM, Rivosecchi M. Fetal cricotracheal manipulation: effects on airway cricoid growth and lung development. Pediatr Surg Int 2003; 19:335–9.

80. Costantino ML, Bagnoli P, Dini G, et al. A numerical and experimental study of compliance and collapsibility of preterm lamb tracheae. J Biomech 2004;37: 183.

9

Cervical Esophagus

Cecille G. Sulman, MD; John Maddalozzo, MD

The esophagus is a muscular tube about 24 cm in length extending from the pharynx to the stomach. It has a cervical, a thoracic, and an abdominal component and is composed of striated and smooth muscle, a submucosa with mucous glands, muscularis mucosa, lamina propria, and a stratified squamous nonkeratinized (mucosal) epithelium. The esophagus varies from other areas of the gut in that there is no distinct serosa layer but is covered by a thin layer of loose connective tissue. The absence of serosa and the longitudinal orientation of the muscle fibers in the esophagus results in a more fragile environment for healing compared with the remaining gastrointestinal tract.

The major steps in esophageal wound healing include inflammation, proliferation, and tissue remodeling. Major factors affecting esophageal wound healing include local and systemic factors, comorbid conditions, and surgical technique. Wound healing problems after esophageal reconstruction include anastomotic leaks, infection, and stricturing. The most common result of significant esophageal injury is stricture formation.

There are many promising options for esophageal wound healing. Strategies may be directed toward decreasing inflammation and scar formation with medications. Tissue remodeling may be encouraged with techniques such as dilation, tissue engineering, or biomaterials. Finally, future technology, such as robotics, may provide a less invasive means to perform reconstructive surgery.

ANATOMY AND PHYSIOLOGY

The esophagus is a hollow muscular tube about 24 cm in length lying ventral to the laryngotracheal airway; it begins proximally at the pharynx at the C6 vertebra with the upper esophageal sphincter (UES) and ends above the stomach at the lower esophageal sphincter (LES) at the T11 vertebra. The UES is the narrowest portion of the esophagus and is composed of cricopharyngeus muscle fibers and the caudal fibers of the inferior pharyngeal constrictor muscles (Figure 1). The LES is located at or just below the diaphragmatic hiatus between the junction of the esophagus and the stomach. When empty, the lumen of the esophagus is slit-like. The proximal third of the esophagus is composed of striated (voluntary) muscle, the middle third is a mixture of both smooth and striated muscle, and the distal third is smooth (involuntary) muscle.

The cricopharyngeus muscle acts in opposition to the function of the constrictor mechanism of the pharynx. At rest, the constrictors are relaxed, and the cricopharyngeus muscle remains in tonic contraction to prevent air intake into the esophagus during inspiration. Backflow from the esophagus into the pharynx is also prevented with tonic contraction of the cricopharyngeus muscle. Peristaltic contraction of the esophageal body in concert with relaxation of the UES and LES allows a food bolus to pass into the stomach.

The inferior thyroid artery supplies the UES and cervical esophagus (Figure 2). Paired aortic esophageal arteries of terminal branches of

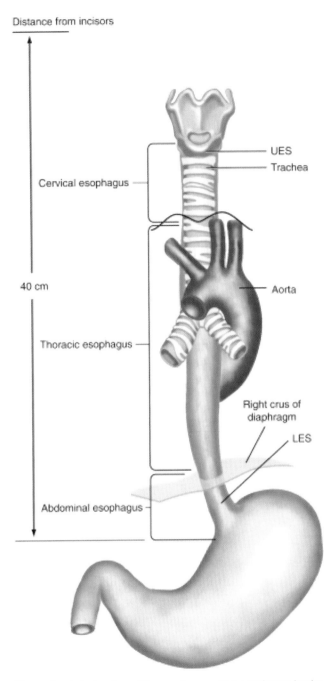

Distance from incisors

Cervical esophagus

UES

Trachea

40 cm

Aorta

Thoracic esophagus

Right crus of
diaphragm

LES

Abdominal esophagus

Figure 1. Anterior view of the esophagus. The esophagus begins approximately at level C6 and ends at the lower esophageal sphincter. The three main components of the esophagus include the cervical, thoracic, and abdominal esophagus.

bronchial arteries supply the thoracic esophagus. The left gastric artery and a branch of the left phrenic artery supply the distal esophagus and LES. Venous drainage is provided by the inferior thyroid vein and a submucosal plexus that drains into the superior vena cava (Figure 3). Midesophageal venous drainage is via the azy-

gous system. The distal esophagus drains via collaterals from the left gastric vein and the azygous vein.

Lymphatic drainage from the cervical esophagus is through the paratracheal lymph nodes and the inferior deep cervical lymph nodes. The midesophageal lymphatic drainage is into the superior and posterior mediastinal nodes. The distal third lymphatics follow the gastric and celiac lymph nodes (Figure 4).

The vagus nerve provides motor innervation to the esophagus (Figure 5). The cell bodies of the vagal efferent fibers innervating the UES and striated muscle originate in the nucleus ambiguus. Efferent fibers innervating the smooth muscle portion of the esophagus and LES originate in the dorsal motor nucleus. Motor and sensory sympathetic nerve supply arises from spinal segments T1 to T10. Sensory innervation is also carried via the vagus nerve and consists of bipolar nerves that have their cell bodies in the nodose ganglion and project to the brainstem.

The cervical esophagus is contained in the visceral space of the neck, which extends from the hyoid bone to the mediastinum (Figure 6). The visceral space also contains the thyroid and parathyroid glands, larynx, trachea, lymph nodes, and recurrent laryngeal nerve. The thyroid gland contacts the esophagus laterally. The recurrent laryngeal nerve traverses the tracheoesophageal groove more intimately on the left. The carotid sheath is lateral to the esophagus and contains the carotid artery, jugular vein, and vagus nerve. The cervical pleura may extend superiorly to contact the cervical esophagus. The major lymphatic drainage system of the head and neck, the thoracic duct, is also in close relation to the esophagus, primarily on the left.

HISTOLOGY

The esophagus is composed of mucosa, submucosa, and muscularis propria (Figure 7). The mucosal surface of the esophagus is composed of a nonkeratinized squamous epithelium, with the exception of the LES, in which there is simple columnar epithelium.[1] The underlying lamina

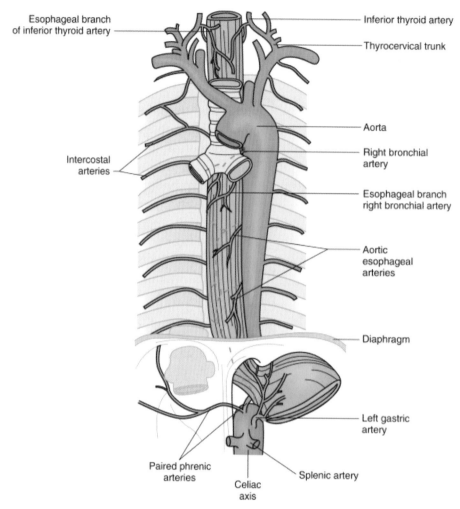

Figure 2.   The arterial system of the esophagus.

propria is highly vascular loose connective tissue, which allows for distention. A prominent muscular mucosa consisting of a scattered longitudinal ring of smooth muscle cells lies between the lamina propria and the submucosa. Lymphocytes, plasma cells, and Meissner's nerve plexus reside in the submucosa, a layer of connective tissue more fibrous than the lamina propria and containing mucus-secreting glands. This is surrounded by the muscularis propria, consisting of an inner circular and an outer longitudinal layer of muscle covered by a thin outer layer of connective tissue. The proximal striated muscularis propria is derived from the branchial arches, whereas the remainder is derived from the foregut. The muscularis propria contains an inner circular muscle layer that provides sequential peristaltic contraction, pro-

pelling the food bolus to the stomach. Between the circular muscle and the outer longitudinal muscle is the myenteric plexus, known as Auerbach's plexus, which mediates much of the intrinsic nervous control of esophageal motor function. The esophagus varies from other areas of the gut in that there is no distinct serosa layer but is covered by a thin layer of loose connective tissue.

MECHANISM OF SWALLOW

Swallowing is a complex process involving the oral cavity, pharynx, larynx, and esophagus. There are four identified stages to swallowing.[2] The first two stages, the oral preparatory and oral stages, are under voluntary control. The second two stages, the pharyngeal and esopha-

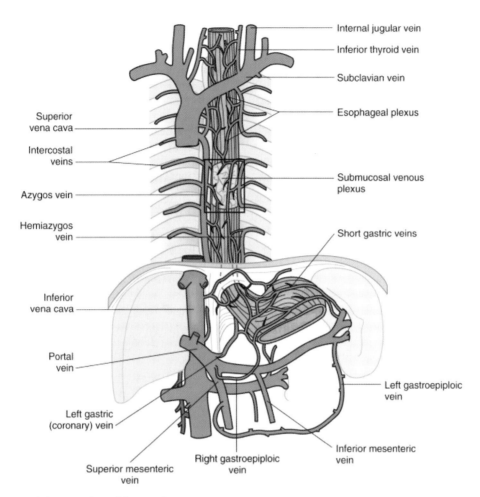

Figure 3. The venous drainage system of the esophagus.

geal stages, are under involuntary control. During the oral preparatory stage, the oral cavity musculature contains the food while the tongue positions the food for mastication and forms a bolus. The soft palate seals the oral cavity posteriorly. In the oral stage, food is moved from the oral cavity to the pharynx, relying primarily on tongue motion to propel the food posteriorly. Once the bolus crosses the tongue base, the pharyngeal swallow is triggered, mediated by cranial nerve IX and the superior laryngeal nerve. Simultaneously, velopharyngeal closure occurs, preventing backflow of material into the nose. The bolus is propelled posteriorly to the pharynx with tongue base retraction, and pharyngeal contraction clears residue from the pharynx. The airway is protected by elevation and closure of the larynx by posterior displacement of the epiglottis, closure of the false and

true vocal cords, and anterior tilting of the arytenoid cartilages. Simultaneously, the cricopharyngeus relaxes and opens to allow the bolus to pass into the esophagus. The duration of the pharyngeal phase of the swallow normally lasts a maximum of 1 second and does not vary dramatically with the consistency of food or with the age or gender of the patient.

The esophageal phase begins when the bolus passes through the UES. Contraction of the circular muscles results in a contractile wave that migrates toward the stomach. The LES then relaxes and opens, allowing the bolus to pass. This sequence of contractions in the esophagus is known as primary peristalsis. Normal esophageal transit time may vary from 8 to 20 seconds. Another type of peristalsis, known as secondary peristalsis, occurs in response to distention of the esophagus. A localized peristaltic wave begins

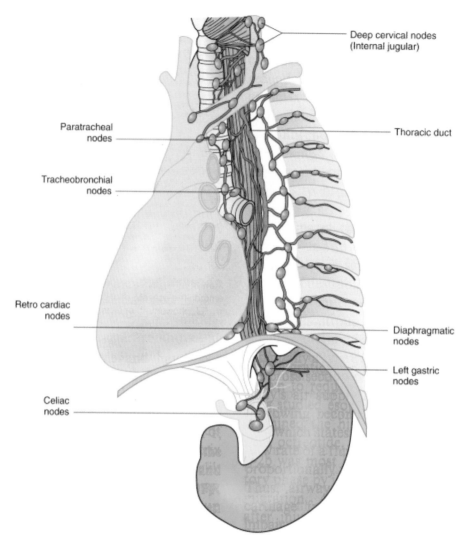

Figure 4. The lymphatic system of the esophagus.

just above an area of distension and is associated with LES relaxation but not UES relaxation.

EVALUATION OF THE ESOPHAGUS

Different methods available to evaluate dysphagia include barium esophagography, esophagoscopy, manometry, videofluoroscopic swallow study (VFSS), ultrasonography, and functional endoscopic evaluation of swallowing (FEES) (Table 9-1).

Barium esophagography is useful for examining structural lesions and evaluating motor disorders and is the best imaging modality for diagnosing an esophageal fistula. It is a non-

invasive procedure but has the disadvantage of radiation exposure.

Manometry evaluates esophageal peristalsis and the adequacy of functioning of the UES and LES with three pressure sensors, located at the UES, the LES, and the body of the esophagus. Manometry can be performed with provocative testing with acid or balloon distention to evoke abnormal contractions and reproduce chest pain.

Esophagoscopy allows visualization of the esophageal mucosa. An advantage of esophagoscopy is the ability to perform therapeutic procedures at the time of evaluation, such as biopsies and dilation. However, esophagoscopy cannot provide reliable information regarding esophageal function. Other drawbacks include

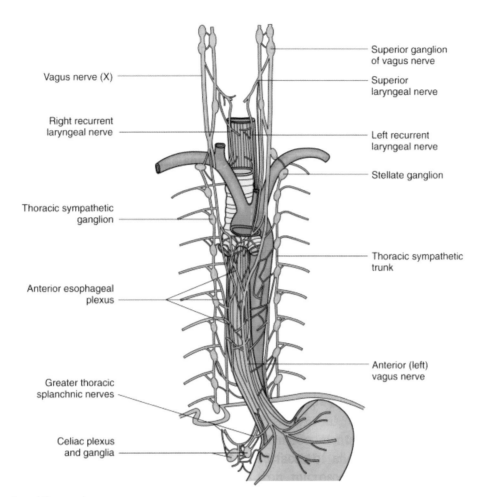

Figure 5. Innervation of the esophagus.

the need for sedation or a general anesthetic and the risk of perforation.

Ultrasound evaluation is limited to detecting the motion of the tongue during swallow and thus is limited to evaluating the oral phase of swallow. FEES may be performed in a clinic setting or at the bedside. FEES is valuable in assessing many aspects of swallowing, including pharyngeal pooling, premature spillage, laryngeal penetration, aspiration, and residue. Also, FEES is therapeutic as well as diagnostic, and patients are provided with feedback during the procedure. Unfortunately, the esophageal phase of swallowing cannot be assessed with this technique.

VFSS is the only study that evaluates all four phases of swallowing. More specifically, aspiration may be detected, oral and pharyngeal motility disorders identified, and the speed of swallowing assessed. Differentiation can be made between food consistencies and the effect of therapy strategies can be followed, such as postural changes, heightened sensory input, and swallowing maneuvers.

HEALING STEPS AFTER INJURY

Three major stages in esophageal healing include inflammation, proliferation, and tissue remodeling.[3] The acute inflammatory phase predominates for the first week and is characterized by cell infiltration and edema formation, mainly confined to the submucosa. Granulocytes predominate in the first 24 hours, and macrophages follow 48 hours after clean surgical injury. Granulocytes are responsible for a significant degree of collagenolytic activity, and their presence is increased by contamination and tissue

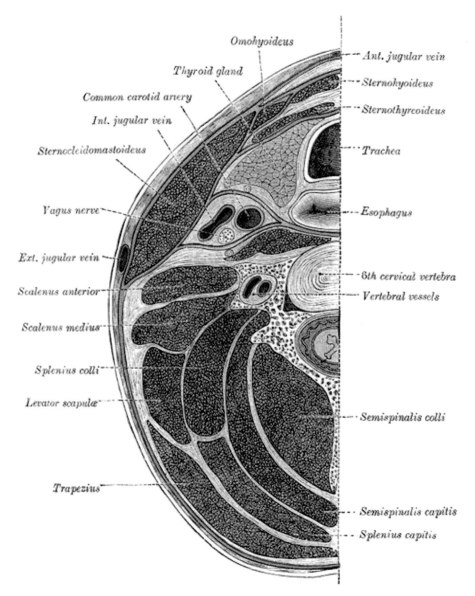

Figure 6. Cross section through the neck below the hyoid bone. Layers of the deep cervical fascia and the structures that are enveloped.

necrosis. Within 2 to 3 days after injury, angiogenesis begins. The second week after injury is the setting for fibroblastic proliferation and collagen formation, which represents the pathophysiologic pathway of stricture formation. Fibroblasts and mainly smooth muscle cells produce matrix proteins, primarily in the submucosa and the subserosa. If injury is limited to the mucosa, it can be reformed by migration and proliferation. Mucosal resurfacing is rapid in the gastrointestinal tract and is accomplished within 1 week. With full-thickness injury, a fibroplastic response occurs, resulting in scar formation. If severe injury is accompanied by tissue destruc-

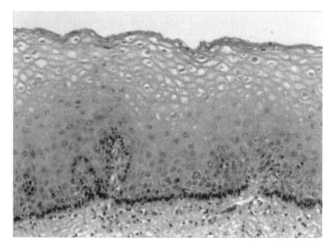

Figure 7. Histology of normal esophagus demonstrating stratified squamous epithelium.

Table 1. METHODS TO EVALUATE THE ESOPHAGUS AND PHARYNX

Method	Indications	Advantages	Disadvantages
Barium esophagography	Structural lesions Strictures Motor disorders Fistulae	Noninvasive Ease of performing	Cannot detect mucosal disease Radiation exposure
Manometry	Esophageal function	Noninvasive Evaluates motility disorders Provocative testing	Radiation exposure
Esophagoscopy	Structural lesions Strictures Fistulae	Ability to perform biopsies Ability to dilate	Invasive Requires general anesthetic/ sedation Risk of perforation Cannot evaluate esophageal function
Videofluoroscopic swallow study	Aspiration Dysphagia	Assessment of oropharyngeal swallow Real-time feedback	Cannot assess esophageal swallow Radiation exposure
Functional endoscopic evaluation of swallowing	Aspiration Dysphagia	Bedside evaluation Real-time feedback Detect anatomic abnormalities	Time consuming Cannot assess esophageal swallow
Ultrasonography	Dysphagia Structural lesions	Noninvasive	Limited to oral phase of swallow

tion or bacterial spillage, the events will last longer and will be more pronounced. Wound contraction is attributable to collagen overproduction and may result in stricture formation.

The absence of serosa and the longitudinal orientation of the muscle fibers in the esophagus result in a more fragile environment for healing. Sutures hold together poorly in the esophagus compared with other visceral organs, such as the stomach.[4] Additionally, the esophagus requires more extensive dissection to mobilize versus the remaining gastrointestinal tract, and anastomosis to another viscus is difficult outside the protective peritoneal cavity.

FACTORS AFFECTING HEALING

Systemic factors influencing the healing process include an adequate blood supply, surgical technique, neoadjuvant therapy, malnutrition, and other comorbid conditions, such as diabetes, cardiovascular diseases, and respiratory insufficiency.[4] Excessive smoking and alcohol use contribute to these comorbid conditions and negatively interfere with the immune system of the patient.[4]

Adequate Blood Supply

Tissue oxygenation is affected by adequate perfusion and blood supply. Hypotension should be avoided because of the potential negative impact on perfusion and tissue oxygenation.[4] Poor oxygenation may contribute to anastomotic leaks, but it is unclear as to the significance of its role versus surgical technique. Additionally, oxygen is a prerequisite to the hydroxylation of lysine and proline during collagen synthesis. Intimate knowledge of esophageal vascular anatomy is a requisite in reconstruction. High intraoperative blood loss has been associated with later development of anastomotic leaks and strictures.[5]

Surgical Technique

Surgical technique plays a vital role in healing. Anastomotic tension should be avoided and sharp dissection performed with fine instrumentation. Hemostasis should be meticulous, without necrosing tissue unnecessarily. Tissues should be handled gently and measures taken to avoid drying of tissue. Everting sutures at the anastomosis carries a greater risk of leakage but a lower incidence of stenosis. Anastomotic leaks have also been associated with a running suture technique.[5] Given the rapid healing rate of intestinal tissue, suture tensile strength is required for a short period only but is critical in the first few days after surgery. After 48 hours, the breaking strength in esophageal anastomoses decreases by 37% from initial values. This loss in strength is a reflection of an imbalance between collagen synthesis and degradation and usually occurs in the first 3 days of healing.

Absorbable suture materials, including chromic catgut, polyglycolic acid, polydioxanone, and polyglyconate, are reasonable to use secondary to the rapid healing rate of intestinal tissue. Additionally, suture absorption eliminates a foreign-body reaction and inflammation. Monofilament sutures have the advantage over multifilament sutures because they do not provide a scaffold for bacterial growth.

Nutrition

The inverse relationship between nutritional status and wound healing potential in experimental animals is well recognized. Both prolonged malnutrition and short-term malnutrition diminish anastomotic healing. The mechanism through which malnutrition affects anastomotic healing is not fully understood and may be due to a lack of amino acids for collagen synthesis or deterioration in patient immunocompetence. As a reflection of poor nutritional status, low serum albumin has been associated with anastomotic leaks (see Chapter 25, "Nutrition and Wound Healing").[5]

Neoadjuvant Therapy

Radiation therapy (RT) causes increased susceptibility to infection by disrupting the normal mucosal barriers to colonization and infection of the upper aerodigestive tract. Direct effects on immune cells include decreased CD8+ and CD4+ lymphocyte counts, impaired lymphocyte response to mitogens, and decreased skin-test positivity to antigens in assays of delayed-type hypersensitivity.[6]

The first symptoms of acute esophagitis start in the second or third week of RT, commonly at doses of 18 to 21 Gy. Radiation doses exceeding 30 Gy to the mediastinum typically cause retrosternal burning and painful swallowing. This is usually mild and limited to the duration of therapy. Esophageal mucosal redness and edema are seen at doses of 40 Gy. Doses of 50 Gy cause a higher incidence and severity of esophageal damage. Moderate to severe esophagitis with strictures, perforations, and fistulae may be seen with doses of 60 to 70 Gy. Late injury may occur up to 8 months, with eventual stricture formation.[7,8] Strictures result from submucosal fibrosis and degenerative changes involving blood vessels.[9] Radiation esophagitis most commonly occurs during treatment of intrathoracic malignancies, particularly lung and esophageal cancers. Endoscopic findings may include erythema, edema, friability of the esophageal mucosa, and ulceration. The frequency and severity of esophagitis increase with radiation dose and with the use of certain chemotherapeutic agents, including doxorubicin, bleomycin, cyclophosphamide, and cisplatin.[10,11]

A single fraction of radiation to the thorax with as little as 20 Gy has demonstrated evidence of mucosal damage to the esophagus. Histologically, vacuolization of the basal cell layer, the absence of mitosis, and submucosal edema are observed.[8] Some regeneration is evident by 1 to 2 weeks with proliferating basal cells and regenerating epithelium. At 3 weeks, regeneration of the esophageal lining is complete, and after 4 weeks, the appearance of the irradiated esophagus normalizes.

If significant injury is present, a barium swallow may demonstrate esophageal dysmotility with a lack of peristalsis and failure of LES relaxation.[8] Patients should be monitored for a change in diet, increased analgesic requirement, weight loss, and the need for intravenous fluids or tube feeds. Odynophagia may be treated with viscous lidocaine during the acute phase. Histamine$_2$ blockers or proton pump inhibitors should be used to prevent further acid-related injury.

Radiation effects on the esophagus may be reduced by exclusion of the esophagus from the treatment field, as in cases of lung cancer. Also, radioprotective agents are promising. Amifostine, which acts as a potent scavenger of oxygen free radicals induced by ionizing radiation, has been demonstrated in a phase III randomized trial to offer radioprotective effects.[12] Also, a future direction involves a plasmid/liposome delivery system to prevent radiation esophagitis.[8]

Gastroesophageal Reflux Disease

The LES resting pressure usually averages between 10 and 30 mm Hg above intragastric pressures. With low LES resting pressures, patients are prone to gastroesophageal reflux disease (GERD). GERD is prevalent, affecting approximately 5 to 10% of the adult world population.[13] The severity of esophageal damage is dependent on the acidity of gastric contents flowing backward into the esophagus, the appropriate clearance of gastric contents from the esophagus, and the time of exposure of the esophagus to reflux contents. Most patients manifest mild disease forms, but severe complications of GERD may result in hemorrhage, ulceration, stenosis, and Barrett's esophagus. Additionally, GERD may play a role in delayed healing after esophageal surgery.

Corticosteroids

Steroids cause immunosuppression of the innate and cell-mediated pathways of the immune system through their effects on phagocyte migration and activation and on T-lymphocyte function. The immunosuppressive effects are dependent on the dosage of steroid used and the duration of therapy. A significant incidence of infection is seen in patients who receive prednisone dosages of 20 to 40 mg daily for more than 6 weeks.[6]

However, steroids have been found to improve surgical outcomes.[14] The preoperative use of steroids in esophageal surgery has resulted in shortened intensive care unit stays,[15] improved postoperative pulmonary function, and early mobilization.[16,17] Steroids reduce inflammation by inhibiting prostaglandin synthesis. Additionally, there is a decrease in interleukin-6 and C-reactive protein, without detrimental effects on wound healing.[16,17]

Comorbid Conditions

Comorbid conditions such as vascular disease and diabetes affect wound healing. The direct effect of diabetes on intestinal wound healing is unknown, but in a diabetic animal model, there is a temporary decrease in bursting pressure in addition to increased abscess formation. Anastomotic complications also increase with age, most likely secondary to disease processes more prevalent in older patients.

ESOPHAGEAL RECONSTRUCTION, COMPLICATIONS, AND MANAGEMENT

Options for Esophageal Reconstruction

Options for reconstruction of the esophagus after esophagectomy with cervical anastomosis include the gastric pull-up and colon or jejunum interposition. The gastric pull-up is a popular reconstructive option secondary to the simplicity of the operation and the need for only one anastomosis.[4] The main blood supply dependent on graft survival is the right gastroepiploic artery and vein, which supplies 60% of the stomach. Approximately 20% of the stomach is vascularized through a dense submucosal and microvascular network and the rest by minute connections between right and left gastroepiploic vessels. Most frequently, the anastomosis is made at the proximal 20% of the gastric fundus.

The colon has consistent vascular anatomy based on arcades connecting the left, middle, and right colic artery.[4] It is popular for reconstructing the esophagus after severe corrosive injury and esophageal atresia. Some argue that leaks and strictures are less common with a colon interposition versus a gastric pull-up.[18] Jejunum is used less frequently because of the technical difficulty of preparing a loop sufficiently long enough to reach the neck for anastomosis. However, the jejunum is a viable option if the stomach and colon are not available.

Anastomotic techniques include hand-sewn or stapled approaches. Some studies have demonstrated no difference in outcome between hand-sewn versus stapled anastomosis; however, the use of semimechanical anastomosis with endostaplers with three rows of staples may result in a reduced leakage rate.[4] Orringer and colleagues reduced the cervical leak rate from 10 to 15% using a hand-sewn technique to 2.7% with a side-to-side stapled anastomosis technique.[19]

Complications of Esophageal Reconstruction

The incidence, mortality, and morbidity of anastomotic complications have substantially decreased in recent years.[4] This decrease is most likely related to refinement in anastomotic techniques and progress in perioperative management.

Postoperative anastomotic leaks are one of the most common complications of esophageal reconstruction, and rates have been reported in up to 53% of patients.[20–22] In more recent series, anastomotic leaks range around 12%. Iannettoni and colleagues reported outcomes in 856 patients after transhiatal esophagectomy with cervical esophagogastric anastomosis.[23] The majority of patients underwent gastric pull-up (94%) versus colon interposition (5%). Approximately 10% of patients had an early postoperative leak, attributed to technical factors. Leaks occurred at the anastomosis or at the site of sutures, suspending the gastric fundus to the cervical prevertebral fascia. It has been reported that there is a higher cervical leak rate with cervical anastomosis versus intrathoracic anastomosis[20]; however, recent studies have not found this to be true.[18,23] In a series of 74 patients, 19 patients underwent cervical anastomosis and 55 underwent thoracic anastomosis. Leaks complicated 5% of patients

in the cervical anastomosis group versus 16% in the thoracic anastomosis group.[20] Anastomotic leaks in the cervical region result in less severe consequences than thoracic leaks, which carry a greater risk of mediastinitis (Table 9-2).[23]

Most leaks can be attributed to conduit ischemia, technical errors, or a combination of the two.[21] The mortality rate may be as high as 37% after esophagectomy and reconstruction.[18,20] Alanezi and Urschel performed a retrospective review of 307 patients who underwent esophageal reconstruction.[21] Esophageal anastomotic leaks developed in 7.5% of patients, and of these patients, 8 (35%) died. Surgical management of esophageal leaks is predictive of subsequent death, but this is most likely linked to the severity of illness requiring surgical intervention.

Graft ischemia is closely related to increased stricture formation and anastomotic leaks. Briel and colleagues reviewed the outcomes of a series of 363 patients.[18] In patients who developed clinical ischemia, one-third healed without complications, one-third developed a stricture without a leak, and one-third developed an anastomotic leak. Half of the patients who developed a leak ultimately developed a stricture.[18] Gastric necrosis was found to be an important predictor of mortality.

Overmanipulation during gastrolysis and the initial compromised blood supply at the apex of the freshly mobilized stomach may result in a cervical anastomotic leak.[23] Vigorous suctioning, tension on the anastomosis, and traction sutures used to facilitate the gastric pull-up maneuver are

Table 2. SIGNS AND SYMPTOMS OF ANASTOMOTIC LEAK
Hematoma
Seroma
Septicemia
Peritonitis
Perianastomotic collection
Leak
Local inflammation
Extravasation of air or saliva
Mediastinitis
Abscess
Emphyema
Pneumothorax

technical factors that may jeopardize the anastomosis. Anatomic factors that may contribute include the lack of serosa of the esophagus, extrinsic compression in neck, and the nonmesothelial environment of the neck. Therefore, surgical experience, technique, and adequacy of gastric conduit vascularity all play a role in healing.

Patients with comorbid conditions, such as diabetes, cardiovascular disorders, and chronic obstructive pulmonary disease, are more likely to develop conduit ischemia.[18] Increased patient body weight is also associated with the occurrence of a stricture. The additional fat in the graft may contribute to compression of the conduit and more technical difficulties with the anastomosis. Malignant infiltration of anastomotic tissues is a rare etiology for anastomotic leakage.

Other reported severe complications of esophageal reconstruction include infectious complications and technical errors. Infections include epidural abscess, perianastomotic collection, mediastinitis, sepsis, and empyema. Technical complications may result in a tracheoesophagogastric anastomotic fistula, major dehiscence, hematoma, seroma, and pneumothorax.[4,23]

Important perioperative factors decreasing the death and complication rates after esophageal resection include the postoperative use of epidural analgesia, bronchoscopy for pulmonary toilet, a history of decreased smoking or nonsmoking, and surgical blood loss less than 1,000 mL. These factors help decrease respiratory failure and positively influence tissue oxygenation.

Management of Complications of Esophageal Reconstruction

Physical findings indicating an anastomotic leak include fever, pain, and drainage. Patients may also have cervical crepitus, erythema, or fluctuance. If a leak is suspected, the cervical wound should be opened at the bedside. The patient should be made nil by mouth, and supplemental nutrition should be begun. Gastric acid secretion should be neutralized with proton pump inhibitors or limited with somatostatin. The patient should be started on broad-spectrum antibiotics. If a patient remains febrile 24 hours after opening the cervical wound and appears to be toxic, without another source of infection, the wound should be explored in the operating room. Treatment goals include adequate drainage of infected fluid collections, resection of necrotic tissue, and prevention of further soilage from the leak.[21] If signs of sepsis continue, thoracotomy with drainage of the abscess and takedown of the anastomosis may be necessary. Diversion is provided with a cervical esophagostomy, and placement of a gastrostomy tube may be necessary. Reconstruction should be delayed until the inflammation has resolved.

Barium esophagography is the best radiologic test for evaluation of an anastomotic leak. However, a normal contrast study does not exclude a leak. The earlier the study is performed, the greater the rate of false negatives. Computed tomography (CT) may be used to rule out a perianastomotic fluid collection and abscess. Esophagoscopy is useful for evaluation of conduit ischemia.

Anastomotic strictures occur after esophagectomy in 22% of patients. Patients who develop strictures respond well to dilatation, with 50% requiring only one dilation procedure.[18] Alternate management after bedside drainage of a cervical wound is early dilation.[23] The patient is maintained on a clear liquid diet. Prior to dressing changes, the patient ingests water to cleanse the wound. Bedside dilation is performed with Maloney dilators ranging from 36 to 46 French. Early dilation is believed to reduce complications of leaks secondary to distal outflow obstruction, resulting in earlier closure and improved swallow.

To improve vascularization of the gastric fundus, gastric ischemic conditioning at the time of laparoscopic cancer staging has been proposed. It is not clear whether such methods indeed result in a decreased incidence of anastomotic complications. Urschel and colleagues used a rodent model of partial gastric devascularization to encourage ischemic conditioning.[22]

Ischemic conditioning performed 3 weeks prior to gastric anastomosis resulted in fewer anastomotic leaks and a higher anastomotic wound breaking strength. Ischemic conditioning results in neovascularization, with the most ischemic parts of the flap showing the greatest vascularity over the delay period. Ischemic conditioning could be performed endoscopically during staging procedures with minimally invasive surgical techniques. This has yet to be applied in the clinical setting.

Burns and Corrosive Esophageal Injury

The most common injuries to the esophagus are secondary to ingestion of caustic substances.[24] The presence and severity of injuries are correlated with the amount of caustic substances ingested, the corrosive properties of the ingested substance, and the duration of mucosal contact. Alkaline caustics and acids are the most common culprits in esophageal burns. Acid injury results in coagulation necrosis, which forms an eschar and thus limits the depth of penetration. Alkalis result in a deeper and more significant injury with liquefactive necrosis. This results in the destruction of cells and cell membranes, with saponification of lipid membranes and denaturation of intracellular proteins.[25] During the reparative phase, between 5 days and 2 weeks, sloughing of the necrotic debris is followed by development of granulation tissue and collagen deposition. Reepithelialization begins with this phase and may persist for many weeks. During this phase, the esophagus is at its thinnest. Scar retraction begins after the second week with collagen deposition and lasts for about 6 months.[26]

Initial patient management should involve airway assessment and volume resuscitation. Laryngeal edema and airway compromise may be assessed at the bedside with flexible laryngoscopy. With significant laryngeal edema, elective intubation or tracheostomy should be considered. The caustic substance should be identified and the ingested amount determined. Emetics and neutralizing agents should be avoided owing to the risk of increased mucosal damage caused by heat production with the neutralizing agent and secondary exposure with emesis. There has been no clear evidence for the use of antibiotics or steroids with caustic injuries,[25] although antibiotics may help decrease infection and steroids may decrease collagen deposition and fibrosis. Proton pump inhibitors may be started to decrease gastric acid production and prevent additional injury and stricture formation.

Esophagoscopy should be performed within 12 to 24 hours to evaluate the extent of injury. The endoscopist should proceed cautiously and terminate the procedure above the first significant area of injury. Esophagoscopy should not be performed more than 5 days from injury secondary to an increased risk of perforation. Contraindications to endoscopy include shock, epiglottic necrosis, respiratory distress, peritonitis, mediastinitis, hypopharyngeal edema, and evidence of perforated viscus. First-degree burns are superficial and produce edema and erythema. Patients with first-degree injuries without strictures may be monitored in the hospital for 48 hours.[27] The esophageal mucosa may slough but does not usually lead to scarring.

Second-degree burns involve the mucosa, submucosa, and muscle layers. Deep ulceration and granulation tissue are produced, followed by collagen deposition and retraction. Third-degree burns are transmural, with deep ulcerations that result in a "black" esophagus. Patients with second- and third-degree burns should be monitored in the intensive care unit. Hydration and antibiotics are begun in addition to proton pump inhibitors. At this point, steroids may not have benefit and may mask mediastinitis. Patients are maintained nil by mouth and monitored for symptoms of perforation. A gastrostomy tube may be placed with passage of a nasogastric string for dilation. Silastic stents may be placed and maintained for several weeks in patients with second-degree and limited third-degree injuries without full-thickness injury. With third-degree burns, there is a 65% mortality rate. Substernal, back, or abdominal pain may suggest perforation.[27] These patients may require esophagectomy.

Clinically apparent esophageal strictures may occur in 10 to 30% of patients with caustic injury, the likelihood increasing with the grade of burn. Patients with circumferential ulceration, blisters, and areas of necrosis tend to develop esophageal strictures. Stricture formation may result in inadequate oral intake, requiring serial dilations. A safe goal for dilation in the adult should be approximately 15 mm.

The presence of ulceration involving more than 50% of the anastomotic circumference is predictive of developing an anastomotic stricture. In more severe strictures in which dilation is not effective, surgical replacement of the esophagus may be required. Owing to continued histologic evidence of continued scar retraction up to 6 months, reconstructive surgery should not be performed less than 6 months after injury. Colon interposition grafts are a popular choice for reconstruction. Han and colleagues believe that the stomach is not ideal for esophageal replacement owing to secondary long-term gastroesophageal reflux, possible ulceration, anastomotic stenosis, and progressive dysfunctional propulsion.[28] The jejunum is seldom used because of thinner blood vessels and is more fragile in the face of acid erosion. It may be used as an option if no other sites are available. The benefit of using the colon is the length of tissue available and fewer complications of esophagitis and stricture because of the resistance to acid. Pivotal keys for a successful surgical procedure are an adequate vascular supply for the esophageal replacement and the absence of tension at the anastomosis. Han and colleagues performed esophageal replacement in 68 patients with severe strictures, primarily using colonic interposition (63), esophagogastrostomy (3), and jejunal interposition (2).[28] There was a 25% complication rate, including cervical anastomotic leakage, cervical wound infection, anastomotic stenosis, intestinal obstruction, pneumothorax, and aspiration pneumonitis. Other complications include an increased risk of cancer by 1,000-fold, tracheoesophageal fistula, hiatal hernia, and reflux (Table 3).

In summary, caustic injury management should begin immediately with assessment of the airway and extent of injury. Endoscopic management should take place within 12 to 24 hours. Delayed assessment should be performed with contrast esophagography. More severe burns result in stricture and perforation. Surgical management should include dilation for stricture. Severe injury and perforation may require esophagectomy and delayed reconstruction.

Esophageal Injury

Less common etiologies for esophageal injuries include iatrogenic, blunt, and penetrating trauma. Iatrogenic causes of perforation are most common, accounting for 33 to 75.5% of cases.[25] Esophageal perforation related to diagnostic is 0.03% and has a mortality rate of 0.001%.[29] The cricopharyngeal area is the most frequently injured.[27] Other infrequent etiologies for cervical esophageal perforation include difficult endotracheal intubation, blind insertion of a minitracheostomy, operations on the cervical spine, thyroidectomy, prolonged intubation, foreign bodies, pills, and infections. The risk of perforation increases if a foreign body is present for more than 24 hours secondary to pressure necrosis.[25] Pill-induced perforation may be caused by antibiotics, antiviral agents, anti-inflammatory agents, quinidine, potassium chloride, and bisphosphonates. Infectious etiologies include *Candida*, herpes simplex virus, and tuberculosis. Risk factors predisposing patients to perforation include anterior cervical osteophytes, Zenker's diverticulum, esophageal strictures, and malignancies.

The primary symptom of esophageal perforation is pain (Table 4). Other symptoms include

Table 3. COMPLICATIONS OF CAUSTIC INGESTION

Respiratory compromise
Esophageal perforation
Gastric perforation
Septicemia
Stricture formation
Increased risk of esophageal cancer
Hiatal hernia
Gastroesophageal reflux
Death

neck ache and stiffness owing to pressure on esophageal attachments to the prevertebral fascia, limiting the spread of oropharyngeal secretions. Tachypnea, fever, and tachycardia are common physical signs. On examination, there may be cervical crepitance or subcutaneous emphysema. In the cervical esophagus, perforation and infection usually remain localized as a periesophageal abscess. However, dissection may spread to the retropharyngeal space and then into the posterior mediastinum. The degree of mediastinal contamination is dependent on the depth and location of the perforation.[25] There may be associated subcutaneous emphysema palpable in 60% of patients and visible in 95% on plain radiography.[25] With mediastinal involvement, the patient may complain of chest or back pain. Thoracic perforations are more likely to develop mediastinitis, which carries a more significant risk of sepsis and shock.

The use of dilation for esophageal strictures has an associated complication rate of 0.3% and may be greater with Maloney dilators versus balloon dilators when used on complex strictures. Dilation of caustic strictures usually affects a greater length and with more luminal compromise may result in perforations in up to 17% of patients. Prevention of perforation may be possible by limiting dilation to less than 15 mm.[29]

The location of a perforation may be evaluated with barium swallow. Water-soluble contrast, such as meglumine diatrizoate, should be used if there is a high degree of suspicion for perforation. A negative examination does not necessarily rule out a perforation and may carry a false-negative rate in 10% of patients.[25] If there is continued suspicion, barium contrast or a CT scan may be pursued. Endoscopic evaluation in a patient with a negative radiologic workup and a continued high index of suspicion carries a sensitivity of 100% and a specificity of 83%. These examinations should be carried out cautiously because insufflated air can convert a small perforation into a large perforation.[25]

Patient outcomes are dependent on the location of the perforation and time lapse between rupture and treatment. A patient may be managed nonoperatively only if there is a well-contained leak in a stable patient without sepsis. If free air is present and the perforation has been present for less than 72 hours, the primary repair should be reinforced with vascularized tissue, such as muscle.[27] With delayed presentation, active infection, or failed conservative management, the esophagus should be excluded with a controlled fistula or esophagostomy and later reconstructed. A gastrostomy should be placed for feeding.

In summary, endoscopy is the main etiology for traumatic perforation of the esophagus. Other etiologies of cervical esophageal perforation include difficult endotracheal intubation, blind insertion of a minitracheostomy tube, operations on the cervical spine, thyroidectomy, prolonged intubation, and stenting of the trachea or esophagus. Management is dependent on patient presentation. Early presentation with an asymptomatic leak may be managed with observation, whereas perforations associated with sepsis should be managed with drainage and diversion.

Table 4. SIGNS AND SYMPTOMS OF ESOPHAGEAL PERFORATION
Pain
Fever
Crepitance
Chest pain
Neck pain
Cervical dysphagia
Leukocytosis
Pleural effusion

Epidermolysis Bullosa

Epidermolysis bullosa is a heterogeneous group of disorders of the stratified squamous epithelium. It is characterized by skin blistering, scarring, and, in some cases, mucosal involvement after minor mechanical trauma.[30] It is presumed that recurrent trauma to the mucosa is precipitated by the ingestion of solid food.

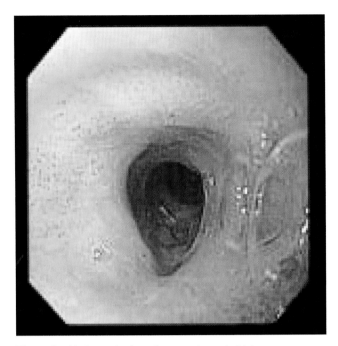

Figure 8. Endoscopic view of an esophageal stricture.

Blistering results, followed by scarring and stricture formation. Fifty percent of strictures occur in the proximal third of the esophagus, usually near the cricoid cartilage and cricopharyngeal muscle, where the esophageal lumen is narrowest. Twenty-five percent are in the distal third of the esophagus, and the rest are in multiple sites. Strictures may be short, 2 to 6 cm, localized in distribution, or longer and more extensive, resulting in shortening of the esophagus.

Management includes bougienage dilation, which carries the risks of perforation and mucosal injury. An alternate technique includes endoscopic balloon dilation. Anderson and colleagues used an endoscopic balloon dilation technique on 60 patients over 10 years, with a median follow-up of 3.5 years.[30] There was a median of two balloon dilatations performed per patient. Fifty-seven of 60 patients had improvement in the dysphagia score, mean weight gain, and body mass index. There were no esophageal perforations, and the only postoperative complication was self-limited odynophagia. The benefits of using balloon dilation include direct visualization, avoiding the need for fluoroscopy and thus radiation to the unstable skin.

PREVENTION OF STRICTURE FORMATION

Dilation

Currently, dilation is the most common means to treat an esophageal stricture and allow patients to continue oral intake. Dilation may be performed with a bougie, such as Maloney dilators or metal olive dilators, or endoscopically with balloon dilators. Endoscopic dilation for esophageal strictures may be performed in both adults and children. Lan and colleagues reviewed endoscopic balloon dilation with fluoroscopic screening in 77 children for strictures related to achalasia, postesophageal atresia repair, reflux esophagitis, postfundoplication, and caustic injury.[31] Esophageal perforation complicated 1.5% of the dilations, requiring one surgical repair for persistent leak. All of the children were asymptomatic at a median follow-up of 6.6 years.

After RT, many esophageal cancer patients present with recurrent dysphagia. Ng and colleagues compared dilation outcomes for patients with esophageal cancer who were treated with

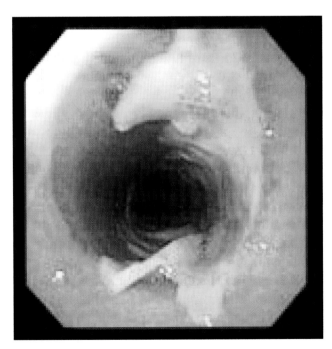

Figure 9. Endoscopic view of radiation esophagitis.

(a)   (b)

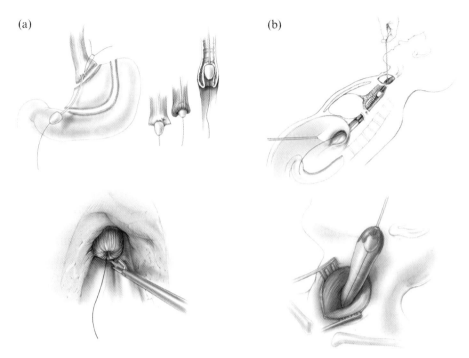

Figure 10. A, Creation of the neo-esophagus after gastric division and inversion of the Esophagus; B, Pullup of gastric conduit.

radiation or no radiation.[9] They found that the perforation rate for dilation in the radiotherapy group was not significantly different from that in controls. Half of the perforations in the control group occurred at the first therapeutic procedure. Endoprostheses were inserted in 48% of radiotherapy patients and 79% of controls at some stage of the illness. The risks of perforation related to esophageal intubation in each group were similar, although tube migration was more frequent in the RT group.

As mentioned previously, early dilation has been used in the management of anastomostic leakage.[4,19] Early postoperative endoscopy with early dilation results in a decreased need for multiple dilations. The rationale for early dilation is to improve esophageal emptying by relieving any esophageal luminal obstruction. Dilation with Maloney esophageal dilators is carried out at the bedside without anesthesia within 3 to 7 days of opening the wound. Fluoroscopic guidance may be helpful if there is a high-grade obstruction or relative tortuosity of the lumen. With this technique, it has been reported that the majority of leaks will close within 1 week of bedside dilation.[32]

Stents

Self-expanding stents, plastic or metal, may be used to treat dysphagia, fistulae, or nonmalignant perforations.[33,34] Complications associated with self-expanding metal stents (SEMS) include migration, tumor ingrowth, and hyperplastic tissue reaction.[33] Self-expanding plastic stents (SEPS) have been reported to have an advantage over SEMS by reducing hyperplasia at the edges of the stent, allowing for easy removal. The rough outer surface and high expansive force minimize dislocation. Evrard and colleagues used SEPS in 21 patients with esophageal stenosis (refractory peptic, caustic, post-RT, anastomotic, and hyperplastic stenosis) and anastomotic leak after esophagectomy.[33] Patients were followed for 8 months after stent removal. Temporary use of the SEPS was curative in the majority of patients, especially those with caustic and hyperplastic strictures and anastomotic fistula. Prior to stent placement, all patients underwent upper gastrointestinal endoscopy and barium esophagography. After dilation, stents were placed under fluoroscopy. Complications included migration of the stent, the need for repeat dilations, or replacement.

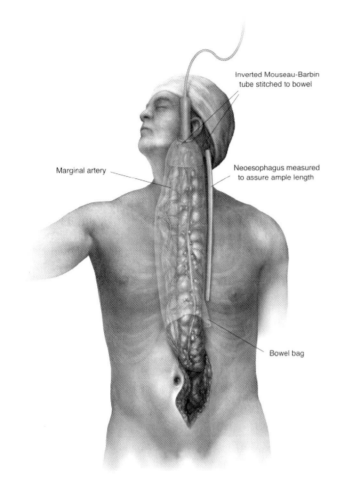

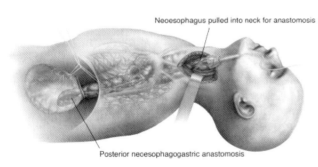

Figure 11.   Pullup of colon interposition graft.

FUTURE PROMISE FOR HEALING

Tissue Engineering

An advantage of tissue engineering is exact replacement of tissue versus using prosthetic materials or tissue type by proxy. The creation of living replacement organs and tissues has the advantages of self-propagation and self-repair. Tissue engineering also saves patients from the morbidity of harvesting a graft, such as the stomach, colon, or jejunum. Additionally, for patients who have had a previous resection or an intestinal disorder, tissue engineering may enable reconstruction even when the usual surgical alternatives are unavailable.[35]

Tissue engineering for esophageal replacement is currently being studied in animal models. Grikscheit and colleagues fabricated a tissue-engineered esophagus and used it to replace the abdominal esophagus in rats.[35] Esophagus organ units were isolated from neonatal and adult rats and paratopically transplanted on biodegradable polymer tubes. These tubes were implanted in syngeneic hosts. Four weeks later, the tissue-engineered esophagus was used as an onlay patch or total interposition graft. To distinguish the tissue-engineered esophagus from native tissue, the tissue-engineered organ units were virally infected to express green fluorescent protein. Histologically, when successfully implanted, the tissue-engineered esophagus resembled native rat esophagus. Fluoroscopy performed at day 42 demonstrated a wide unobstructed lumen in animals that underwent onlay patch grafting. Rats with interposition grafts demonstrated stenosis at the upper anastomosis and dilation at the lower anastomosis.

Tissue engineering demonstrates promise for esophageal reconstruction, particularly when used as an onlay graft, and may save patients significant morbidity from using tissue grafts.

Biomaterials

Biomaterials may be an essential component for successful growth of new organs by its many properties as a scaffold, a delivery vehicle, and a depot.[36] As a scaffold, biomaterials guide tissue growth and provide a transient base for cellular generation. Biomaterials mimic natural extracellular matrix function by eliciting cellular responses that promote tissue growth and may aid in tissue organization. The biomaterial may be fashioned into a three-dimensional structure to guide tissue growth to fit a particular need. Biomaterials also may be used as a delivery

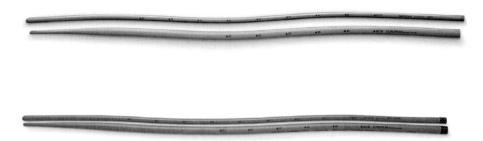

Figure 12. Maloney Esophageal Dilators.

vehicle for cells or bioactive factors. Direct injection of cell suspensions without biomaterials is difficult to control because localization and organization of the transplanted cells are unpredictable. Another use of biomaterials is to serve as a depot for the local release of growth factors.

Ideally, biomaterials must be biocompatible, nontoxic, and biodegradable. The material must support tissue growth and yet be readily absorbed so that minimal inflammation and foreign-body response are elicited. Degradation products should be nontoxic and readily metabolized. Another ideal property would be promotion of cellular interaction, growth, and tissue development. Prosthetic materials that have been used include Dacron, polyglycolic acid mesh, and polytetrafluoroethylene. Unfortunately, Dacron has had a tendency to extrude. Neomucosal growth has not been noted, and poor growth is observed with architectural disarray of the regenerated tissue.[37]

Small intestinal submucosa (SIS) and urinary bladder submucosa (UBS) are biologic materials collected from porcine organs that are decellularized and processed to preserve native extra-

cellular matrix and soluble mediators. They have been studied in dermal, cardiovascular, dura mater, and urinary bladder applications in animal models and in human clinical studies including orthopedic, urogenital, and dermatologic wound repair. SIS has also been used for abdominal wall defects, diaphragmatic hernias, and tendon repairs and as a coverage graft for compromised wounds.[36]

Animal models have demonstrated the efficacy of SIS. Chen and Beierle used SIS harvested from porcine small intestine to patch defects on the wall of the small bowel and esophagus.[36] After several weeks, the SIS scaffold dissolved and new growth of esophagus and small bowel was demonstrated. The SIS patch allowed the bowel to grow over the scaffold and maintain a normal diameter rather than a likely stricture with primary healing. Grossly, the specimens showed that the patched bowel had no narrowing, and, histologically, the neointestine resembled native bowel with minimal architectural disarray.

Badylak and colleagues used porcine-derived, xenogeneic extracellular matrix derived either from the SIS or the UBS to patch 5 cm defects in female dogs or replace a circumferential defect.[37] The SIS and UBS grafts contained angiogenic factors, such as basic fibroblast growth factor and vascular endothelial growth factor (VEGF). These scaffolds have been shown to be excellent substrates for epithelial cell growth. Early histologic examination of the grafted regions revealed neovascularization, collagen deposition, and early spindle cell deposition. After 50 days, only a small amount of collagenous material remained at the graft site, with the majority of

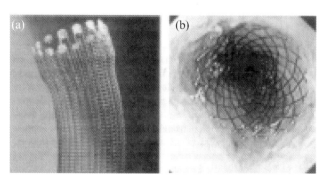

Figure 13. A, Esophageal stent; B, Endoscopic view of expanded stent in the esophagus.

the patch graft site replaced by organized bundles of skeletal muscle. The graft material was resorbed and could not be identified by light microscopy. Additionally, the graft surfaces were completely covered by squamous epithelium. There was no stenosis in dogs with patch grafts. However, there was a 50% stenosis with dogs that had circumferential replacement grafts. The stenosis in the circumferential grafts may be explained by the low intraluminal pressure in the esophagus. When these bioscaffold materials have been used for venous and arterial tubal patch grafts, there is a high patency rate, most likely owing to the presence of intraluminal pressure. Given that the intraluminal pressure is low in the esophagus, this may result in stricture formation for the tubed grafts.

A collagen sponge processed from porcine skin has been used as a scaffold for regeneration of stomach and small bowel in a dog model. The luminal side of the sponge was covered with a sheet of silicone to prevent digestion from acidic fluid. At 16 weeks, the tissue-engineered stomach wall was highly organized with the presence of the proton pumps and a thin muscle layer.[38]

Komuro and colleagues used a piglet experimental model in which myectomy or myotomy to the submucosa was performed in the cervical or thoracic esophagus.[38] A collagen sponge scaffold extracted and prepared from porcine skin was used to repair the muscular defect. Two months later, gross and histologic examinations were performed. On gross examination, no strictures were diagnosed. The collagen scaffold was replaced by loose connective tissue containing vessels and nerves, although there was no muscle regeneration.

Biomaterials may serve as an important vehicle in the future for tissue growth and delivery of growth factors. Animal models demonstrate success; however, with circumferential replacement, there tends to be anastomotic stricturing.

AlloDerm

AlloDerm (LifeCell Corporation, Branchburg, NJ) is human skin that has been processed to removal all epidermal and dermal cells while preserving the remaining biologic dermal matrix. Sinha and colleagues used AlloDerm to reconstruct through-and-through pharyngeal defects after resection of cancer in 14 patients.[39] The majority of patients had reinforcement of the AlloDerm graft with a superiorly based sternocleidomastoid flap. Two patients, one with and one without a muscle flap, developed a fistula. There were no graft contractures or stricture formation.

Esophagoplasty was performed by patching defects in the cervical esophagus in a dog with AlloDerm. All of the dogs survived, without any leak or stricture formation. Histologically, there was partial reepithelialization of the patch with neovascularization at 1 month. By 2 months, the mucosa was completely regenerated and the collagen framework absorbed. AlloDerm may serve as a patch material without the mobidity of harvesting organs.

Growth Factors

Use of growth factors in a concentrated and directed form may accelerate the healing of esophageal injuries while preventing stricture formation (see Chapter 30, "Growth Factors: Modulators of Wound Healing"). Transforming growth factor β is a physiologic component of platelet α-granules and is released during the early events of the healing process. It is chemotactic for both fibroblasts and macrophages, increases the production of collagen by both intestinal smooth muscle cells and fibroblasts, and modulates the expression of collagenase. Topical application has been shown to accelerate intestinal wound healing. As mentioned previously, interferon-α-2b has been shown to decrease the severity of inflammation and fibrosis.

Epidermal growth factor (EGF) is a trophic factor with indirect effects on the protection and repair of esophageal and gastric mucosa after injuries. EGF is naturally found in saliva, gastric juice, urine, and α-granules of platelets. In injured tissue, EGF induces cell proliferation via increased deoxyribonucleic acid (DNA) synthesis, as well as stimulates fibroblasts and improves local vascular conditions. EGF has also demonstrated a beneficial effect in rats in preventing stricture formation and decreasing the presence of hydroxyproline, a marker for collagen.

Tissue hypoxia also induces expression of growth factors. Baatar and colleagues induced esophageal ulcers in rats and concluded that hypoxia induces expression of hypoxia-inducible transcription factor 1α, an activator of VEGF.[40] VEGF is a major mediator of angiogenesis. Additionally, rats injected with plasmid-encoded rhVEGF had an increase in the formation of microvessels compared with controls. This study may have future implications for gene therapy to accelerate the healing of esophageal ulcers.

Halofuginone

Stricture formation is ultimately the product of collagen deposition and wound contraction. Halofuginone, isolated from the plant *Dishroa febrifuga*, is a specific inhibitor of the synthesis of collagen type I, which is the major matrix constituent produced during fibrosis.[41] Ozcelik divided 60 rats into four groups: a control group, a sham laparotomy group, a caustic injury group induced with 50% NaOH without treatment, and a caustic injury group treated with halofuginone.[41] Halofuginone was administered by intraperitoneal injection on the first postoperative day. Histologic examination revealed that halofuginone inhibited collagen deposition and resulted in a lower stricture formation rate. Halofuginone may prove to be a more specific means to decrease collagen production and thus stricture formation.

Sphingosylphosphorylcholine

Sphingosylphosphorylcholine (SPC) is an intracellular second messenger with a wide spectrum of activity in cell growth regulation and signal transduction. It is the most powerful stimulator of cell proliferation and DNA synthesis. When SPC is induced, the number of mitotic cells increases, resulting in a smaller cross-sectional scar area and more normal-appearing tissue in the wound sites. Yagmurlu and colleagues compared a control group of rats with esophageal burns with a group in which SPC was applied by gavage for 7 days.[42] At 28 days, contrast esophagography demonstrated prevention of strictures with SPC treatment. Histologically, there was decreased collagen deposition in the SPC group versus the control group, as well as minimal muscular atrophy. SPC may then serve to enhance healing following caustic esophageal burns without deleterious effects on wound strength.

Octreotide

Octreotide is a somatostatin analog that inhibits cell migration and proliferation and has been shown to reduce fibrosis. Kaygusuz and colleagues studied esophageal burns in 63 rabbits and examined the histologic effects of no intervention, octreotide, or interferon-α-2b.[43] Interferon-α-2b was most beneficial in the acute inflammatory phase by inhibiting cell proliferation and cell migration. A histologic examination 20 days after injury revealed that octreotide depressed fibrotic activity in the second phase of wound healing. Hydroxyproline levels, an indicator of collagen production, were found to be significantly lower in the octreotide group versus controls. Octreotide may have a worthwhile future application for reducing stricture formation following corrosive injury of the esophagus secondary to low cost and morbidity compared with surgical treatment, as well as good patient tolerance.[42]

Caffeine Acid Phenethyl Ester

Caffeine acid phenethyl ester (CAPE) is a natural product extracted from the propolis of honeybees. CAPE has strong antioxidant, antimitotic, anti-inflammatory, immunomodulatory, and wound healing properties. It inhibits lipoxygenase activity, preventing tissue infiltration of human leukocytes, thus suppressing inflammation and modulating immune reactions.

Koltuksuz and colleagues subjected 76 rats to corrosive esophageal injury induced with NaOH and divided them into four groups: sham, control, CAPE, and EGF.[44] The rats were evaluated with contrast esophagography and histologic analysis at day 28. Subcutaneous administration of CAPE to rats with caustic burns resulted in mild stenosis compared with severe esophageal stenosis in the control groups. Additionally, hydroxyproline levels were statistically lower. Use of CAPE has promise for accelerating healing and limiting fibrosis and stenosis.

Lathyrogens

Lathyrogen compounds interfere with collagen cross-linking by inhibiting the enzyme lysyl oxidase (beta-aminoproprionitrile) or altering the biochemical structure of collagen (D-penicillamine). D-Penicillamine does not influence bursting strength, collagen content, or solubility in gastrointestinal anastomosis. Lower doses have been shown to decrease cutaneous wound strength and increase its collagen solubility.

N-Acetylcysteine is another lathyrogen that interferes with collagen cross-linking by stimulating glutathione synthesis, promoting detoxification, and acting directly as a free radical scavenger. Applications of *N*-acetylcysteine have included use as a mucolytic agent for respiratory illness and as a chelating agent in heavy metal poisoning. In animals exposed to caustic injury with alkaline agents, *N*-acetylcysteine was found to decrease the rate of stricture formation and lessen the severity of stenosis.[45]

Fibrin Glue

Fibrin glue components are natural biologic factors that include fibrinogen, thrombin, calcium chloride, and fibrinolysis inhibitor, which, when mixed together in different ratios, produce a liquid that can be applied to tissue surfaces and that undergoes controlled polymerization to form an adherent fibrin matrix. Applied to wounds in situ,

it produces rapid formation of granulation tissue and early epithelialization. Fibrin glue has been used to obliterate recurrent tracheoesophageal fistulae by an endoscopic approach.[46] Recurrent tracheoesophageal fistula repair involving a thoracotomy with esophageal replacement or interposition of tissue (pericardium, pleura, or muscle) has been associated with a high rate of recurrent fistula formation.[47] An endoscopic approach with closure of the fistula with fibrin glue via the trachea has been successful in closing persistent tracheoesophageal fistulae but does require multiple applications. Use of fibrin glue for closure of recurrent tracheoesophageal fistulae has promise as a procedure with low morbidity compared with open repair.

Aerosolized fibrin glue has also been used as a delivery vehicle for gene transfer into epithelial cells on a mucosal surface.[48] This technique was developed for the therapy of malignant or premalignant lesions but, as a component of the normal wound healing response, may have applications for the delivery of growth factors and other soluble mediators to promote healing.

CO$_2$ Laser

A novel use of the CO$_2$ laser as a soldering system has been tested on rats with esophageal perforation. Nageris and colleagues used a CO$_2$ laser consisting of an infrared detector and two optical silver halide fibers.[49] One fiber delivered the CO$_2$ laser beam to a small target and a second fiber transmitted infrared radiation to the heated target. Longitudinal incisions experimentally created in the esophagus were repaired with CO$_2$ laser soldering or a two-layer closure with polyglactin suture. Bovine serum albumin 50% was applied to the edges of the perforation, and a CO$_2$ laser was used to solder the entire length of the incision. There was a 75% success rate for rats treated with laser-assisted closure and an 80% success rate for rats closed with suture. Complications in the CO$_2$ laser group that resulted in death included total breakdown of the wound, esophageal fistula, and neck abscess. Histologic analysis demonstrated mucosal surface reepithelialization and fibrotic changes in the submucosa and muscular layer, with no difference between the two groups 1 month after repair. The advantages of using a CO_2 laser soldering technique include short procedure time, less foreign-body reaction, and the potential for endoscopic application.

Robotics

The use of robotics has been increasing in recent years with urologic and thoracic applications. The computer-assisted surgical system was approved by the US federal government and is available as the daVinci Surgical System (Intuitive Surgical, Inc., Sunnyvale, CA). The daVinci system is composed of three separate components. The robotic arm is a videoscope-mounted chassis with three to four arms on which operative instruments may be interchanged. A surgeon console contains the control panel for precise robotic manipulation, and an integrative control cart provides communication between the surgeon console and the robotic arms.[50] Most of the endorobotic instruments have seven degrees of freedom, referred to as the EndoWrist, simulating normal wrist movements, differentiating it from laparoscopic procedures. Few institutions have reviewed the use of robotics in esophageal surgery via a thoracic approach. Use of the robotic system is technically challenging in a confined chest wall with cardiac and respiratory movements. The robotic technique has been used for mobilization of the esophagus and resection of esophageal masses.[51] Additionally, the robotic system has been used in patients who underwent esophagectomy and gastric tubulization with a left cervical anastomosis.[52] As this technology evolves the speed of patient recovery, discomfort, cost of the procedure, and long-term operative quality may improve, making its use more widely accepted.

REFERENCES

1. Burkett HG, Yang B, Heath JW. Wheater's functional histology. New York: Churchill Livingstone; 1993.

2. Woodson GE. Laryngeal and pharyngeal function. In: RobertHurley, editor. Otolaryngology, head and neck surgery. Vol 3. 3rd ed. St. Louis: Mosby-Year Book; 1998. p. 1844–53.

3. Witte MB, Barbul A. Repair of full-thickness bowel injury. Crit Care Med 2003;31 (8 Suppl):S538–46.

4. Lerut T, Coosemans W, Decker G, et al. Anastomotic complications after esophagectomy. Dig Surg 2002;19: 92–8.

5. Dewar L. Factors affecting cervical anastomotic leak and stricture formation following esophagogastrectomy and gastric tube interposition. Am J Surg 1992;163:484–9.

6. Sikora AG. Otolaryngologic manifestations of immunodeficiency. Otol Clin North Am 2003;36:647–72.

7. Silverstein FE, Tytgat GNJ. Gastrointestinal endoscopy. 3rd ed. London: Mosby-Wolfe; 1997.

8. Werner-Wasik M, Yu X, Marks LB, et al. Normal-tissue toxicities of thoracic radiation therapy: esophagus, lung, and spinal cord as organs at risk. Hematol Oncol Clin North Am 2004;18:131–60.

9. Ng TM, Spencer GM, Sargeant IR, et al. Management of strictures after radiotherapy for esophageal cancer. Gastrointest Endosc 1996;43:584–90.

10. Maguire PD, Sibley GS, Zhou SM, et al. Clinical and dosimetric predictors of radiation-induced esophageal toxicity. Int J Radiat Oncol Biol Phys 1999;45: 97–103.

11. Byhardt RW, Scott C, Sause WT, et al. Response, toxicity, failure patterns, and survival in five Radiation Therapy Oncology Group (RTOG) trials of sequential and/or concurrent chemotherapy and radiotherapy for locally advanced non-small-cell carcinoma of the lung. Int J Radiat Oncol Biol Phys 1998;42:469–78.

12. Brizel DM, Wasserman TH, Henke M, et al. Phase III randomized trial of amifostine as a radioprotector in head and neck cancer. J Clin Oncol 2000;18:3339–45.

13. Moretzsohn LD, de Brito EM, Reis MS, et al. Assessment of effectiveness of different dosage regimens of pantoprazole in controlling symptoms and healing esophageal lesions of patients with mild erosive esophagitis. Arq Gastroenterol 2002;39:123–5.

14. Holte K, Kehlet H. Perioperative single-dose glucocorticoid administration: pathophysiologic effects and clinical implications. J Am Coll Surg 2002;195:694–712.

15. Takeda S, Ogawa R, Nakanishi K, et al. The effect of preoperative high dose methylprednisolone in attenuating the metabolic response after oesophageal resection. Eur J Surg 1997;163:511–7.

16. Schulze S, Andersen J, Overgaard H, et al. Effect of prednisolone on the systemic response and wound healing after colonic surgery. Arch Surg 1997;132:129–35.

17. Nagelschmidt M, Fu ZX, Saad S, et al. Preoperative high dose methylprednisolone improves patient outcome after abdominal surgery. Eur J Surg 1999;165:971–8.

18. Briel JW, Tamhankar AP, Hagen JA, et al. Prevalence and risk factors for ischemia, leak, and stricture of esophageal anastomosis, gastric pull-up versus colon interposition. J Am Coll Surg 2004;198:536–42.

19. Orringer MB, Marshal B, Iannettoni MD. Eliminating the cervical esophagogastric anastomotic leak with a side-to-side stapled anastamosis. J Thorac Cardiovasc Surg 2000;119:277–88.

20. Blewett CJ, Miller JD, Young EM, et al. Anastomotic leaks after esophagectomy for esophageal cancer: a comparison of thoracic and cervical anastomoses. Ann Thorac Cardiovasc Surg 2001;7:75–8.

21. Alanezi K, Urschel JD. Mortality secondary to esophageal anastomotic leak. Ann Thorac Cardiovasc Surg 2004; 10:71–5.

22. Urschel JD, Antkowiak JG, Delacure MD, et al. Ischemic conditioning (delay phenomenon) improves esophago-gastric anastomotic wound healing in the rat. J Surg Oncol 1997;66:254–6.

23. Iannettoni MD, Whyte RI, Orringer MB. Catastrophic complications of the cervical esophagogastric anasto-mosis. J Thorac Cardiovasc Surg 1995;110:1493–501.

24. Schaefer SD. Laryngeal and esophageal trauma. In: RobertHurley, editor. Otolaryngology, head and neck surgery. Vol 3. 3rd ed. St. Louis: Mosby-Year Book; 1998. p. 2011–2.

25. Duncan M, Wong RKH. Esophageal emergencies: things that will wake you from a sound sleep. Gastroenterol Clin North Am 2003;32:1035–52.

26. Bassiouny IE, Al-Ramadan SA, Al-Nady A. Long-term functional results of transhiatal oesophagectomy and colonic interposition for caustic oesophageal stricture. Eur J Pediatr Surg 2002;12:243–7.

27. Zwischenberger JB, Savage C, Bidani A. Surgical aspects of esophageal disease—perforation and caustic injury. Am J Respir Crit Care Med 2001;164:1037–40.

28. Han Y, Cheng QS, Li XF, et al. Surgical management of esophageal strictures after caustic burns: 30 years of experience. World J Gastroenterol 2004;10:2648–9.

29. Eisen GM. Complications of upper GI endoscopy. Gastrointest Endosc 2002;55:783–93.

30. Anderson SHC, Meenan J, Williams KN, et al. Efficacy and safety of endoscopic dilation of esophageal strictures in epidermolysis bullosa. Gastrointest Endosc 2004;59:28–32.

31. Lan LC, Wong KK, Lin SC, et al. Endoscopic balloon dilation of esophageal strictures in infants and children: 17 years' experience and a literature review. J Pediatr Surg 2003;38:1712–5.

32. Orringer MB, Lemmer JH. Early dilation in the treatment of esophageal disruption. Ann Thorac Surg 1993;56: 1432–3.

33. Evrard S, Le Moine O, Lazaraki G. Self-expanding plastic stents for benign esophageal lesions. Gastrointest Endosc 2004;60:894–900.

34. Adler DG, Pleskow DK. Closure of a benign tracheoeso-phageal fistula by using a coated, self-expanding plastic stent in a patient with a history of esophageal atresia. Gastrointest Endosc 2005;61:765–8.

35. Grikscheit T, Ochoa ER, Srinivsan A, et al. Tissue-engineered esophagus: experimental substitution by only patch or interposition. J Thorac Cardiovasc Surg 2003;126:537–44.

36. Chen MK, Beierle EA. Animal models for intestinal tissue engineering. Biomaterials 2004;25:1676–81.

37. Badylak S, Meurling S, Chen M, et al. Resorbable bioscaffold for esophageal repair in a dog model. J Pediatr Surg 2000;35:1097–103.

38. Komuro H, Nakamura T, Kaneko M, et al. Application of collagen sponge scaffold to muscular defects of the esophagus: an experimental study in piglets. J Pediatr Surg 2002;37:1409–13.

39. Sinha UK, Chang KE, Shih CW. Reconstruction of pharyngeal defects using AlloDerm and sternocleido-mastoid muscle flaps. Laryngoscope 2001;111:1910–6.

40. Baatar D, Jones MK, Tsugawa K, et al. Esophageal ulceration triggers expression of hypoxia-inducible factor-1α and activates vascular endothelial growth factor gene. Am J Pathol 2002;161:1449–57.

41. Ozcelik MF, Pekmezci S, Saribeyoglu K, et al. The effect of halofuginone, a specific inhibitor of collagen type 1 synthesis, in the prevention of esophageal strictures related to caustic injury. Am J Surg 2004;187: 257–60.

42. Yagmurlu A, Burhan A, Bingol-Kologlu M, et al. A novel approach for preventing esophageal stricture forma-tion: sphingosylphosphorylcholine-enhanced tissue remodeling. Pediatr Surg Int 2004;20:778–82.

43. Kaygusuz I, Irfan MD, Celik O, et al. Effects of interferon-alpha-2b and octreotide on healing of esophageal corrosive burns. Laryngoscope 2001;111 (11 Pt 1):1999–2004.

44. Koltuksuz U, Mutus HM, Kutlu R, et al. Effects of caffeic acid phenethyl ester and epidermal growth factor on the development of caustic esophageal stricture in rats. J Pediatr Surg 2001;36:1504–9.

45. Liu AJ, Richardson MA. Effects of N-acetylcystine on experimentally induced esophageal injury. Ann Otol Rhinol Laryngol 1985;94:477–82.

46. Willets IE, Dudley NE, Tam PKH. Endoscopic treatment of recurrent tracheo-oesophageal fistulae: long-term results. Pediatr Surg Int 1998;13:256–8.

47. McGahren ED, Rodgers BM. Bronchoscopic obliteration of recurrent tracheoesophageal fistula in an infant. Pediatric Endosurgery and Innovative Techniques 2001;5:37–42.

48. Teraishi F, Umeoka T, Saito T. A novel method for gene delivery and expression in esophageal epithelium with fibrin glues containing replication-deficient adenovirus vector. Surg Endosc 2003;17(11):1845–8.

49. Nageris BI, Zilker Z, Zilker M, et al. Esophageal incisions repair by CO2 laser soldering. Otolaryngol Head Neck Surg 2004;131:856–9.

50. Kernstine KH. Robotics in thoracic surgery. Am J Surg 2004;188 (4A Suppl):895–975.

51. Elli E, Espat NG, Berger R, et al. Robotic-assisted thoracoscopic resection of esophageal leiomyoma. Surg Endosc 2004;18:713–6.

52. Giulianotti PC, Coratti A, Angelini M, et al. personal experience in a large community hospital. Arch Surg 2003;138:777–84.

10

Salient Healing Features of the Tympanic Membrane

Sten Hellström, MD, PhD

UNIQUE HISTOLOGY AND HEALING PHYSIOLOGY

The tympanic membrane is a unique structure suspended in air. Its major acoustic portion, the pars tensa, consists of an outer layer of a keratinizing squamous epithelium, a middle layer—lamina propria—of mainly densely packed collagenous fibers, and an inner layer of a thin mucosal epithelium. When perforated, the healing of a healthy tympanic membrane starts with the migration of the keratinizing squamous epithelium. The advancing squamous epithelium is guided by a spur of keratin. Below the epithelium, a loose connective tissue, rich in active fibroblasts, is formed. In an inflamed middle ear, the inflammatory reaction will speed up the healing of a perforation. Obviously, the healing of a tympanic membrane differs from that of a healing skin wound in that the epithelium will close the wound without the need to migrate on a bed of granulation tissue.

MAJOR STEPS IN HEALING OVER TIME

Analysis of the events involved in healing of a tympanic membrane perforation obtained in an animal model shows that (1) during the first days after the perforation, there is an ingrowth of blood vessels toward the perforated area; (2) a simultaneous accumulation of inflammatory cells starts to occur in the vicinity of the perforation border; (3) after 3 to 4 days, the extremely thickened keratinizing squamous epithelium begins to migrate and reduce the size of the perforation border; (4) secondary to the migrating epithelium, the connective tissue layer will start to expand and now contains large amounts of the glycosaminoglycan hyaluronan; (5) a perforation occupying one quadrant will close within 10 to 12 days, and almost immediately after the closure, the thickened keratinizing squamous epithelium starts to normalize; and (6) after 3 to 6 months, the initial loose connective tissue of lamina propria will change to a layer with densely packed collagen fibers.

COMMON WOUND HEALING PROBLEMS

The majority, about 80 to 90%, of tympanic membrane perforations will heal spontaneously. The challenge is to elucidate why some perforations become persistent or permanent, whereas others will heal spontaneously.

FUTURE PROMISE FOR HEALING IMPROVEMENT

Knowledge is accumulating that characterizes the components involved in the healing mechanisms, such as extracellular matrix components and growth factors. Findings in genetically altered animals indicate, for example, that the presence of plasminogen in the perforated area is crucial for the closure of a perforated tympanic membrane. So far, surgical techniques using tissue transplants have been requested for closure of a tympanic membrane perforation. However, increasing knowledge of the healing mechanisms may well lead to a scientific breakthrough, which means that a specific mixture of components can be manufactured with the ability to heal a perforated tympanic membrane without surgery.

Tympanic membrane perforation is a common condition that is estimated to affect 1 to 3% of the US population and 1% of the population worldwide.[1] Tympanic membrane perforations are primarily the result of middle ear infection, trauma, eustachian tube dysfunction, barotrauma, and iatrogenic injury. Fortunately, most perforations heal spontaneously, thus avoiding sequelae such as hearing loss and infection. Traditionally, chronic perforations have been managed by tympanoplasty, which is successful in > 90% of patients.[2] To understand the healing properties of the tympanic membrane, one needs to understand its structure and physiology.

When vertebrates started to live on land, one important function for survival was to recognize airborne sound. The sense organs used in water, designed to recognize vibrations, had to be modified for detection of sound transmitted in air. This is a difficult task as 99% of the energy is lost when sound is airborne. The vertebrates on land developed tympanic membranes and middle ears with ossicles. Functionally, we associate tympanic membranes with sound transmission, but as doctors and physicians, we should not forget that it is a very helpful window toward the middle ear, which will help diagnose a variety of middle ear conditions. In this chapter, the structure of the tympanic membrane and its healing properties when it is traumatized or diseased are reviewed.

TYMPANIC MEMBRANE STRUCTURE

The tympanic membrane is a unique structure suspended in air and consists of two portions, the pars tensa and the pars flaccida. The tense portion is mainly devoted to sound transmission, but the function of the smaller area, representing the flaccid portion, is still an enigma. Similar to many other organs and diseases, Hippocrates was the first to describe the tympanic membrane in 400 BC.[3] Since, many researchers have studied the tympanic membrane's structure. As depicted by Lim in the 1960s, the tense portion of the tympanic membrane consists of an outer layer of a keratinising squamous epithelium, a middle layer consisting of mainly densely packed collagenous fibers, but with narrow subepithelial connective tissue layers and an inner layer of a thin mucosal epithelium (Figure 1).[4,5] In contrast, the flaccid portion is composed of a thick lamina propria consisting of a loose connective tissue surrounded by an outer keratinising squamous epithelial layer and an inner mucosal epithelial lining. Blood vessels and nerves are mainly located subepithelial to the outer layer. The tympanic membrane can also be characterized as being built up by a mucosal layer facing the middle ear cavity and a layer of skin toward the external ear canal. The origin of these two different tissues refers to the embryology of the tympanic membrane as it develops from an endodermal layer forming the mucosa-covered middle ear cavity and an outer ectodermal skin covering the external ear canal.[6] The flaccid portion differs from the tense portion because it lacks the densely packed collagenous fiber layer.[7] In contrast, it is composed of a loose connective tissue. In our studies of the tympanic membrane and its healing properties, the rat has been used as an animal model, which is referred to in the following text for a more detailed description of the tense portion and the flaccid portion.

The rat tympanic membrane is about 5 mm in diameter and has a rather large flaccid portion.[8–10] In fact, most mammals have a relatively larger pars flaccida compared with the pars tensa than the human has.[9,10] The thickness of the pars tensa of the rat tympanic membrane is fairly thin, approximately 5 μm, which should be compared with a 60 μm–thick human tympanic membrane.[5,8,11] The membrane thickens toward the annulus. The outer keratinizing squamous epithelium of the pars tensa rests on a very dense layer of collagenous fibers. These collagenous fibers are arranged in mainly two directions, radially and circularly. The radial fibers are in the majority,

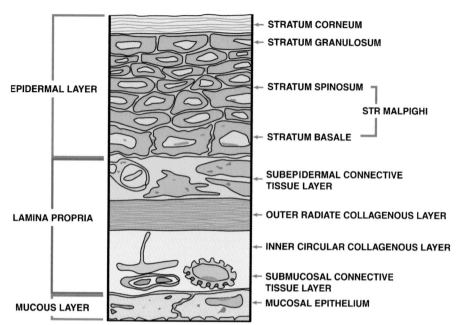

EPIDERMAL LAYER

LAMINA PROPRIA

MUCOUS LAYER

← STRATUM CORNEUM
← STRATUM GRANULOSUM

← STRATUM SPINOSUM ⌉
                    ⎸ STR MALPIGHI
← STRATUM BASALE ⌋

← SUBEPIDERMAL CONNECTIVE
   TISSUE LAYER

← OUTER RADIATE COLLAGENOUS LAYER

← INNER CIRCULAR COLLAGENOUS LAYER

← SUBMUCOSAL CONNECTIVE
   TISSUE LAYER
← MUCOSAL EPITHELIUM

Figure 1. The classic illustration of the tympanic membrane. Reproduced with permission from Lim DJ.[4]

but in the periphery, toward the inner surface, there are fibers that are mainly circular. The very thin inner layer of epithelial cells contrasts to the rest of the epithelial coat of the middle ear cavity as ciliated cells and goblet cells are lacking (Figure 2A). Immunohistochemical studies of the collagen fibers made by Hussl and colleagues and more recently by Stenfeldt and colleagues on normal tympanic membranes show that collagen types II and III predominate, with a minor occurrence of type I collagen.[12,13]

The pars flaccida has a substantially different morphology compared with that of the pars tensa in that the fibrous or connective tissue layer consists of a loose connective tissue (Figure 2B).[7] Close to the outer epithelium, the connective tissue

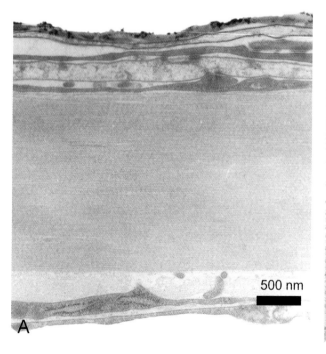

500 nm

A

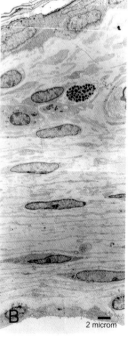

B

2 microm

Figure 2. Electron micrographs of a normal pars tensa (*A*) and a normal pars flaccida (*B*).

layer holds blood vessels and bundles of nerves. However, the most conspicuous element of the pars flaccida is the abundance of mast cells.[14,15]

If stained in vivo for mast cells, by use of toluidine blue, the pars flaccida exhibits a great number of mast cells scattered at random throughout the whole pars flaccida area. In comparison, the pars tensa only contains mast cells along the malleal blood vessels. In fact, counted as the number of mast cells per square millimeter of tissue, the pars flaccida is one of the most mast cell–rich compartments of the body. The abundance of mast cells originally discovered in the rat pars flaccida has also been verified in the human tympanic membrane.[15]

The role that pars flaccida mast cells play in middle ear physiology and pathophysiology remains still to be elucidated. Not only do mast cells contain classic inflammatory mediators, such as histamine, and preformed mediators, such as leukotrienes, they also contain other cytokines and chemokines.[16] A release of products from mast cells will start repair processes of, for example, collagen, and it may well be that the mast cells in normal middle ear physiology will have the role of restoring the pars tensa after microdamage of the fibrous tissue caused by sound transmission. Moreover, activated mast cells initiate an effusion production, which fills the attic compartment of the pars flaccida in a couple of hours,[17] a secretion response that might be part of the mucosal defense system. Fluid collected from the attic space, when analyzed, was found to contain histamine and metabolites from both the lipoxygenase and the cyclooxygenase pathways.

The vascular and nerve supplies of the tympanic membrane also deserve comment. Tympanic membrane specimens stained for erythrocytes, by bensidine, exhibit a dense network of blood vessels along the annulus of the pars tensa. Some vessels are located along the handle of the malleus, but the semitransparent portions of the pars tensa are devoid of vessels.[18] In comparison, the pars flaccida is more richly vascularized than the pars tensa, and several vessels cross and branch in the pars flaccida. It is feasible that the sparse vascularity of the acoustic portions of pars tensa is physiologically important because the minute vibration of the tympanic membrane, when stimulated by sound, might be affected by passing erythrocytes disturbing the sound transmission. Recent investigations have shown that some thin vessels also cross the semitransparent portions of the pars tensa from the handle of the malleus to the annulus area.[19] However, in normal conditions, these blood vessels are too narrow to allow erythrocytes to pass and thus may only allow plasma to pass.

In contrast, during inflammatory conditions, the blood vessels dilate considerably within hours after the start of an episode of otitis media. It appears that there are some preformed blood vessels also in the semitransparent portions of pars tensa that will immediately open for the passage of blood cells when an inflammatory reaction starts.[19]

It is well known that it is very painful to touch the tympanic membrane, and this is because the tympanic membrane is richly innervated. Immunohistochemistry has shown that several neuropeptidergic nerves are located in the flaccid portion, whereas they are more sparsely distributed in the tense portion.[20] Thus, substance P and vasoactive intestinal polypeptide have been shown to occur in the pars flaccida but not in the pars tensa. This observation contrasts to that of the occurrence of catecholaminergic nerve fibers, which occur in both the annulus area and the thinner portion of the pars tensa.[20] In fact, these catecholaminergic fibers seem to run adjacent to the fine-caliper vessels revealed in the semitransparent portion of the pars tensa.[19]

STRUCTURE OF THE TYMPANIC MEMBRANE IN AN INFLAMED MIDDLE EAR

The tympanic membrane is the diagnostic window, and it has the ability to mirror ongoing processes in the middle ear cavity. Already a few hours after the start of an episode of otitis media, there are typical signs of the acute inflammatory changes, including increased vascularity, less opacity, and reduced mobility. It has also been shown that irrespective of the evoking agent, for example, microorganisms, mechanical trauma, or irradiation, the earliest changes will appear in the pars flaccida.[21]

The sequence of the early inflammatory changes has been followed in a pneumococcal acute otitis media model.[22] If pneumococci are introduced into the rat middle ear cavity and the tympanic membrane status is monitored otomicroscopically every 3 hours, the pars tensa of the tympanic membrane will become richly vascularized within 6 hours. Furthermore, it will bulge, and a pus-like fluid will start to appear medial to the tympanic membrane. Within 48 hours, roughly 50% of the tympanic membranes will spontaneously perforate owing to increased pressure. Histologically, striking changes in the pars flaccida structure appear already after 3 hours.[22] The stroma of the connective tissue of the pars flaccida becomes swollen and edematous, and abundant polymorphonuclear leukocytes, expelled from the blood vessels, will traverse the connective tissue and accumulate in the middle ear cavity.[22,23] During the next few hours, an amorphous substance, immunochemically identified as fibrin or fibrinogen, will accumulate in the connective tissue layer. At 48 hours after the inoculation of pneumococci, the pars flaccida will be completely infiltrated with inflammatory cells, mainly leukocytes. The simple squamous inner epithelium will change to a cuboidal or columnar profile containing ciliated cells and goblet cells.

HEALING PROPERTIES OF THE TYMPANIC MEMBRANE

The healing properties of perforated tympanic membranes have been mainly studied in animal models.[24–29] In these models, it has been rather easy to perform perforations standardized in size, the healing pattern of which can be monitored by various microscopic techniques until closure. The results, which follow, have mainly been obtained by studies in the rat.

A perforation, standardized in size in a healthy tympanic membrane and performed by a myringotomy lancet, will close very uniformly.[30,31] In such a model, all perforations occupying one quadrant of the tense portion close or heal within 10 to 12 days. The immediate closure is followed by the formation of scar tissue, and still, 3 months later, the collagenous fiber layer is not completely reorganized. In a perforation of a healthy tympanic membrane, the healing process starts with the migration of the keratinizing squamous epithelium.[28–31] The advancing squamous epithelium is guided by a spur of keratin, protruding like a nail. Below the epithelium, a loose connective tissue, rich in active fibroblasts, is formed. This is a mechanism completely different from normal skin wound healing, in which the closing squamous epithelium will migrate on a bed of granulation tissue (see Chapter 1). At the time of closure, the multilayered migrating epithelium and the connective tissue meet each other roughly simultaneously (Figure 3). One day later, the squamous epithelium will start to diminish in thickness, and the major thickness of the healed area will be due to an increased, unorganized connective tissue layer.

One matrix substance has been of certain interest in general wound healing and in particular in healing of tympanic membrane perforations: the glycosaminoglycan hyaluronan. With access to a hyaluronan binding protein probe, it has been possible to follow the occurrence and

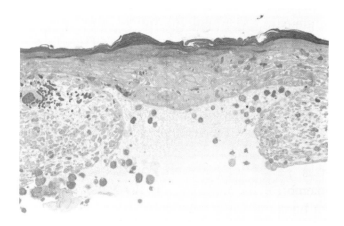

Figure 3. Light micrograph showing the healing of a tympanic membrane perforation. The keratinizing squamous epithelium is closing the perforation ahead of the connective tissue layer.

participation of this extracellular matrix component during the healing process.[30,32] In the normal pars tensa, there is hardly any detectable hyaluronan. However, within the first 2 to 3 days after a tympanic membrane perforation, there is a heavy accumulation of hyaluronan in the perforation borders. The intense presence of hyaluronan will persist in the advancing borders until the tympanic membrane is closed at days 10 to 12. Already 2 to 3 days later, the occurrence of hyaluronan has diminished, and 1 week later, hardly any staining of hyaluronan will be seen. This observation led to the assumption that hyaluronan is of importance for the early healing pattern of a tympanic membrane perforation.

EXTRACELLULAR MATRIX COMPONENTS

In a series of experiments, hyaluronan was applied to the tympanic membrane perforation and the healing rate of saline-treated and untreated perforations was compared.[30,32] Interestingly, there was faster healing of the tympanic membrane when the perforation was treated with hyaluronan compared with the untreated or saline-treated perforations. The hyaluronan-treated perforations not only closed faster, but the collagenous fiber layer also showed a faster reconstitution. In the hyaluronan-treated tympanic membranes, the keratinizing squamous epithelium appeared to migrate in the hyaluronan layer to cover the perforation much more quickly. The results initiated a clinical study in which hyaluronan was tested for closure of chronic tympanic membrane perforations in humans.[33] This clinical study could not show significant benefit of hyaluronan treatment to favor healing of tympanic membrane perforations compared with the traditional paper patch technique. However, one has to consider that the testing of hyaluronan in the animal model was performed on closure of acute tympanic membrane perforations. Persistent perforations in humans, which are chronic wounds, may have a completely different healing capacity.

The promising experimental results of the hyaluronan studies led us also to investigate other extracellular matrix components and, in particular, the glycosaminoglycans: chondroitin-4-sulfate, unsulfated chondroitin, chondroitin-6-sulfate, native chondroitin, and dermatan sulfate.[34] The various monoclonal antibodies used to detect the different chondroitin sulfate oligosaccharides rendered less prominent staining reactions compared with that of the hyaluronan. Unsulfated chondroitin, chondroitin-4-sulfate, and chondrotin-6-sulfate were constantly present in small amounts during the whole healing process. In contrast, unsulfated chondroitin, native chondroitin, and dermatan sulfate seemed to increase in the healed area of the tympanic membrane after closure of the perforation.

Another extracellular matrix component, fibronectin, was shown to appear in the perforation border on the first day after tympanic membrane perforation.[34] Fibronectin was also present in the advancing edge of migrating epithelial cells and in relation to collagen bundles and fibroblasts in the annulus fibrosus. The fibronectin results lead to the speculation that fibronectin provides a favorable microenvironment for cell migration and proliferation and acts as a stimulus for the reepithelialization process in the perforated tympanic membrane, as also suggested for fibronectin in healing of skin wounds in rats.[35,36] However, exogenously applied to the rat tympanic membrane model, fibronectin was not able to enhance the healing rate.[31]

Other constituents have been investigated in attempts to identify tissue components with the ability to improve healing of tympanic membrane perforations. Heparin, an acidic mucopolysaccharide that can activate the plasminogen system, did not close the tympanic membrane perforations more rapidly, but the healed tympanic membranes regained their original structure, in particular the collagenous layer, much more quickly by topical application of increasing concentrations of heparin.[37] This observation was somewhat unexpected because high concentrations of heparin caused very heavy bleeding at the perforation border. Despite the formation of large crusts covering the perforation, the perforations healed, and after 1 month, the scar tissue was excellent, showing an almost normal tympanic membrane appearance.

The results of the heparin study are interesting in view of recent results from ongoing experimental studies in genetically altered animals. These studies show that a lack of plasminogen, an activator of proteases, will arrest the healing in tympanic membrane perforations and cause persistent perforations.[38] Even more exciting is that when systemically substituting plasminogen to this genetically plasminogen-deficient species, the perforation will heal.[38] It becomes evident that in the remodeling phase of the healing tympanic membrane, a degradation of the extracellular matrix components is mandatory before the migration of the keratinizing squamous epithelial cells and the formation of a new connective tissue will occur.

GROWTH FACTORS

Growth factors are members of a large functional group of polypeptide regulatory molecules secreted by different cells. They are important players in orchestrating all stages of wound healing, exerting their influence through autocrine and paracrine fashions within sites of injury and repair (see Chapter 29, "Growth Factors: Modulators of Wound Healing"). Polypeptide growth factors and matrix moieties have also been suggested to have the ability to accelerate the healing of tympanic perforations.[39–42] Reports on topically applied epidermal growth factor (EGF) onto experimental tympanic membrane perforations have shown varying results.[39,43,44] In a human trial on chronic tympanic membrane perforations, no benefit was shown by use of topical application of EGF.[45] Fibroblast growth factors (FGFs) applied to tympanic membrane perforations have been extensively studied. Neither basic FGF (FGF-2) nor acidic FGF (FGF-1) has produced a statistically significantly higher TM closure rate compared with control treatment.[46,47] Similar results have been obtained in studies testing platelet-derived growth factor, transforming growth factor-β, and keratinocyte growth factor.[2,48,49] However, one has to consider that most investigations on growth factors and their ability to heal tympanic membrane perforations have been performed in animal models with acute perforations. Only a few experimental studies involve topical application of polypeptide growth factors in chronic perforations,[50–52] and so far, there is no clear-cut evidence that any of these substances may affect healing in the clinical situation. A clinical concern when using growth factors is the possibility of adverse cell activation, leading to excess scarring, cholesteatoma formation, or malignant transformation.[1] There is also the theoretical risk that topical agents reaching the middle ear may diffuse through the round window membrane and injure the cochlea. Fortunately, these problems have not been demonstrated in short-term applications.[1]

BIOENGINEERED TISSUES

Several experimental studies have evaluated the beneficial effects of biologic matrices as graft materials for myringoplasty of chronic tympanic membrane perforations. Using a preserved allograft commercial product (AlloDerm, LifeCell Corporation, Branchburg, NJ) in controlled animal studies, several groups have reported successful closure of chronic tympanic membrane perforations comparable to closures with autologous fascia, with excellent gross and histologic outcomes.[53,54] The allograft showed histologic evidence of ingrowth of fibroblasts and vasculature compared with the fascial graft. A recent report described similar use of acellular porcine small intestine submucosa (Surgisis, Cook Biotech, West Lafayette, IN) versus cartilage graft in tympanoplasty repair of chronic tympanic membrane in the chinchilla model. In tympanoplasties performed in five chinchillas with small intestine submucosa, five of five (100%) remained healed 6 weeks postoperatively, whereas three of five (60%) remained healed with cartilage repair; both compared favorably with the untreated controls, which showed no healing.[55]

STEM CELLS

Recently, attempts to use embryonic stem cells for healing of tympanic membrane perforations have been undertaken. Limited animal experiments showed that these stem cells enhance healing, possibly by differentiation and integration into tympanic membrane tissue.[56] However, further experimental studies are needed to evaluate the clinical potential of applying stem cells onto chronic perforations of the tympanic membrane.

HEALING OF MYRINGOTOMIZED TYMPANIC MEMBRANES IN OTITIS MEDIA

Clinically, ears with acute otitis media close their spontaneously perforated tympanic membranes even more rapidly than a perforated normal drum head. Early structural tympanic membrane reactions to a myringotomy were studied in an acute otitis media model.[57,58] In an inflamed middle ear infected by *Streptococcus pneumoniae*, the keratinocyte layer at the perforation border reacted and increased in thickness 6 hours after the myringotomy. At 9 hours after the perforation, abundant inflammatory cells, mainly polymorphonuclear leukocytes, macrophages, and small lymphocytes, infiltrated the richly vascularized connective tissue layer. Four days after the myringotomy, most of the perforations were completely closed, and at 1 week, the tympanic membrane structure was almost normalized. An identical myringotomy in a tympanic membrane in a noninflamed middle ear showed a similar healing pattern but with a delayed response. Inflammatory cells did not occur within the perforation border until 1 to 2 days after the myringotomy, which compared with 6 to 12 hours in the infected middle ear. That the tympanic membrane perforations seem to close faster in acute otitis media was also shown in an earlier experimental study.[59] These studies suggest that a traumatized tympanic membrane tissue in acute otitis has a strong healing capacity, and that, therefore, the risk of development of a residual perforation is low.

FORMATION OF SCLEROTIC INLAYS IN THE HEALING TYMPANIC MEMBRANE

One of the peculiar elements developing in a number of tympanic membranes that have been perforated is the formation of sclerotic inlays, which is called myringosclerosis. Myringosclerosis is a pathologic condition characterized by thickening and hyalinization of the connective tissue layer—lamina propria—of the tympanic membrane. Clinically, myringosclerosis is noted as being a sequela of inflammatory conditions of the middle ear but will also occur in a certain number of perforated tympanic membranes of a healthy middle ear. In particular, these sclerotic inlays will appear in a tympanic membrane that has been subjected to an open perforation and that has remained open or nonhealed for a long time, as, for example, in a tympanostomy tube–treated tympanic membrane.[60] The myringosclerotic deposits consist of a combination of calcium and phosphorus, resembling hydroxyapatite, which accumulate close to the collagen fibers.[61] In a perforated but healed tympanic membrane, myringosclerosis occurs not only in the scar area but also more commonly in the quadrant contralateral to the perforated quadrant.[62] From experimental studies, it has been suggested that the development of myringosclerosis depends, at least partially, on increased production of oxygen-derived free radicals in the perforated or traumatized tissue.[63] Reactive oxygen species are generated through changes in the concentration of oxygen in the middle ear cavity, produced by perforating the tympanic membrane and exposing the middle ear cavity to room air, causing a relatively hyperoxic environment (21% O_2). Normally, the middle ear space is in equilibrium with blood gas oxygen levels of around 7% O_2.

EXPERIMENTAL CHRONIC PERFORATIONS

The interest in studying the healing pattern of a perforated tympanic membrane mainly emanates from the expectation to be able to initiate healing and replace surgical myringoplasty by medical therapy. In a search for such remedies, one of the major setbacks in most experimental models for studying the healing pattern of a tympanic membrane perforation has been that almost all have involved acute and not chronic perforations, the latter representing the clinical challenge. Experimental models for chronic tympanic membrane perforations described in the literature are few.[50–52,64] It has been shown that hydrocortisone topically applied onto a perforated tympanic membrane will retard healing almost completely. An experimental hydrocortisone-induced chronic perforation will need months to heal compared with the 10 to 12 days for closure of a perforated nontreated tympanic membrane.[51] Retarded healing of TM perforations has also been observed after application of mitomycin C, an antineoplastic chemotherapeutic agent widely used in ophthalmology because of its ability to prevent closure of the trabeculectomy site in patients with glaucoma.[64,65] Mitomycin C selectively interrupts deoxyribonucleic acid (DNA) replication and will inhibit mitosis and protein synthesis, which means that it could act through mechanisms similar to those in plasminogen deficiency, a lack of activation of proteases. A chronic model of TM perforation has been created in the chinchilla by undermining and surgical manipulation of the wound margins to prevent reepithelialization.[43] This model has been used to evaluate the efficacy of various therapeutic approaches to promote healing of the tympanic membrane.[2,53–55] However, none of these models fully recapitulates the clinical condition of chronic TM perforations, and more clinically comparable models are needed.

CONCLUSION

In summary, the tympanic membrane is a unique structure that land-living animals need for the transmission of sound to aural receptors in the inner ear. The tympanic membrane is very useful for physicians because it can reveal ongoing disease processes in the middle ear cavity. The tympanic membrane is an extremely fast-reacting tissue of the middle ear, which makes it helpful when we want to detect early inflammatory changes in the middle ear cavity. Furthermore, the tympanic membrane has a unique healing capacity. A perforation is closed by migrating epithelial cells guided by a spur of keratin prior to definite closure by connective tissue elements. In inflammatory conditions, the healing capacity is further increased. However, under certain conditions, the perforated tympanic membrane will remain open and become a chronic or persistent perforation that requires closure by certain surgical techniques. Increased knowledge, obtained through investigating and characterizing the physiologic and biochemical events at a molecular level of a healing perforated tympanic membrane, might well lead to a scientific breakthrough for the discovery of a specific mixture of components with the ability to heal, or ideally regenerate, a perforated tympanic membrane.

REFERENCES

1. Ma Y, Zhao H, Zhou X, Topical treatment with growth factors for tympanic membrane perforations. Progess towards clinical application. Acta Otolaryngol (Stockh) 2002;122:586–99.
2. Soumekh B, Hom DB, Levine S, et al. Treatment of chronic tympanic-membrane perforations with a platelet derived releasate. Am J Otol 1996;17:506–11.
3. Weir N. Otolaryngology. An illustrated history. Cambridge (UK): Butterworths & Co; 1990.
4. Lim DJ. Tympanic membrane. Electron microscopic observation.Part I: Pars tensa. Acta Otolaryngol (Stockh) 1968;66:188–98.
5. Lim DJ. Human tympanic membrane. An ultrastructural observation. Acta Otolaryngol (Stockh) 1970;70:176–86.
6. Hammar JA. Studien über die Entwicklung des Vorderdarms und einiger angrenzenden Organe. Arch Mikr Anat 1902;59:471–628.
7. Lim DJ. Tympanic membrane. Electron microscopic observation. Part II: Pars flaccida. Acta Otolaryngol (Stockh) 1968;66:512–32.
8. Schmidt SH, Hellström S. Tympanic membrane structure—new views. A comparative study. ORL J Otorhinolaryngol Relat Spec 1991;53:32–6.
9. Shrapnell HJ. On the form and structure of the tympanic membrane. Lond Med Gazette 1832;10:120–4.
10. Stenfors L-E, Hellström S. The original description of Shrapnell's membrane reviewed in the light of recent experimental studies. J Laryngol Otol 1983;97:985–9.

11. Lim DJ. Structure and function of the tympanic membrane: a review. Acta Otorhinolaryngol Belg 1995;49: 101–15.

12. Hussl B, Timpl R, Lim DJ, et al. Immunohistochemical analysis of connective tissue components in tympanosclerosis. In: Lim DJ, Bluestone CD, Klein JO, Nelson JD, editors. Recent advances in otitis media: proceedings of the Fourth International Symposium Hamilton, Ontario: BC Decker; 1988. p. 402–6.

13. Stenfeldt K, Johansson C, Hellström S. Collagen structure of the tympanic membrane; collagen I, II and III in the healthy tympanic membrane, during healing of a perforation, and during infection. Arch Otolaryngol Head Neck Surg 2006;132:293–8.

14. Alm PE, Bloom GD, Hellström S, et al. Mast cells in the pars flaccida of the tympanic membrane. A quantitative morphological and biochemical study in the rat. Experientia 1983;39:287–9.

15. Widemar L, Hellström S, Stenfors LE, Bloom GD. An overlooked site of tissue mast cells—the human tympanic membrane. Implications for middle ear affections. Acta Otolaryngol (Stockh) 1986;102:391–5.

16. Metcalfe DD, Baram D, Mekori YA. Mast cells. Physiol Rev 1997;77:1033–79.

17. Alm P, Bloom GD, Hellström S, et al. The release of histamine from the pars flaccida mast cells—one cause of otitis media with effusion? Acta Otolaryngol (Stockh) 1982;94:517–22.

18. Albiin N, Hellström S, Salén B, et al. The vascular supply of the rat tympanic membrane. Anat Rec 1985;212:17–22.

19. Hellström S, Spratley J, Eriksson PO. Tympanic membrane vessel revisited: a study in an animal model. Otol Neurotol 2003;24:494–9.

20. Widemar L, Hellström S, Schultzberg M, et al. Autonomic innervation of the tympanic membrane. An immunocytochemical and histofluorescence study. Acta Otolaryngol (Stockh) 1985;100:58–65.

21. Magnuson K, Hellström S. Early structural changes in the rat tympanic membrane during pneumococcal otitis media. Eur Arch Otorhinolaryngol 1994;251:393–8.

22. Eriksson PO, Mattsson C, Hellström S. First forty-eight hours of developing otitis media: an experimental study. Ann Otol Rhinol Laryngol 2003;112:558–66.

23. Eriksson PO, Johansson C, Hellström S. Inflammatory cells during developing otitis media. An experimental sequential study. [Submitted].

24. McIntire C, Benitez JT. Spontaneous repair of the tympanic membrane: histopathological studies in the cat. Ann Otol (St. Louis) 1970;79:1129–31.

25. McMinn RMH, Taylor M. The cytology of repair in experimental perforations of the tympanic membrane. Br J Surg 1966;53:222–32.

26. Reynen C, Kuypers W. The healing pattern of the drum membrane. Acta Otolaryngol Suppl (Stockh) 1971; Suppl 287:1–74.

27. Reeve DRE. Repair of large experimental perforations of the tympanic membrane. J Laryngol 1977;91:767–78.

28. Boedts D. The tympanic epithelium in normal and pathological conditions. Acta Otorhinolaryngol Belg 1978;32:295–420.

29. Stenfors LE, Carlsöö B, Salén B, Winblad B. Repair of experimental tympanic membrane perforations. Acta Otolaryngol (Stockh) 1980;90:332–41.

30. Laurent C, Hellström S, Fellenius E. Hyaluronan improves the healing of experimental tympanic membrane perforations. A comparison of preparations with different rheologic properties. Arch Otolaryngol Head Neck Surg 1988;114:1435–41.

31. Hellström S, Bloom GD, Berghem L, et al. A comparison of hyaluronan and fibronectin in the healing of tympanic membrane perforations. Eur Arch Otorhinolaryngol 1991;248:230–5.

32. Hellström S, Laurent C. Hyaluronan and healing of tympanic membrane perforations. An experimental study. Acta Otolaryngol Suppl (Stockh) 1987;442:54–61.

33. Laurent C, Söderberg O, Anniko M, Hartwig S. Repair of chronic tympanic membrane perforations using applications of hyaluronan or rice paper prostheses. ORL J Otorhinolaryngol Relat 1991;53:37–40.

34. Laurent C, Hellström S. Extracellular matrix components reflect the dynamics of a healing tympanic membrane perforation—a histochemical study. Int J Biochem Cell Biol 1997;29:221–9.

35. Grinnell F, Billingham RE, Burgess L. Distribution of fibronection during wound healing in vivo. J Invest Dermatol 1981;76:181–9.

36. Cheng CY, Martin DE, Leggett CG, et al. Fibronectin enhances healing of excised wounds in rats. Arch Dermatol 1988;124:221–5.

37. Hellström S, Spandow O. Exogenous heparin, topically administered, aids the remodelling of connective tissue in the healing of experimental tympanic membrane perforations. ORL J Otorhinolaryngol Relat Spec 1994; 56:45–50.

38. Li J, Eriksson PO, Hansson A, et al. Plasmin is essential for the healing of tympanic membrane perforations. Tromb Haemost 2006;96:512–9.

39. Amoils CP, Jackler RK, Lusting LR. Repair of chronic tympanic membrane perforations using epidermal growth factor. Otolaryngol Head Neck Surg 1992;107: 669–83.

40. Mondain M, Saffiedine S, Uziel A. Fibroblast growth factor improves the healing of experimental tympanic membrane perforations. Acta Otolaryngol (Stockh) 1991;111:337–41.

41. Fina M, Baird A, Ryan A. Direct application of basic fibroblast growth factor improves tympanic membrane perforation healing. Laryngoscope 1993;103:804–9.

42. Mondain M, Ryan A. Histological study of the healing of traumatic tympanic membrane perforation after basic fibroblast growth factor application. Laryngoscope 1993;103:312–8.

43. Lee AJ, Jackler RK, Kato BM, et al. Repair of chronic tympanic membrane perforation using epidermal

growth factor: progress toward clinical application. Am J Otol 1994;15:10–8.

44. Dvorak DW, Abbas G, Ali T. Repair of chronic tympanic membrane perforations with long-term epidermal growth factor. Laryngoscope 1995;105:1300–4.

45. Ramsay HA, Hekkoinen EJ, Laurila PK. Effect of epidermal growth factor on tympanic membranes with chronic perforations: a clinical trial. Otolaryngol Head Neck Surg 1995;113:375–9.

46. Chauvin K, Bratton C, Parkins C. Healing large tympanic membrane perforations using hyaluronic acid, basic fibroblast growth factor, and epidermal growth factor. Otolaryngol Head Neck Surg 1999;121:43–7.

47. Goldman SA, Siegfried J, Scoleri P, et al. The effect of acidic fibroblast growth factor and live yeast cell derivative on tympanic membrane regeneration in a rat model. Otolaryngol Head Neck Surg 1997;117:616–21.

48. Yeo SE, Kim SW, Suh BD, et al. Effects of platelet-derived growth factor-AA on the healing process of tympanic membrane perforation. Am J Otolaryngol 2000;21:153–60.

49. Clymer MA, Schwaber MK, Davidson JM. The effects of keratinocyte growth factor on healing of tympanic membrane perforations. Laryngoscope 1996;106:280–5.

50. Amoils CP, Jackler RK, Milczuk H, et al. An animal model of chronic tympanic membrane perforation. Otolaryngol Head Neck Surg 1992;106:47–55.

51. Spandow O, Hellström S. Animal model for persistent tympanic membrane perforations. Ann Otol Rhinol Laryngol 1993;102:467–72.

52. Truy E, Disant F, Morgon A. Chronic tympanic membrane perforation: an animal model. Am J Otol 1995;16:222–5.

53. McFeely WJ Jr, Bojrab DI. Kartush JM. Tympanic membrane perforation repair using AlloDerm. Otolaryngol Head Neck Surg 2000;123(1 Pt 1):17–21.

54. Laidlaw DW, Costantino PD, Govindaraj S, et al. Tympanic membrane repair with a dermal allograft. Laryngoscope 2001;111(4 Pt 1):702–7.

55. Spiegel JH. Kessler JL. Tympanic membrane perforation repair with acellular porcine submucosa. Otol Neurotol 2005;26:563–6.

56. von Unge M, Dirckx JJJ, Olivius NP. Embryonic stem cells enhance the healing of tympanic membrane perforations. Int J Pediatr Otorhinolaryngol 2003;76:215–9.

57. Spratley J, Hellström S, Eriksson P-E, Pais-Clemente M. Myringotomy delays the tympanic membrane recovery in acute otitis media: a study in the rat model. Laryngoscope 2001;112:1474–81.

58. Spratley J, Hellström S, Eriksson P-O, Pais-Clemente M. Early structural tympanic membrane reactions to myringotomy: a study in an acute otitis media model. Acta Otolaryngol (Stockh) 2002;122:479–87.

59. Magnuson K, Hermansson A, Hellström S. Healing of tympanic membrane after myringotomy during *Streptococcus pneumoniae* otitis media. An otomicroscopic and histologic study in the rat. Ann Otol Rhinol Laryngol 1996;105:397–404.

60. Mattsson C. Myringosclerosis—an experimental basis for a theory of its etiology [thesis]. Umeå: Umeå University; 1997.

61. Buyanover GW, Joyce A, Ingold KU. The biochemical composition of tympanosclerotic deposits. Arch Otorhinolaryngol 1987;243:366–9.

62. Lesser THJ, Williams KR, Skinner DW. Tympanosclerosis, grommets and shear stresses. Clin Otolaryngol 1988;13:375–80.

63. Mattsson C, Magnuson K, Hellström S. Myringosclerosis caused by increased oxygen concentration in traumatized tympanic membranes. Experimental study. Ann Otol Rhinol Laryngol 1995;104:625–32.

64. Estrem SA, Batra PS. Preventing myringotomy closure with topical mitomycin C in rats. Otolaryngol Head Neck Surg 1999;120:794–8.

65. Kupin TH, Juzych MS, Shin DH, et al. Adjunctive mitomycin C in primary trabeculetomy in phakic eyes. Am J Ophthalmol 1995;119:30–9.

11

Sinonasal Mucosal Wound Healing: Implications for Contemporary Rhinologic Surgery

Taha Z. Shipchandler, MD; Pete S. Batra, MD; Martin J. Citardi, MD

Optimizing the environment for healing in inflamed and infected postoperative nasal and sinus cavities is the keystone for sinonasal medicine and surgery. Rhinologic surgeons, as well as basic scientists and other clinical investigators, have sought to define the processes of wound healing of sinonasal mucosa. Although considerable knowledge has been gained, the precise mechanisms that drive sinonasal mucosal wound healing have been incompletely elucidated, and, as a result, management of the sinonasal mucosa after rhinologic surgery remains controversial because much of clinical practice is based on anecdotal experiences and incomplete scientific data. This chapter describes the current state of knowledge of wound healing of sinonasal mucosa; more importantly, this chapter places that information within a clinical context that highlights current clinical practices.

ANATOMY AND PHYSIOLOGY

Knowledge of anatomy, physiology, and histology is essential to understanding the healing processes of the sinonasal mucosa; this information supports the rationale for perioperative decision-making, as well as areas of research. This chapter does not serve as an all-inclusive source for paranasal sinus anatomy, histology, and physiology, but it does highlight the unique and salient aspects of anatomy, histology, and physiology that affect the healing of these tissues. Thus, this information serves as a guideline on which surgical decisions are based.

Anatomy of the Nose and Paranasal Sinuses

Internal Nasal Valve

A brief discussion of the internal nasal valve is important because it is essential to preserve the function of this structure to promote airflow after nasal surgery. Adverse effects on the internal nasal valve can negate the improved cross-sectional area obtained during nasal surgery. Since, by definition, a valve can vary the flow that passes through it, the internal nasal valve is not a valve at all because it is always open. The valve is the narrowest part of the nasal cavity and the narrowest part of the upper airway during nasal breathing. The superior border of each nasal valve consists of the limen nasi, which is formed by the junction between the upper lateral cartilages where they overly the lower lateral cartilages. This junction can be easily noted during manual nasal tip elevation. The nasal valve is bordered medially by the nasal septum, laterally by the head of the inferior turbinate, and inferiorly by the nasal floor. Congestion caused by inflammatory processes may greatly increase airway resistance through the internal nasal valve. In addition, surgical alterations to this area from rhinoplasty and/or septoplasty can result in poor surgical outcomes.

Turbinates and Meatus

Detailed knowledge of the precise location of the superior, middle, and inferior turbinates and their corresponding meatus is necessary when treating diseases of the sinonasal cavities. A fourth turbinate, the supreme turbinate, located superiorly to the superior turbinate, is rare, and when it occurs, it is typically quite small. The middle, superior, and supreme turbinates are extensions of the ethmoid bone, whereas the inferior turbinate is a separate bone unto itself. Each inferior turbinate is anchored into the lateral nasal wall formed by the inner surfaces of the lacrimal bones and maxilla. The air space underlying each turbinate is known as a meatus, and each meatus is named for the turbinate above it. Thus, the inferior turbinate, middle turbinate, and superior turbinate are above the inferior meatus, middle meatus, and superior meatus, respectively. The inferior meatus contains the opening of the nasolacrimal duct. This duct is located approximately 1 cm posterior to the head of the inferior turbinate. Damage to this structure can result in unilateral epiphora following surgery. The superior meatus contains the opening to the drainage pathway of the posterior ethmoidal cells.

The middle meatus serves as the drainage conduit for the anterior ethmoidal, maxillary, and frontal sinuses (Figure 1). These sinuses drain initially into the infundibulum, a funnel-shaped trough bordered medially by the uncinate process and laterally by the orbit. The secretions drain from the infundibulum to the middle meatus through the hiatus semilunaris, a crescent-shaped cleft bordered anteriorly by the uncinate process and posteriorly by the ethmoid bulla.

Ostiomeatal Complex

The common drainage pathway for the anterior ethmoid, frontal, and maxillary sinuses is known as the ostiomeatal complex (OMC). The OMC is not a true anatomic structure; rather, the OMC is a functional designation and refers to the physiologic concept of the mucociliary clearance of these sinuses through this narrow region. Any

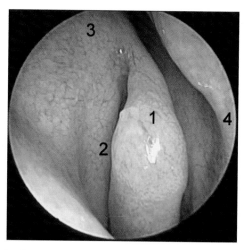

Figure 1. Endoscopic view of a normal left middle meatus. 1 = middle turbinate; 2 = uncinate process; 3 = agger nasi region; 4 = septum.

adverse manipulation to this area will have profound effects on paranasal sinus function. Blockage of the OMC region can lead to edema and inflammation, which subsequently obstructs the "upstream" sinuses that must drain through the OMC region. Stasis and accumulation of secretions in the sinuses will result in sinusitis. Numerous factors may initiate this sequence of events. Surprisingly, anatomic variations have not been consistently associated with OMC compromise. On the other hand, viral rhinitis, inhalant allergies, and numerous other factors may trigger the initial events of OMC obstruction. Functional endoscopic sinus surgery (FESS) focuses on alleviating the obstruction in the OMC region while preserving as much healthy native tissue as possible.[1,2]

Maxillary Sinus

The maxillary sinuses, the largest sinuses of the paranasal sinuses, occupy a large portion of the body of each maxilla (Figure 2). They are bordered superiorly by the orbital floor, the central portion of which is traversed by the infraorbital nerve, which may be dehiscent. The alveolar process of the maxilla forms the inferior border of the maxillary sinus. The close association of the first and second molars with the floor of the maxillary sinus provides an easy route of superior spread for dental infections. As a result, isolated maxillary sinusitis may be due to a

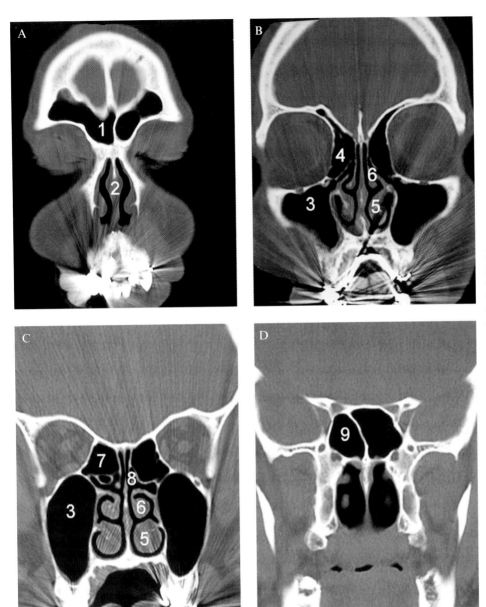

Figure 2. *A–D,* Coronal sinus computed tomographic scans demonstrating relevant paranasal sinus anatomy. 1 = frontal sinus; 2 = nasal septum; 3 = maxillary sinus; 4 = anterior ethmoid; 5 = inferior turbinate; 6 = middle turbinate; 7 = posterior ethmoid; 8 = superior turbinate; 9 = sphenoid sinus.

dental infection that has eroded the maxilla. The lacrimal duct is located anteromedially along the medial maxillary wall. The pterygomaxillary space is behind the posterior wall of the maxillary sinus.

The ostium of the maxillary sinus is at the superior aspect of its medial wall. Accessory ostia may occur at areas of natural bony dehiscence, or fontanelles, along the medial maxillary sinus wall (the lateral nasal wall). These can form accessory drainage pathways and have been implicated in the phenomenon of mucus recirculation. In this clinical scenario, the mucus from the maxillary

sinus is expelled through the natural ostium, which then falls back into the maxillary sinus through an accessory ostium. The mucus simply recirculates between the natural and accessory ostia. Mucus recirculation may also result from inappropriate placement of the maxillary antrostomy during FESS (Figure 3).

Ethmoidal Sinuses

The ethmoidal sinuses (also known as the ethmoidal labyrinth) are a complex group of cells with great variability (see Figure 2). They are bordered by the lamina papyracea laterally

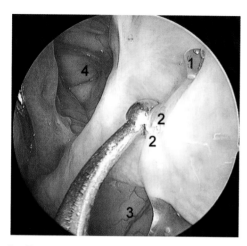

Figure 3. Endoscopic view of maxillary mucus recirculation after incorrect placement of the surgical maxillary antrostomy. 1 = natural maxillary ostium; 2 = mucus; 3 = surgical maxillary antrostomy; 4 = open ethmoid cavity.

and the middle and superior turbinates medially. The ethmoid bone is open above; the roof of the ethmoidal cells is formed by the horizontal or orbital process of the frontal bone. The basal lamella of the middle turbinate anatomically divides the ethmoidal labyrinth into anterior and posterior ethmoidal cells. The anterior group drains into the infundibulum of the middle meatus, whereas the posterior group drains into the superior meatus. Both the anterior and posterior groups are subdivided into many different types of cells based on anatomic location and embryologic origin. A concha bullosa is pneumatization of an ethmoidal cell into the middle turbinate. This enlargement of the middle turbinate may cause obstruction of the middle meatus.

Frontal Sinus

The frontal sinus develops as an extension of anterior ethmoidal pneumatization on each side. The frontal sinuses are bordered posteriorly by the anterior cranial fossa, anteriorly by the skin and soft tissues of the forehead, and inferiorly by the roof of the orbit. The frontal sinus forms from a superior evagination of the antero-superior ethmoidal cells through the area of the frontal recess. The frontal recess is a complex structure that is bordered by the middle turbinate medially, the lamina papyracea laterally,

and the agger nasi region anteriorly. The posterior boundary of the frontal recess has been arbitrarily set at the anterior ethmoidal artery. Depending on the degree of pneumatization of the ethmoidal cells, the frontal recess can be wide or narrow. Description of the patterns of frontal recess pneumatization[3] is beyond the scope of this chapter. The frontal sinuses drain from lateral to medial through the frontal ostium and then through the frontal recess and into the middle meatus. A small amount of the mucus will naturally recirculate in the inferior part of the medial frontal sinus. Great variability exists in regard to the size and shape of the frontal sinus from person to person. Complete agenesis, either unilateral or bilateral, as well as extremely large frontal sinuses with pneumatization to the lateralmost portion of the orbit, may occur.

Sphenoidal Sinus

The sphenoidal sinus is formed by pneumatization of the sphenoid bone. Although a sphenoidal sinus is present on both sides, an intersinus bony septum typically divides pneumatization asymmetrically. The degree of pneumatization of the sphenoidal sinus also varies greatly among individuals. Occasionally, the sphenoid pneumatization may be rudimentary or the sphenoidal sinus may be completely absent. In contrast, the pneumatization may be extensive and has been observed into the pterygoid plates, the palatine bone, and the vomer.

The sphenoidal sinus is surrounded by many vital structures whose indentations in the sphenoid walls may be visualized during sphenoid endoscopy. The bulge for the sella turcica lies medially in the posteromedial wall. The cavernous sinus is just beyond the lateral wall of the sphenoidal sinus. An indentation for the internal carotid artery and the optic nerve may be seen inferolaterally and superolaterally. The vidian nerve, or nerve of the pterygoid canal, runs along the floor of the sphenoidal sinus. The sphenoid os, predominantly a membranous os, is located approximately 10 mm superior to the floor of the sinus and drains into the sphenoethmoidal recess.

Sinonasal Mucosal Histology

Van Cauwenberge and colleagues described the histology of the nasal cavity as containing several different types of epithelium.[4] The nasal vestibule is lined with keratinized squamous epithelium with vibrissae, sweat glands, and sebaceous glands. The anterior third of the nasal cavity, along with the anterior portions of the inferior and middle turbinates, is lined predominantly with squamous and transitional cell epithelium. Cuboidal cells with microvilli are the primary cell type found in this region. A pseudostratified columnar epithelium covers the posterior two-thirds of the nasal cavity and contains ciliated and nonciliated columnar cells, mucin-secreting goblet cells, and basal cells (Figure 4). This epithelium serves to protect the upper and lower airways via mucociliary clearance activity. The columnar to goblet cell ratio is around 5:1. Each ciliated cell contains from 50 to 200 cilia. The ultrastructure of the cilia is the standard "nine plus two" organization of microtubules arranged in doublets. Each doublet has dynein arms extending outward between peripheral doublets; the dynein arms provide motion to the cilia. Cilia beat on average from 10 to 20 times per second in a coordinated fashion with a fast forward beat

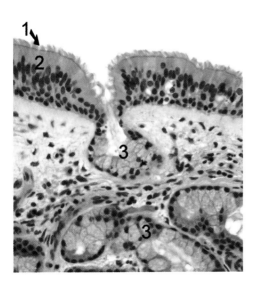

Figure 4. Light microscopy (hematoxylin-eosin stain; ×20 original magnification) of normal sinonasal mucosa. 1 = ciliated surface; 2 = pseudostratified respiratory epithelium; 3 = seromucinous glands. Courtesy of Aaron Hoscar, MD.

and a slower return beat. The microvilli along the surface of the epithelium help expand the surface area, thus improving air humidification and warming. Goblet cells produce thick mucus, which traps the irritants and particulates. This mucus is propelled and cleared by the action of the cilia. The nasal epithelium lies on the basement membrane and lamina propria. Unique to the nasal mucosa is that the basement membrane is penetrated by capillaries that allow fluids to readily pass from these vessels to the nasal mucosa.[5] The glandular, nervous, and vascular structures are contained within the lamina propria. Serous and mucinous glands also penetrate into the lamina propria and basement membrane and are controlled by the sympathetic and parasympathetic nervous systems for thin and thick mucus secretion, respectively.

Olfactory epithelium lines the superomedial part of the superior turbinate, superior septum, and nasal roof. This pseudostratified epithelium contains olfactory cells, which are bipolar neurons, basal cells, and Bowman's glands (serous tubuloalveolar glands). Basal cells are stem cells that can differentiate to reconstitute the olfactory epithelium after damage.

Sinonasal Physiology

The mucous blanket of sinonasal cavities is composed of two layers, the gel and sol phases (Figure 5). The gel phase, or the superficial layer, is produced by goblet and submucosal glands and provides an environment that traps foreign particulate matter, which can then be cleared through the mucociliary clearance actions of the cilia. The sol phase, or the deep layer, is produced by microvilli and provides a fluid that facilitates ciliary motility and movement of the gel layer. The mucous blanket consists of mucoglycoproteins, immunoglobulins, interferon, anti-inflammatory cells, and a variety of other immunologic substances. Together, these substances and the mucous blanket, in concert with the active beating of the cilia, form the mucociliary clearance system. Cilia move mucus

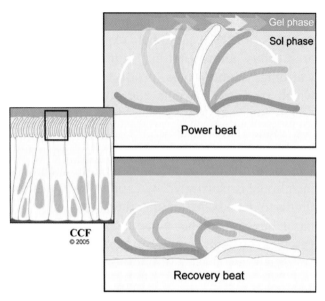

Figure 5. Schematic representation of the ciliary beat cycle.

at a rate of 3 to 25 mm/min toward natural sinus ostia and ultimately to the nasopharynx and oropharynx, where the transported mucus is swallowed (Figure 6).

Many factors can slow mucociliary clearance. Primary ciliary dyskinesia, Kartagener's syndrome, decreased humidity and temperature, topical drugs, wood dust, tobacco smoke, inhaled gases, scar tissue, granulation tissue, and infection all have been associated with disruption of ciliary motility. In addition, ciliary beating in vitro seems to cease between 7 and 12°C. Disruption of mucociliary clearance

mechanisms can precipitate the sinusitis cycle (Figure 7).[6]

Nasal airflow resistance is affected by a variety of factors. The internal nasal valve, as mentioned earlier, is the narrowest part of the nasal airway; thus, air passing through this segment of the airway is moving at the fastest speed. This creates turbulent airflow, which serves to more effectively humidify and cleanse the air. Airflow resistance is also controlled greatly by the parasympathetic and sympathetic nervous systems. The vasculature is under constant sympathetic tone. When this tone decreases, the nasal vessels engorge much like erectile tissue, and the mucosa thickens. This results in increased airflow resistance. This change in tone is noted in the normal nasal cycle, which occurs every 2 to 7 hours in approximately 80% of the population. Other factors influencing the relative engorgement of the nasal mucosa include age, exercise, posture, hormones, pharmacotherapy, trauma, and emotional and psychological responses.[7]

SINONASAL MUCOSAL WOUND HEALING PROCESSES

Normal Wound Healing

Wound healing is a well-studied dynamic process in which various cells, in a highly complex

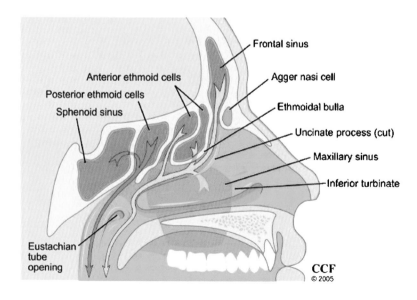

Figure 6. Schematic representation of the mucociliary clearance pattern of the lateral nasal wall. Note that the mucus from the anterior ethmoidal cells, frontal sinus, and maxillary sinus is transported posteriorly in a path inferior to the eustachian tube opening, whereas the mucus from the posterior ethmoidal cells and sphenoid sinus is transported above the eustachian tube opening.

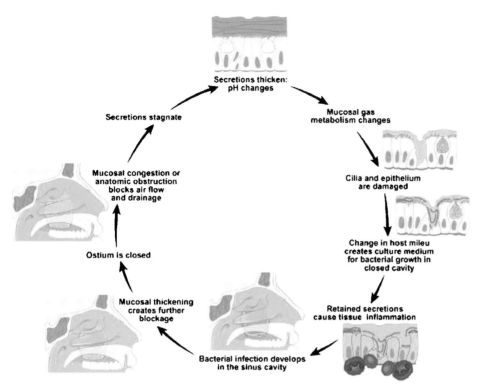

Figure 7. The sinusitis cycle. Adapted from Reilly JS.[6]

interaction, secrete a variety of substances that ultimately interact with the extracellular matrix (ECM) to either recreate normal tissue or create scar tissue that replaces the native tissue but does not provide the same function. Most investigations of sinonasal mucosal wound healing share the ultimate goal of understanding and describing healing processes that are most likely to lead to a restoration of normal mucociliary clearance.

Watelet and colleagues divided sinonasal mucosal wound healing into four overlapping phases: inflammation, cell proliferation, matrix deposition, and tissue remodeling.[8] Regulation of these phases occurs by the interaction of numerous growth factors, cytokines, and immunogenic substances with a variety of cells and the ECM.

Phase of Inflammation
Injury to nasal mucosa results in immediate bleeding with exposure of underlying connective tissue to circulating platelets. The platelets then release a variety of vasoactive substances that cause temporary vasoconstriction with primary clot formation. Through interaction with platelets, damaged endothelium releases a variety of growth factors, including platelet-derived growth

factor, transforming growth factor α, and transforming growth factor β. Fibrin acts as a temporary matrix to which other cells adhere. Simultaneously, polymorphonuclear leukocytes (PMNs) infiltrate the ECM after release of elastase and collagenase, which together are necessary for the transit of PMNs through the lamina propria. PMNs predominate during the first 24 to 48 hours of the inflammatory phase, followed by monocytes, which predominate from days 3 to 5. Monocytes and macrophages help in microscopic wound débridement via phagocytosis and secrete additional growth factors, including epidermal growth factor and fibroblast growth factor. Lymphocytes also play a role by linking the immune response to wound healing. In a clean surgical wound, the inflammatory phase lasts several days; however, the process may persist for weeks in a contaminated wound.

Phases of Cell Proliferation and Matrix Deposition
New tissue formation can be noted approximately 3 to 5 days after injury through the formation of granulation tissue. Fibroblast migration plays an important role in the phase

of cell proliferation and ECM deposition. Various growth factors secreted by both fibroblasts and other inflammatory cells stimulate fibroblast proliferation. Increased ECM deposition provides a structural network that facilitates the interactions of fibroblasts, which regulate cell proliferation and matrix deposition. Once a large number of fibroblasts have reached the wound, they synthesize protein and release growth factors. Angiogenesis occurs through the proliferation of local endothelial cells. The endothelial cells secrete additional growth factors, which promote neovascularization and subsequent delivery of oxygen. Reepithelialization occurs a few hours after initial injury. One proposed theory is that nearby undamaged respiratory cells lose their orientation and start to migrate to the wound bed. Alternatively, undifferentiated respiratory basal cells may undergo proliferation, migration, and subsequent differentiation to form the natural sinonasal mucosal lining.

Phase of Tissue Remodeling

Tissue remodeling takes place over a 6-month period after initial injury. During this time, the inflammatory, angiogenesis, and fibroblast proliferation phases diminish. The composition of the ECM changes during this time from predominantly hyaluronic acid, fibronectin, and collagen types I, III, and V to predominantly collagen type I as the main ECM component. Wound maturation is marked by a delicate balance between collagen synthesis and lysis to create well-healed scar tissue. This phase produces the greatest increase in wound tensile strength.

Healing after Surgical Intervention

Weber and colleagues described four overlapping phases of sinonasal mucosal wound healing.[9] Observations provided by video-endoscopy after sinus surgery served as the basis for these phases. During the first 7 to 12 days, bloody crusts covered the entire wound (phase 1), followed by the formation of granulation tissue (phase 2) over the next 2 to 4 weeks. The third phase, the edematous phase, was marked by increasing swelling of the healing tissue, whereas the fourth phase was characterized by normalization to native tissues between weeks 12 and 18. Several patients in this study were also treated intranasally with topical budesonide, which seemed to shorten the duration of the wound healing phases and reduce both granulation tissue and edema. On the other hand, its overall effect on mucosal function was unclear. Functional tests, such as mucociliary clearance, were not performed.

Alterations in the previously discussed healing patterns can occur for a variety of reasons, including environmental factors, application of topical substances and medications, the presence of infection, and the depth or mechanism of injury. The most well-studied healing patterns are based on observations of wound healing after injury of various depths. When the basement membrane is undamaged, normal epithelial height has been observed as soon as 3 days after injury. On the other hand, the healing process can take weeks if the basement membrane is removed; removal of the basement membrane leads to the development of a transitional cell epithelium rather than a normal nasal respiratory epithelium, whereas the healing process takes weeks if the basement membrane is removed.[10] In the later scenario, healing leads to the formation of transitional cell epithelium rather than normal nasal respiratory epithelium.

Moriyama and colleagues proposed removal of a minimal amount of sinonasal tissue to optimize wound healing of sinonasal mucosa.[11] In this view, reversibly "diseased" mucosa should be preserved; aeration and drainage will lead to normalization of these tissues. Thus, transformation from diseased mucosa to normal mucosa takes place with proper care as long as the mucosa is still viable. Importantly, complete removal of the mucosa and periosteum may create a wound that takes longer than a year to heal completely, and even after healing, the mucosal structure and function may be irretrievably altered.

Sinonasal mucosal healing patterns following surgery have been studied in rabbits 10 weeks after maxillary sinus mucosa removal.[12] Histologic changes included a decrease in both the number and the ultrastructural pattern of ciliary regeneration. A decrease in seromucinous glands was also observed when compared with the unoperated contralateral maxillary sinus mucosa, which served as the control in this study. In addition, an increase in inflammation, scarring, fibrous bands, and mucus viscosity was noted after mucosal stripping. A similar study also showed a decrease in the size of the operated maxillary sinus owing to increased scarring, fibrosis and bone degradation, and neogenesis.[13] Epithelialization was noted 2 weeks after mucosal injury; however, the lamina propria was far from healed.

Monitoring Wound Healing

Both clinical assessments of postoperative sinonasal mucosal healing and research into these healing processes are hampered by the lack of objective measurements of the healing process. Ideally, biochemical markers, rather than visual inspection by endoscopy (in the clinic) and microscopy (for research), would provide a foundation for better understanding of the status of wound healing.

Watelet and colleagues examined the presence of matrix metalloproteinase 9 (MMP-9) both preoperatively and postoperatively in patients who underwent FESS for chronic rhinosinusitis or sinonasal polyposis.[14] MMP-9 levels were shown to be dramatically increased in all patients immediately postoperatively; however, the healing quality after 6 months, as determined by inspection and the use of a visual analog scale, significantly and independently correlated with preoperative MMP-9 levels, the severity of the initial disease, and previous sinus surgery. Patients with favorable healing had significantly lower MMP-9 levels between 3 weeks and 6 months. Thus, MMP-9 may serve as an independent variable for monitoring postoperative healing status.

Asai and colleagues examined the time interval for postoperative FESS patients to taste the sweetness from a saccharin granule placed on the floor of the maxillary sinus.[15] Increased time was noted in patients with greater edema and inflammation was noted during nasal endoscopy compared with patients in whom endoscopy showed minimal edema and inflammation. The saccharin test serves as a potential test for the function of mucociliary clearance following sinonasal mucosal injury.

PERIOPERATIVE MANAGEMENT OF SINONASAL MUCOSAL WOUND HEALING

The primary goal of FESS is the restoration of normal mucociliary clearance to chronically infected paranasal sinuses (Figure 8). Secondary objectives include preservation of mucosa and normal structures. In fact, these secondary objectives are intrinsic to the primary goal. Since the introduction of FESS in the United States two decades ago, there has been much discussion about appropriate postoperative care. As surgical techniques have evolved, the strategies for postoperative care have also improved. Although much of the discussion focuses on postoperative care, it is more appropriate to talk about perioperative management because optimization of the final surgical results occurs before the surgical procedure commences. Thus, preoperative, intraoperative, and postoperative

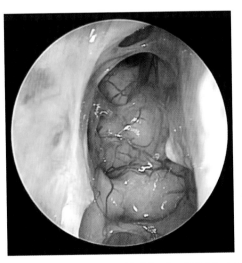

Figure 8. Endoscopic view provided by the 30° telescope of a healthy middle meatus after functional endoscopic sinus surgery.

management are all critical to achieving a successful result.[16]

Preoperative Care

Preoperative care aims to minimize inflammation and active infection present in the sinonasal cavities prior to surgery. The objective is to create an ideal environment for both intraoperative manipulation and postoperative healing. Use of culture-directed antimicrobial agents for several weeks preoperatively, along with nasal irrigations, topical nasal steroids, and/or systemic steroids, minimizes both infection and inflammation within the sinonasal tissues before surgery. Inflammation and edema of sinonasal mucosa respond readily to such treatments, which allows for several advantages during surgery, including improved visualization of key structures, decreased bleeding, and decreased intraoperative swelling.

Careful preoperative surgical planning through the use of computer-aided surgery technology can also improve postoperative healing and, ultimately, surgical success.[17–19] Although much of the focus for computer-aided surgery in rhinology is on intraoperative navigation, these systems also facilitate the software-enabled review of preoperative imaging and serve as powerful platforms for preoperative planning. Detailed examination of the paranasal sinuses provided by high-resolution computed tomography at a computer workstation provides superb information about the patient's anatomy; this knowledge can then guide surgical planning.

The preoperative phase also provides a platform for patient education. During this time, patients should learn about the anticipated course of their treatments, including the important postoperative care measures. It is critical that patients understand that for many individuals, inflammatory disease of the paranasal sinuses is a chronic, lifelong condition that will likely require some degree of long-term medical treatment. Although surgery may serve to dramatically reduce symptoms and therefore be considered "curative," surgery cannot reverse the genetically programmed tendency for sinonasal mucosal inflammation in many of these patients. Thus, the surgery should be viewed as a component of a comprehensive treatment algorithm. Patients must understand this important point, and the time to convey this point is before the decision for surgery is confirmed.

Preoperative planning also aims to counsel patients to adjust their environments to maximize the chance for success of FESS. In addition to limiting exposure to allergens and other environmental irritants, patients must be aware that both preoperative and postoperative tobacco smoke exposure may lead to decreased improvement following FESS. Smoke impairs mucociliary clearance and ciliary function. Smoke exposure in adults has been well documented as a negative predictor of success.[20,21] More recently, smoke exposure in children has been shown to have a significant effect on the overall success of surgery 12 months postoperatively: Twenty percent of children with reported smoke exposure perioperatively needed repeat procedures compared with the nonexposed group.[22]

Intraoperative Care

Several measures and techniques may be employed intraoperatively to optimize surgical outcome. Both scar prevention and avoidance of middle meatal collapse are important factors in achieving good functional results after FESS. Thus, intraoperative maneuvers must seek to minimize both scarring and middle meatal collapse.

Excessive mucous membrane removal leads to granulation tissue formation and scar development. Regenerated mucosa lacks normal ciliary ultrastructure and does not provide the same function as native mucosa.[12] Thus, preservation of mucosa and minimizing collateral mucosal injury are paramount. In addition, denuded bone may stimulate unwanted osteogenesis. This can lead to obstruction in narrow areas, such as the frontal recess, as well as bony overgrowth of ostia and other sinonasal recesses.

Therefore, blood clots present in the middle meatus, damaged mucosa, and areas of exposed bone must be addressed intraoperatively.

The use of predominantly through-cutting forceps as opposed to grasping forceps facilitates greater surgical precision. These through-cutting instruments minimize mucosal stripping and thereby reduce the potential for leaving exposed bone. In addition, through-cutting forceps cause less pulling on delicate structures. Soft tissue shavers (microdébriders), when used judiciously, also remove diseased mucosa and bony fragments in an organized fashion with minimal mucosal loss and minimal exposure of intact bony fragments. However, aggressive and injudicious use of shaver technology has been reported with significant skull base and orbital injury.[23,24]

A recent study with rabbits compared healing of sinonasal mucosa after full-thickness mucosal removal (including periosteum) and partial-thickness mucosal removal with a soft tissue shaver.[25] Partial-thickness mucosal loss was associated with a faster rate of reepithelialization and a significant increase in ciliary regeneration, and full-thickness mucosal loss was associated with greater mucosal crusting. This study lends support to the importance of mucosal preservation during FESS. Clinically, careful mucous membrane preservation can allow ethmoid cavity healing in 10 to 12 days and mucociliary function return within 2 weeks.

Prevention of middle meatus collapse is imperative during surgery because postoperative middle turbinate lateralization can lead to complete blockage of the frontal, ethmoidal, and maxillary sinuses and thus iatrogenic sinusitis and even mucocele formation. Middle meatal collapse will also preclude endoscopic monitoring of the postoperative cavity. Excessive removal of the middle turbinate basal lamella and middle turbinate fracture result in collapse. Scar contracture and healing naturally pull the middle turbinate laterally against the lateral nasal wall, especially after removal of the inferior portion of the basal lamella. In addition, destabilization of the middle turbinate superiorly will foster the tendency for middle turbinate lateralization. The creation of deliberate adhesions between the middle turbinate and septum (known as the controlled synechia technique) will serve to counteract the tendency for middle meatal collapse.[26] The adhesions may be created by deliberately traumatizing the medial aspect of the middle turbinate and the corresponding portion of the septum. A middle meatal spacer will be necessary for 3 weeks postoperatively as the adhesions mature; the spacer should be replaced every 5 to 7 days during this time. If necessary, delayed lysis of the adhesion may be completed in the office at a later date.

Topical intraoperative agents may adversely affect wound healing. One study examined the effect of topical cocaine in a sheep model.[27] Approximately 50% ciliated mucosal loss occurred after just 10 minutes of contact with cocaine, whereas the corresponding level of mucosal loss in the control group was only 15%. Vasoconstricting agents must be used with caution, although the need for topical decongestants for tissue vasoconstriction and hemostasis is great.

Middle meatal blood clots should be cautiously suctioned intraoperatively to decrease postoperative fibrin clots and eventual scar formation. The use of middle meatal spacers, which may be placed intraoperatively, dramatically reduces clot formation in the middle meatus postoperatively. A well-placed sponge covered by a latex glove finger (finger cot) provides a nonadherent spacer that does not allow clot to build in the middle meatus. It should be emphasized that this spacer is neither a stent nor a hemostatic device; instead, the stent simply occupies space that otherwise may be occupied by bloody clots. The spacer can easily be removed 5 to 7 days postoperatively during routine office débridement.

Absorbable materials, which are selected so that they do not elicit a dramatic proinflammatory response (discussed below), may also serve a similar purpose. Surgicel Fibrillar (Johnson & Johnson, Piscataway, NJ), an oxidized, regenerated cellulose product that resembles fluffy cotton in its dry state, provides a substrate for hemostasis, offers some bactericidal and bacteriostatic effects, and resorbs rapidly. Thus, it offers many of the properties of an ideal intrasinus dressing after FESS. Anecdotal experiences suggest that placement of Surgicel Fibrillar after FESS (Figure 9) is beneficial, but this observation has not been confirmed in formal clinical trials.

A more selective approach may be employed for use of nasal packing after FESS. In cases with minimal intraoperative bleeding and mild to moderate inflammation, one may be able to forgo placement of all packing agents and reserve packing for cases with extensive inflammation and/or bleeding. Orlandi and Lanza reported on 165 cases managed in a selective fashion; 147 patients (85%) were able to avoid packing altogether.[28] The median estimated blood loss during surgery was 50 mL, whereas no bleeding complications were reported postoperatively. Importantly, this selective approach does not obviate the commitment to the postoperative débridement process; the surgeon assumes the responsibility of meticulous postoperative care, including comprehensive removal of clots during office-based endoscopic débridement.

Postoperative Care

During the postoperative period, a comprehensive regimen is warranted to achieve an optimal result. The typical postoperative office visit includes a problem-focused but detailed medical history and nasal endoscopy. Although the central issue for these visits is sinonasal health, it is important not to overlook concomitant diseases, including asthma, which is quite prevalent in this patient population. Patient education, which will enhance compliance with the treatment recommendations, can be reinforced.

Components of postoperative care include

- Validated measures of clinical outcomes (such as the 20-Item Sinonasal Outcome Test [SNOT-20],[29] the 31-Item Rhinosinusitis Outcome Measure [RSOM-31],[30] or other validated outcomes measures[31])
- Standardized questionnaires
- Nasal endoscopy
- Meticulous endoscopic débridement
- Culture-directed antibiotics
- Systemic and topical nasal steroids
- Nasal irrigations
- Antiallergy measures (for patients with confirmed inhalant allergy)
- Aspirin desensitization (for acetylsalicylic acid [ASA] triad patients)
- Antifungal treatments (for patients with confirmed fungal rhinosinusitis)

The first office débridement usually is scheduled for 5 to 7 days after the procedure. Patients are then asked to return in 5 to 10 days for a second office visit. Thus, there are approximately two office visits in the first 2 to 3 weeks after surgery. The third office visit is usually scheduled 6 to 10 weeks after surgery. Of course, additional office visits may be necessary depending on the individual healing process.

Office-based endoscopic débridement strikes a delicate balance between complete manual cleansing of the sinus cavities and the creation of additional trauma, which leads to fresh bleeding and additional crusting. Débridement aims to clean the sinonasal cavities and promote healthy tissue healing by removing blood clots, fibrin debris, devitalized bone fragments, and early polyps. This helps prevent unwanted scar formation and removes potential sources of

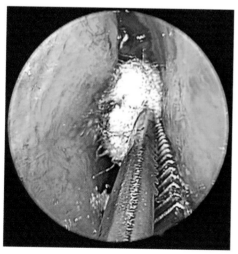

Figure 9.   Endoscopic placement of a tuft of Surgicel Fibrillar.

infection and inflammation. Endoscopic débridement is performed with the same finesse as a procedure in the operating room. Topical anesthesia and decongestants, supplemented by the infiltration of local anesthetics with dilute epinephrine, may be applied; however, such measures may not be necessary in all patients. Appropriate instrumentation must be available in the office. At a minimum, 0 and 30° telescopes, straight and curved suctions, and grasping and through-cutting forceps may serve as a basic instrument set. A video tower and an image archive are desirable. If frontal sinus surgery was performed, then additional instruments, including a 45 or 70° telescope and giraffe forceps, will be necessary for débridement.

The use of postoperative antibiotics is dependent on several factors. If active infection is present during the time of surgery, then antibiotics based on intraoperative culture are appropriate. If no active infection is present, then postoperative antibiotics may be required only for 1 to 2 weeks until the majority of the healing has taken place. Acute suppurative infections require cultures, which will serve as the rationale basis for antibiotic selection. Most commonly, oral antibiotics are selected. Selected patient populations with immunocompromise, cystic fibrosis, and/or ciliary dysmotility commonly harbor multidrug-resistant organisms and thus may benefit from intravenous antibiotics. Routine use of intravenous antibiotics is discouraged in light of the costs and associated risk factors of this administration route, including venous thrombosis, catheter dislodgment, and line sepsis.[32] The healed sinus cavity that develops an acute bacterial infection may be the ideal site for nebulized antibiotics.[33] Topical ceftazidime, gentamicin, and/or tobramycin irrigations are helpful for confirmed *Pseudomonas* rhinosinusitis.[34] Topical mupirocin irrigations may be used for confirmed infection with methicillin-resistant *Staphylococcus aureus*.[35]

Numerous irrigation regimens are in clinical practice. The consensus favors irrigation for postoperative débridement and cleansing starting on the first postoperative day. Irrigations reduce crusting and edema and help remove the fibrin clot, which may lead to scarring. Isotonic saline irrigations offer the theoretical advantage that they are less likely to have a direct injurious effect on mucosa cilia. On the other hand, hypertonic irrigations may reduce tissue edema by drawing free water from edematous tissues through osmosis. Hypotonic irrigations should be discouraged. A disposable piston syringe with a catheter tip may be used for the irrigations. The syringe should be discarded when it becomes dirty.

The use of nasal irrigations has been shown to be beneficial both in terms of time free of disease and patient symptoms. Side effects are minimal and include local irritation, burning, otalgia, and pooling in the sinuses. Nasal irrigation solutions differ in their tonicity, pH, and buffering agents, and numerous delivery systems are in clinical practice. Brown and Graham reviewed the use of nasal irrigations in a variety of clinical settings and noted several studies showing that hypertonic saline may be more beneficial than isotonic saline, as measured by the patients' degree of cough and radiology scores.[36] The use of buffering agents, such as baking soda, may serve to minimize local irritation and burning and thus improve compliance. However, no literature currently confirms this approach. The impact of the various formulations for saline irrigations on mucociliary clearance and ciliary beat frequency remains controversial.

The administration of corticosteroids will reduce sinonasal inflammation. As a result, steroids are included in most postoperative care plans. Topical nasal steroids are best studied for allergic rhinitis, and clinical studies for this indication note a risk of acute rhinitis and acute sinusitis.[37] In addition, the standard nasal spray bottles are not designed to deliver medication directly to the sinuses. Nonetheless, many patients receive topical nasal steroids via nasal spray. Topical steroids may also be administered via nasal drops if the patient assumes an appropriate head position.[38–44] Topical steroids may also be directly instilled into a frontal sinus occluded by swollen mucosa at the frontal recess.[45] For patients with severe eosinophilic inflammation of the sinus mucosa (ie, "hyperplastic" sinusitis or polyposis), systemic steroids seem to have a significant beneficial impact because they reduce inflammation and thus the tendency for early polyp recurrence. By reducing edema, the steroids improve sinus aeration, which seems to be important for the restoration of sinonasal health.

Patients with the ASA triad (Samter's triad, which is sensitivity to ASA with a history of having nasal polyps and asthma) may be candidates for postoperative ASA desensitization. Although ASA desensitization will tend to stabilize the level of sinonasal inflammation, it will not reverse mature sinonasal polyposis. Thus, it is appropriate to proceed with desensitization approximately 3 to 4 weeks after surgery, when the immediate benefits of the procedure are still substantial and the risk of polyposis recurrence is low. Evaluation for possible ASA desensitization should be coordinated carefully with an experienced allergist or immunologist in the preoperative period. ASA desensitization has demonstrated efficacy in ameliorating asthma and sinonasal symptoms in this challenging patient group.[46,47]

Management styles for postoperative care differ greatly among practicing otorhinolaryngologists. Thaler examined the pros and cons of "frequent" versus "less frequent" endoscopic débridements following FESS.[48] The advantages attained by frequent débridement of crust, clot, and fibrin debris include decreasing scar formation, maintaining the patency of sinus drainage pathways, and removing potential niduses for infection. No case-controlled studies, however, confirm this practice. On the other hand, the clinical experiences with healing after pediatric sinus surgery suggest that endoscopic débridements should be relatively "infrequent" for all patients. Some otorhinolaryngologists have extended this practice to the adult population and report synechiae formation in 1.3 to 11% of patients following FESS without any office débridements.[49,50] When débridements are not performed, patients are typically advised to perform frequent nasal saline irrigations. In addition, Kuhnel and colleagues found that mucosal biopsies taken from underneath crusts that were removed 1 week after FESS showed avulsion of mucosa in 23% of cases, but this was not observed if the endoscopic débridement was postponed until 2 weeks after surgery.[51] These observations suggest that less frequent débridement may allow more time for healing. Ultimately, the ideal frequency of débridement cannot be established through a universal rule; instead, the amount of débridement should reflect the clinical situation. Important factors include concomitant infection, underlying inflammatory etiology, and the extent of surgery, as well as the surgeon's personal technique and management style.

PACKING MATERIALS

The ideal nasal and sinus packing material would provide hemostasis, act as a spacer, support the turbinate, and maximize patient comfort, whereas it would have limited potential for the generation of a foreign body reaction and granulation tissue. The ideal pack would thus act as a dressing that would promote and even accelerate patient healing. Simultaneously, the ideal pack would suppress the growth of bacteria and accelerate mucosal healing. Unfortunately, the ideal pack has not been developed to date.

The use of bioabsorbable materials for nasal packing and mucosal dressings has become increasingly popular over the past 5 to 10 years. These materials interpose a viscous and elastic biomaterial between denuded areas of mucosa, in a process known as viscoseparation; this maneuver in theory should prevent fibrin synechiae formation and maximize patient comfort. Much uncertainty surrounds the use of newer bioabsorbable packing materials for hemostasis, spacers, and stents, especially in comparison with traditional nonabsorbable material (gauze and expandable sponges), and even the avoidance of all packing materials altogether.

Patient Comfort

Postoperative comfort and pain with the use of traditional packs have been well studied. Kuo and colleagues showed that significant patient discomfort resulted from both the presence of a traditional pack and the removal of the pack.[52] Topical packing impregnated with lidocaine decreased the use of oral analgesics in their patient population. Other literature supports the contention that packing removal is the most disliked portion of perioperative care in patients after FESS.[53] The disadvantages of traditional nasal packing include patient discomfort and damage to the nasal mucosa from packing placement and removal, as well as from the mere presence of the packing material.[54]

Absorbable Agents

Several studies examine the use of various bioabsorbable materials as packing materials. In general, these studies support only limited conclusions.

Gelfilm (Pharmacia Upjohn, Kalamazoo, MI), a thin gelatin derived from porcine skin, has been used as a middle meatal stent. In one study of FESS in children, granulation tissue and adhesions were more common when a Gelfilm middle meatal stent was used.[55] For this study, the postoperative middle meatus without Gelfilm served as the control group. The authors did not comment on the patency of the middle meatus. These data support the concept that bioabsorbable materials may provoke inflammatory reactions. Although bioabsorbable materials seem less disruptive from a wound healing perspective, their in vivo breakdown requires an inflammatory reaction that may adversely impact wound healing.

Materials consisting of hyaluronic acid derivatives have recently gained favor and are a topic for research in both animal models and human trials. Hyaluronic acid is found in the healing tissues of fetuses who show no scar formation, and its derivatives have been developed for use in the peritoneal cavity following abdominopelvic

surgery for the prevention of adhesions and scarring. In addition, hyaluronic acid has been shown to have bacteriostatic effects. Kimmelman and colleagues compared Sepragel (Genzyme Biosurgery, Cambridge, MA), a cross-linked hyaluronic acid polymer, to no packing in patients who underwent bilateral endoscopic ethmoidectomies.[56] They noted improvement in primary outcome measures, including a reduction in synechiae and middle meatal stenosis starting at 2 weeks postoperatively. In addition, pain was reportedly less on the Sepragel side. Only 9% and 3% of Sepragel remained 2 and 3 weeks after surgery, respectively. McIntosh and colleagues studied a similar substance, Merogel (Medtronic Xomed, Jacksonville, FL), a hyaluronic acid ester, in an uninfected sheep model in which full-thickness mucosal removal was performed, and noted that significant increases in reepithelialization and epithelial height beginning 84 days postoperatively were present when Merogel was placed on the wound.[57] No differences in ciliary regeneration were noted under electron microscopy. Further studies are planned in sheep whose sinuses have been infected with fungi to assess whether these findings would be similar in acutely or chronically inflamed sinuses. Jacob and colleagues studied the effects of Merogel in a mouse model.[58] They noted significant osteogenesis when Merogel was compared with Merocel sponges (Medtronic Xomed) and no packing at all. This finding was discovered when implanting Merogel into both the sinonasal cavity and calvarial bone. It should be noted that the amount of Merogel was large relative to the size of the mouse sinonasal cavity. In addition, the investigators did not soak the Merogel before placement; thus, the Merogel had to pull water from nearby tissues, and the low volume of water may impair Merogel's spontaneous chemical breakdown. As water is pulled from the tissues, the resultant drying of the surrounding mucosa may promote scar tissue formation and possibly osteogenesis. This study suggests important limitations for the clinical use of Merogel. Use of large amounts of Merogel should probably be discouraged because the undesirable osteogenesis could narrow sinus drainage pathways, despite appropriate surgical technique.

Merogel may also be used as a drug delivery system. Rajapaksa and colleagues reported on the impact of the incorporation of insulin-like growth factor 1 (IGF-1) into Merogel packing in an animal model of wound healing in healthy sheep and sheep with chronic sinusitis.[59] Merogel with IGF-1 was associated with an improvement in mucosal reepithelialization at day 28 in the healthy sheep but not the sheep with sinusitis. There were no other differences in mucosal reepithelialization between the two groups over the 4-month study period. Interestingly, Merogel with IGF-1 was associated with reduced ciliary recovery in the sheep with sinusitis at days 56 and 112.

Maccabee and colleagues examined the effects of Merogel and FloSeal (Fusion Medical Technologies, Mountain View, CA), a bovine-derived gelatin matrix with thrombin, and compared their use to no packing after stripping of mucosa in the maxillary sinuses of rabbits.[60] After maxillary sinus stripping, sinus cavities were filled with Merogel, FloSeal, or nothing. After 14 days, a histologic study of maxillary sinus mucosa showed marked fibrosis of the basal lamina and lamina propria, loss of the mucociliary blanket, and incorporation of the Merogel fibers into the regenerated epithelium. In addition, neo-osteogenesis was found, consistent with the findings of Jacob and colleagues.[58] The FloSeal group showed similar changes but to a lesser degree compared with the Merogel group. Lymphocytosis occurred in both groups surrounding the areas of mucosa infiltrated with Merogel and FloSeal; the presence of lymphocytes suggested an inflammatory process. The study also noted that both materials were still present after 14 days. In the clinical realm, large amounts of FloSeal and Merogel are not used, and any material that persists after the early postoperative period can be removed through office-based endoscopic débridement. Of course, if the material is eliciting a large inflammatory reaction, then the surgeon's ability to achieve meaningful endoscopic débridement will be compromised.

Chondroitin sulfate, like hyaluronan, is an ECM glycosaminoglycan. Chondroitin sulfate has recently been produced in a gel-like form and has shown promise for treatment of full- and partial-thickness cutaneous wounds. Gilbert and colleagues assessed the impact of a chondroitin sulfate hydrogel in the rabbit model.[61] After removal of a 6 mm area of maxillary sinus mucosa bilaterally, one randomly chosen side was impregnated with a chondroitin sulfate hydrogel disk. The other side received no treatment. On postoperative day 4, the chondroitin sulfate–treated side showed evidence of fibrinous exudates covering the entire wound, whereas the control side showed only exposed bone. On postoperative day 14, both sides appeared to be similar under histologic examination. A foreign body reaction to chondroitin sulfate was not observed during the course of the experiment.

Limited studies have been done comparing one bioabsorbable agent with another; however, this is the focus of much ongoing research in the field of sinonasal wound healing. Chandra and colleagues compared the use of FloSeal with thrombin-soaked Gelfoam (Upjohn Pharm), a porcine skin gelatin, in the ethmoid cavities of patients.[62] FloSeal was associated with increased amounts of granulation tissue and adhesion formation compared with thrombin-soaked Gelfoam over the first 6 to 8 weeks after surgery. Both agents were equally effective at achieving hemostasis and optimizing patient comfort. More recently, these authors have provided an update on this cohort: after a minimum of 1 year of follow-up and a mean follow-up of 21 months, the incidence of adhesions and adhesions requiring lysis was significantly greater in those patients who had received FloSeal.[63] The authors also were able to detect evidence of retained FloSeal within a mucosal adhesion 25 months after surgery.

Few studies compare absorbable agents with traditional packing in the healing of sinonasal mucosa. Miller and colleagues performed a prospective, randomized, controlled study that compared Merogel with Merocel in the middle meatus following FESS.[64] The Merocel was removed on postoperative days 5 to 7. The results showed that there was no significant difference at the longest follow-up time (8 weeks postoperatively) between the two groups regarding scarring, synechiae, edema, or infection. There was no formal evaluation of patient comfort performed during the study, nor was there histopathologic examination of mucosa over time. The use of Merogel obviated the need for packing removal in this study; thus, the authors favored Merogel over Merocel, which must be removed.

Retinoic Acid

Topical retinoic acid solution has been tested in rabbits as a potential material to promote healing of sinonasal mucosa. It has been shown that topical retinoic acid can promote regeneration of damaged tracheal mucosa to its original respiratory type instead of reverting by metaplastic changes to a squamous epithelium. Two different concentrations of retinoic acid applied to rabbit maxillary sinuses that had been stripped of their mucosa led to improved mucosal and ciliary regeneration with less cellular atypia and fibrosis when compared with stripped, nontreated controls.[65] In addition, the low-concentration group showed less cellular atypia and less heterogeneity in the cellular layer when compared with the high-concentration group. No effects on scar formation, middle meatal stenosis, or mucosal functionality, however, were examined in this study.

FUTURE DEVELOPMENTS

The management of wound healing after FESS has changed dramatically since this technique was introduced to the United States two decades ago. With enhanced understanding of the postoperative healing process and the advent of more biocompatible materials, additional changes are likely over the next decade.

Clearly, the current science of wound healing is limited by the lack of an appropriate animal model for assessment of the basic processes of wound healing of sinonasal mucosa. Although the rabbit model has been commonly used, this approach does not seem to closely resemble human physiology. Importantly, relatively little is known about rabbit immunology; thus, it is difficult to assess the impact of the observations made in the rabbit sinuses on the unique and complex immunology in humans. Larger animals, such as sheep, have also been used, but, again, the immunology of these animals is not well studied. On the other hand, mouse immunology is well studied, but the animal's small size makes surgical manipulations problematic. Alternatively, the study of in vitro mucosal explants may allow investigation of the impact of alterations in the chemical microenvironment on mucosal function; however, this information will indicate little about healing within an intact paranasal sinus cavity. Despite these important issues, animal models can provide critical information that can be extrapolated to surgical care of patients.

Since the beginnings of sinus surgery, rhinologists have debated the appropriateness of nasal packing. Recently, two trends have emerged. On the one hand, the routine use of nasal packing seems less common, whereas more resorbable materials for nasal packing are now available. It is likely that this debate will continue and will remain unresolved, at least in the near future. Also, the notion that a biomaterial is automatically preferable has been called into question as certain biomaterials have been associated with granulation tissue, scarring, etc. Additional efforts for the development of the ideal biomaterial for nasal packing continue. Over the long run, the rationale for the use of nasal packing is likely to shift from epistaxis prevention and stenting toward the application of a surgical dressing that will support and facilitate appropriate wound healing. If this concept takes hold, then it may be more appropriate to discuss mucosal dressings rather than nasal packing. In theory, a nasal dressing may provide a platform for the delivery of agents that can facilitate or modify wound healing and thus optimize the final surgical outcome.

CONCLUSIONS

The mucosa that lines the nose and paranasal sinuses serves an active barrier function that cleanses this gateway to the lower respiratory tree through the complex process of mucociliary clearance. Disruption of mucociliary clearance leads to multiple disease states, including rhinosinusitis. After injury, sinonasal mucosa progresses through the stages of inflammation, cell proliferation, matrix deposition, and tissue remodeling. It is appropriate to consider perioperative management principles that form a comprehensive approach that incorporates preoperative, intraoperative, and postoperative interventions. Throughout this integrated management strategy, medical treatment seeks to optimize the conditions for good wound healing. In recent years, numerous bioabsorbable agents have been proposed as packing materials, but on close examination, most of these products seem to carry significant disadvantages. Regardless of packing material (and in the absence of packing material), removal of old blood during postoperative débridements is critical because that old blood may mature into fibrinous material, which, ultimately, will lead to frank scarring. Investigations into sinonasal mucosal wound healing continue, and it is anticipated that they will form the basis of a clinical strategy that will permit scientifically based interventions that will direct rapid and physiologically functional healing.

REFERENCES

1. Kennedy DW. Functional endoscopic sinus surgery (technique). Arch Otolaryngol Head Neck Surg 1985; 111:643–9.
2. Kennedy DW, Zinreich SJ, Rosenbaum AE, Johns ME. Functional endoscopic sinus surgery (theory and diagnostic evaluation). Arch Otolaryngol Head Neck Surg 1985;111:576–82.
3. Lee WT, Kuhn FA, Citardi MJ. 3D CT analysis of frontal recess anatomy in patients without frontal sinusitis. Otolaryngol Head Neck Surg 2004;131:164–73.
4. Van Cauwenberge P, Lien S, De Belder T, Watelet J. Anatomy and physiology of the nose and the paranasal sinuses. Immunol Allergy Clin North Am 2004;24:1–17.
5. Munzel M. The permeability of intercellular spaces of the nasal mucosa. J Laryngol Rhinol Otol 1974;51:794–8.
6. Reilly JS. The sinusitis cycle. Otolaryngol Head Neck Surg 1990;103:856–62.
7. Williams T. Walsh, Robert C. Kern. Sinonasal Anatomy, Function, and Evaluation, Chapter 22. In: Byron J. Bailey, Jonas T. Johnson, editors, Lippincott Williams & Wilkins; 2006;307–18.
8. Watelet J, Bachert C, Gevaert P, Van Cauwenberge P. Wound healing of the nasal and paranasal mucosa: a review. Am J Rhinol 2002;16:77–84.
9. Weber R, Keerl R, Jaspersen D, et al. Computer-assisted documentation and analysis of wound healing of the nasal and oesophageal mucosa. J Laryngol Otol 1996; 110:1017–21.
10. Hilding DA, Hilding AC. Ultrastructure of tracheal cilia and cells during regeneration. Ann Otol Rhinol Laryngol 1966;75:281–94.
11. Moriyama H, Yanagi K, Ohtori N, et al. Healing process of sinus mucosa after endoscopic sinus surgery. Am J Rhinol 1996;10:61–6.
12. Benninger MS, Schmidt JL, Crissman JD, et al. Mucociliary function following sinus mucosal regeneration. Otolaryngol Head Neck Surg 1991;105:641–8.
13. Forsgren K, Stierna P, Kumlien J, Carlsoo B. Regeneration of maxillary sinus mucosa following surgical removal: experimental study in rabbits. Ann Otol Rhinol Laryngol 1993;102:459–66.
14. Watelet J, Claeys C, Van Cauwenberge P, Bachert C. Predictive and monitoring value of matrix metalloproteinase-9 for healing quality after sinus surgery. Wound Repair Regen 2004;12:412–8.
15. Asai K, Haruna S, Otori N, et al. Saccharin test of maxillary mucociliary function after endoscopic sinus surgery. Laryngoscope 2000;110:117–22.
16. Kuhn FA, Citardi MJ. Advances in postoperative care following functional endoscopic sinus surgery. Otolaryngol Clin North Am 1997;30:479–90.
17. Citardi MJ. Computer-aided frontal sinus surgery. Otolaryngol Clin North Am 2001;34:111–22.
18. Citardi MJ, Batra PS. Image-guided sinus surgery: current concepts and technology. Otolaryngol Clin North Am 2005;38:439–52.
19. Olson G, Citardi MJ. Image-guided functional endoscopic sinus surgery. Otolaryngol Head Neck Surg 2000;123: 188–94.
20. Briggs RD, Wright ST, Cordes S, Calhoun KH. Smoking in chronic rhinosinusitis: a predictor of poor long-term outcome after endoscopic sinus surgery. Laryngoscope 2004;114:126–8.
21. Senior BA, Kennedy DW, Tanabodee J, et al. Long-term results of functional endoscopic sinus surgery. Laryngoscope 1998;108:151–7.

22. Ramadan HH, Hinerman RA. Smoke exposure and outcome of endoscopic sinus surgery in children. Otolaryngol Head Neck Surg 2002;127:546–8.

23. Church CA, Chiu AG, Vaughan WC. Endoscopic repair of large skull base defects after powered sinus surgery. Otolaryngol Head Neck Surg 2003;129:204–9.

24. Graham SM, Nerad JA. Orbital complications in endoscopic sinus surgery using powered instrumentation. Laryngoscope 2003;113:874–8.

25. Shaw CL, Cowin A, Wormald PJ. A study of the normal healing pattern and mucociliary transport after endoscopic partial and full-thickness removal of nasal mucosa in sheep. Immunol Cell Biol 2001;79:145–8.

26. Bolger WE, Kuhn FA, Kennedy DW. Middle turbinate stabilization after functional endoscopic sinus surgery: the controlled synechiae technique. Laryngoscope 1999;109:1852–3.

27. Shaw CL, Dymock RB, Cowin A, Wormald PJ. Effect of packing on nasal mucosa of sheep. J Laryngol Otol 2000;114:506–9.

28. Orlandi RR, Lanza DC. Is nasal packing necessary following endoscopic sinus surgery? Laryngoscope 2004;114:1541–4.

29. Piccirillo JF, Merrit MG, Richards RL. Psychometric and clinometric validity of the 20-Item Sinonasal Outcome Test (SNOT-20). Otolaryngol Head Neck Surg 2002;126:41–7.

30. Piccirillo JF, Edwards D, Haiduk A, et al. Psychometric and clinometric validity of the 31-Item Rhinosinusitis Outcome Measure (RSOM-31). Am J Rhinol 1995;9:297–306.

31. Leopold D, Ferguson BJ, Piccirillo JF. Outcomes assessment. Otolaryngol Head Neck Surg 1997;117(Suppl 2):S58–68.

32. Gross ND, McInnes RJ, Hwang PH. Outpatient intravenous antibiotics for chronic rhinosinusitis. Laryngoscope 2002;112:1758–61.

33. Vaughan WC, Carvalho G. Use of nebulized antibiotics for acute infections in chronic sinusitis. Otolaryngol Head Neck Surg 2002;127:558–68.

34. Leonard DW, Bolger WE. Topical antibiotic therapy for recalcitrant sinusitis. Laryngoscope 1999;109:668–70.

35. Solares CA, Batra PS, Hall GS, Citardi MJ. Treatment of chronic rhinosinusitis exacerbations due to methicillin-resistant *Staphylococcus aureus* with mupirocin irrigations. Am J Otolaryngol 2006;27:161–5.

36. Brown CL, Graham SM. Nasal irrigations: good or bad? Curr Opin Otolaryngol Head Neck Surg 2004;12:9–13.

37. Benninger MS, Ahmad N, Marple B. The safety of intranasal steroids. Otolaryngol Head Neck Surg 2003;129:739–50.

38. Moffet AJ. Postural instillation. A new method of inducing local anesthesia in the nose. J Laryngol Otol 1941;56:429–36.

39. Wilson R, Sykes DA, Chan KL, et al. Effect of head position on the efficacy of topical treatment of chronic mucopurulent rhinosinusitis. Thorax 1987;42:631–2.

40. Moren F, Fjorneck K, Klint T, et al. A comparative distribution study of two procedures for administration of nose drops. Acta Otol (Stockh) 1988;106:286–90.

41. Raghavan U, Logan BM. New method for instillation of nasal drops. J Laryngol Otol 2000;114:456–9.

42. Karagama YG, Lancaster JL, Karkenevatos A, et al. Delivery of nasal drops to the middle meatus: which is the best head position? Rhinology 2001;26:226–9.

43. Cannady SB, Batra PS, Citardi MJ, Lanza DC. "Vertex-to-floor" position delivers topical nasal drops to the olfactory cleft after FESS. Am J Rhinol 2006;133:735–40.

44. Mygind N. Topical steroid treatment for allergic rhinitis and allied conditions. Clin Otolaryngol 1982;7:343–52.

45. Citardi MJ, Kuhn FA. Endoscopically guided frontal sinus beclomethasone instillation for refractory frontal sinus/recess mucosal edema and polyposis. Am J Rhinol 1998;12:179–82.

46. Stevenson DD, Hankammer MA, Mathison DA, et al. Aspirin desensitization treatment of aspirin-sensitive patients with rhinosinusitis-asthma: long term outcomes. J Allergy Clin Immunol 1996;98:751–8.

47. Berges-Gimeno MP, Simon RA, Stevenson DD. The natural history and clinical characteristics of aspirin-exacerbated respiratory disease. Ann Allergy Asthma Immunol 2002;89:474–8.

48. Thaler ER. Postoperative care after endoscopic sinus surgery. Arch Otolaryngol Head Neck Surg 2002;128:1204–6.

49. Brennan L. Minimizing postoperative care and adhesions following endoscopic sinus surgery. Ear Nose Throat J 1996;75:45–8.

50. Fernandes S. Postoperative care in functional endoscopic sinus surgery. Laryngoscope 1999;109:945–8.

51. Kuhnel T, Hoseman W, Wagner W, Fayad K. How traumatizing is mechanical mucous membrane care after interventions on paransal sinuses? A histological immunohistochemical study. Laryngorhinootologie 1996;75:575–9.

52. Kuo MJ, Zeitoun H, Macnamara M, et al. The use of topical 5% lidocaine ointment for relief of pain associated with post-operative nasal packing. Clin Otolaryngol 1995;20:357–9.

53. Von Schoenberg M, Robinson P, Ryan R. Nasal packing after routine nasal surgery: is it justified? J Laryngol Otol 1993;107:902–5.

54. Chandra RK, Kern RC. Advantages and disadvantages of topical packing in endoscopic sinus surgery. Curr Opin Otolaryngol Head Neck Surg 2004;12:21–6.

55. Tom LW, Palasti S, Potsic WP, et al. The effects of gelatin film stents in the middle meatus. Am J Rhinol 1997;11:229–32.

56. Kimmelman CP, Edelstein D, Cheng HJ. Sepragel (hylan B) as a postsurgical dressing for endoscopic sinus surgery. Otolaryngol Head Neck Surg 2001;125:603–8.

57. McIntosh MB, Cowin A, Adams D, et al. The effect of dissolvable hyaluronic acid-based pack on the healing of the nasal mucosa of sheep. Am J Rhinol 2002;16:85–90.

58. Jacob A, Faddis BT, Chole RA. MeroGel hyaluronic acid sinonasal implants: osteogenic implications. Laryngoscope 2002;112:37–42.

59. Rajapaksa S, McIntosh D, Cowin A, et al. The effect of insulin-like growth factor 1 incorporated into hyaluronic acid-based nasal pack on nasal mucosa healing in a healthy sheep model and sheep model of chronic sinusitis. Am J Rhinol 2005;19:251–6.

60. Maccabee MS, Trune DR, Hwang PH. Effects of topically applied biomaterials on paranasal sinus mucosal healing. Am J Rhinol 2003;17:203–7.

61. Gilbert EM, Kirker KR, Gray SD, et al. Chondroitin sulfate hydrogel and wound healing in rabbit maxillary sinus mucosa. Laryngoscope 2004;114:1406–9.

62. Chandra RK, Conley DB, Kern RC. The effect of FloSeal on mucosal healing after endoscopic sinus surgery: a comparison with thrombin-soaked gelatin foam. Am J Rhinol 2003;17:51–5.

63. Chandra R, Conley DB, Haines K, Kern RC. Long-term effects of FloSeal packing after endoscopic sinus surgery. Am J Rhinol 2005;19:240–3.

64. Miller RS, Steward DL, Tami TA, et al. The clinical effects of hyaluronic acid ester nasal dressing (Merogel) on intranasal wound healing after functional endoscopic sinus surgery. Otolaryngol Head Neck Surg 2003;128:862–9.

65. Maccabee MS, Trune DR, Hwang PH. Paranasal sinus mucosal regeneration: the effect of topical retinoic acid. Am J Rhinol 2003;17:133–7.

12

Burned Facial Skin

Dipan Das, MD; Arun K. Gosain, MD

Burn injuries place a huge toll on our medical system and are the second most common cause of accidental death after automobile accidents. With the advancements in trauma and burn management over the past three decades, there has been a significant improvement in survival from major burns. Better resuscitation and a multidisciplinary burn team approach have facilitated the reduction in mortality and improvement of care. This has led to the increase in the number of people who survive the initial injury and require further care for the effects of their burn injuries. Management of facial burn injuries does not stop after acute resuscitation but begins with careful planning of long-term wound management and reconstruction to obtain optimal esthetic and functional outcomes.

Burns affect approximately 1.1 million people in the United States, of whom approximately 45,000 sustain injuries that require hospitalization.[1] Not only has there been a decrease in the incidence of thermal injuries in the past decade owing to better safety measures and domestic smoke alarms, there has also been a decline in the associated mortality owing to better resuscitation, control of infections, and better wound care with early excision and wound closure.[1] Successful management of burn patients involves a multidisciplinary approach. Thermal injury not only requires prompt resuscitation and acute care but also needs proper planning for possible future reconstructions to achieve optimal long-term outcomes, that is, adequate function, comfort, and appearance. The goals of managing a burned face are similar to those of burns elsewhere in the body; however, the outcome of facial burns has significant social and functional implication. Our aim in this chapter is to identify healing problems of burn wounds and to describe techniques to treat and overcome such problems, particularly with facial burns.

PATHOPHYSIOLOGY OF BURNS

General principles apply to burn wound care, whether it be in the face or elsewhere. To understand and treat burn wounds, one must understand the pathophysiology of such injuries. Burns involve destruction of exposed and underlying tissue owing to extreme temperatures. Injury occurs when tissue absorbs more energy than it can dissipate, leading to damage and coagulation of cellular proteins and organelles. Cellular damage leads to release of cytokines and an increase in microvascular permeability, producing a loss of intravascular plasma volume into the tissue interstitium in the form of edema.[2–5]

Burn wounds show three distinct zones of histologic injury.[6] The central region, composed of nonviable tissue, is the zone of coagulation. Surrounding this region is the zone of stasis, where blood flow is initially present but ultimately becomes ischemic and requires excision. Beyond the zone of stasis is the zone of hyperemia, where there is increased vascular permeability and an inflammatory response (Figure 12-1). Recognition of this zone is important because the tissue is viable and does not warrant excision. Preservation of native

PARTIAL THICKNESS BURN

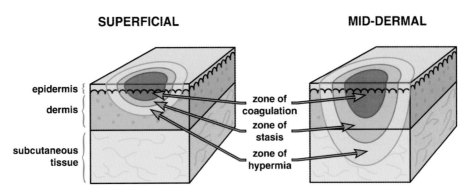

Figure 1. Zones of thermal damage.

tissue plays a vital role in burn care and reconstruction.

Burns are categorized by the depth of thermal tissue injury in terms of relative thickness (Figure 12-2). Although there have been studies using various modalities in the determination of the depth of thermal wounds, visual assessment has so far been the most feasible and common way.[7] Recognizing the depth of injury helps not only in determining the initial resuscitation and patient outcome but also in planning treatment options later. The change in perfusion in the zone of stasis, progression of inflammation and edema,

and nonuniformity of the injury contribute to difficulty in accurate assessment of burn depth by physicians in the first 24 to 48 hours. A superficial or first-degree burn involves the epidermis, commonly caused by a scald, flash flame, or sunburn. It is light pink in appearance, without blisters, and very painful. Hair follicles and sweat glands are not destroyed, and the wound heals with peeling and no permanent scarring and can be treated with topical antibiotic ointments. A partial-thickness or second-degree burn involves the entire epidermis and variable portions of the dermal layer. The appearance is hyperemic but

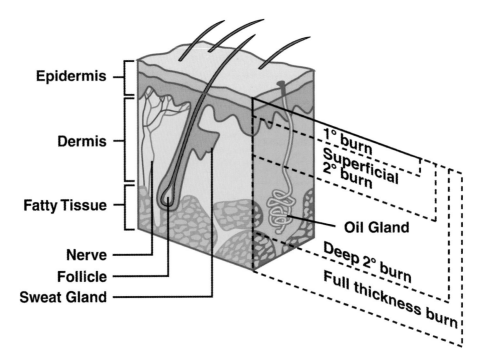

Figure 2.   Cross Section of the different layers of skin with different degrees of thermal injury.

may be pale, moist with blisters, and tender. Second-degree burns can be divided into superficial and deep. Superficial second-degree burns heal in 10 to 14 days and usually do not require grafting. The healed skin is thin and hairless. When the thermal injury extends well into the dermis, it is known as a deep second-degree burn. These wounds take more than 30 days to heal and can convert to full-thickness burns if they become infected; hence, early tangential excision and grafting are required. Full-thickness or third-degree burns involve the entire epidermal and dermal layer, leaving no epidermal cell reservoirs to repopulate and reepithelialize the wound. These wounds appear waxy white and leathery and are insensate. The underlying subcutaneous tissue may also be involved. These wounds fail to heal and require excision and grafting. When the underlying muscle and/or bone are involved, it is classified as a fourth-degree burn. Owing to significant tissue loss, these injuries may require tissue transfers along with grafting.

CLINICAL HEALING PROBLEMS

Thermal injury in general, including the face, requires identifying and anticipating wound healing problems early in the management to help in the proper care of these wounds. Several problems affect proper burn wound healing:

Degree of Tissue Damage

Early assessment of the extent and depth of the burn wound is essential not only in planning surgical care but also in adequate resuscitation. Adequate circulation is critical for the patient's survival and for adequate perfusion of the injured tissue. Inadequate tissue perfusion may lead to progression in the depth and extent of thermal damage.[8,9] Surgical management is dependent on the depth of the wound. First-degree and superficial second-degree burns may be managed conservatively with topical wound care. Deep second- and third-degree burns require surgical care in the form of wound

débridement, early excision, and wound coverage. An inadequate wound bed after débridement poses difficulties in adequate wound healing that may require a different approach in surgical management. Depth of injury and the total body surface area burned are crucial factors in the prognosis of the patient and in determining the amount of normal tissue available for wound coverage.

Wound Coverage

First described by Janzekovic[10] in the 1970's, thermal wounds, both partial and full thickness, are managed by early excision and skin grafting. The thermally damaged tissue is surgically debrided within 3 to 7 days after initial resuscitation followed by wound coverage with skin grafts.[11,12] Wounds left to heal without excision for longer than 2 to 3 weeks result in hypertrophic scarring and poorer prognosis compared with early burn excision and grafting. The latter approach leads to improved survival, better cosmetic results, a shorter hospital stay, earlier rehabilitation, lower metabolic complications, and reduced risk of wound infections.[13,14] The caveat to early excision is that the wound must not be excised unless it can be immediately closed or covered. The availability of adequate autograft must be determined depending on the total body surface area burned. Skin substitute for temporary coverage and tissue expanders have been useful for attaining adequate tissue coverage in complicated burn wounds.

Infection

Infection is the leading cause of death in burn patients, especially when the total body surface area involved is $> 30\%$.[15] Burn wounds are an ideal media for bacterial growth and provide a portal for microbial invasion. Microbial colonization of these wounds occurs by the end of the first week. Wounds with bacterial counts $> 10^5$ microorganisms per gram of tissue have poor skin graft uptake and delay in wound closure (see Chapter 26, "Controlling Infection"). Use of prophylactic antibiotics offers no protection, but adequate wound débridement and topical wound care with antimicrobial agents or biologic dressings minimize the microbial load within the burn wound (see Chapters 27 and 32).

Metabolism and Nutrition

Burn victims are in a hypermetabolic state, and the increase in the metabolic rate is proportional to the extent of the burn injury.[16] Optimal nutrition is essential in proper wound healing. Successful management of the postburn hypermetabolic response requires providing adequate nutritional support with a high-protein and high-calorie diet. Malnutrition leads to poor healing and graft uptake, as well as poor immunogenic protection from wound infection and sepsis (see Chapter 25, "Nutrition and Wound Healing").

Maintenance of Function

The goal of secondary burn reconstruction is to restore function and appearance. The body heals burn wounds by hypertrophic scar formation, which leads to disfigurement and contractures. Scar formation, although a normal healing process, may lead to poor functional and aesthetic outcomes. Techniques to minimize postburn scar formation must be kept in mind while managing thermal wounds, even after wound closure and reconstruction.

Maintenance of Aesthetic Units

Maintaining aesthetic units is vital in managing facial burns. Respecting the aesthetic units of the face provides optimal outcomes both visually and functionally. Facial reconstruction preserving the facial aesthetic units (Figure 12-3) and using cutaneous grafts of the same thickness, shape, and size of a unit helps prevent a patchy appearance and provides the optimal aesthetic appearance. Each facial region has a different cutaneous thickness and texture, which may warrant specific donor tissue. Scar formation

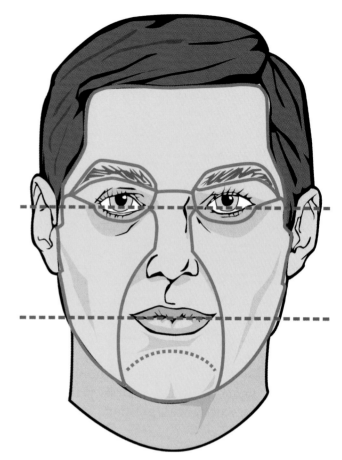

Figure 3. Regional esthetic units of the face. (Modified from Gonzalez-Ulloa M: Restoration of the face covering by means of selected skin in regional aesthetic units. Br J Plast Surg 1956;9:212.)

between each unit may be hidden within skin folds or natural shadow lines.[17–19]

APPROACH TO CLINICAL HEALING PROBLEMS

With consideration of the common healing problems outlined above, the management of facial burns should be planned to overcome such healing problems to achieve optimal results. Guidelines to keep in mind while approaching facial burn wounds are as follows[20]:

1.   Assess and analyze the deformity. Missing or displaced tissues or structures should be documented preoperatively.
2.   Develop a long-term plan. Stage the procedure depending on the defect and the availability of donor tissue and resources. Functional needs have a higher priority than aesthetic ones.

3. Discuss surgical plans with patients and have them actively involved in care.

4. Consider early excision and grafting to avoid primary healing with hypertrophic scars.

5. Delay reconstruction until scars and grafts mature.

6. Consider the use of splints, external pressure stockings, or elastic masks to minimize scar hypertrophy.

7. Release extrinsic contractures before intrinsic contractures. Contractures of adjacent structures are extrinsic whereas contracture of the part itself is an intrinsic contracture. Extrinsic contractures should be dealt with before correcting intrinsic deformities or else the deformity maybe over corrected with poor esthetic outcomes.

8. Hide scars behind hairlines and orient scars along relaxed skin tension lines.

9. Use donor tissue that closely matches the skin surrounding the deformity in color and thickness.

10. Resurface according to the regional aesthetic units.

11. While resurfacing an aesthetic unit, try to incorporate excised scar to contour adjacent areas such as the nasal tip, columella, and philtrum.

12. Use full-thickness skin grafts to limit contractures and achieve better surface texture.

13. Protect new scars and grafts from ultraviolet radiation. Have patients protect their faces with shades or sunscreen to avoid hyperpigmentation.

14. Educate patients in the appropriate use of cosmetics to camouflage deformities.

After acute resuscitation, facial burn care may be divided into initial acute management and delayed facial reconstruction.

Acute Management

Although primary excision and grafting of burns elsewhere in the body have become the standard management, a conservative approach is recommended for facial burns.[10–14] A less aggressive surgical approach is taken to allow viable tissue to heal, which helps in the accurate assessment of the depth of facial burns.[20] Facial burns are managed with topical antimicrobial agents, eschar or dead tissue débridement, and eventual skin grafting of granulating wounds. Conservative management may last from 10 days to 3 weeks. Open wounds after eschar débridement may be covered with autografts or temporarily covered with skin substitutes until definitive wound closure is attained.

First-degree or superficial second-degree burns may be expected to heal with minimal scarring or deformity after conservative management. Deep second-degree burns that are allowed to heal within 3 weeks have a lower incidence of hypertrophic scar formation compared with burns that require more than 3 weeks to heal. Some authors advise early excision and skin grafting for these wounds to prevent scarring and contractures. Third-degree burns require excision within a week to 10 days once facial edema has resolved and viable tissue is demarcated.

Topical Agents

Topical antimicrobial agents are not necessary if immediate burn wound excision is performed, but if conservative management is chosen, daily application on burn wounds is recommended for the first 7 to 10 days to prevent wound infections. A variety of topical antimicrobial agents are available and are used for the conservative management of facial burns (Table 12-1). Silver impregnated dressings (Acticoat, Smith and Nephew, Largo, FL) have recently come into use, which avoids the need for frequent dressing changes, thereby reducing patient discomfort, labor, and potential cross-contamination of wounds. Acticoat dressings can be changed every 3 to 5 days and need to be kept moist with sterile water. Such dressings improve wound care and have been shown to decrease burn wound infections compared with silver nitrate but have shown no significant difference in the rate of wound reepithelialization.[21]

Table 1. COMMONLY USED TOPICAL ANTIMICROBIAL BURN WOUND AGENTS		
	Mafenide acetate	**Silver nitrate soaks**	**Silver sulfadiazine cream**
Form of treatment	Topical application	Occlusive dressing	Topical application or single-layer dressing
Concentration of active agent (%)	11.1	0.5	1.0
Advantages	Penetrates eschar; wound is readily visible; no gram negative resistance	No hypersensitivity; painless, except at time of dressing change; no gram-negative resistance; reduces heat loss from wound	Painless on application; wound is readily visible when cream is applied
Limitations	Painful on application for 20–30 min; accentuates postburn hyperventilation; hypersensitivity in 7% of patients; delays spontaneous eschar separation	No penetration of eschar; marked electrolyte abnormalities: Na^+, K^+, Ca^{++}, and Cl^-; methemoglobin; dressing limits joint movement	Poor penetration of eschar; bone marrow suppression with neutropenia; hypersensitivity; resistance in *Enterobacter cloacae* and some *Pseudomonas* species

Skin Substitutes

Temporary wound coverage is achieved with skin substitutes and is commonly used in three circumstances. The first and most important indication is as a temporary biologic covering of excised wounds while awaiting healing of donor sites. Second, they are used as a temporary cover on clean superficial wounds to alleviate pain and accelerate epithelialization. Lastly, they may be used to cover wounds to assess the viability of the wound.

An ideal skin substitute is nonantigenic, nontoxic, impermeable to exogenous microorganisms, flexible, pliable, and biodegradable. It adheres to the wound, resists shear stress, and allows fibroblast ingrowth.[22] No such biologic dressing meets all of these criteria, but clinical situations, cost, and availability each play a major role in determining the dressing to be used. The three types of skin substitutes currently in clinical use are allografts, xenografts, and synthetic membranes.

Allografts are harvested from cadaveric donors screened for malignant and infectious diseases. These grafts are considered to be the gold standard for temporary burn wound coverage. Allografts vascularize and heal similarly to autografts until immunologic rejection occurs. Rejection typically occurs after 2 to 3 weeks in immunosuppressed burn patients.[23,24]

Xenografts are split-thickness grafts harvested from a variety of species but most commonly from the domestic pig. Porcine xenografts are reconstituted nonviable dermis fashioned into sheets. This xenograft does not vascularize but adheres to the wound coagulum and provides protection while the underlying wound epithelializes.

With advances in technology and bioengineering, improved synthetic skin substitutes are available to try to reproduce the properties of an ideal skin substitute. Synthetic membranes are available with different compositions and properties and have variable applications depending on the condition of the burn wound (Table 12-2).

Integra (Integra Life Sciences, Plainsboro, NJ), a bilaminate skin substitute composed of a porous matrix of cross-linked bovine tendon collagen and glycosaminoglycan and an outer semipermeable silicon layer, has played an increasing role as a dermal substitute in the management of facial burns.[25,26] AlloDerm (LifeCell Corporation, Branchburg, NJ), an acellular dermal matrix derived from donated human skin, also provides a similar scaffold for new dermis to form. It is prepared by removing the epidermis and cellular components of the dermis responsible for the immune response and graft rejection. In the pediatric burn literature, the use of TransCyte (Advanced Tissue Sciences, La Jolla, CA) has resulted in improved outcomes and decreased length of hospitalization.[27,28] Although temporary wound coverage is attempted with some of the above skin substitutes, definitive coverage is achieved either by autografts or by surgical flaps.

Table 2. SKIN SUBSTITUTES		
Material	Composition	Use
Biobrane®	Bilayer synthetic membrane: inner nylon mesh embedded with collagen (porcine), outer Silastic layer.	Temporary skin substitute; facilitates reepithelialization
TransCyte	Bilayer membrane: inner nylon mesh with cultured newborn human fibroblast cells, outer semipermeable silicone layer	Temporary skin substitute; facilitates reepithelialization
Integra	Bilaminate membrane: inner matrix of cross-linked bovine tendon collagen and glycosaminoglycan, outer semipermeable silicone layer	Dermal substitute with integrated silicone epidermal analog
AlloDerm	Acellular nonimmunogenic dermal matrix derived from donated human skin	Dermal substitute; requires a superficial autograft

Delayed Facial Reconstruction

Once the facial burn wound is acutely managed and wound coverage is attained, definitive correction of facial burn deformities is delayed for a minimum of 12 months or longer after the initial injury to allow scars and grafts to mature. During this period, adequate nutritional support and prevention of scar hypertrophy and wound infection should be stressed. Early reconstructive procedures may be required for reasons of function and comfort, that is, eyelid reconstruction to protect an exposed cornea, lip release for disabling perioral contractures, or severe restrictive neck scarring.

To prevent hypertrophic scarring and wound contractures, external splints and elasticized masks are used during the interim between acute burn care and delayed reconstruction. Constant pressure on wounds leads to softer and thinner scars.[29] Pressure of about 25 mm Hg has been found to inhibit hypertrophic scarring and is required constantly during the period of scar maturation. Intralesional injection of triamcinolone and topical silicone gel sheets can also be used on burn scars to prevent hypertrophic scarring.[30–32]

Reconstructive goals consist of improving functionality, minimizing disfigurement, and restoring facial symmetry. The head and neck area, which is commonly unprotected, is highly vulnerable to burn injury. The presence of unique and distinct structures in the face makes it particularly difficult to reconstruct, and imperfections are difficult to conceal. Maintaining the aesthetic units and orienting scars along skin creases or hairlines must be kept in mind while reconstructing the face. Acquiring tissue that may replace injured structures of the face is a challenge, and variable techniques can be used to reconstruct the face, which is beyond the scope of the present chapter. General techniques used to manage facial burns and application of these techniques to specific areas of the face are discussed.

TECHNIQUES IN FACIAL BURN RECONSTRUCTION

Most of facial burn reconstruction involves either correcting deformities produced by hypertrophic scarring or reconstructing lost tissue. Initially, the facial deformity must be analyzed and a long-term plan formulated to stage reconstruction. A combination of different techniques may be required to achieve optimal functional and aesthetic outcome. Burn wounds allowed to heal by secondary intention tend to form scar tissue. Waiting for scars to mature (ie, to present as pale, flat, and soft scar tissue) before correcting the deformity yields better and permanent results. Surgical repair of burn scars involves scar incision or scar excision. Scar incision consists of incision within the scar to intrinsically release the contracture. Scar excision involves the complete removal of a burn scar, leaving healthy, nonscarred tissue at the wound edges. If open wounds that result from scar excision are large, a skin graft or transposition of surrounding tissue in the form of flaps may be required for wound coverage; if these open wounds are smaller, they may be closed primarily.

Respecting the aesthetic units of the face, skin grafts or flaps applied to the face for resurfacing should cover the entire aesthetic unit. As described by Gonzalez-Ulloa, various regions of the face with skin of variable color, texture, mobility, and thickness exist (see Figure 12-3).[18] To achieve optimal cosmesis, these factors should be kept in mind when resurfacing facial burns. Whether skin grafts or flaps yield better results remains debatable. Skin grafts are less bulky and do not mask facial expression but tend to contract and undergo hyperpigmentation over time. Flaps, on the other hand, maintain a more normal skin quality and do not shrink; however, they can be bulky and mask facial expression. Hence, while resurfacing facial burns, the selection should be made to match as closely as possible the surrounding tissue. A combination of flaps and grafts may be required in some situations. As a general guideline, if a portion of the face needs to be resurfaced, grafts should be used in a field of grafts or scars. If a single area of the face is burnt, resurface with a regional flap, if available.

Grafting

Full-thickness or thick split-thickness skin grafts are preferred for resurfacing an aesthetic unit owing to less contracture and better surface texture. Grafts are commonly used in resurfacing the eyelids, forehead, and lips. Split-thickness skin grafts tend to contract and hyperpigment, leading to poor cosmesis. Graft donor sites should be selected to closely match the texture, color, and thickness of native skin in the recipient site. To aid in donor-site selection, the normal skin thicknesses of each region of the face are provided in Table 12-3.

Although skin grafts are commonly used in other parts of the body, matching the graft with the native tissue tends to be a challenge in the face and tends to produce a patchy appearance if aesthetic units are not preserved. The scalp is the preferred donor site to attain better color match. Hypertrophic graft junctures, ectropion, or a

Table 3. REGIONAL AESTHETIC UNITS (THICKNESS AND SOURCE OF SKIN FOR TRANSPLANTATION)		
Type of Aesthetic Unit	Diameter	Donor Sites
Thick skin	0.048 in (1,200 μ)	
Cheek		Dorsal region
Mental region		Costal region
Nose		Medial thigh
Upper lip		Lumbar region
Medium-thickness skin	0.024 in (600 μ)	
Lower lip		The above mentioned plus
Neck		Thigh (exterior)
Nose (dorsum)		Thigh (anterior)
Ear (anterior-exterior)		Thigh (posterior)
Forehead		Infrascapular region
Thin skin	0.015 in (375 μ)	
Upper eyelid		Arm (interior)
Lower eyelid		Ear (posterior-interior)
Ear (posterior-interior)		Supraclavicular region

Adapted from Gonzalez-Ulloa M.[18]

deformed or retracted nasal tip may require subsequent revision.

Flaps

Flaps are useful not only in resurfacing burn wounds but also in reconstructing damaged structures of the face. Transposition flaps in the form of Z-plasties and pedicled flaps in nose and eyebrow reconstruction are just a few examples of how extensively flaps can be used in facial burn reconstruction. Flaps carry their own blood supply and heal better with less contracture formation but tend to be bulky. Flaps are classified based on their vascular pattern.

Cutaneous or Random Pattern Flaps

Cutaneous flaps in the form of local flaps help in scar lengthening and wound coverage. V-Y advancement flaps, Z-plasties, and W-plasties are commonly used to lengthen scars and release contractures to reestablish function to facial structures, especially in the perioral and neck regions (Figure 12-4). Surrounding healthy tissue can be expanded with tissue expanders (discussed below) implanted into the subcutaneous tissue, and the surplus tissue generated can be subse-

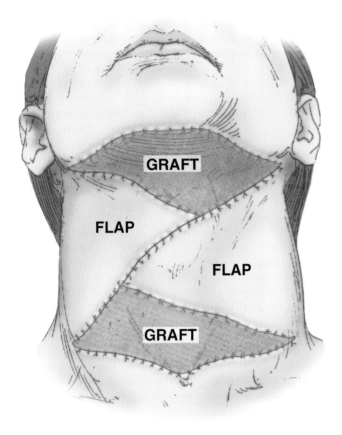

Figure 4. Neck release and resurfacing with a combination of local flaps and skin grafts.

quently transposed over excised burn scars to attain better cosmesis.

Axial or Arterial Pattern Flaps

An axial flap is one with blood supply derived from an artery contained in its long axis. Axial flaps are useful in burn reconstruction and require a clear understanding of the anatomy of the cutaneous arterial supply of the transferring tissue. These flaps are commonly used in constructing the eyebrows and the ear. A vascularized island pedicle flap from the temporal scalp based on the superficial temporal vessels can be used to reconstruct the eyebrows (Figure 12-5). Forehead or retroauricular flaps for the nose, temporoparietal fascia flaps for the ear, and dorsal scapular island flaps for the neck or scalp are also examples of axial pattern flaps.[32]

Free Flaps

Free flaps prove to be very useful in attaining tissue for burns when local tissue is not available or in the reconstruction of facial structures such as the nose and ears in the form of composite grafts or when adjacent tissues are not sufficient

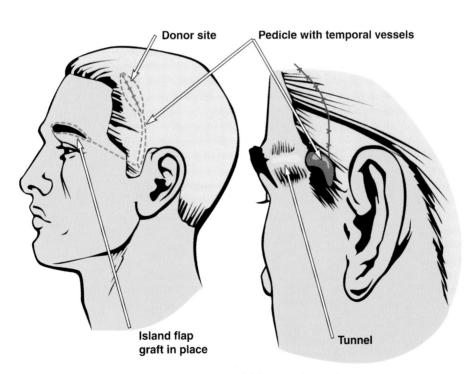

Figure 5. Eyebrow reconstruction with scalp flap based on the superficial temporal vessels.

for release of scar contracture. Preexpanded free flaps from the groin and scapular regions are also used for reconstructing wide defects in the neck (Figure 12-6). Tissue expanders in the free flap donor sites are useful both to thin the donor-site tissues so that they are a better match in thickness to the tissues of the face and neck and to allow primary closure of the free flap donor site. Free flaps can be tailored to the exact size, shape, or bulk required for reconstruction.

Tissue Expanders

Tissue expansion provides optimal tissue replacement when adjacent tissues are insufficient for direct advancement to resurface a burn defect. The utility of this procedure is broad and helps not only in burn wound closure but also in donor-site closure. Tissue expansion requires multiple office visits, and patients often object to their appearance during the expansion process. However, the benefits of tissue expansion outweigh the disadvantages. The advantages of tissue expansion include good texture and color-matched tissue, preservation of hair-bearing quality and skin sensation, avoidance of distant flaps, and increased vascularity of the expanded

tissue with improved flap survival. Tissue expansion yields superior aesthetic results and hence is commonly used in burn reconstruction in our unit.

Tissue expanders were introduced into clinical practice by Radovan in 1976.[33] Tissue expanders have since gone through gradual modifications to improve expansion, longevity, and handling capabilities. Tissue expanders are presently made out of a silicone shell that is serially expanded with periodic injections of saline. Injection ports may be integrated into the expander or be remote; remote ports may be implanted beneath the tissues (internal) and injected percutaneously or left external to avoid the need for percutaneous injection. Our preference is the use of tissue expanders with remote internal ports to minimize the chance of accidental port avulsion or implant puncture during port injection. Different expander sizes and shapes are available to allow the expanders to be tailored to fit the site of expansion and the amount of tissue required. It is recommended that the diameter of the tissue expander should be 2.5 to 3 times the width of the defect to allow for closure of the defect and the donor site; however, if limited donor tissue is available for

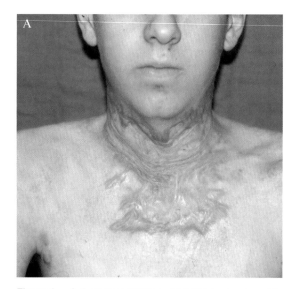
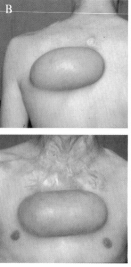
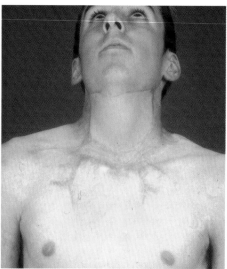

Figure 6.   *A,* A 14-year-old boy with limited extension of the neck owing to burn scar contractures extending from infraclavicular to submental skin. *B,* A tissue expander was placed in the left upper back to expand the donor site for a free scapular flap (*top, left*), and another tissue expander was placed in the mid–upper chest for direct advancement of the adjacent skin (*bottom, left*). Following transfer of the preexpanded free scapular flap to resurface the upper and midportions of the neck and transfer of the expanded chest skin to resurface the lower portion of the neck, the patient has regained full extension to the neck, with a much improved aesthetic outcome (*right*).

expansion, the tissue expander should be sized to maximize expansion of the available donor site. Expanders are placed in a subcutaneous pocket adjacent to the burn scar, and a separate pocket is made for the inflation port. Wounds are closed in two layers and allowed to heal prior to expansion to prevent wound dehiscence and expander extrusion. In addition, placement of the incision at least 2 cm away from the tissue expander minimizes the risk of expander extrusion. Expansion is usually started within 3 weeks following expander placement, and the expander is inflated weekly or biweekly, depending on the tissue quality and the patient's comfort.

Tissue expanders can be used to expand normal skin to obtain skin for expanded full-thickness skin grafts, to preexpand distant donor sites for preexpanded microvascular free flaps, or to expand tissue adjacent to the burn wound to resurface the defect with advancement of adjacent flaps.

Complications from tissue expansion can be categorized into major and minor complications. Major complications are those that lead to loss of the expander or an additional unplanned surgery; these complications include implant extrusion, wound dehiscence, deflation, device failure, and infection. Minor complications are those that do not result in unplanned surgical intervention, such as seroma formation, port leakage, or early infection that can be treated with antibiotic therapy. In addition, atrophy or pressure necrosis of underlying muscle and bone may occur from tissue expansion.[34]

Some salient points to consider while using tissue expanders include the following:

1. *Patient selection.* Tissue expansion is an elective procedure. Tissue that is expanded should be healthy, well vascularized, and free from contamination. Optimal expansion can be obtained only by patients who are compliant and adhere to a regular expansion schedule.
2. *Preoperative planning.* The amount of tissue required, the size and shape of the tissue expander, and optimal placement of the

expander must be determined. Incisions for expander placement should be made adjacent to the lesion and at least 2 cm away from the expander to decrease the chances of wound dehiscence.

Reconstruction of neck burns is usually dealt with earlier in burn wound management. Neck contractures may compromise access to the airway and exert an extrinsic pull on the rest of the face; hence, addressing neck contractures is useful prior to addressing lip and eyelid ectropion. Expanders can be inserted in the subcutaneous plane superficial to the platysma to produce thinner flaps. However, if vascularity is in question, the expanders can be placed deep to the platysma, dissecting the pocket carefully to avoid injury to the facial nerve branches. To avoid airway compromise, expanders should not be placed over the midline structures of the neck. Instead, expanded tissue can be transposed medially to cover median neck wounds.

Tissue expanders are particularly helpful in scalp burns. This technique provides hair-bearing scalp tissue to close burn wounds and cover areas of burn alopecia. Scalp expansion is usually avoided in children below 1 year of age to prevent molding of the soft calvarial bone. Expanders are placed below the galea aponeurotica for scalp expansion with port sites located distant to the pocket to prevent expander extrusion. Advancement of expanded scalp tissue in a sagittal plane toward the midline provides more advancement than that in an anterior to posterior direction and produces less eyebrow elevation and facial distortion.[35–37] Figure 12-7 illustrates the use of tissue expansion to resurface the neck, lower face, and scalp in a 6-year-old girl following burn injury.

POTENTIAL FUTURE THERAPIES

Aesthetic outcome is paramount in assessing the reconstructive result of facial burns. Techniques employed should focus on minimizing scarring, attaining tissue that may closely replicate the native facial tissue that is to be replaced. Owing

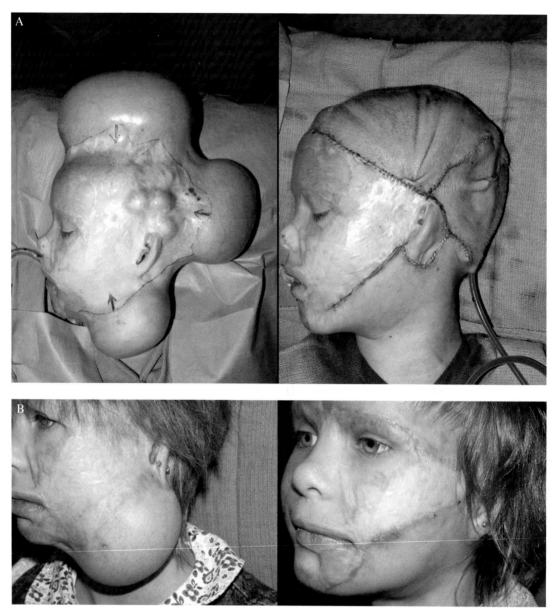

Figure 7.   *A,* A 6-year-old girl has had three tissue expanders placed for expansion of the frontoparietal scalp, the occipital scalp, and the neck to advance the adjacent tissues in the direction of the respective arrows (*left*). The expanded frontoparietal scalp is advanced to restore the normal frontal hairline; the expanded occipital scalp is advanced to restore the postauricular hairline; the expanded neck skin is advanced to provide non-hair-bearing tissue to the postauricular sulcus and the lower face (*right*). *B,* The neck and lower facial skin are reexpanded to advance uninjured skin to the level of the lateral commissure of the mouth (*top*); a full-thickness skin graft has been applied beneath the left side of the lower lip to further lift the lateral commissure and better define the vermilion-cutaneous junction of the lower lip (*bottom*).

to differences in thickness, texture, and color of the native skin in different aesthetic units of the face, developing aesthetically compatible skin substitutes for the reconstruction of facial burns represents a formidable challenge. With advancements in molecular and cell biology, growing dermal cells or tissue cultures to use for wound coverage has become an attainable option in burn management. However, owing to differ-

ences in aesthetic outcome, we would caution that skin substitutes should currently be used for the reconstruction of facial burns only if no native donor sites are available.

Facial transplantation has received a lot of media coverage lately with the recent face transplant performed in Amiens University Hospital, Lyons, France, by Dr. Bernard Devauchelle. Now that research has made the concept of facial transplant a reality, one must weigh the benefit of this form of reconstruction compared with autogenous tissue, given the sequelae of long-term immunosuppression required with the former.

SUMMARY

Burn injuries take a huge toll in global health care and may represent the greatest worldwide need for reconstructive surgery. With the advancements in trauma and burn management over the past three decades, there has been a significant improvement in survival from major burns. Better resuscitation and a multidisciplinary burn team approach have facilitated the reduction in mortality and improved care; hence, there is an increased need for burn reconstruction. Without question, access to health care and available resources for reconstruction are the limiting steps in providing adequate reconstruction of burn injuries worldwide. Whereas the problems of global health care delivery are beyond the scope of this chapter, it is imperative that health care centers in the developed world be familiar with current techniques in reconstruction of facial burns. At present, the mainstay of this treatment centers around the proper selection and transfer of autogenous tissue. However, over time, transfer of allografts, xenografts, cultured autogenous cells, skin substitutes, and face transplant will undoubtedly receive increasing attention for reconstruction of facial burns. Although many of these breakthroughs will be developed in the research laboratories, the challenge for the clinician will be to determine which form of reconstruction is most appropriate for which injury. Our goal should not be to provide the simplest or the most novel form of reconstruction but rather to provide the form of reconstruction that will best serve each individual patient.

REFERENCES

1. Centers for Disease Control and Prevention. Deaths resulting from residential fires and the prevalence of smoke alarms—United States 1991–1995. Morbidity and Mortality Weekly Report 1998;47(38):803–6.

2. Lund T, Onarheim H, Wiig H, Reed RK. Mechanisms behind increased dermal imbibition pressure in acute burn edema. Am J Physiol 2989;256(4 Pt 2):H940–8.

3. Yurt RW, Pruitt BA Jr. Base-line and postthermal injury plasma histamine in rats. J Appl Physiol 1986;60:1782–8.

4. Gibran NS, Heimbach DM. Current status of burn wound pathophysiology. Clin Plast Surg 2000;27:11–22.

5. Shirani KZ, Vaughan GM, Mason AD Jr, Pruitt BA Jr. Update on current therapeutic approaches in burns. Shock 1996;5:4–16.

6. Arturson MG. The pathophysiology of severe thermal injury. J Burn Care Rehabil 1985;6:129–46.

7. Atiyeh BS, Gunn SW, Hayek SN. State of the art in burn treatment. World J Surg 2005;29:131–48.

8. Kloppenberg FW, Beerthuizen GI, Ten Duis HJ. Perfusion of burn wounds assessed by laser Doppler imaging is related to burn depth and healing time. Burns 2001;27:359–63.

9. Kim DE, Phillips TM, Jeng JC, et al. Microvascular assessment of burn depth conversion during varying resuscitation conditions. J Burn Care Rehabil 2001;22:406–16.

10. Janzekovic Z. A new concept in the early excision and immediate grafting of burns. J Trauma 1970;10:1103–8.

11. Heimbach DM. Early burn excision and grafting. Surg Clin North Am 1987;67:93–107.

12. Tompkins RG, Remensnyder JP, Burke JF, et al. Significant reductions in mortality for children with burn injuries through the use of prompt eschar excision. Ann Surg 1988;208:577–85.

13. Fraulin FO, Illmayer SJ, Tredget EE. Assessment of cosmetic and functional results of conservative versus surgical management of facial burns. J Burn Care Rehabil 1996;17:19–29.

14. Engrav LH, Heimbach DM, Walkinshaw MD, Marvin JA. Excision of burns of the face. Plast Reconstr Surg 1986;77:744–51.

15. Pruitt BA Jr. The diagnosis and treatment of infection in the burn patient. Burns Incl Therm Injury 1984;11:79–91.

16. Waymack JP, Herndon DN. Nutritional support of the burned patient. World J Surg 1992;16:80.

17. Gonzalez-Ulloa M, Castillo A, Stevens E, et al. Preliminary study of the total restoration of the facial skin. Plast Reconstr Surg 1954;13(3):151–61.

18. Gonzalez-Ulloa M. Restoration of the face covering by means of selected skin in regional aesthetic units. Br J Plast Surg 1956;9:212.

19. Maillard GF, Clavel PR. Aesthetic units in skin grafting of the face. Ann Plast Surg 1991;26:347.

20. Feldman JJ. Reconstruction of the burned face in children. In: Serafin D, Georgiades NG, editors. Pediatric plastic surgery. Vol 1. St Louis: Mosby; 1984.

21. Tredget EE, Shankowsky HA, Groeneveld A, Burrell R. A matched-pair, randomized study evaluating the efficacy and safety of Acticoat silver-coated dressing for the

treatment of burn wounds. J Burn Care Rehabil 1998; 19:531–7.

22. Pruitt BA Jr, Levine NS. Characteristics and uses of biologic dressings and skin substitutes. Arch Surg 1984; 119:312–22.

23. Sheridan RL, Tompkins RG, Burke JF. Management of burn wounds with prompt excision and immediate closure. J Intensive Care Med 1994;9:6–17.

24. Sheridan RL, Tompkins RG. Skin substitutes in burns. Burns 1999;25:97–103.

25. Klein MB, Engrav LH, Holmes JH, et al. Management of facial burns with a collagen/glycosaminoglycan skin substitute—prospective experience with 12 consecutive patients with large, deep facial burns. Burns 2005;31: 257–61.

26. Griffin JE, Johnson DL. Management of the maxillofacial burn patient: current therapy. J Oral Maxillofac Surg 2005;63:247–52.

27. Kumar RJ, Kimble RM, Boots R, Pegg SP. Treatment of partial-thickness burns: a prospective, randomized trial using TransCyte. Aust N Z J Surg 2004;74: 622–6.

28. Lukish JR, Eichelberger MR, Newman KD, et al. The use of a bioactive skin substitute decreases length of stay for pediatric burn patients. J Pediatr Surg 2001;36: 1118–21.

29. Larson DL, Abston S, Evans EB, et al. Techniques for decreasing scar formation and contractures in the burned patient. J Trauma 1971;11:807–23.

30. Quinn KJ. Silicone gel in scar treatment. Burns Incl Therm Inj 1987;13 Suppl:S33–40.

31. Ahn ST, Monafo WW, Mustoe TA. Topical silicone gel: a new treatment for hypertrophic scars. Surgery 1989; 106:781–6; discussion 786–7.

32. Musgrave MA, Umraw N, Fish JS, et al. The effect of silicone gel sheets on perfusion of hypertrophic burn scars. J Burn Care Rehabil 2002;23:208–14.

33. Radovan C. Tissue expansion in soft-tissue reconstruction. Plastic & Reconstructive Surgery 1984;74(4):482–92.

34. MacLennan SE, Corcoran JF, Neale HW. Tissue expansion in head and neck burn reconstruction. Clin Plast Surg 2000;27:121–32.

35. Ninkovic M, Moser-Rumer A, Ninkovic M, et al. Anterior neck reconstruction with pre-expanded free groin and scapular flaps. Plast Reconstr Surg 2004;113:61–8.

36. Angrigiani C, Grilli D, Karanas YL, et al. The dorsal scapular island flap: an alternative for head, neck, and chest reconstruction. Plast Reconstr Surg 2003;111:67–78.

37. Beasley NJ, Gilbert RW, Gullane PJ, et al. Scalp and forehead reconstruction using free revascularized tissue transfer. Arch Facial Plast Surg 2004;6:16–20.

13

Keloids and Hypertrophic Scarring

Harvey Chim, MBBS, MRCS, MMed; Mark Boon Yang Tang, MBBS, MRCP, MMed, FAMS

OUTLINE

Clinical Healing Problem

Keloids and hypertrophic scars are benign skin abnormalities characterized by an overgrowth of scar tissue with excessive deposition of collagen in the dermis and subcutaneous tissues. The pathogenesis of keloids and hypertrophic scars represents a derangement in the wound healing process, with aberrations occurring at all stages of wound healing.

Approach to Management of Keloids and Hypertrophic Scars

Differentiation between keloids and hypertrophic scars is essential as the treatment and prognosis of each condition may be different. Differential diagnoses of scar-like lesions in the head and neck include dermatofibroma and scar sarcoidosis, as well as more sinister lesions, such as morpheic basal cell carcinoma, metastatic skin nodules, and dermatofibrosarcoma protruberans. Inflammatory conditions such as pseudofolliculitis barbae, acne keloidalis nuchae, and folliculitis decalvans should also be considered.

Treatment Modalities

Numerous modalities of treatment are available, and these can be divided into medical, surgical, and physical therapies. Treatment protocols may vary between different centers and should be individualized for each patient.

Pearls and Pitfalls

Different conditions may mimic keloids. When in doubt, a diagnostic skin biopsy may be appropriate. Treatment should always be tailored toward patient expectations, which may range from cosmesis to symptom relief.

Potential Future Therapies

Many new therapies are currently being tested in the laboratory or in the clinical setting. Promising modalities include topical imiquimod and transforming growth factor β (TGF-β) inhibitors.

CLINICAL HEALING PROBLEM

Definition

Keloids and hypertrophic scars are benign skin abnormalities caused by aberrant wound healing and characterized by an overgrowth of scar tissue with excessive deposition of collagen in the dermis and subcutaneous tissues. Hypertrophic scars remain within the confines of the original lesion (Figure 1A), but keloids extend laterally beyond the original site of injury, often with claw-like extensions (Figure 1B)—hence the derivation of the term *keloid* from the Greek word *chele*, meaning *crab claw*.

Epidemiology and Risk Factors

Numerous factors have been described in the etiology of keloids and hypertrophic scars. These

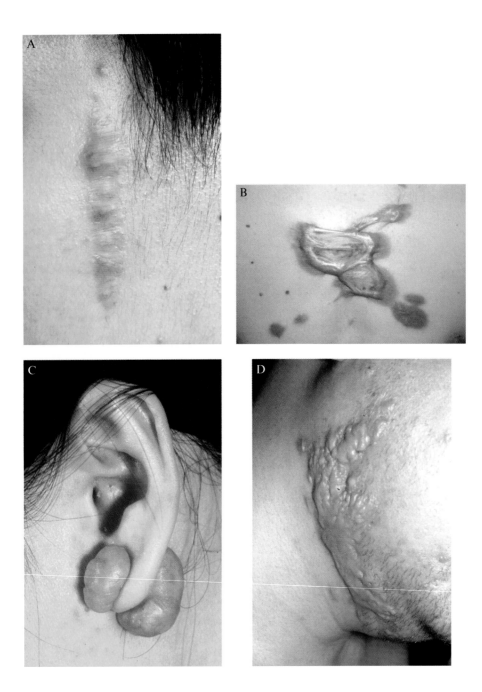

Figure 1. Keloids and hypertrophic scars represent a benign overgrowth of scar tissue. A, Hypertrophic scars are confined to the site of the initial injury, with a smooth, shiny, atrophic epidermal surface. B, Keloids typically extend beyond the site of initial injury, with characteristic claw-like extensions. In the head and neck, keloids are prone to develop at the earlobe (C) and jawline (D), in these patients secondary to relatively minor trauma, such as ear piercing and acne, respectively, as shown here.

can be conveniently divided into epidemiologic, exogenous, genetic, and immunologic factors (Table 1). Generally, keloids are prevalent among the darker-pigmented races, inclusive of Africans and Asians, with a reported incidence of between 4.5 and 16%.[1] The incidence of hypertrophic scarring has been reported to be approximately 39 to 68% after surgery and 33 to 91% after burns, depending on the depth of the wound.[1] Keloids tend to occur during and after puberty, with a peak incidence in the second

decade of life. There is no gender predilection. In addition, the influence of hormonal factors appears to be significant owing to observations that keloids appear during puberty, enlarge during pregnancy, and resolve after menopause.

Exogenous factors such as trauma and skin or wound tension have been implicated as significant factors in the development of keloids and hypertrophic scars. Significantly, however, large keloids often result from minor dermatologic insults, such as ear piercing, varicella infec-

Table 1. RISK FACTORS FOR KELOIDS AND HYPERTROPHIC SCARS
Risk factors for keloids and hypertrophic scars
Epidemiology
Darker pigmented races
Age during and after puberty
Exogenous
Traumatic skin injury: surgical incisions, laser therapy, burns
Wound infection
Unfavorable surgical technique
Unfavorable wound placement (not aligned along skin creases)
Unfavorable approximation of wounds
Wounds closed under tension
Wound contamination
Recent systemic isotretinoin treatment (past 6–12 mo)
Specific for keloids
Genetic
Hereditary (autosomal dominant or recessive)
Dermatologic diseases: acne vulgaris, acne conglobata, hidradenitis suppurativa, pilonidal cysts
Syndromes: Rubinstein-Taybi syndrome, pachydermoperiostosis, Goeminne syndrome
Immunologic
Cell membrane proteins: HLA B14, B21, BW16, BW35, DR5, DQW3
Increased serum immunoglobulin E, M, and G levels
Decreased serum immunoglobulin A levels
Increased C3, decreased C4 levels
Hormonal
Keloids enlarge during puberty and pregnancy

HLA = human leukocyte antigen.

tion, and postvaccination or acne lesions. Conversely, injury to the deep dermis is often required for the development of hypertrophic scars, with size commensurate with the extent of injury. Surrounding undamaged skin is not involved in hypertrophic scars, unlike keloids, which are defined by growth of scar tissue beyond the confines of the original injury. Other genetic and immunologic factors have been implicated and may predispose certain individuals to the formation of keloids.

Etiology and Pathogenesis

The pathogenesis of keloids and hypertrophic scars represents a derangement in the wound healing process, with aberrations at all stages of wound healing contributing to the etiology of these phenomena. To adequately describe the pathogenesis of these conditions, it would be relevant to first examine the normal wound healing process.[2] Wound healing consists of three main phases: inflammation, repair, and tissue remodeling. In the inflammatory phase, bleeding is arrested by platelet aggregation and activation of the complement cascade. Vasoactive cytokines such as platelet-derived growth factor (PDGF) and monocyte chemoattractant protein 1 cause vasodilatation and pain and stimulate chemotaxis of leukocytes. The result is a fibrin clot. Repair follows inflammation, with reepithelialization of wounds beginning hours after injury, followed by the growth of epithelium over the sealed wound within 24 to 48 hours. Subsequently, growth factors, especially PDGF and transforming growth factor β (TGF-β), stimulate the migration of fibroblasts, macrophages, and endothelial cells into the wound space to form granulation tissue approximately 4 days after injury. Neovascularization and epithelial proliferation are maximal, and collagen fibrils begin to appear. The production of collagen, fibronectin, elastin, and proteoglycans results in deposition of the extracellular matrix (ECM) and strengthening of the wound. This is followed by tissue remodeling, in which collagen deposition and remodeling result in transformation of the provisional ECM into a collagenous matrix and subsequently into an acellular scar. The wound softens and flattens, and the underlying inflammation resolves. Continued collagen synthesis and degradation result in increasing wound strength, with final scar maturation occurring up to 12 months after injury.

Inflammation

Keloid fibroblasts have difficulty in degrading the initial fibrin clot because they exhibit a low level of plasminogen activator and a high level of inhibitor activity, leading to lower plasmin concentrations and therefore defective fibrinolysis.[3] Burns or infected wounds predispose individuals to keloid and hypertrophic scar formation by exaggerating the inflammatory phase, leading to an increase in the concentration of profibrotic cytokines, such as insulin-like growth factor 1 (IGF-1), TGF-β, and PDGF, which are secreted by degranulating platelets and macrophages.[4]

These cytokines, when produced in excess, lead to derailed ECM formation and production of excessive scar tissue.

Repair

Excessive fibroplasia, mediated through abnormal growth factor activity and aberrant fibroblasts, is largely responsible for the excessive scarring of keloids and hypertrophic scars. Several mechanisms are responsible for this. One of the most important pathogenetic growth factors identified is TGF-β, ?which is pivotal in the transformation of granulation tissue into a collagenous matrix.[1] During formation of granulation tissue, neovascular endothelial cells express the TGF-β_1 gene, leading to activation of adjacent fibroblasts, which express markedly elevated levels of TGF-β_1, as well as collagen types I and VI. Lesional fibroblasts derived from hypertrophic scars and keloids, however, have been found to be more sensitive to TGF-β stimulation and respond to a lower concentration of TGF-β compared with normal fibroblasts. Excessive TGF-β production in the inflammatory phase, when present, further contributes to stimulation of fibroblasts, leading to increased ECM production and subsequent exuberant scarring. TGF-β also stimulates production of ECM indirectly through the induction of other profibrotic cytokines, such as PDGF, connective tissue growth factor, and epidermal growth factor. PDGF has been shown to promote granulation tissue formation and collagen production during the later stages of wound healing. Connective tissue growth factor has been associated with skin sclerosis. Finally, TGF-β has a synergistic effect on growth stimulation of keloidal fibroblasts by epidermal growth factor. Keloidal fibroblasts have been found in vitro to produce high levels of collagen, elastin, proteoglycan, and fibronectin and show abnormal responses, compared with normal fibroblasts, to metabolic agents such as glucocorticoids, phorbol esters, and growth factors.[5] Fibroblasts from hypertrophic scars exhibit a moderate elevation in collagen production in vitro; however, their response to metabolic agents is similar to that of normal fibroblasts. Another important difference between keloids and hypertrophic scars is that scar contracture is mediated by fibroblasts found in hypertrophic scars, unlike keloids, in which this does not occur. Keloidal fibroblasts demonstrate increased production of fibronectin for months to years after the original wound, as opposed to normal scars, in which fibronectin formation stops within a few days after the wound closes. Fibronectin acts as a matrix for the organization of the ECM during wound healing.

In addition, excessive neovascularization has been noted in the granulation tissue of keloids and hypertrophic scars when compared with normal scars. These show occlusion of their lumina owing to an excess of endothelial cells and excessive collagen deposition. The resultant tissue hypoxia leads to further stimulation of angiogenesis by macrophages through mediators such as vascular endothelial growth factor and further hyperproliferation of fibroblasts, with increased collagen deposition, leading to excessive scarring.

Tissue Remodeling

Aberrant growth factor and fibroblast activity continues throughout after the phase of tissue remodeling. In normal scars, collagen synthesis peaks about 6 months after injury, declining to normal levels 2 to 3 years after wounding. In keloids, however, collagen synthesis continues for several years.[6] Excessive collagen deposition may result not only from increased collagen synthesis but also decreased collagen degradation during scar remodeling.

APPROACH TO MANAGEMENT OF KELOIDS AND HYPERTROPHIC SCARS

Clinical Presentation

Differentiation between keloids and hypertrophic scars is essential because they respond differently to treatment and have different prognoses (Table

2). Hypertrophic scars usually appear within 4 weeks after trauma or surgery as an elevated, wider, or thickened scar confined to the site of the initial injury. They often appear bright red initially, with a smooth, shiny, atrophic epidermal covering, overlying fine telangiectatic blood vessels.

Conversely, keloids may appear months to years after the initial injury, which may be trivial, such as acne or small wounds. In some cases, the patient may not recall any preceding trauma; spontaneous keloids have been known to develop on the midchest area. They have varying morphology, appearing as papules, pedunculated lesions (on the ears and neck), or firm, elevated, fibrotic plaques. Characteristically, the lesions extend beyond the site of initial injury, extending both vertically upward or laterally with typical claw-like prolongations. Certain head and neck locations, such as the earlobe (Figure 1C) and jawline (Figure 1D), are predisposed to developing keloids (see Table 2). A keloid may initially be soft and pink but demonstrates rapid growth over the next few months, resulting in a firm, protruberant, dense lesion that may be erythematous or slightly violaceous in color. Older lesions tend to be hyperpigmented or, less commonly, even hypopigmented. They usually lack hair follicles and other appendages, such as sebaceous glands.

Although many patients are most concerned about the cosmesis of their scars, keloids can be associated with significant physical symptoms, such as pain, tenderness, and pruritus, which also can have a major impact on their quality of life. A recent study found that up to 86% of patients experienced itch, 46% experienced keloid-related pain, and 43% reported mechanical allodynia.[7] Itch was localized more frequently to the edge of their keloids, in contrast to pain, which was

Table 2. DIFFERENCES BETWEEN KELOIDS AND HYPERTROPHIC SCARS		
	Keloids	**Hypertrophic Scars**
Characteristics		
Onset	Appear after 3 mo and can be delayed up to several yr after trauma or surgery	Appear within 4 wk after trauma or surgery
Location	Regional susceptibility: anterior chest, shoulders, earlobes, chin, upper arms, and lower legs. Rare at eyelids, genitalia, palms, soles, cornea, and mucous membranes	Flexor surfaces of joints, abdomen
Areas of predilection	Areas of high tension on healing wounds	Described to be related to forces opposite to areas of skin tension
Appearance	Extend beyond site of original wound Usually raised, thick, and firm protuberant growths with claw-like extensions	Raised scars that remain within the boundaries of the wound
Progression	Tend to persist without regression and usually continue to grow vertically and laterally Do not exhibit scar contracture	Frequently regress spontaneously Exhibit scar contracture
Response to treatment	High recurrence after surgery	May undergo spontaneous regression Respond well to intralesional corticosteroids Less recurrence after surgery
Histology[26]		
General/collagen	Swirling whorls and nodules of thick hyalinized collagen bundles (keloidal collagen) diagnostic	Less compact, smaller collagen fibrils arranged in a wavy pattern
Hyaluronic acid	Found mainly in the thickened granular and spinous layers of the epidermis	Found mainly as a narrow strip in the papillary dermis
Diagnostic markers	Keloidal collagen arranged in swirling nodular pattern High expression of α-SMA	Absence of typical keloidal collagen α-SMA present
Other distinguishing features	Nonflattened epidermis Nonfibrotic papillary dermis Tongue-like advancing edge Horizontal cellular fibrous band in upper reticular dermis Prominent fascia-like band	Prominent vertical blood vessels

SMA = smooth muscle actin.

reported more commonly at the center of the lesion. Despite these differences between keloids and hypertrophic scars, in clinical practice, it may still be difficult to distinguish between them owing to similar morphology and behavior. Occasionally, a skin biopsy may be helpful in distinguishing between both conditions, although further skin injury may induce fresh scarring.

Differential Diagnoses of Keloids in the Head and Neck

The differential diagnoses of keloids (Table 3) include benign skin conditions such as dermatofibroma, scar sarcoidosis, keloidal scleroderma, and more sinister lesions, such as morpheic or pigmented basal cell carcinoma, metastatic skin nodules, and dermatofibrosarcoma protruberans (Figure 2). Dermatologic conditions with keloid-like scarring specific to the head, neck, and upper trunk region include pseudofolliculitis barbae, acne keloidalis nuchae, and folliculitis decalvans. It is important to recognize these inflammatory conditions because treatment of the secondary scarring process without managing the primary underlying cause will only predispose the individual to even further scarring and morbidity.

Acne Keloidalis Nuchae

This condition appears as keloid-like papules or plaques over the occiput and posterior neck (Figure 3A), which may be preceded by localized folliculitis. The papules may subsequently coalesce into thickened plaques that usually form a horizontal keloidal band across the occipital scalp or nape of the neck, associated with scarring alopecia. These large, hairless plaques may be fringed by tufted hairs at their borders, with characteristic polytrichia emerging from a single follicular opening ("doll's hair–like picture"). This condition is most commonly seen in black men. Symptoms include pruritus, burning, and pain. Prevention and early intervention are essential to management of this condition. Hair should be allowed to grow long in the affected areas, and mechanical irritation by tight collars or helmets should be avoided. Topical and intralesional corticosteroids, topical and systemic antibiotics, and oral isotretinoin may be used to attenuate the underlying inflammation. Secondary bacterial infection should be treated early. Primary surgical excision or shaving of large lesions with adjuvant corticosteroids and radiotherapy may be attempted in severe recalcitrant cases.

Pseudofolliculitis Barbae

This condition has a predilection for black and Hispanic men who have tightly curled hair. It is precipitated by frequent shaving, which results in the new hair curving back to penetrate the skin, causing a foreign body inflammatory response with subsequent dermal fibrosis and scarring. Clinically, the condition presents with multiple inflamed papules on the neck, chin, lower jaw, and submandibular area. On close inspection, an

Table 3. DIFFERENTIAL DIAGNOSIS OF KELOIDS AND HYPERTROPHIC SCARS	
Differential Diagnosis	Key Distinguishing Features
Dermatofibroma	Solitary, firm, raised, dome-shaped dermal papule or nodule
	Exhibits the "dimple sign": "dimpling" or depression of the central part of the lesion when compressed between two fingers
Scar sarcoidosis	Sarcoidal infiltration usually occurs in old scars
	Manifests as translucent, violaceous to brown papules or nodules
Keloidal scleroderma	Indurated nontender, well-demarcated plaques with a predilection for the superior part of the thorax, sparing the face and hands
Basal cell carcinoma	Firm papules or nodules with rolled pearly edges and peripheral telangiectasia
	Pigmented variant more commonly seen in Asian patients
Metastatic carcinomatous skin nodules	Asymptomatic, hard, infiltrated skin nodules that may ulcerate with a predilection for the scalp and trunk.
	May present as multiple nodules over the operative scar for the primary tumor
Dermatofibrosarcoma protuberans	Locally invasive, reddish brown, indurated plaque
	Ill-defined, irregular edges and protuberant nodules

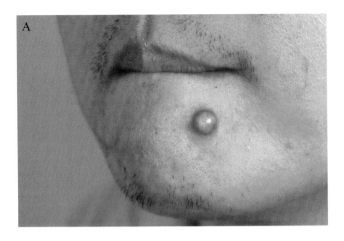
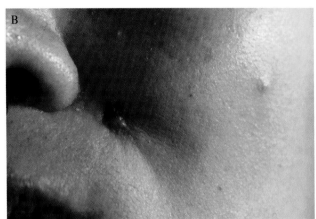
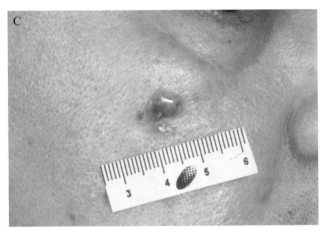

Figure 2. Differential diagnoses of keloids. *A,* Dermatofibroma: appears as a well-circumscribed, dome-shaped, tan dermal nodule. *B,* Dermatofibrosarcoma protruberans: puckering of skin suggests significant local invasion and extension to surrounding structures. *C,* Basal cell carcinoma: characteristic pearly edges and telangiectasias are evident.

embedded hair shaft may be seen at the center of the papule. Secondary bacterial infection is a common complication that can lead to abscesses or cellulitis, with consequent scarring and keloid formation. The mainstay of therapy is prevention by minimizing shaving and allowing the beard to grow so that embedded hairs will detach. Laser hair removal or electrolysis may be an effective option for hair reduction. Topical and systemic antibiotics may be needed for secondary infection.

Folliculitis Decalvans

This is a form of neutrophilic scarring alopecia that presents with follicular papules and pustules on the scalp and beard areas associated with tufting of hairs (Figure 3B). Severe cases can result in keloidal plaques and nodules with sinus track formation, which may sometimes be referred to as "folliculitis keloidalis." It is

postulated that these patients may have an abnormal host response to staphylococcal super-antigens, resulting in an aberrant inflammatory response. Treatment is difficult owing to a high relapse rate. Long-term systemic combination antibiotics, isotretinoin, and intralesional corti-costeroids have been used for treatment.

TREATMENT MODALITIES

Medical Therapies

Corticosteroids

Overview. Intralesional corticosteroids have been accepted as a mainstay of therapy for treatment of keloids and hypertrophic scars since the mid-1960s. The main advantage of this modality is its relative ease of administration, good safety profile, and inexpensive cost. When

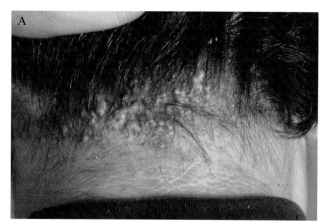

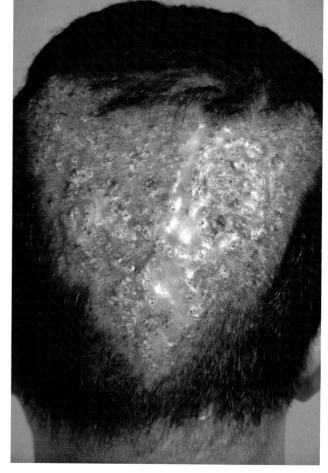

Figure 3.   Inflammatory conditions predisposing to keloidal scarring in the head and neck. *A*, Acne keloidalis nuchae. This patient has keloid-like papules and plaques over the posterior neck, with characteristic scarring, alopecia, and polytrichia. *B*, Follicultis decalvans. Severe scarring alopecia has resulted, with sinus track formation, keloidal plaques, and nodules over the posterior scalp.

used alone, this modality tends to be more efficacious for younger hypertrophic scars that may flatten completely. However, patients should be counseled that older hypertrophic scars and keloids treated with steroids may soften and flatten only to a certain extent but not regress completely. Keloid-related pain and itch, however, may improve with therapy. Intralesional corticosteroids can also be used in combination with other modalities, such as cryotherapy and surgery. Highly variable response rates of 50 to 100% with recurrence rates of 9 to 50% have been described for intralesional corticosteroids alone.[1,8,9]

Mechanism of Action.   Steroids inhibit α_2-macroglobulin, which inhibits collagenase. When this pathway is blocked, collagenase production increases, thus enabling collagen degradation. In addition, steroids have also been described to act by decreasing collagen and glycosaminoglycan synthesis, decreasing fibroblast proliferation, reducing inflammation in the wound, increasing hypoxia, and decreasing TGF-β and IGF-1 levels in scar tissue.

Technique.   The most common steroid used for intralesional injection is triamcinolone acetonide. Because injection often causes significant pain, topical anesthetics such as EMLA (AstraZenaca, USA) or ELA-Max (Ferndale Laboratories, USA) cream can be applied to the lesion 30 minutes to 1 hour prior to the injection. This is especially useful in pediatric patients. Alternatively, lidocaine can be mixed with triamcinolone for intralesional injection, but this will result in dilution of the steroid concentration. A concentration of 10 to 40 mg/mL of triamcinolone may be used, depending on the thickness and clinical response of the lesions. Injections should be given at an interval of 3 to 6 weeks. Beware of using large amounts of high-potency steroids or giving injections at too frequent intervals as this may lead to skin atrophy. Steroids can be injected using a syringe equipped with a Luer-Lok device (Becton Dickson and Company, USA) through a fine 30-gauge needle. The needle should be injected from the lateral borders of the lesion rather than perpendicularly and should be passed back and forth through the scar tissue to ensure an even distribution of steroid. Injections at 5 to 10 mm intervals are suitable for large keloids. The steroid should be injected fairly deeply into the central fibrous bulk of lesion and should not extend into the subcutaneous tissue as this may lead to subcutaneous fat atrophy. Blanching of the lesion is often noted during the injections.

Side Effects.
These include hypopigmentation, skin and subcutaneous fat atrophy (Figure 4), telangiectasias, necrosis, and ulceration. Rarely, iatrogenic Cushing's syndrome may occur if excessive amounts of steroids are used indiscriminately. Although reversible, effects such as hypopigmentation may last from 6 to 12 months. Subcutaneous fat atrophy may be permanent and usually manifest as a depressed area at or around the treated scar. The risk of side effects increases when steroids are injected into the surrounding normal skin or underlying subcutaneous tissue or if large volumes of steroids are used, owing to increased diffusion of the medication into the surrounding dermis.

Adjunctive Therapies.
The use of very light cryotherapy prior to the injection may faciliate intralesional steroid injections by inducing tissue edema with subsequent cellular and collagen disruption. This leads to "softening" of the lesion and may be helpful in very hard and fibrotic

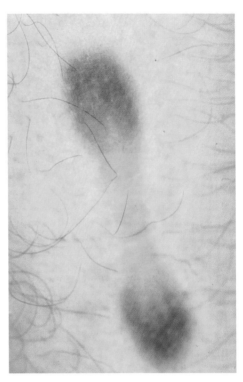

Figure 4. Skin atrophy and hypopigmentation at the periphery are noted at the periphery of this keloid treated by intralesional corticosteroids. Often the response to treatment may not be uniform, with a better response seen at the central portion of the keloid.

lesions, which are difficult to inject otherwise. Pressure or silicone gel sheeting used in conjunction with intralesional corticosteroids has been found to be more efficacious than when either modality is used as a monotherapy.[1] Steroids may also be infiltrated into the wound following excision of a keloid, and this has been shown to reduce the recurrence rate of keloids (to less than 50%) compared with surgery alone (45–100%). The first injection should be given immediately after wound closure or 1 week postoperatively, with injections every 2 to 3 weeks for another 3 to 6 months to prevent recurrence. Finally, injection with a mixture of 5-fluorouracil (5-FU) and triamcinolone acetonide (9:1 dilution of 50 mg/mL 5-FU to 10 mg/mL triamcinolone) has been successful in management of keloids. Unfortunately, this combination is associated with more pain than steroids alone.

Interferon Therapy
Overview. The use of intralesional interferon has been shown to be effective for treatment of

keloids both as monotherapy and for postsurgical prophylaxis, for which it was reported to be significantly better than triamcinolone acetonide injections for preventing keloid recurrence.[10] However, the main problems associated with its use include pain and high cost.

Mechanism of Action. Interferons α, β, and γ inhibit the synthesis of collagen types I, III, and VI and also enhance keloidal collagenase activity, therefore promoting collagen breakdown. Interferons α and β also reduce glycosaminoglycan synthesis.

Technique. One million units of interferon-α is injected into each linear centimeter of the keloid or along the postoperative site. The frequency of injection has been reported from three times a week to every 2 weeks.

Side Effects. Intralesional interferon reportedly causes more pain than corticosteroids. Systemic side effects in the form of influenza-like symptoms, such as fever and myalgia, are frequently encountered, especially if large areas are treated. Premedication with acetaminophen is useful in countering these adverse side effects.

Other Intralesional Agents

These include 5-FU and bleomycin. 5-FU alone or in combination with triamcinolone has been used, but side effects include pain at the injection site, hyperpigmentation, and tissue sloughing. In a recent study involving 20 patients, 95% responded favorably to treatment.[11] With 0.01% bleomycin injected every 3 to 4 weeks, patients experienced flattening of keloids and hypertrophic scars.[12] A multiple-needle puncture method can be used. However, larger-scale prospective studies with proper follow-up are needed before this agent can be used as standard therapy.

Topical Retinoids

Overview. Topical retinoids have been reported to be effective in reducing the size, weight, and hardness of keloids and hypertrophic scars, as well as alleviating symptoms such as pruritus.[13] However, the total volume reduction was less than 20% in treated keloids.[14]

Mechanism of Action. Retinoids were shown in vitro to reduce collagen metabolism in fibroblasts derived from keloids.

Technique. Tretinoin cream can be used initially at lower concentrations of 0.01% once a day, subsequently increasing in frequency to twice a day, and concentrations from 0.025 to 0.05% twice daily. It should be used for at least 8 to 12 months.

Side Effects. These may include irritant contact dermatitis, erythema, dryness, and scaling.

Surgical Therapies

Surgery for Keloids

Overview. The principal aim in the management of keloids is prevention. Nonessential cosmetic surgery should be avoided for patients with epidemiologic risk factors for keloid formation (see Table 1), and exogenous risk factors must be minimized through good surgical technique if surgery is essential. Surgery should be avoided on keloid-prone anatomic sites, and if absolutely indicated, incisions must follow skin creases or relaxed skin tension lines if possible. Surgical excision of keloids should be considered only when medical therapy has failed or is unacceptable owing to the high recurrence rate after excision. This has been reported to range from 45 to 100% in different series.[15] To prevent the recurrence of keloids, surgery is often performed in combination with other adjunctive measures, such as intralesional corticosteroids and silicone sheeting.

Technique. Many surgical techniques have been described, and these vary according to the expertise and preference of the surgeon. These include simple elliptical incision with primary closure, pedicle flaps, rotation and transposition flaps, or even excision and grafting with a full-thickness skin graft for large keloids. Small pedunculated earlobe keloids can be excised primarily; however, large, nonpedunculated earlobe keloids may need closure with a tongue-like flap derived from the flattest part of the lesion. Generally, wounds should be closed without tension and should follow skin creases. Leaving a rim of keloid around the excision site (intramarginal excision) may be a useful technique to debulk a large, disfiguring keloid by avoiding further injury to adjacent unaffected but keloid-prone skin (Figure 5). However, other authors have claimed that this method does not help prevent recurrences.[16]

Adjunctive Therapies. These are essential owing to the high recurrence rate from primary excision. The use of adjunctive medical therapy in the form of intralesional corticosteroids or interferon injections, as well as topical imiquimod, has been described. When intralesional steroids are

used, sutures should be left in 3 to 5 days more than usual to prevent wound dehiscence. Other useful therapeutic adjuncts include pressure, silicone gel sheeting, and radiotherapy. For earlobe keloids, pressure earrings or clips are available for use postoperatively. These should be applied at least 2 weeks after suture removal to reduce the risk of wound dehiscence immediately after surgery. Patients should be advised that adjunctive postoperative therapies are an essential part of surgical excision and often require a prolonged period of treatment and follow-up.

Surgery for Hypertrophic Scars

Overview. Surgery offers a much better prognosis for hypertrophic scars compared with keloids. The key to surgery is correction of underlying exogenous factors, which may have precipitated formation of the hypertrophic scar. As such, surgery is directed toward excision of

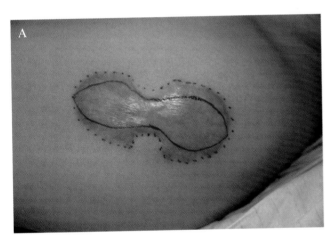
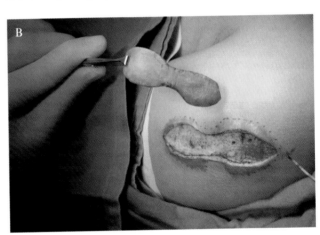
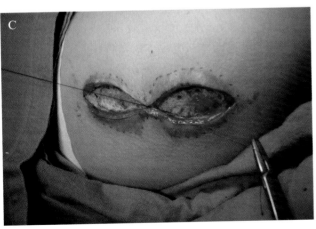
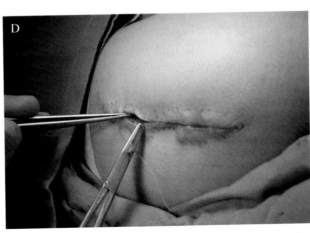

Figure 5. Intramarginal excision of keloids. *A,* The *dotted line* denotes the boundary of the keloid, whereas the *continuous line* shows the planned incision. *B,* The keloid is excised en bloc, and the wound is closed without tension by subcutaneous (*C*) and subcuticular (*D*) sutures.

scars, or techniques, such as Z- and W-plasty, to reorient the scar along the relaxed tension lines. Good surgical technique is also essential to prevent recurrence. Wounds should be closed without tension, dead space should be obliterated, and all foreign or inflammatory tissue should be removed.

Technique. For facial scars, W-plasties are preferred to Z-plasties, with the exception of scars close to the vermilion border of the lip or on the eyelids.[17] The converse is true for scars outside the face. Subcuticular sutures may also be used to splint scars subject to tension for periods ranging from 6 weeks to 6 months.

Adjunctive Therapies. Adjuncts such as silicone gel sheeting, pressure garments, and surgical taping may be used. However, modalities such as radiation or corticosteroids may not be indicated owing to the risk of side effects and substantially better prognosis when compared with keloids.

Cryosurgery

Overview. Cryotherapy is a simple, in-office procedure that can be used alone or in combination with other adjunctive therapies, such as intralesional corticosteroid injections. When used as monotherapy, it is best reserved for small lesions such as acne or small earlobe keloids. A response rate of 51 to 76% for cryosurgery used as monotherapy has been reported, increasing to 84% when used in conjunction with corticosteroids.[1,8,18]

Mechanism of Action. Cryosurgery acts through direct cell damage and microvascular injury leading to ischemic tissue necrosis and sloughing, with resultant scar volume reduction. At a cellular level, it may also act by modifying collagen synthesis and differentiation of keloidal fibroblasts.

Technique. Liquid nitrogen cryotherapy using a handheld cryospray unit (Figure 6) is the most favored means of administration because it can achieve a deeper freezing depth than the dipstick method. With the spray

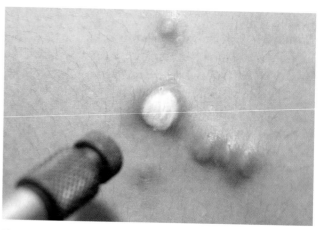

Figure 6. Liquid nitrogen cryotherapy. The nozzle of the cryospray unit is seen in the foreground, with the treated lesion in the center of the picture.

technique, a direct spray is administered to the lesion either in zigzag fashion across the lesion or in a centripetal fashion, spraying from the center of the lesion and spiraling outward. Freeze times ranging from 10 to 30 seconds have been used. Two to three freeze-thaw cycles may be necessary depending on the depth of the scar.

Side Effects. Immediate side effects include pain, edema, and even bullae formation. Treatment of lesions on the forehead and temples and in front of the ears may produce headache. Long-term side effects include permanent hypopigmentation, especially in pigmented patients. Postinflammatory hyperpigmentation may also result and may last for several months.

Laser Surgery

Overview. The use of lasers as a treatment modality for keloids is not well established owing to the lack of large, prospective, controlled studies. Previous trials showed high recurrence rates ranging from 45 to 93% after CO_2 laser excision of keloids and hypertrophic scars, respectively, with no distinct advantage over conventional surgical excision.[8] However, it may still have a role in the excision of small earlobe keloids or when debulking large lesions, in which wound closure may be more difficult otherwise. The 1,064 nm neodymium:yttrium-aluminum-garnet (Nd:YAG) laser has been reported to cause flattening and softening of lesions, but follow-up studies have shown a variable high recurrence rate of 0 to 100%. More recently, the 585 nm flashlamp pumped pulsed dye laser (PDL) has been reported to improve scar-related pruritus, erythema, and structure (surface texture and height). Cosmetically, this may be a useful modality in patients who find scar erythema unacceptable. Improved cosmesis, relief of pruritus, and flattening of keloids and hypertrophic scars were reported in 57 to 83% of patients treated with PDL, with improvement lasting at least 6 months.[19,20]

Mechanism of Action. CO_2 lasers cause direct cell damage through thermal injury. The Nd:YAG laser is postulated to act by inhibition of collagen synthesis and deposition. The PDL works through selective photothermolysis, leading to localized thermal injury of cutaneous blood vessels, collagen breakdown, and tissue ischemia.

Adjunctive Therapies. When used in combination with intralesional corticosteroids, laser therapy was found to be more efficacious.[8]

Physical Therapies and Radiation

Pressure
Overview. Pressure therapy is considered first-line therapy in many centers, particularly for the treatment of hypertrophic scars following burns and earlobe keloids postexcision. It may be applied as monotherapy through devices such as customized pressure garments, compressive and adhesive bandages, or pressure earrings or used postoperatively. Previous studies have demonstrated that external compression leads to softening and flattening of hypertrophic scars; however, a recent randomized, controlled trial by Chang and colleagues showed no benefit in patients with burn scars.[21] Nevertheless, this noninvasive option continues to be an important modality for treatment of keloids and hypertrophic scars. Scars older than 6 to 12 months also respond poorly to pressure therapy.

Mechanism of Action. Pressure causes microvascular occlusion, leading to local hypoxia. As a result, cohesiveness between collagen fibrils decreases, and there is decreased tissue metabolism and increased collagenase activity. The result is degeneration and apoptosis of fibroblasts, with concomitant shrinking of collagen nodules and scar tissue. In addition, collagen fibrils become more parallel to the epidermis, with increased formation of normal collagen bundles. Pressure also seems to decrease α-macroglobulins, which inhibit breakdown of collagen by collagenase. Also, a decrease in scar hydration leads to mast cell stabilization and decreased neovascularization, both of which are involved in abnormal ECM production.[1]

Technique. To be effective, pressure garments need to be worn 18 to 24 hours a day for at least 6 to 12 months, until scar maturation. The pressure exerted should be at least 24 mm Hg, so as to exceed capillary pressure and cause microvascular occlusion, but must be less than 30 mm Hg to avoid compromise of the peripheral blood circulation. Early release of the garments may lead to rebound hypertrophy of scars. Therapy should commence once reepithelialization occurs.

Side Effects. Patient adherence is the main difficulty with the use of pressure garments as the elastic garments are uncomfortable and must be worn continuously for prolonged periods of time. In tropical climates, owing to heat and humidity, pressure garments are often not a practical treatment modality. Pressure garments may not exert therapeutic pressure levels at specific anatomic areas, particularly during movement.

Adjunctive Therapies. Surgery followed by pressure therapy has shown good response rates of 90 to 100%, particularly for earlobe keloids, for which pressure earrings are often applied after surgery.[22] Prophylactic pressure garments are recommended for wounds taking 14 to 21 days to heal and necessitated in wounds taking more than 21 days to heal as wounds healing poorly often develop keloids subsequently.[22]

Silicone Gel Sheeting and Other Occlusive Dressings

Overview. Silicone gel sheeting was introduced in the 1980s and has since become standard therapy in many centers. This treatment works best for young hypertrophic scars compared with keloids of longer duration. Its role in scar prophylaxis is unclear. The lack of significant side effects, good tolerability, and proven efficacy in scar improvement and symptom relief from pain and pruritus has led to its wide use.[15,23] This painless modality is particularly suitable for use in children. It can also be combined with other treatment modalities, such as intralesional injections. Other occlusive dressings include polyurethane dressings.

Mechanism of Action. This appears to be related to occlusion and hydration. Hydration of the skin leads to reduced capillary activity, reduced collagen deposition, and down-regulation of fibroblast collagen and glycosaminoglycan production by keratinocytes. Pressure is not required. The therapeutic effect has also been shown to be unrelated to temperature, a difference in oxygen tension, or silicone permeation.

Technique. Silicone gel sheets are cut to size and placed directly over the lesion (Figure 7). Most sheets are self-adhesive and do not require secondary dressings. Patients should be advised that the lesion and its surrounding area should be cleansed and completely dry before application. They should be worn continuously for at least 12 to 18 hours a day and usually need to be applied for 6 to 12 months to exert a therapeutic effect. Silicone can also be applied as a gel formulation, which solidifies into a transparent film, which may be more cosmetically acceptable for facial scars or useful in difficult areas that require high conformability, such as the elbow.

Side Effects. Minor complications, such as occlusive dermatitis, maceration, and secondary

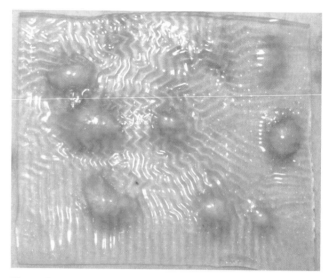

Figure 7. Treatment of multiple keloids with adhesive silicone gel sheeting. Patients should be advised that these should be worn continuously for at least 12 to 18 hours a day and usually need to be applied for 6 to 12 months to exert a therapeutic effect.

bacterial infection, are uncommon and preventable with proper hygiene and shorter wear duration. The key disadvantage is patient nonadherence owing to the inconvenience of prolonged therapy and slow mode of action.

Adjunctive Therapies. Silastic conformers may be used in combination with pressure garments to treat concave regions or areas in which pressure is not effectively applied.

Radiation Therapy

Overview. The use of radiation therapy has been a controversial issue owing to the potential risk of iatrogenic malignancy, which may be unacceptable in the treatment of a seemingly benign skin condition such as keloids. However, only limited case reports of malignancy (an example being medullary thyroid carcinoma) have been reported, but the causal association has been questioned.[24] Radiotherapy is used mainly after surgical excision, with control rates of 72 to 92% reported and even a low recurrence rate of 13% for one series of earlobe keloids. Monotherapy is usually not favored owing to its highly variable response rate of 10 to 94% and a high recurrence rate of 50 to 100%.[1,15] In general, radiotherapy should be reserved as a final option for very resistant keloids. Contraindications include keloids near the neck area and other vital structures. It is relatively contraindicated in children and adolescents.

Mechanism of Action. Irradiation destroys fibroblasts irreversibly and may also cause damage to tissue stem cells and affect ECM gene expression.

Technique. The source, frequency, and dosage of radiotherapy used vary from center to center. However, there is a general consensus that radiotherapy should commence in the very early postoperative period, with some centers starting immediately after surgery. The appropriate use of treatment portals will prevent scatter from affecting other body areas.

Side Effects. These include pain, erythema, radiation dermatitis, hyperpigmentation, paresthesias, and the long-term risk of malignancy. Growth interference may also be an unacceptable complication in children, as reported in a case of an infant who developed generalized atrophy and bone hypoplasia of the entire hand and forearm after receiving radiotherapy for keloids on his hand.[25]

PEARLS AND PITFALLS

Pearls and Pitfalls in Diagnosis

Although the diagnosis of keloids and hypertrophic scars is straightforward in the vast majority of cases, one should be aware of the various dermatologic conditions in the head and neck that can clinically mimic keloids. These were described earlier (see Table 3). This is especially so in solitary, spontaneously arising "scars" in which the history of skin trauma is unclear or in which the patient notes that there has been a recent change in or enlargement of an old surgical scar. Although keloids per se do not have malignant potential, squamous cell carcinoma has been described to coexist in facial scars containing keloidal collagen.[26] One should always be wary if there are atypical clinical features, such as ulceration or tethering to the underlying deep structures, or if there is an unexpected poor response to repeated therapeutic measures. A diagnostic skin biopsy may be indicated whenever the diagnosis is in doubt, with the primary aim of ruling out scar sarcoidosis, locally invasive lesions such as dermatofibrosarcoma protuberans, and, rarely, malignancy.

Pearls and Pitfalls in Treatment

The treatment of keloids and hypertrophic scars is challenging owing to the high relapse rate and long treatment duration. This underscores the need for the clinician to develop a strong therapeutic relationship with the patient and to fully understand and address the specific primary concern of the patient. Treatment should be tailored specifically to meet these patient expectations with regard to cosmesis, symptomatology, duration, cost, and side effects of each treatment option. The use of camouflage cosmetics to conceal unsightly bright red scars is an important adjunctive modality, especially for facial scars. The use of photography to document pre- and post-treatment results is an invaluable part of good medical record keeping and allows both the physician and the patient to visually track the lesion during follow-up consultations. Treatment of keloids may take months to years, and patients must be made aware of this, including the expected end points. For large lesions, staged procedures or multimodality combination therapies may be appropriate. Measures to prevent iatrogenic keloid formation cannot be overemphasized. Apart from good surgical techniques that have been mentioned previously, a noteworthy risk factor for facial keloidal scarring is concurrent or recent isotretinoin therapy, often prescribed for severe acne. Retinoids are postulated to enhance keloid formation through a modulatory effect on connective tissue metabolism, including suppression of collagenase. It is important to delay scar revision procedures, such as laser resurfacing or dermabrasion, at least 6 months to 1 year in such patients. Owing to the high risk of recurrence, surgical excision should not be undertaken for keloids, particularly in the face and neck, unless other modalities have failed.

POTENTIAL FUTURE THERAPIES

With continuing research into the pathophysiology of keloids and hypertrophic scars, new medical, immunologic, or surgical therapies will continue to emerge.

Medical Therapies

Imiquimod Therapy

Overview. Some limited studies have found that postoperative application of imiquimod cream was associated with a decrease in the recurrence rate of keloids after excision.[27] More controlled studies with a longer follow-up are needed to evaluate the role of this agent in secondary keloid prevention and as a possible primary prophylactic measure in keloid-prone patients.

Mechanism of Action. Imiquimod 5% cream acts through inducing local production of interferon-α, which inhibits excessive collagen and glycosaminoglycan production by keloidal fibroblasts. It may also act by altering the aberrant expression of apoptotic genes that may be responsible for keloid formation.

Technique. Topical imiquimod should be applied immediately following keloid excision and continued daily for 8 weeks.

Side Effects. These include erythema, skin irritation, and postinflammatory hyperpigmentation. The effect of imiquimod on wound healing is not precisely known, and it has been recommended that patients with large wounds closed under tension or with grafts and flaps should not start imiquimod for 4 to 6 weeks postoperatively owing to the risk of wound dehiscence.

Calcium Channel Blockers

Intralesional verapamil and nifedipine have been shown to inhibit the incorporation of proline into ECM proteins, leading to altered cytoskeletal reorganization and a change in the shape of fibroblasts; with consequent increased collagenase activity and decreased collagen synthesis by fibroblasts. The result is ECM degradation in dermal scars. Tacrolimus mutes the *gli-1* oncogene. Research has shown that there is increased expression of the *gli-1* oncogene in keloids but not normal scar tissue. More in vitro studies are needed to study this therapy.[28] Methotrexate used after surgical excision was found to prevent recurrence of keloids. The dose used was 15 to 20 mg every 4 days starting a week before surgery and continuing for 3 to 4 months after wound healing. Botulinum toxin, when injected into the muscles underlying a facial wound, was reported to improve cosmesis and maturity of the resultant scar.[29] This may have promise in preventing formation of keloids.

Pentoxifylline (Trental) inhibits the proliferation of fibroblasts derived from keloids and reduces production of collagen, fibronectin, and glycosaminoglycans. Its mechanism is unclear but may be due to improved circulation, with consequent removal of fibroblast growth factors.

Collagen Synthesis Inhibitors

These work variously through microtubular disruption, stimulation of collagenase, and inhibition of collagen synthesis, with promising results in animal trials. Drugs investigated include colchicines and topical putrescine. Nonspecific inhibitors of collagen synthesis, such as penicillamine, showed unacceptable toxicity. Quercetin, a flavonol, was found to inhibit fibroblast proliferation, collagen production, and contraction of keloid and hypertrophic scar–derived fibroblasts. The mechanism of action was found in vitro to be due to blockade of the TGF-β-Smad signaling pathway.[30]

Histamine$_1$ Blockers

Antihistamines have been used to prevent excessive scarring by reducing fibroblast proliferation and collagen synthesis.

Immunologic Therapies

TGF-β Inhibitors

TGF-β plays a major role in fibroplasia and was also shown to be responsible for scarring in glomerulonephritis and pulmonary fibrosis. Antibodies against TGF-β were shown in animal models to result in reduced scarring and improved wound healing.[15,31] Currently, a number of strategies for TGF-β modulation are undergoing investigation in animal and early human trials. These include TGF-β antibodies, manipulation of binding proteins, such as α_2-macroglobulin, and blocking TGF-β activation through the mannose 6-phosphate receptor. Tranilast inhibits the release of histamine and prostaglandins from mast cells, as well as collagen synthesis by hypertrophic scar and keloid fibroblasts. This was found to be through release of TGF-β_1, which is not found in normal skin fibroblasts. Long-wavelength ultra-violet A (340–400 nm; UVA1) may prevent keloid recurrence postsurgery through reducing mast cells and stimulation of collagenase production.[28] Prostaglandin E_2 (dinoprostone) appears to restore normal wound healing.

Surgical Adjuncts

Tissue-Engineered Skin

Skin substitutes have been available commercially for some time. Recently developed bilayered skin products, such as Apligraf (Organogenesis Inc., USA) and Orcel (Ortec Inc., USA), can help in closure of difficult wounds after excision of keloids or hypertrophic burn scars, as well as increasing the availability and decreasing the morbidity of donor sites for split- and full-thickness skin grafts.

ACKNOWLEDGMENTS

We would like to thank Professor Walter Tan from Raffles Hospital for use of his intraoperative photographs and considerable valuable advice. We are also indebted to colleagues at the National Skin Center for providing many clinical photographs.

REFERENCES

1. Niessen MD, Spauwen PHM, Schalkwijk J, Kon M. On the nature of hypertrophic scars and keloids: a review. Plast Reconstr Surg 1999;104:1435–58.
2. Singer AJ, Clark RAF. Cutaneous wound healing. N Engl J Med 1999;341:738–46.
3. Tuan TL, Zhu JY, Sun B, et al. Elevated levels of plasminogen activator inhibitor-1 may account for the altered fibrinolysis by keloid fibroblasts. J Invest Dermatol 1996;106:1007–11.
4. Tredget EE, Nedelec B, Scott PG, Ghahary A. Hypertrophic scars, keloids, and contractures. The cellular and molecular basis for therapy. Surg Clin North Am 1997;77:701–30.
5. Tuan TL, Nichter LS. The molecular basis of keloid and hypertrophic scar formation. Mol Med Today 1998;4:19–24.
6. Diegelmann RF, Cohen IK, McCoy BJ. Growth kinetics and collagen synthesis of normal skin, normal scar and keloid fibroblasts in nitro. J Cell Physiol 1979;98:341–6.
7. Lee SS, Yosipovitch G, Chan YH, Goh CL. Pruritus, pain and small nerve fibre function in keloids: a controlled study. J Am Acad Dermatol 2004;51:1002–6.
8. Berman B, Bieley HC. Keloids. J Am Acad Dermatol 1995;33:117–23.
9. Lawrence WT. In search of the optimal treatment of keloids: report of a series and a review of the literature. Ann Plast Surg 1991;27:164–78.
10. Berman B, Flores F. Recurrence rates of excised keloids treated with postoperative triamcinolone acetonide injections or interferon alfa-2b injections. J Am Acad Dermatol 1997;37:755–57.
11. Kontochristopoulos G, Stefanaki C, Panagiotopoulos A, et al. Intralesional 5-fluorouracil in the treatment of keloids: an open clinical and histopathologic study. J Am Acad Dermatol 2005;52:474–9.
12. Espana A, Solano T, Quintanilla E. Bleomycin in the treatment of keloids and hypertrophic scars by multiple needle punctures. Dermatol Surg 2001;115:1158–60.
13. De Limpens JAM. The local treatment of hypertrophic scars and keloids with topical retinoic acid. Br J Dermatol 1980;103:319–23.
14. Daly TJ, Weston WL. Retinoid effects on fibroblast proliferation and collagen synthesis in vitro and on fibrotic disease in vivo. J Am Acad Dermatol 1986;15:900–2.
15. Mustoe TA, Cooter RD, Gold MH, et al. International clinical recommendations on scar management. Plast Reconstr Surg 2002;110:560–71.
16. Lindsey WH, Davis PT. Facial keloids: a 15-year experience. Arch Otolaryngol Head Neck Surg 1997;123:397–400.
17. Borges AF. The W-plasty versus the Z-plasty scar revision. Plast Reconstr Surg 1969;44:58–62.
18. Zouboulis CC, Blume U, Buttner P, Orfanos CE. Outcomes of cryosurgery in keloids and hypertrophic scars: a prospective consecutive trial of case series. Arch Dermatol 1993;9:1146–51.

19. Alster TS, Williams CM. Treatment of keloid sternotomy scars with 585 nm flashlamp-pumped pulsed-dye laser. Lancet 1995;8959:1198–2000.

20. Dierickx C, Goldman MP, Fitzpatrick RE. Laser treatment of erythematous/hypertrophic and pigmented scars in 26 patients. Plast Reconstr Surg 1995;95:84–90.

21. Chang P, Laubenthal KN, Lewis RW II, et al. Prospective, randomized comparison of two types of pressure therapy garments. J Burn Care Rehabil 1995;16:473–5.

22. Rahban SR, Garner WL. Fibroproliferative scars. Clin Plast Surg 2003;30:77–89.

23. Poston J. The use of silicone gel sheeting in the management of hypertrophic and keloid scars. J Wound Care 2000;9:10–6.

24. Hoffman S. Radiotherapy for keloids [letter]? Am Plast Surg 1982;9:205.

25. Kovalic JJ, Perez CA. Radiation therapy following keloidectomy: a 20-year experience. Int J Radiat Oncol Bio Phys 1989;17:77–80.

26. Lee JYY, Yang CC, Chao SC, et al. Histopathological differential diagnosis of keloid and hypertrophic scar. Am J Dermatopathol 2004;26:379–84.

27. Berman B, Kaufman J. Pilot study of the effect of postoperative imiquimod 5% cream on the recurrence rate of excised keloids. J Am Acad Dermatol 2002;47 Suppl:S209–11.

28. Kelly AP. Medical and surgical therapies for keloids. Dermatol Ther 2004;17:212–8.

29. Sherris DA, Gassner HG. Botulinum toxin to minimize facial scarring. Facial Plast Surg 2002;18:35–9.

30. Phan TT, Lim IJ, Chan SY, et al. Suppression of transforming growth factor beta/Smad signaling in keloid-derived fibroblasts by quercetin: implications for the treatment of excessive scars. J Trauma 2004;57:1032–7.

31. Tyrone JW, Marcus JR, Bonamo SR, et al. Transforming growth factor beta3 promotes fascial wound healing in a new animal model. Arch Surg 2000;135:1154–9.

14

Laser-Resurfaced Facial Skin: Clinical Problems and Issues of Healing Tissues: Pearls and Pitfalls

R. James Koch, MD; Vishal Banthia, MD

Laser skin resurfacing has become an integral component of rejuvenation surgery. It has emerged as the dominant modality for the treatment of the common characteristics of photoaged skin—facial rhytids, dyschromias, scarring, actinic changes—and allows for more precision and control than its resurfacing counterparts in dermabrasion and chemical peeling. The laser permits control of ablation depth and allows for varying these depths as needed. In addition to such precision, there is a favorable heating of the dermis, which ultimately tightens collagen fibers and stimulates neocollagen secretion by fibroblasts.

Currently, two laser wavelengths are commonly used for facial skin resurfacing: pulsed CO_2 and erbium:yttrium-aluminum-garnet (Er:YAG). Early laser systems were developed in the 1960s and used continuous-wave CO_2, which was associated with a high risk of scarring because the long exposure of tissue to laser energy produced uncontrollable and unpredictable thermal damage.[1,2] In efforts to decrease thermal injury and subsequent complications, pulsed CO_2 systems were developed to deliver high-energy pulses that were shorter than the thermal relaxation time of the absorbed tissue components. The pulsed Er:YAG laser system was pioneered in the 1990s and generated less thermal damage and fewer side effects than the pulsed CO_2 laser but was limited by poor intraoperative hemostasis

and suboptimal clinical results in comparison. Combination CO_2 and Er:YAG laser systems were then developed to combat these limitations by improving intraoperative hemostasis and clinical results. Using clinical and histologic analyses, the senior author (R.J.K.) demonstrated that blended CO_2-Er:YAG regimens yielded skin tightening effects somewhere between that of the CO_2 laser and the Er:YAG laser, with healing times closer to that of the Er:YAG laser.[3]

We evaluated the long-term histologic response to five common resurfacing modalities: (1) CO_2, (2) CO_2 followed by Er:YAG, (3) Er:YAG, (4) blended CO_2-Er:YAG (Derma-K, ESC Medical Systems, Yokoam, Israel), and (5) phenol peeling (Figure 1). Facial skin biopsies were performed 4 to 6 months after treatment. Overall, examination of histologic samples demonstrated differences among the various treatments. CO_2 treatment resulted in long-term development of the greatest increase in collagenesis and a decrease in solar elastosis. CO_2 treatment followed by Er:YAG and blended CO_2-Er:YAG treatment seemed to be intermediate in these effects. Phenol treatment produced similar neocollagen density and elastosis treatment but a thinner band of neocollagen. Er:YAG treatment alone produced the least visible long-term improvement in collagenesis.

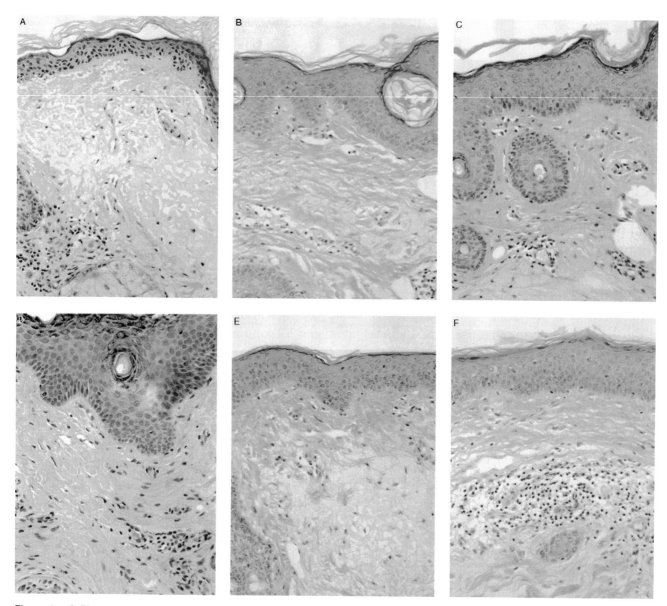

Figure 1. *A*, Photomicrograph of a nontreated (control) facial skin specimen demonstrating marked dermal elastosis and mild to moderate melanocyte atypia and hypertrophy ($\times$400 original magnification). *B*, Photomicrograph of CO_2 laser–treated skin 6 months after treatment. The degree of solar elastosis is substantially improved, and a 0.27 mm band of neocollagen is visible. Melanocytic and keratinocytic atypia are likewise improved ($\times$400 original magnification). *C*, Photomicrograph of skin treated with a CO_2 laser followed by an erbium:yttrium-aluminum-garnet (Er:YAG) laser. A band of neocollagen has developed with a mean of 0.21 mm. Moderate improvement in elastosis is seen. These findings are intermediate between CO_2 and Er:YAG treatment alone ($\times$400 original magnification). *D*, Photomicrograph of skin treated with the Derma-K laser (combined CO_2 and Er:YAG). A band of neocollagen has developed with a mean of 0.20 mm. Moderate improvement in elastosis is seen. These findings are intermediate between CO_2 and Er:YAG alone ($\times$400 original magnification). *E*, Photomicrograph of skin treated with phenol 53%. A limited band of neocollagen has developed with a mean of 0.15 mm. Moderate improvement in elastosis is seen. These findings are intermediate between CO_2 and Er:YAG treatment alone ($\times$400 original magnification). *F*, Photomicrograph of a representative specimen of skin treated with an Er:YAG laser. A small but identifiable band of neocollagen with a mean of 0.08 mm is present. Minimal improvement in elastosis is seen. These changes are the smallest of the tested resurfacing modalities.

Although laser technology has evolved to render cutaneous resurfacing safe, some morbidity is to be expected regardless of which laser system is used. Additionally, the potential for developing serious complications is real. It is therefore important for laser practitioners to be cognizant of potential complications and their causes, which can often be associated with poor patient selection, intraoperative technique, and postoperative wound care. Implementation of sound principles

TISSUE EFFECTS

Understanding the complications of resurfaced skin warrants an overview of the normal tissue effects and healing process occurring after laser resurfacing. Each laser pass imparts zones of thermal injury, some of which are reversible and irreversible. It is imperative to minimize thermal injury as a large zone of thermal necrosis has been implicated as an etiology for complications associated with laser resurfacing.[4–6] The CO_2 laser imposes greater thermal injury to a greater wound depth in comparison with the Er:YAG laser and, hence, has a higher likelihood of generating potential complications. Laser energy for the Er:YAG is produced in the infrared spectrum at 2,940 nm, which is absorbed by water approximately 10 times greater than that of CO_2 at 10,600 nm. The tissue interaction provides true ablation with minimal thermal damage. Each Er:YAG pulse removes only 25 to 30 μm of tissue compared with the CO_2 pulse at 50 to 100 μm.[3] There is less collateral dermal energy because the thermal conduction is approximately 5 μm with Er:YAG. In contrast, pulsed CO_2 generates a significantly greater degree of collateral thermal injury because it generates 30 to 50 μm of thermal conduction. The laser output of Er:YAG is directly absorbed by collagen and dermal proteins, whereas the CO_2 laser vaporizes extracellular water in the dermis. Each Er:YAG pass generates the same amount of ablation, whereas the pulsed CO_2 generates a decreased vaporization depth with each successive pass. There also is a small additive effect of increasing thermal damage with the number of passes, and the pulsed CO_2 has proportionately more energy contributing to thermal damage per pass.

Irreversible areas of thermal injury are extruded from the wound before reepithelialization occurs, and this manifests as tissue seeping from the wound. The average time to reepithelialization is 8.5 and 5.5 days for the CO_2 and Er:YAG lasers, respectively.[7,8] Areas with reversible damage have the ability to recover but are especially susceptible in the reepithelialization period to potential complications in the form of infection and dermatitis, which can generate a prolonged inflammatory and unfavorable wound healing response.

The wound produced by laser resurfacing undergoes a healing response similar to that of any wound. The laser can be thought of as a biostimulator that initiates the well-characterized phases of wound healing: inflammation, proliferation, and remodeling. Heat-induced immediate collagen tightening and initiation of the wound healing response to injury may result, in part, from cytokine secretion at the cellular level. Nowak and colleagues evaluated the effect of pulsed CO_2 laser energy on keloid and normal dermal fibroblast secretion of growth factors in an in vitro model.[9] Secretion of basic fibroblast growth factor was stimulated and that of transforming growth factor β_1 (TGF-β_1) was inhibited in keloid-producing and normal dermal fibroblasts. The known ability of basic fibroblast growth factor to promote organized collagen bundles may account for the observed clinical and histologic effects of increased collagen density and reorganization seen with laser resurfacing. The inhibition of TGF-β_1, which causes tissue fibrosis, also may play a protective role in minimizing scar production during the healing process. Future research into further elucidating and precisely controlling the wound healing response, for example, by way of manipulating growth factors, may potentially minimize complications.

AVOIDING COMPLICATIONS: GENERAL PRINCIPLES

Although the incidence of severe complications after laser resurfacing remains low, some general principles relevant to preoperative, perioperative, and postoperative management help avoid unwanted outcomes. Laser surgeons must uphold the overriding tenet of maintaining a healthy balance between optimizing results and minimizing morbidity (ie, error on the conservative side). The balance begins with appropriate and rigorous patient selection. Those patients at higher risk of developing complications should be either not treated or treated conservatively with appropriate preoperative counseling and expectations. As a general rule, patients with higher sun-reactive skin types are at greater risk especially of developing pigmentary complications, and those with type VI skin are generally not considered resurfacing candidates. Table 1 details the Fitzpatrick skin types, and Figure 2 demonstrates a typical result after CO_2 laser resurfacing.

A thorough history and physical examination should be performed to identify patients with contraindications for resurfacing. Absolute contraindications include active acne, deep acne pits or picks, systemic lupus erythematosus, sclero-

derma, keloid formers, and isotretinoin (Accutane, Roche Pharmaceuticals, Nutley, NJ) use in the past 2 years. Isotretinoin is effective for cystic acne because it targets the sebaceous glands but causes a compromise in gland function, which results in impaired skin reepithelialization and a propensity for scar formation. Relative contraindications include a history of herpetic infections, diabetes mellitus, smoking, hypertrophic scar formation, skin hypersensitivity (to topical sunscreen, makeup, and ointments), and previous chemotherapy, radiation exposure, or chemical or laser peels. A small area behind an ear may be lasered to serve as a test patch if uncertainty to treat exists.

Minimizing thermal injury to tissue is paramount in the perioperative arena. Although there is an evolving trend toward using less energy and fewer laser passes, the laser surgeon should never use watts (CO_2) or joules (Er:YAG) per pulse setting below the amount recommended for the handpiece being used. Sufficient energy is required to reach the fluence necessary for char-free ablation. Turning the power too low forces heat into the tissue instead of the laser vapor. Tailoring the energy level and number of passes to the skin type is also helpful in preventing complications. For pulsed CO_2 treatment, we advocate reducing the energy, density, and passes toward the jawline and neck and

Table 1. FITZPATRICK SUN-REACTIVE SKIN TYPES		
Skin Type	Skin Color	Tanning Response
I	White	Always burns; never tans
II	White	Usually burns; tans with difficulty
III	White	Sometimes mild burn; tan average
IV	Brown	Rarely burns; tans easily
V	Dark brown	Very rarely burns; tans very easily
VI	Black	No burn; tans very easily

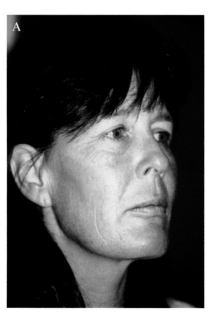
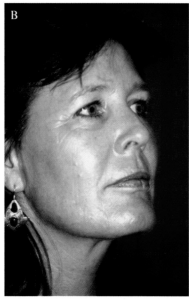

Figure 2. Typical result with pulsed CO_2 laser skin resurfacing. Preprocedure (*A*) and 1 year after treatment (*B*).

eyelid regions because the skin is thinner and harbors fewer sebaceous glands. Additionally, overlap of pulses should be minimized (less than 10%).

Combining laser resurfacing with botulinum toxin A (Botox, Allergan, Irvine, CA), filler substances, or surgery may be useful as an adjunct procedure. Botulinum toxin A is helpful for hyperdynamic facial lines, especially in the area of glabellar furrows (currugator and procerus muscles) and crow's feet (orbicularis oculi muscle) regions. Filling agents, such as hyaluronic acid in the form of Restylane (Medicis, Scottsdale, AZ), can help blunt deeper rhytids and nasolabial and labiomandibular folds. We recommend injecting a filling agent after a few weeks following laser resurfacing to allow for complete reepithelialization.

Blepharoplasty should be considered if there is significant dermatochalasis because eyelid skin is thin, and caution should be exercised to avoid a full-thickness injury or cicatricial ectropion with the laser. Transconjunctival blepharoplasty and periorbital laser resurfacing are an excellent combination because they address the two most common problems of the aging lower eyelid: pseudoherniated fat and mild skin laxity. Because the skin-muscle complex is undisturbed when retroseptal transconjunctival blepharoplasty is performed, it is safe to resurface the lower eyelid skin immediately. Furthermore, it is safe to perform a concurrent subgaleal or subperiosteal brow-lift procedure (eg, endoscopic brow-lift). Rhytidectomy should be performed in those patients with severe facial elastosis, and the combination can be performed by first performing the surgery followed by laser resurfacing after 3 to 4 months. This sequence allows for the resurfacing of the rhytidectomy scars. Concomitant rhytidectomy is not recommended because resurfacing skin that has just been undermined carries a risk of flap necrosis, especially when using a non–deep plane rhytidectomy approach.

The postoperative period is perhaps most important in terms of preventing and detecting potential complications early. Postoperative wound care regimens vary. Some prefer the application of closed, occlusive dressings, whereas others prefer open wound care. The senior author (R.J.K.) evaluated several wound dressings and discovered no differences with efficacy but demonstrated a quicker healing time and decreased erythema and pain when a closed dressing was applied.[10] Other groups have reported an increased incidence of wound infection associated with closed dressings.[11] We recommend using a closed biosynthetic dressing (eg, Vigilon (C.R. Bard, Inc., Murray Hill, New Jersey), N-terface (Winfield Laboratories, Inc., Richardson, Texas)) for 2 to 3 days followed by an open wound care regimen using acetic acid soaks (1 tablespoon of white vinegar in 1 pint of tap water) with applicaton of petroleum jelly (Vaseline) or Aquaphor (Beiersdorf-Futuro, Inc., Cincinnati, Ohio) four times per day until reepithelialization is complete. Regardless of the postoperative wound care regimen used, patients must be closely followed and monitored (at least on postoperative days 1, 7, 14, and 28) for the complications described below.

PROLONGED ERYTHEMA

Erythema after laser resurfacing is an expected side effect that occurs in all patients regardless of their sun-reactive Fitzpatrick skin type. Patients with type I skin, however, tend to be most susceptible to persistent erythema. As with most complications, the severity of erythema depends on the degree of tissue insult; the risk of prolonged erythema is higher with multiple laser passes and/or considerable pulse overlapping. Specifically, the amount of residual thermally damaged tissue is the prime correlate to the degree and duration of erythema. In other words, the depth of the peel is not as important as the amount of remaining dermal thermal necrosis when it comes to predicting erythema.[3]

Erythema is predictably more pronounced after CO_2 laser resurfacing than after Er:YAG. After CO_2 laser resurfacing, erythema usually subsides within 4 weeks but may persist 6 months or longer.[12] Erythema after Er:YAG laser resurfacing is usually less severe and of shorter duration. In our experience, the average duration of postprocedure erythema associated with CO_2 and Er:YAG treatment is 3 to 6 weeks and 1 to 2 weeks, respectively.

Hydrocortisone 2.5% can be used twice a day for 3 to 4 weeks for persistent erythema, but its application should not begin until 4 to 6 weeks after reepithelialization so that the normal wound healing process is not retarded. Topical application of ascorbic acid has also been shown to mitigate protracted erythema.[13] In addition, patients should adhere to strict sun precautions (sun avoidance, hats, and sunscreen) and avoidance of all potentially irritating topical compounds except those prescribed. A green-based makeup can be used and seems to offer the best camouflage.

An acute change in erythema in the immediate postresurfacing period is worrisome. An increase in the intensity of erythema may herald contact dermatitis or infection. In the early postresurfacing period, the nonepithelialized skin without its native protective epidermal coating is sensitive to irritative stimuli, which can yield a contact dermatitis. Afflicting up to 65% of patients, signs of contact dermatitis include diffuse and intense facial erythema with possible associated pruritis.[4,5,12,14–16] Hypersensitivity to topical substances is one of the most common causes of severe erythema in the postoperative period. Fragrances or allergens within topical ointments, soaps, moisturizers, or cosmetics are the usual culprits; as a result, it is essential that all topical agents (makeup, sunscreens, moisturizers) are hypoallergenic and without fragrance, aloe, vitamins, or other potentially sensitizing agents. Of special note, antibiotic ointments (Bacitracin, Neosporin, Polysporin) are often cited as generating hypersenstivity reactions.[1] As a result, many laser practitioners use only occlusive ointments such as Aquaphor or Vaseline in the postoperative period until reepithelialization occurs.

One must first differentiate contact dermatitis from infection as the etiology of the hyperintense erythema. Early identification of dermatitis and

infection is imperative because untreated areas may result in scarring. Once infection has been ruled out by culture, the offending agent must be discontinued. Topical corticosteroids (eg, desonide cream, Temovate (GlaxoSmithKline, Pittsburgh, Pennsylvania)), cool compresses, and oral antihistamines can hasten recovery and alleviate pruritis.[1] Severe cases may require a brief course of systemic steroids (eg, methylprednisolone [Solu-Medrol] dose pack, methylprednisolone, Pharmacia & Upjohn Co., Kalamazoo, Michigan). Protracted, focal areas of erythema with induration and tenderness may herald incipient scar formation and should be promptly and aggressively treated with topical corticosteroid preparations or pulsed dye laser irradiation as described below.

ACNE AND MILIA

As for any type of resurfacing procedure, acne and milia are common but minor side effects that can occur after laser resurfacing. Acne has been reported to afflict as many as 80% of patients, and milia has been reported to afflict 14% of patients after resurfacing.[14] Abnormal follicular epithelialization and the use of occlusive healing ointments and dressings are thought to account for such skin blemishes, which usually occur within 2 weeks after resurfacing. Patients with a history of acne are at heightened risk.

Although lesions resolve spontaneously, especially after occlusive ointments and dressings are discontinued, short courses of oral (ie, minocycline) and topical antibiotics may be used for persistent acne flares.[7,12] Topical antibiotic application (ie, clindamycin) may also help hasten acne resolution but should be used once reepithelialization is complete. Persistent milia may be treated with topical retinoic acid or manual unroofing using an 18-gauge needle or cotton-tipped applicators.

INFECTION

Although the incidence of infection following laser resurfacing is reportedly low (0.4–4.5%), it is important to rapidly identify and treat infection to avoid potential scarring.[11,12,14] Significant pain more than 2 days after treatment may indicate a bacterial, fungal, or viral infection. Focal areas of erythema, crusting, and yellow-green discharge after the second postoperative day are signs of infection. A high degree of vigilance and suspicion is necessary because examination findings may be subclinical and the patient may be dismissed as having a low pain threshold. Crusting and discharge can be sent for Gram stain, KOH smear, and cultures as appropriate.

Although bacterial and fungal infections rarely occur, many laser practitioners treat patients prophylactically with antibiotics. Routine prophylaxis in all healthy patients without high risk (ie, diabetics) remains controversial. Fungal infections may reveal satellite lesions with an erythematous base and slow reepithelialization. For *Candida* treatment, 100 to 200 mg of fluconazole per day is used. If infection occurs in the presence of prophylactic antibiotic administration, *Pseudomonas* or resistant staphylococcal or streptococcal infections must be considered. Antibiotic therapy should be guided accordingly and based on cultures and sensitivities if resistance is suspected. In addition to medical therapy, the facial wound should be kept clean with frequent dressing changes and dilute acetic acid washes.

Reactivation of the herpes simplex virus (HSV) is not an uncommon postresurfacing phenomenon.[12,14,15,17] An assumption should be made that all patients are carriers of HSV and should be pretreated with antiviral prophylaxis. Perkins and Sklarew found that patients with a negative history of cold or canker sores had an almost 7% chance of developing herpetic infection after resurfacing without pretreatment with antiviral medications.[18] In contrast, 50 to 100% of those patients with a positive history developed herpetic infection without pretreatment. We use valacyclovir 500 mg twice per day beginning 2 days before the laser procedure and continuing for a total of 10 days. The use of acyclovir and famciclovir is acceptable and has been described.[1,17] Despite adequate prophylaxis, however, 2 to 7% of patients may develop herpetic outbreaks.[12,17]

The diagnosis of HSV infection is essentially clinical. Characteristic findings include vesico-pustules, punctate erosions, and crusting associated with pain and possible paresthesias. Cultures and smears may be helpful in definitive diagnosis if uncertainty exists. As with all types of infection, herpetic lesions should be treated promptly and aggressively because untreated infection may yield prolonged erythema and permanent unsightly scarring.

SKIN DYSCHROMIA

The incidence of skin dyschromia in the form of hypo- or hyperpigmentation is related to sun-reactive Fitzpatrick skin type. The risk of hyperpigmentation increases with higher skin types, but the risk of hypopigmentation is greater in those patients with type VI skin. Because of the higher risk of pigmentary alterations, patients with skin types III to VI are not considered candidates for laser resurfacing by some laser practitioners. Postinflammatory hyperpigmentation, in particular, occurs more frequently than hypopigmentation and almost universally in skin types IV to VI but can occur in almost a third of patients of all skin types.[7,12,14–16,19] In addition to having higher skin types, patients with a history of melasma and those with pigment changes associated with hormonal changes (ie, pregnancy, oral contraceptive use) have a higher chance of developing hyperpigmentation. Those patients with a current suntan are additionally at risk of hyperpigmentation because melanocytes are already hyperstimulated and laser resurfacing should be delayed.[1]

The incidence of postinflammatory hyperpigmentation is nonintuitively the same after CO_2 and Er:YAG laser resurfacing, despite the latter causing less thermal damage.[1] Hyperpigmentation occurs 3 to 4 weeks after resurfacing and can persist for several months if treatment is not begun. Exposure to direct sunlight (including that through glass) can stimulate melanocyte activity and precipitate postinflammatory hyperpigmentation. Figure 3 demonstrates postinflammatory hyperpigmentation after exposure to direct sunlight 10 days after resurfacing. Avoiding sunlight and using protective covering (ie, hats, umbrella shade) and potent sunscreens are, therefore, key in the postresurfacing period. We prefer to use ultraviolet (UV)A- and UVB-protective sunscreens with zinc or titanium oxide with an associated sun protection factor of 30 or greater.

Persistent hyperpigmentation is treated with a cream mixture of hydrocortisone 1%, hydroquinone 5%, and tretinoin 0.05% twice a day for 1 month on and 1 month off until resolved. The problem usually resolves in 6 to 8 weeks, so we are slow to begin such a regimen. The hydroquinone can be increased to 8% in severe cases, and tretinoin can be increased to 0.1% for thick, sebaceous skin. Both should not be increased at the same time because this can cause significant skin irritation, which can generate a cyclical course of persistent erythema and pigment changes. In addition, one must be cautious in the use of higher-strength hydroquinones because patients may develop paradoxical onchronosis. Other lightening agents (kojic acid), as well as azelaic acid, glycolic acid, and ascorbic compounds, can also be used.[1] The use of sequential micropeels (30–50% glycolic acid) at

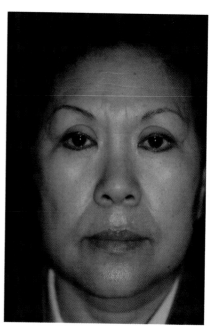

Figure 4. Splotchy hyperpigmentation in an Asian patient 3 months after laser skin resurfacing. The expected hyperpigmentation resolved with bleaching agents.

2- to 4-week intervals may help normalize pigmentary alterations.[15,20]

As mentioned, laser skin resurfacing of sun-reactive Fitzpatrick skin types IV and V is likely to precipitate hyperpigmentation, yet this is manageable. We do not consider this a complication in these patients and do not hesitate to resurface them if they are pretreated and understand the protracted course. Figure 4 demonstrates expected hyperpigmentation after laser resurfacing in an Asian patient with skin type IV. Although no conclusive evidence regarding pretreatment with topical bleaching agents and retinoic acid compounds demonstrates a reduction in postresurfacing hyperpigmentation, we continue to pretreat and resurface patients of higher skin types with success. A combination topical cream formula of hydroquinone 5 to 8%, plus hydrocortisone 1%, plus tretinoin 0.05 to 0.1% applied twice a day for 4 to 6 weeks is recommended prior to resurfacing these patients. Such a regimen not only helps quiesce melanocyte stimulation but also instills a rigorous ethic of good skin care in the postresurfacing period.

Hypopigmentation is an uncommon but usually serious and permanent complication

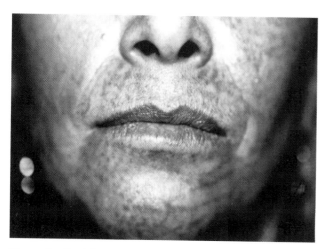

Figure 3. Postinflammatory hyperpigmentation in a patient who exposed her skin to direct sunlight 10 days after full-face laser skin resurfacing.

following laser resurfacing. Although the incidence of hypopigmentation is decreasing with the trend toward more conservative laser resurfacing, its occurrence in as many as 20% of patients undergoing multiple-pass pulsed CO_2 laser treatment has been noted in the past.[14] The phenomenon is delayed and noticeable usually after 4 to 12 months, once erythema and hyperpigmentation have subsided.[12,14] Patients with a history of resurfacing procedures (ie, laser or chemical peels, dermabrasion) may have an increased risk of developing hypopigmentation. True hypopigmentation is rare because most involved areas are pale relative to adjacent nontreated photodamaged skin. Thus, resurfacing multiple adjacent cosmetic facial units or perhaps the entire face may best prevent resulting lines of demarcation around sites of relative hypopigmentation.

Treatment of hypopigmentation involves blending the pigment gradient. Light peels with glycolic or trichloroacetic acid may help blunt the contrasting areas and awkward lines of demarcation. Other management schemes involve exposure to sunlight and topical psoralen application with controlled UV light therapy to stimulate melanocyte production.[1] Given the recalcitrant nature of hypopigmentation, however, patients may need to embrace a lifetime application of camouflaging makeup.

SCARRING

Hypertrophic scarring represents another rare but feared complication, which may stem from both intraoperative and postoperative events. Intraoperative causes of excessive thermal necrosis—extensive overlap of pulses, the use of inappropriately high densities, or failing to wipe off lasered tissue—may yield future scarring.[7,14,15,19] Postoperatively, patients with wound infection or contact dermatitis are at risk. Additionally, patients with a history of keloid formation, who have used isotretinoin within the previous 6 months, or with a history of radiation therapy to the facial area are at increased risk of scarring and should not be resurfaced with the

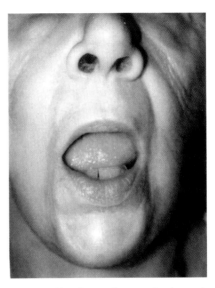

Figure 5. Patient with trismus from perioral scarring following pulsed CO_2 laser skin resurfacing 9 months previously.

laser.[21] Figure 5 reveals a patient who developed perioral scarring after laser resurfacing.

Erythema and associated induration are often precursors to hypertrophic scarring and should be treated early. One should have suspicion when noting such findings after infection or contact dermatitis. Potent class I topical corticosteroids (ie, Temovate 0.05%) can be applied twice a day for 2 weeks. Caution must be exercised to not exceed 50 g per week, and the treatment course should not extend beyond 2 weeks. Intralesional corticosteroid plus silicone gel or sheeting can also improve scarring. The gel is easier to use

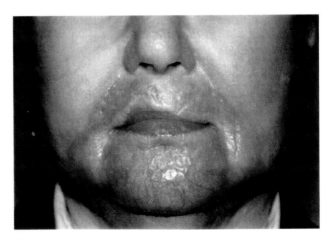

Figure 6. Patient with severe perioral scarring likely resulting from overlapping of pulsed CO_2 laser passes. Patient is 1 year postprocedure and has improved from her original condition using treatment with silicone gel, intralesional steroids, and a pulsed dye laser.

than the sheets and is applied twice a day. The exact mechanism of action of silicone sheets or gel remains unknown, but it may be related to autocrine fibroblast growth factor production.[22] The use of the 585 nm pulsed dye laser has been described to treat erythematous and persistent scars but requires multiple sessions.[23–25] Figure 6 shows a patient's final result using such modalities.

LOWER EYELID ECTROPION

Lower lid ectropion is a rare complication after laser resurfacing because a careful history and physical examination will help prevent its occurrence. Patients with a previous blepharoplasty or other lid surgeries and those with findings of lid laxity via the snap test are at risk. In such cases, fewer laser passes with lower energy densities around the lower lid are advised. Although ectropion usually improves with conservative management by way of taping and massage over time, surgical correction may be warranted for refractory cases. The rare surgical intervention involves lid suspension procedures, placement of mucosal grafts, or midface lifts.

CONCLUSIONS

Laser skin resurfacing plays a safe and effective role in aesthetic surgery. A substantial recovery period and some morbidity are expected sequelae, but most patients ultimately have very good to excellent results in terms of skin tightening and resolution of rhytids. Fortunately, the more common side effects (acne or milia formation, erythema) are minor and self-resolving, whereas serious complications (scarring, lid ectropion, hypopigmentation) occur only rarely. Avoiding complications is key and depends primarily on meticulous patient selection, conservative intraoperative technique, and close postoperative monitoring of patients.

Despite the established safety of current laser resurfacing systems, patients demand less downtime and risk of complications while still maintaining high expectations. Newer laser systems

are being designed to address these concerns. The Fraxel SR (Reliant Technologies, Palo Alto, CA) laser is a 1,550 nm erbium-doped fiber laser that deposits microscopic thermal zones of injury in the skin. Each laser pass impacts a fractional volume of tissue while sparing adjacent tissue and effectively treats 20% of the relevant area. Unlike the traditional CO_2 and Er:YAG laser systems, the Fraxel laser spares the stratum corneum, which results in a rapid healing response in which reepithelialization occurs within 24 hours. Several treatment sessions spaced 1 to 2 weeks apart are necessary to achieve optimal results. Nonablative technologies to tighten the dermis without peeling the surface were also recently introduced. Thus far, the results of the Fraxel laser are pending, and existing nonablative technologies show only minimal clinical efficacy in improving skin texture. With long-term studies of and potential improvements in these new laser systems, the future of skin rejuvenation will likely lie in these minimally ablative to nonablative realms.

REFERENCES

1. Alster TS, Lupton JR. Prevention and treatment of side effects and complications of cutaneous laser resurfacing. Plast Reconstr Surg 2002;109:308–16.
2. Lanzafame RJ, Naim JO, Rogers DW, et al. Comparison of continuous wave, chop-wave and superpulse laser wounds. Lasers Surg Med 1988;8:119–24.
3. Greene D, Egbert BM, Utley DS, Koch RJ. In vivo model of histologic changes after treatment with the superpulsed CO_2 laser, erbium:YAG laser, and blended lasers: a 4 to 6-month prospective histologic and clinical study. Lasers Surg Med 2000;27:362–72.
4. Stuzin JM, Baker TJ, Baker TM, et al. Histologic effects of the high-energy pulsed CO_2 laser on photoaged facial skin. Plast Reconstr Surg 1997;99:2036–50.
5. Cotton J, Hood AF, Gonin R, et al. Histologic evaluation of preauricular and postauricular skin after high-energy short-pulsed carbon dioxide laser. Arch Dermatol 1996;132:425–8.
6. Trelles MA, Mordon S, Svaasand LO, et al. The origin and role of erythema after carbon dioxide laser resurfacing: a clinical and histological study. Dermatol Surg 1998;24:25–9.
7. Alster TS. Cutaneous resurfacing with CO_2 and erbium:YAG lasers: preoperative, intraoperative, and postoperative considerations. Plast Reconstr Surg 1999;103:619–32.

8. Ziering CL. Cutaneous laser resurfacing with the erbium:YAG laser and the char-free carbon dioxide laser: a clinical comparison of 100 patients. Int J Aesthetic Restor Surg 1997;5:29.

9. Nowak KC, McCormack MC, Koch RJ. The effect of superpulsed carbon dioxide laser energy on keloid and normal dermal fibroblast secretion of growth factors: a serum-free study. Plast Reconstr Surg 2000; 105:2039–48.

10. Koch RJ, Newman JP, Goode RL. Closed dressings after laser skin resurfacing. Arch Otolaryngol Head Neck Surg 1998;124:751–7.

11. Sriprachya-Anunt S, Fitzpatrick RE, Goldman MP, et al. Infections complicating pulsed carbon dioxide laser resurfacing for photoaged facial skin. Dermatol Surg 1997;23:527–35.

12. Nanni CA, Alster TS. Complications of carbon dioxide laser resurfacing: an evaluation of 500 patients. Dermatol Surg 1998;24:315–20.

13. Alster TS, West TB. Effect of topical vitamin C on postoperative carbon dioxide laser resurfacing erythema. Dermatol Surg 1998;24:331–4.

14. Bernstein LJ, Kauvar ANB, Grossman MC, et al. The short- and long-term side effects of carbon dioxide laser resurfacing. Dermatol Surg 1997;23:519–25.

15. Lowe NJ, Lask G, Griffin ME. Laser skin resurfacing: pre- and posttreatment guidelines. Dermatol Surg 1995;21: 1017–9.

16. Keller GS, Lacombe VG. Laser resurfacing: An overview. In: Keller GS, Lacombe VG, Lee P, et al, editors. Lasers in aesthetic surgery. Thieme; 2001. p. 41–66.

17. Alster TS, Nanni CA. Famciclovir prophylaxis of herpes simplex virus reactivation after laser skin resurfacing. Dermatol Surg 1999;25:242–6.

18. Perkins SW, Sklarew EC. Prevention of facial herpetic infections after chemical peel and dermabrasion: new treatment strategies in the prophylaxis of patients undergoing procedures of the perioral area. Plast Reconstr Surg 1996;98:427–33.

19. Nanni CA. Handling complications of laser treatment. Dermatol Ther 2000;13:127.

20. Horton S, Alster TS. Preoperative and postoperative considerations for carbon dioxide laser resurfacing. Cutis 1999;64:399–406.

21. Katz BE, MacFarlane DF. Atypical facial scarring after isotretinoin therapy in a patient with a previous dermabrasion. J Am Acad Dermatol 1994;30: 852–3.

22. Hanasono MW, Lum J, Carroll LA, et al. The effect of silicone gel on basic fibroblast growth factor levels in fibroblast cell culture. Arch Facial Plast Surg 2004;6: 88–93.

23. Alster TS, Nanni CA. Pulsed dye laser treatment of hypertrophic burn scars. Plast Reconstr Surg 1998;102: 2190–5.

24. Alster TS. Improvement of erythematous and hypertrophic scars by the 585 nm flashlamp-pumped pulsed dye laser. Ann Plast Surg 1994;32:186–90.

25. Dierickx C, Goldman MP, Fitzpatrick RE. Laser treatment of erythematous/hypertrophic and pigmented scars in 26 patients. Plast Reconstr Surg 1995;95: 84–90.

15

Irradiated Skin and Its Postsurgical Management

David B. Hom, MD; Vu Ho, MD; Chung Lee, MD

Radiation combined with surgery is a common modality for treating head and neck cancer. Poor soft tissue wound healing after surgery in a previously irradiated patient continues to be a significant clinical problem. Postoperative wound complication rates following radiation exposure can occur in up to 67% of cases.[1,2] Poor wound healing after surgery can result in patient death from carotid artery rupture or in prolonged morbidity from fistula formation, wound dehiscence, skin flap reconstructive failure, and skin necrosis. Trauma, infection, and surgery to irradiated skin can precipitate into a major nonhealing wound.[3,4]

The healing of a surgical wound is influenced by radiation because radiation affects all cells (endothelial, mesenchymal, and fibroblast cells) within its treatment field. For the wound to heal, the normal steps of wound healing must take place: hemostasis, inflammation, angiogenesis, collagen synthesis and turnover, epithelialization, and contraction. Delay in any of these steps can result in a poorly healing wound (Figure 1).

If healing impairment occurs during the earlier phase of healing, interference with the subsequent stages of wound healing also occurs. Radiation to soft tissue induces soft tissue damage by obliteration of the microvasculature, increasing fibrosis and causing an aberration of cellular replication.

Radiation injury to soft tissue can be divided into early and late radiation injury (Figure 2). Early radiation injury occurs during the first several weeks of treatment and results from the depletion of rapidly dividing cells suffering mitotic deaths from radiation deoxyribonucleic acid (DNA) damage (early-responding tissues). To respond to this injury, stem cells go into a state of accelerated repopulation to attempt to heal the injured tissue. If the stem cell compart-

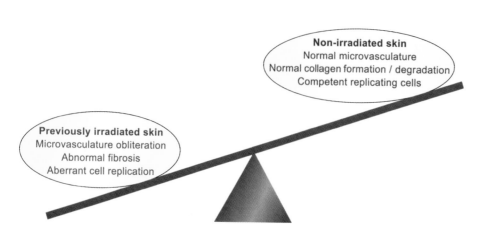

Figure 1. Cellular environment of previously irradiated skin versus non-irradiated skin.

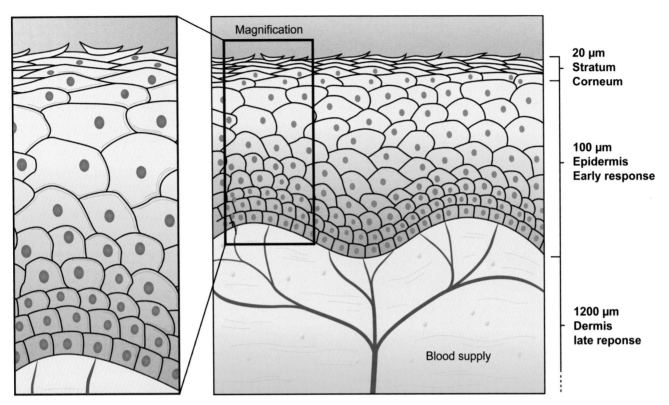

Figure 2. Early and late responses of skin from irradiation.

ment is eradicated by the radiation, nonhealing acute radiation injury occurs. During acute radiation injury, epithelial tissues with rapid cellular replication rates, such as skin, mucosa, and salivary glands, are most vulnerable to injury. Thus, unavoidable acute side effects from irradiation include mucositis, dry mouth, and decreased taste.

Late radiation injury occurs in slowly or nonproliferating tissues (late-responding tissues). Given that vascular and connective tissues do not rapidly proliferate, their major changes are not evident until months to years after treatment. The mechanism of late radiation injury is thought to be due to damage to the microvasculature and the direct depletion of slowly dividing cells. Radiation injury to the microvascular endothelium is a critical event in the pathogenesis of poor healing by inducing DNA damage and apoptosis of microvascular endothelial cells.[5–10] This delayed tissue injury is manifest as fibrosis and damage to capillaries, small arteries, and medium-sized arteries (Figure 3).

RADIATION MODALITIES

Modalities for delivering radiation include external beam (radiation administered through planned portals to a specified anatomic area), interstitial brachytherapy (radioisotopes within a tube implanted into tissue temporarily or permanently), and intracavitary brachytherapy (radioisotopes contained in an applicator, which is placed in a body lumen such as the esophagus or trachea). External beams are either beams of high-energy electron particles or high-energy x-rays. The mechanism of biologic damage caused by x-rays versus electron beams is similar. Electron beams directly produce free radicals, whereas x-rays ionize tissue molecules, producing electrons, which form free radicals. These free radicals damage DNA.

Radioisotopes emit gamma or beta rays. Gamma rays emitted from cesium 137, iridium 192, or iodine 125 are high-energy x-rays similar to external beam treatments. Beta rays are electrons. Electron beams have limited tissue penetration, with virtually no deposition of dose

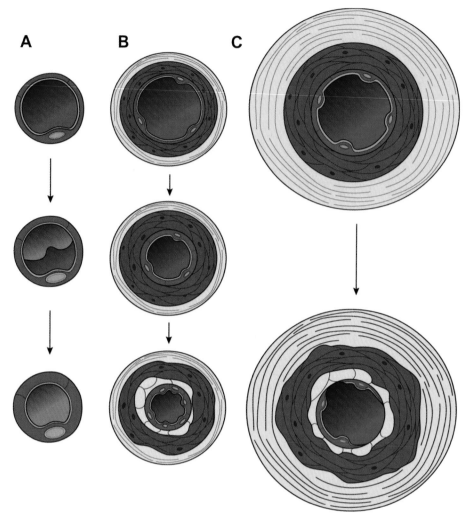

Figure 3. Radiation affects capillaries, arterioles, and small arteries. *A*, With the capillary, the lumen narrows over time from swelling from the endothelial cells and sclerosis of the vessel wall. A thrombus can form, occluding the vessel. *B*, With the arteriole, edema occurs with the endothelium and smooth muscle, thus narrowing the lumen. Degenerative changes (endothelial proliferation, subendothelial deposition of a hyaline-like substance, focal destruction of smooth muscle cells) develop within the vessel wall. *C*, With the small artery, progressive damage of the endothelium and media occurs. Radiation changes (fragmentation of the internal elastic lamella, degeneration of the smooth muscle media with accumulations of a hyaline-like substance, fibrosis of the adventitia) occur. Reproduced with permission from Anderson WAD, Kissane JM, editors.. Pathology. St Louis: CV Mosby; 1977.

beyond a few centimeters. Electron beams are useful for treating superficial target sites.

DOSE–TUMOR CONTROL RELATIONSHIPS

Certain assumptions are made about the relationship between total dose and daily dose to tumor control and tumor-bearing volume. One assumption is that the highest total dose tolerated by normal tissues is the most appropriate dose. However, this belief is not consistent among clinicians. Some reports have suggested

advantages with particular fractionation regimens. Unfortunately, in these studies, little is mentioned in the volume irradiated and whether a reduction in tumor volume was achieved during the course of treatment.[11]

RADIOBIOLOGIC BASIS OF FRACTIONATION

The use of multiple fractions over many weeks of radiation therapy is based on the principle of improving the therapeutic ratio between normal tissues and tumors. The goal is to maximize the cell death of tumors and to minimize unacceptable damage to normal cells. This is accomplished through the use of multiple fractions and is explained by the four radiobiologic processes: (1) repair, (2) reoxygenation, (3) redistribution, and (4) repopulation.[12]

Neoplastic cells behave as early-responding tissues owing to their increased replication rate. Attempts to increase damage to neoplastic cells that are vulnerable to early injury have been made by modifying radiation fractionation regimens. These alternative fractional regimens attempt to increase the chance of damage to early-responding tissues (which include the tumor and, unfortunately, early-responding normal tissue) without increasing the risk of damage to late-responding tissues. Such regimen examples are accelerated fractionation, hyperfractionation, or a combination of both regimens, accelerated hyperfractionation. Standard or conventional fractionation denotes a regimen delivering 180 to 200 cGy per fraction, once a day, five times per week to a total dose of 6,500 to 7,000 cGy in 6.5 to 7 weeks.

Hyperfractionation refers to schedules in which the patient is treated twice daily at least 6 hours apart. The dose per fraction is reduced, the total dose is increased, the number of dose fractions is increased, and the overall time is relatively unchanged. The basic rationale of hyperfractionation is that the use of small-dose fractions allows for higher total doses to be administered within the tolerance of late-responding normal tissues and that this translates into a higher biologically effective dose to the tumor.[11]

Another twice-daily treatment is accelerated fractionation. Accelerated fractionation describes a radiation regimen in which the overall time is reduced, but the number of dose fractions, total dose, and size of dose per fraction are either unchanged or somewhat reduced, depending on the extent of overall time reduction. Accelerated hyperfractionation refers to a fractionation schedule that incorporates features of both hyperfractionation and accelerated fractionation.

Chemotherapy has become a common addition to radiation therapy in the treatment of head and neck cancer. Chemoradiation is primarily an attempt to increase cure rates, preserve organ function, and improve cosmesis.

Almost all studies have shown more toxicity with the combined chemoradiation treatments. However, there is increased consensus among clinicians that the addition of chemotherapy to radiation therapy offers the most promise in the treatment of locally advanced head and neck cancers. Newer drug combinations, along with altered radiation fractionation regimens, are currently being evaluated.

SOFT TISSUE RESPONSE TO RADIATION

The soft tissue biologic response from radiation is a function of the total dose, dose per fraction, and the time interval over which the total dose is given. Other factors affecting tissue are the size of the irradiated field and time between treatment fractions. Radiation dose is defined as a measure of the physical energy deposited per unit mass of tissue (1 Gy = 1 joule per kilogram; 100 Gy = 1 cGy = 1 rad).

The tolerance of normal tissues to conventionally fractionated radiation is described as the minimum tolerance dose and the maximum tolerance dose. The minimum tolerance dose is the dose that causes complications in 5% of patients within 5 years. The maximum tolerance dose is the dose that causes complications in 50% of patients within 5 years (Table 15-1). Therapeutic ratio is defined as the normal tissue tolerance dose divided by the tumor lethal dose.[4]

Radiation oncologists are keenly aware of the doses and dose fractionation schemes beyond which there is an unacceptable incidence of damage to a given tissue or organ and plan treatment accordingly. In fact, many radiation therapy centers treat malignant tumors to the maximum doses that can be tolerated by the normal tissue(s) containing the tumor.

Chronic radiation injury occurs 4 to 6 months after radiation therapy. Changes clinically stabilize over many months and do not

Table 1. TOLERANCE DOSES OF SOFT TISSUE IN THE HEAD AND NECK			
	TD 5/5 (cGy)	TD 50/5	Complication
Skin	5,500	7,000	Ulceration/ necrosis
Larynx	5,000	7,000	Edema, cartilage, necrosis
Esophagus	5,500	6,800	Stricture, perforation
Spinal cord	4,700	7,000	Myelitis/necrosis
Thyroid	4,500	8,000	Thyroiditis, hypothyroidism
Brain	4,500	6,000	Necrosis

TD 5/5 = minimum tolerance dose; TD 50/5 = maximum tolerance dose.

usually cause major problems unless the tolerance dose of the tissues has been exceeded. In the tissues, capillaries progressively dilate and diminish, resulting in decreased capillary numbers. Injuries to small vessels occur by 6 months after radiation. Injury to larger vessels can continuously occur several years later.[6] In skin, although much vascular damage is evident, normal intact microvasculature can still be evident.[13] Several months following radiation, fibrous tissue gradually increases within the submucosal and subcutaneous tissue planes. This avascularity and fibrosis are progressive, dose dependent, and permanent.[14] It is important to note that the skin always "remembers" its previous radiation exposure and its tolerance for any future radiation is compromised in most circumstances. Owing to its decreased vascularity and increased fibrosis, previously irradiated tissue is more susceptible to trauma, infection, irritation, and slower healing.

Tissue ischemia is the most common cause of radiation-induced complications. Latent complications or injury from radiation can include skin atrophy, muscle fibrosis, telangiectasia, friable mucosa, xerostomia, trismus, neuropathy, retinopathy, cataract formation, myelitis, hypothyroidism, lymphatic obstruction, and osteonecrosis. Poor nutrition, sepsis, and hypotension can further exacerbate the healing of damaged irradiated tissue. Any localized trauma or infection to previously irradiated skin or mucosa can precipitate into a major nonhealing wound. Patients with a compromised vasculature system (diabetes, hypertension) are more susceptible to significant radiation-induced injury.[15]

EARLY AND LATE RADIATION INJURY

The risk of radiation injury in normal tissue increases with age, low hemoglobin, smoking, collagen, vascular disease, diabetes, and poor nutrition.[16] In addition, one can roughly approximate the total dose administered to a patient by calculating the nominal standard dose (NSD) from the radiation prescription (total dose, fraction NSD Total radiaton dose, treatment overall time):

$$NSD = \frac{\text{Total radiation dose}}{N^{0.24}T^{0.11}}$$

where N = the number of fractions and T = the overall treatment time in days. This formula was derived empirically so that all parameters with the NSD (with units called "rets") would have the same risk of early skin reaction. The volume of treatment also influences the degree of radiation injury.[17,18]

Early Injury

For tissues vulnerable to early injury, a critical factor is the overall time of treatment. Cellular death from radiation damage occurs during mitosis. In rapidly dividing cells, mitosis and death occur quickly. During radiation treatment, rapidly dividing cells are depleted quickly, resulting in a homeostatic response of the cell population to accelerate its rate of repopulation. Therefore, injury to tissues vulnerable to early injury will be increased when the overall duration of treatment is lengthened. This is in contrast to slowly proliferating cells, which live longer before they undergo mitoses and die. In some instances, the entire course of radiation is completed before the slowly proliferating cells are depleted, thus not requiring an induction of a repopulation response.

Late Injury

For tissues vulnerable to late injury (late-responding tissues), a critical factor is the fraction size or dose of the treatment fraction. Slowly dividing cells survive small doses of radiation better than early-responding tissues. However, as the dose is increased, the surviving portion of late-responding tissues drops off much more rapidly than that of early-responding tissues, until at higher radiation doses, early-responding tissues have a proportionally higher survival rate than late-responding tissues. Thus, the damage to late-responding tissues is higher at higher fraction doses. Cellular repair from radiation injury usually occurs within 6 hours after irradiation.

Vascular injury is the predominant factor responsible for the manifestation of late effects following irradiation.[6] Capillaries progressively dilate, become obliterated, and decrease in number. Despite the cutaneous vascular damage, normal microvasculature is maintained.

Radiation necrosis can develop with high doses of radiation. This is characterized by an early erythematous and bullous reaction, followed by epidermal necrosis, which is then superseded by ulceration. Radionecrotic ulceration often occurs in the most poorly vascularized areas of the irradiated field and can develop by moisture and trauma.[19] Early-radiation ulceration as a result of epidermal necrosis may heal but can persist or recur if dermal necrosis and vascular occlusion are involved. Small areas may heal with conservative treatment; however, management of extensive radionecrosis often requires excision and flap reconstruction or grafting.[19] In contrast, late-radiation ulcers are more common and may develop years following radiation exposure. These lesions can occur spontaneously but are often precipitated by trauma, chronic irritation or pressure, infection, and actinic exposure. Predisposing factors include epidermal atrophy and deep-vessel occlusion with ischemia. Often painful, these ulcers heal slowly and can persist for years or indefinitely. Chronic radiation skin ulcers must be differentiated from neoplastic recurrence by biopsy. Cutaneous changes include epidermal atrophy, dryness, hyperkeratosis, loss of skin appendages, telangiectasia, dyschromia, hypopigmentation and hyperpigmentation, and marked fibrosis.

One of the most common delayed radiation-induced cutaneous changes is the development of fibrosis or subcutaneous induration. The typical manifestation of fibrosis is nonhomogeneous, with areas of dense, acellular collagen.[20] Characteristically, fibrin is present in the stroma as a fibrinous exudate consisting of a network of acidophilic fibrils surrounded by collagen and fibroblasts.[20] This fibrinous exudate can be found months to years following radiation exposure, suggesting that its persistence in the stroma is the result of decreased fibrinolysis or increased fibrin formation or the result of both mechanisms.[20] The fibrotic changes can cause crippling and deforming skin retraction.

The treatment of chronic radiation dermatitis consists of ameliorating symptoms. Appropriate antibiotic treatment of infections is paramount. Topical creams are helpful, and the occasional use of topical glucocorticoids may reduce inflammation and pruritus. Of note, it is essential that patients be kept under long-term supervision for detection and appropriate treatment of potential malignant changes.

RADIATION INJURY TO CELLS

At the molecular level, radiation causes cellular injury by damaging DNA, leading to cell death.[17] The DNA damage is induced by photon and electron beam irradiation by creating hydroxyl free radicals. With the presence of oxygen, more hydroxyl free radicals are produced. Low oxygen conditions decrease the lifetime of these free radicals and consequently decrease the degree of DNA damage.[17]

The response of normal tissue to radiation (radiosensitivity) is dependent on (1) the degree to which the targeted cell repairs the DNA damage and (2) the ability of the targeted cell population to regenerate (repopulate) among the damaged target cells around them.

Cells are most radiosensitive when in the G_2 and M phases of the cell cycle.[21] Most repair of radiation damage occurs within 6 hours after irradiation, and cell death usually follows one to five postradiation division cycles.[21]

COMMON HEALING PROBLEMS FOLLOWING RADIOTHERAPY

Acute Radiation Injury: Mucositis and Dermatitis

Within 3 to 4 weeks after the initiation of radiation, mild to severe mucositis develops, along with skin erythema. Frequent mouth and pharyngeal rinsing with saline or saline soda solutions may mitigate painful mucosal irritation. Within the oral cavity, *Candida* superinfection can occur and can be treated with nystatin oral rinses, miconazole troches, or a systemic antifungal agent, such as fluconazole. To diminish oral pain while eating, topical anesthetic mouth rinses can be helpful. If oral nutritional supplements are not adequate, nutritional support by nasogastric feeding or parenteral hyperalimentation may be necessary. In certain circumstances, intubation or tracheotomy may be required for severe acute mucosa edema from radiation (Table 2).

Following the completion of full-course radiation (6,000–7,000 cGy), taste usually returns within several months. If the salivary glands received a high dose (5,000–6,000 cGy), xerostomia will likely be permanent. Ethyol amifostine (Ethyol, WR-2721) has been tested and used as a cytoprotective agent to prevent xerostomia and/or mucositis.[22] Pilocarpine (Salagen) is also helpful in treating radiation-associated xerostomia.[23,24]

Similar general principles of wound care management apply in the irradiated wound except that adhesives should be used sparingly to prevent epithelial injury. The major tenets of wound care summarized in Table 3 should be followed to achieve optimal healing.[25]

If significant wet desquamation develops on the skin, cessation of radiation therapy may be required with treatment with moist dressings. Moist dermal reactions may need to be rinsed with a wound cleanser to reduce bacterial colonization and any necrotic debris removed. Antibiotic ointments or creams (ie, silver sulfadiazine) can act as a temporary occlusive barrier to encourage reepithelialization and reduce bacterial colonization. It is imperative to avoid wound desiccation (Table 4).[26]

Despite this skin care, if the wounds increase in size and become more painful, wound excision is indicated with coverage with well-vascularized skin flaps. Well-vascularized tissue outside the irradiated field is recommended because the ischemic bed of the resected irradiated ulcers is unlikely to revascularize a skin graft. Owing to damaged microvasculature, deep skin ulcers from radiation are less likely to heal spontaneously and only have a scant granulation tissue response. In addition, irradiated skin wounds have a decreased ability to contract and epithelialize.[27] Whenever a persistent nonhealing skin ulcer is evident, one should always be aware that a malignant recurrence could be present, and a repeat biopsy is indicated.

Table 2. GRADES OF MUCOSITIS SEVERITY		
Grade	Clinical Examination	Functional or Symptomatic
1	Erythema of the mucosa	Minimal symptoms, normal diet
2	Patchy ulcerations or pseudomembranes	Symptomatic but can eat and swallow modified diet
3	Confluent ulcerations or pseudomembranes; bleeding with minor trauma	Symptomatic and unable to adequately aliment or hydrate orally
4	Tissue necrosis; significant spontaneous bleeding; life-threatening consequences	Symptoms associated with life-threatening consequences
5	Death	Death

Adapted from National Cancer Institute Common Toxicity Criteria, from MacDonald J, Haller D, Mayer R: Grading of toxicity, in MacDonald J, Haller D, Mayer R (eds): Manual of Oncologic Therapeutics. Philadelphia, PA, Lippincott, 1995, pp 519–523.

Table 3. PRINCIPLES OF OPTIMAL WOUND CARE IN IRRADIATED SKIN
Débride necrotic tissue
Identify and treat infection
Pack dead spaces lightly
Divert any salivary drainage away from the wound
Drain any excess fluid collection
Absorb excess exudate
Maintain a moist wound surface
Maintain open fresh epithelial wound edges
Protect the wound from trauma
Maximize nutritional status
Protect the fragile irradiated skin from trauma by
Avoiding excessive cold, heat, and sun
Not using adhesive tape
Avoiding shaving with a razor
Maintaining meticulous skin hygiene to maintain maximal skin integrity

Adapted from Hom DB et al.[26]

To create a moist wound healing environment, six major moisture-retentive categories exist, encompassing a large number of products (gauzes, hydrogels, hydrocolloids, alginates, foams, and transparent films). These dressings are discussed in more detail in Chapter 31 of this book.

A chronic wound, which is made clean, should show signs of healing within 4 weeks.[28] If adequate healing does not proceed, then the wound must be properly reevaluated for (1) adequate nutrition, (2) sufficient blood supply, (3) proper wound management, (4) wound pressure relief, and (5) bacteria contamination.

Chronic Radiation Injury

During chronic radiation injury, deeper soft tissue structures can also be involved.[29] Chronic wound complications can result in patient death from carotid artery rupture or cause prolonged morbidity from fistula formation, wound dehiscence, skin flap reconstructive failure, or skin necrosis. The management of these deeper wound complications (carotid artery exposure, fistulae, esophageal strictures) is addressed in Chapter 16 of this book.

Unfortunately, oral cutaneous and pharyngocutaneous fistulae are common occurrences following combined radiation and surgical therapy. The risk of fistula formation increases with increasing irradiation dose.[27] When radiation is given preoperatively, fistula healing may be more prolonged. The highest risk of carotid artery rupture is when a fistula forms in close proximity to the carotid artery within an irradiated field. This circumstance may arise when a previously irradiated patient undergoes surgery for a recurrent tumor.[30,31]

In managing fistulae, local débridement and wound care are required to remove necrotic tissue and to ensure that salivary flow is not contaminating the wound. Nutritional status must also be maximized to encourage wound healing. Diversion of salivary flow away from the carotid artery is paramount with wide drainage of infected areas. If a fistula is present above a stricture, it will not heal until the stricture is corrected. No local or regional flaps should be transposed until the infection is under control and granulation tissue has developed. A nasogastric tube is useful for feeding and maintaining a tract to help prevent stenosis. Whenever transferring vascularized tissue (ie, regional or free tissue flap), the flap must be firmly sutured

Table 4. TYPES OF RADIATION TOXICITY TO SKIN				
Symptom/Sign	Degree 1	Degree 2	Degree 3	Degree 4
Erythema	Minimal, transient	Moderate < 10% BSA	Marked 10–40% BSA	Severe > 40% BSA
Sensation/itching	Pruritus	Slight, intermittent pain	Moderate persistent pain	Severe persistent pain
Blistering	Rare	Rare Hemorrhage	Bullae	Bullae Hemorrhage
Desquamation	Absent	Patchy, dry	Patchy, moist	Confluent, moist
Ulcer/necrosis	Epidermal only	Dermal	Subcutaneous	Muscle or bone
Onycholysis	Absent	Partial	Partial	Complete

Adapted from Waselenko JK, MacVittie TJ, Blakely WF, et al. Medical management of the acute radiation syndrome: recommendations of the Strategic National Stockpile Radiation Working Group. Ann Intern Med 2004;140:1039.
BSA = body surface area.

and anchored to deep fascia to resist its gravitational pull causing incisional line dehiscence. Skin breakdown beside the mandible may also be part of the orocutaneous fistula. If the exposed mandible has been previously irradiated, an increased risk of developing osteomyelitis is evident. Management of poor bone healing mandible is described in Chapter 17 of this book.

When a fistula develops from poor healing before radiation therapy, a decision must be made to either postpone radiation or to proceed with radiation, realizing that it may delay wound healing further. Radiation therapy can be instituted if the wound can be stabilized safely, with no undue exposure risk (ie, carotid artery). Once the acute postradiotherapy inflammatory process has subsided, definitive treatment for the fistula can proceed.

RADIATION TIMING AND ITS EFFECTS ON WOUND HEALING

The time when radiation is given in relation to wounding determines the ultimate wound healing effects. When radiation is given after wounding, healing is most affected several days after wounding, resulting in decreased incisional tensile strength.[29,32] If radiation is given later, soft tissue healing becomes less vulnerable to irradiation.[31]

If radiation is given before wounding, radiation dose and time of administration are major parameters that affect healing. The higher the radiation dose, the more impact it will have on wound healing. Radiation maximally delays wound healing when administered within several days before wounding. In lengthening this time, the effects of radiation to healing decrease. It has been recommended to wait 4 to 6 weeks after preoperative radiation before surgery to allow acute radiation effects (mucositis) to resolve.[29]

PLANNED PREOPERATIVE RADIATION

Most agree that wound healing is affected by previous radiation. However, it remains controversial as to what degree preoperative irradiation contributes to surgical morbidity.[33] Some studies state that moderate doses of preoperative radiation do not significantly increase surgical morbidity.[33,34] A modest dose of preoperative irradiation (3,000–5,000 cGy) fractionated over 3 to 5 weeks and given 3 to 6 weeks prior to surgery has not been proven to significantly decrease wound healing clinically.[35] On the other hand, other studies have demonstrated significant increases in surgical complications with preoperative radiation.[35,36] Doses greater than 5,000 cGy in 5 weeks can cause delayed healing and increased wound complications, especially when administered just before surgery.[29]

Surgical complications increase especially when sutured sites are closed under extreme tension, resulting in tissue ischemia and dehiscence. For this reason, it may explain the higher rate of wound complications following pharyngeal wall cancer excision treated with preoperative radiation and surgery because a tighter closure often results. This is supported by the finding that surgical resection at the pharyngeal region can result in a 3 to 14% incidence of carotid artery rupture.[37,38] Radiation decreases vascularization and increases fibrosis, and an additional ischemic insult, such as a tight closure, can further compromise tissue survival.[25]

PLANNED POSTOPERATIVE RADIATION

Most studies indicate that the best time to institute postoperative irradiation is at least 3 weeks after surgery to allow normal wound healing to occur. However, delaying the administration of radiation longer than 6 weeks can decrease the oncologic benefit of radiation treatment.[39] A major argument against postoperative radiation has been the delay in initiating radiation therapy if a wound dehiscence or complication develops.[40] However, with appropriate precautions and nutritional support, it has been shown that radiation therapy can be safely administered to patients with an open wound.[39]

More recently, patients with head and neck cancer are receiving the combination of radiation and chemotherapy during their treatment protocols. With this combined regimen, the risk of a poor healing wound increases even further.

SURGICAL CONSIDERATIONS IN A PATIENT WITH A HISTORY OF IRRADIATION

The incidence of serious complication is very high (greater than 50%) when surgery is performed on tissues previously irradiated at high doses (greater than 6,000 cGy).[41] Such complications of infection, tissue necrosis, and fistulization are common and require months to heal. Because of this higher incidence of complications, a controlled salivary pharyngostome could be created to help divert the salivary drainage preferentially away from the carotid artery. More limited surgical excisions and modest radiation doses (5,000 cGy less) have less severe complications.[30]

Precautions are necessary to minimize trauma to previously irradiated skin. Careful preoperative planning and a preventive approach are critical to minimize complications. Close attention must be made for optimizing conditions for wound healing (see Table 3). Maintaining a positive nitrogen balance and body weight should be achieved either by nutritional supplements, tube feeding, or parenteral nutrition.[42,43] Specific vitamin, mineral, or nutrient deficiencies should also be corrected by supplementation. Vitamins such as A and E have been implicated to improve healing in irradiated wounds.[44,45]

With any history of radiation to the neck, hypothyroidism should be ruled out with thyroid function tests and corrective thyroid medication given to maximize healing.[46] When mucosa barriers are violated during a clean contaminated procedure, preoperative antibiotics should be given to minimize infection.[47]

Incisions must be tailored so that if they should ever become dehiscent, the exposed tissue (ie, carotid artery) would not endanger the patient. Tight closures of the pharynx are to be avoided because dehiscence could lead to carotid exposure. Well-vascularized tissue outside the irradiated field should be used for coverage of the carotid and mandible. Local skin flaps and skin grafts that normally are adequate in nonirradiated areas become precarious in previously irradiated wounds.[48] Skin flap necrosis occurs more frequently in previously irradiated reconstructive sites, suggesting that neovascularization is impaired in previously irradiated skin.[49] Further details of the management of irradiated deep soft tissue wounds are described in chapter 16.

An important aspect in managing irradiated skin is to prevent its breakdown and to promptly institute conservative treatment whenever skin injury is evident. Avoidance of trauma and irritation to the skin (ie, shaving with a razor, using harsh soaps, having excessive sun exposure) is recommended. Patients with a compromised vasculature system (diabetes, hypertension) are more susceptible to significant radiation-induced injury.[15]

Dental care of the previously irradiated patient must be carefully considered. Nonessential dental procedures should be avoided. Essential dental work must be accomplished aseptically. Perioperative administration of antibiotics is appropriate in all irradiated patients requiring dental extractions. Hyperbaric oxygen (HBO) should be considered for major procedures.

HYPERBARIC OXYGEN

At present, HBO is used to attempt to improve healing of previously irradiated wounds.[50,51] The goal of HBO is to enhance neovascularization and granulation tissue formation within a hypoxic and hypocellular irradiated wound.[52–55] The mechanism of how HBO improves the healing of previously irradiated tissue is not completely understood. In vascular compromised tissue, HBO can increase tissue oxygen partial pressure and stimulate angiogenesis, granulation tissue formation, and reepithelialization.[56,57] It is thought that HBO generates an oxygen gradient that is lacking in irradiated tissue to induce angiogenesis.[53] On HBO exposure, an increased capillary density from neovascularization is created in irradiated tissue, raising the tissue oxygen level over time.[58] This increased angiogenesis from HBO is believed to be long-lasting.[52] In animal models, increased neovascularization and viability were observed when HBO was administered to ischemic skin flaps.[59]

HBO has been used preoperatively and postoperatively in irradiated wounds to attempt to reduce poor healing. When surgical wounding is planned within irradiated tissues, Marx and colleagues proposed that HBO can be administered as a preventive means to minimize wound healing complications.[60] Specifically, mandibular bone necrosis was reduced following dental extractions in a randomized controlled study using HBO. The Marx protocol consists of 20 treatments at 2.4 atmospheres absolute pressure for 90 minutes before the procedure and 10 HBO treatments after the procedure. In the study, the HBO group had a 5.4% incidence of mandibular necrosis versus the control group of 29.9%.

For soft tissue healing, HBO was of benefit in patients who received preoperative radiation and laryngeal or pharyngeal cancer resection. Specifically, 12 of 15 patients in the HBO group healed completely compared with 7 of 15 in the control group. In the control group, two patients had severe postoperative bleeding and one of these patients succumbed from the hemorrhage.[61] Using HBO to treat poorly healing wounds is discussed in more detail in Chapter 27 of this book.

FUTURE APPROACHES

Therapy to Protect Tissue from Ionizing Radiation

Different approaches to protect tissues from ionizing radiation include (1) administering radioprotective agents prior to irradiation, (2) administering agents to prevent secondary toxicity during or following irradiation, and (3) administering rescue agents, such as bone marrow colony-stimulating factors or hyperbaric oxygen. Several substances have been reported to yield cellular radioprotection. These agents include vitamin C, beta-carotene, vitamin E , ribose-cysteine, glutamine, $MgCl_2$ /adenosine triphosphate, and WR-2721 (amifostine).[62]

Potential of Growth Factor Therapy

Recombinant human platelet-derived growth factor BB (rhPDGF, becaplermin) was the first growth factor approved by the US Food and Drug Administration (FDA) to treat chronic wounds in 1998 for diabetic neuropathic ulcers.[63,64] Since then, the off-label use of rhPDGF has been reported to be beneficial to improve the healing of recalcitrant irradiated chronic dermal ulcers and postlaryngectomy fistulae.[65,66] Specifically, in these cases, rhPDGF was used to induce further granulation formation (Figures 4 and 5). The off-label use of rhPDGF is not recommended for treating routine poorly healing irradiated wounds. However, it has future potential use in refractory poor healing wounds. If such growth factor treatment is planned, the patient should be informed and willing to accept its possible theoretical risks. These possible risks are the development of malignancy or excessive scarring. In addition, a biopsy should be considered before growth factor treatment in the previously irradiated patient.

In 2004, palifermin recombinant keratinucyte growth factor (rKGF-2) (Kepivance) received FDA approval to prevent and treat oral mucositis in patients with bloodborne malignancies (ie, leukemias and lymphomas) receiving chemotherapy and radiation. At the present time, phase 3 studies are being conducted with rKGF-2 to treat oral mucositis in head and neck cancer patients.[67]

A common concern about using growth factors to improve poor wound healing is the possibility of the risk of malignant transformation or recurrence in patients who have had previous neoplasms. However, no studies to date have provided evidence of malignant transformation resulting from the use of supplemental

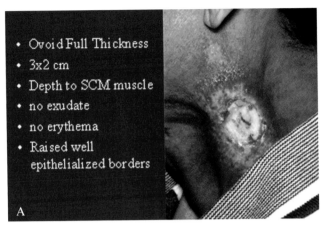

- Ovoid Full Thickness
- 3x2 cm
- Depth to SCM muscle
- no exudate
- no erythema
- Raised well epithelialized borders

A

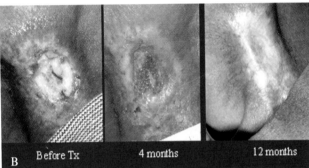

B   Before Tx   4 months   12 months

Figure 4. *A*, A 47-year-old male with a 12-year, refractory, painful, nonhealing, full-thickness dermal wound on his left neck following external beam radiation, radium needle implants, and chemotherapy for a T2N2bM0 nasopharyngeal carcinoma. He has been tumor free for 12 years. Despite multiple conventional therapies (moist hydrogel dressings, topical and oral antibiotics, serial débridements, hyperbaric oxygen), the wound did not heal. The depth of full-thickness dermal ulcer was down to the sternocleidomastoid muscle (SCM), with raised rolled epithelialized edges present. *B*, Dermal ulcer before treatment, at 4 months after recombinant human platelet-derived growth factor BB topical treatment showing increased granulation tissue in the wound bed, and 1 year later after a split-thickness skin graft was successfully grafted (Reproduced with permission from Hom D and Manivel C.[68]).

growth factors when no preexisting genetic mutation exists.

Over the last decade, clinical trials have studied the effects of other recombinant growth factors (epidermal growth factor, transforming growth factor β [TGF-β) on chronic extremity skin wounds from diabetes and vascular insufficiency. These clinical studies have been mixed. These studies demonstrate that wound healing is dependent not only on the growth factor environment but also on other parameters, such as wound care, bacteria count, tissue oxygen level, and nutrition.[68] In clinical studies using

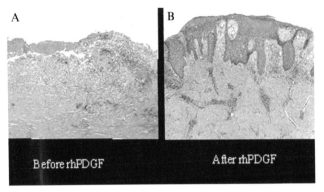

Before rhPDGF   After rhPDGF

Figure 5. Serial histology skin biopsies from the patient in figure 4 before and after recombinant human platelet-derived growth factor BB (rhPDGF) treatment confirm the wound transformation from a chronic state to an acute healing state. *A*, Skin biopsy before rhPDGF treatment shows complete coagulative necrosis and denudation of the epidermis (hematoxylin-eosin stain; ×40 original magnification). *B*, Skin biopsy obtained 6 months following treatment with rhPDGF shows viable skin, a thickened epidermis with irregular acanthosis, and a thickened papillary and reticular dermis with markedly hyalinized collagen fibers and perivascular inflammatory infiltrate (hematoxylin-eosin stain; ×40 original magnification). Reproduced with permission from Hom D and Manivel C.[68]

rhPDGF, it should be emphasized that growth factor therapy should be considered as an adjunctive mode of therapy and is not a replacement for standard wound care (ie, proper dressing changes, control of infection, and débridement).[64,69]

Previously irradiated surgical wounds are considered to heal more like chronic wounds with the presence of increased proteases and proinflammatory cytokines and decreased protease inhibitors and growth factors.[70] In chronic wounds, fibroblast growth factor (FGF) and TGF-β) concentrations are down-regulated and significantly lower when compared with acute wounds.[71,72]

Supplemental basic FGF may also have the potential to improve wound healing and skin flap survival in previously irradiated soft tissue.[72] Supplemental basic FGF has also been shown to reduce radiation damage to endothelial cells in the pulmonary microvasculature, lower gastrointestinal tract, and central nervous system.[5,10,73–75] These studies suggest that it may be possible to improve surgical wound healing of previously irradiated dermal tissue with growth factors.

CONCLUSION

Previous radiation to soft tissue increases the risk of postoperative tissue breakdown because of transformation of the tissue into a hypocellular, hypovascular, and hypoxic tissue state. During early radiation injury, rapidly dividing cells are susceptible to cell death because they are undergoing rapid mitosis. As the cell population becomes depleted, their stem cells go into a state of accelerated repopulation to attempt to replenish the injured tissue. However, if the stem cell population is eradicated by the radiation, nonhealing acute radiation injury results. Several months after radiation, late radiation injury occurs. During this time, the slow or nonproliferating tissues are vulnerable to injury owing to the direct depletion of the slowly dividing cells. Clinically, at this latent phase, fibrosis and microvasculature damage become apparent.

An important aspect in managing irradiated skin is to give close attention to prevent its breakdown and to promptly begin treatment whenever skin injury is evident. Careful preoperative planning and a preventive approach are crucial to minimize complications in the irradiated patient to optimize healing.

REFERENCES

1. Girod D, McCulloch, Tsue T, et al. Risk factors for complications in clean-contaminated head and neck surgical procedures. Head Neck 1995;17:7–12.
2. Habel D. Surgical complications in irradiated patients. Arch Otolaryngol 1967;82:382–6.
3. Hom D, et al. Choices of wound care management for irradiated soft tissue wounds. Otolaryngol Head Neck Surg 1999;121:591–8.
4. Coleman JJ. Management of radiation-induced soft tissue injury to the head and neck. Clin Plast Surg 1993;491–505.
5. Pena L, Fuks Z, Kolesnick R. Radiation-induced apoptosis of endothelial cell in the murine central nervous system: protection by fibroblast growth factor and sphingomyelinase deficiency. Cancer Res 2000;60:321–7.
6. Hopewell JW, Calvo W, Reinhold HS. Radiation effects on blood vessels: role in late normal tissue damage. In: Steel G, Adams GE, Horwich A, editors. The biological basis of radiotherapy. 2nd ed. New York: Elsevier; 1989. p. 223–4.
7. Reinhold H, Fajardo L, Hopewell J. The vascular system. Adv Radiat Biol 1990;14:177–226.
8. Tibbs M. Wound healing following radiation therapy. Radiother Oncol 1997;42:99–106.
9. Langley RE, et al. Radiation-induced apoptosis in microvascular endothelial cells. Br J Cancer 1997;75:666–72.
10. Fuks Z, et al. Basic fibroblast growth factor protects endothelial cells against radiation-induced programmed cell death in vitro and in vivo. Cancer Res 1994;54:2582–90.
11. Cox J. Clinical perspectives of recent developments in fractionation. Semin Radiat Oncol 1992;2:10–5.
12. Thames H. On the origin of dose fractionation regimens in radiotherapy. Semin Radiat Oncol 1992;2:3–9.
13. Roswit B, Wisham L, Sorrentino J. The circulation of radiation damaged skin. AJR Am J Roentgenol 1953;69:980–90.
14. Bernstein E, et al. Biology of chronic radiation effect on tissues and wound healing. Clin Plast Surg 1993;20:435–53.
15. Mustoe T, Porras-Reyes B. Modulation of wound healing response in chronic irradiated tissues. Clin Plast Surg 1993;20:465–72.
16. Bentzen S, Overgaard J. Patient-to-patient variability in the expression of radiation-induced normal tissue injury. Semin Radiat Oncol 1994;4:68–80.
17. Withers H. Biologic basis of radiation therapy. In: Perez C, Brady L. Principles and practice of radiation oncology. Philadelphia: JB Lippincott Company; 1992. p. 64–96.
18. Hall E. Radiobiology for the radiobiologist. 5th ed. Philadelphia: Lippincott Williams & Wilkins; 2000.
19. Spittle MF, Kelly CG. Radiotherapy and Reactions to Ionizing Radiation. In: Burns T, Breathnach S, Cox N, Griffiths C, editors. Rook's textbook of dermatology. Malden, MA: Blackwell Science 2004;4:76.1–76.8.
20. Fajardo L. Morphology of radiation effects on normal tissues. In: Perez C, Brady L, editors. Principles and practice of radiation oncology. Philadelphia: J.B. Lippincott; 1992; p. 114–23.
21. Malkinson FD. Radiobiology of the skin. In: Freedberg IM, Eisen AZ, Wolff K, Austen K, Goldsmith L, Katz S, Fitzparitck T, editors. Fitzpatrick's dermatology in general medicine. New York: McGraw-Hill; 1999. p. 1514–23.
22. Brizel DM, et al. Phase III randomized trial of amifostine as a radioprotector in head and neck cancer. J Clin Oncol 2000;18:3339–45.
23. Johnson J, et al. Oral pilocarpine for post-irradiation xerostomia in patients with head and neck cancer. N Engl J Med 1993;329:390–5.
24. Valdez I, et al. Use of pilocarpine during head and neck radiation therapy to reduce xerostomia and salivary dysfunction. Cancer 1993;71:1848–51.
25. Hom DB, Adams G, Koreis M, Maisel R. Choosing the optimal wound dressing for irradiated soft tissue wounds. Otolaryngol Head Neck Surg 1999;121:591–8.
26. Coleman J. Management of radiation-induced soft tissue injury to the head and neck. Clin Plast Surg 1993;20:491.

27. Johansen L, Overgaard J, Elbrond O. Pharyngo-cutaneous fistulae after laryngectomy: influence of previous radiotherapy and prophylactic metronidazole. Cancer 1988; 61:673–8.

28. Rijswijk LV. Wound assessment and documentation. In: Krasner DK, Rodeheaver GT, Sibbald R, editors. . Chronic wound care: a clinical source book for healthcare professionals. Wayne (PA): HMP Communications; 2001. p. 101–15.

29. Moore M. The effect of radiation on connective tissue. Otolaryngol Clin North Am 1984;17:389–99.

30. Joseph D, Shumrick D. Risks of head and neck surgery in previously irradiated patients. Arch Otolaryngol 1973; 97:381–4.

31. Trible W. The effect of preoperative radiation on subsequent surgery in carcinoma of the larynx. Ann Otol Rhinol Laryngol 1957;66:953–62.

32. Gorodetsky R, et al. Effect of fibroblast implants on wound healing of irradiated skin: assay of wound strength and quantitative immunohistology of collagen. Radiat Res 1991;125:181–6.

33. Snow J, et al. Randomized preoperative and postoperative radiation therapy for patients with carcinoma of the head and neck: preliminary report. Laryngoscope 1980; 90:930–45.

34. Mascial V, et al. Does preoperative irradiation increase the rate of survival complications in carcinoma of the head and neck? Cancer 1982;49:1297–301.

35. Van der Brenk H, Orton C, Stone M, et al. Effects of x-radiation on growth and function of report blastema (granulation tissue). Int J Radiat Oncol Biol Phys 1974; 25:1–19.

36. Ketcham A, Hoye R, Chretien P. Irradiation twenty-four hours preoperatively. Am J Surg 1969;118: 691–7.

37. Everts E. Surgical complications (oral cavity, oropharynx, nasopharynx). In: Cummings C, et al, editors. Otolaryngology-head and neck surgery. St Louis: CV Mosby; 1986. p. 1141–28.

38. Marks J, et al. Pharyngeal wall cancer: an analysis of treatment results, complications and patterns of failure. Int J Radiat Oncol Biol Phys 1978;4:587–93.

39. Issacs J, et al. Postoperative radiation of open head and neck wounds. Laryngoscope 1987;97:267–70.

40. Vikram B. Importance of the time interval between surgery and postoperative radiation therapy in the combined management of head and neck cancer. Int J Radiat Oncol Biol Phys 1979;5:1837–49.

41. Marchetta F, Sako K, Maxwell W. Complications after radical head and neck surgery performed through previously irradiated tissues. Am J Surg 1967;114: 835.

42. Gullane P, et al. Correlation of pharyngeal fistulization with preoperative radiotherapy, reduced serum albumen and dietary obstruction. Otolaryngol Head Neck Surg 1979;87:311–7.

43. Donald P. Complications of combined therapy in head and neck carcinoma. Arch Otolaryngol 1978;104: 329–33.

44. Levenson S, et al. Supplemental vitamin A prevents the acute radiation-induced defect in wound healing. Ann Surg 1984;200:494–512.

45. Taren D, Chvapil M, Weber C. Increasing the breaking strength of wounds exposed to preoperative irradiation using vitamin E supplementation. Int J Nutr Res 1987; 57:133–7.

46. Alexander M, Zajtchuk J, Henderson R. Hypothyroidism and wound healing. Arch Otolaryngol 1982;108:289–91.

47. Johnson J, et al. Efficacy of two third-generation cephalosporins in prophylaxis for head and neck surgery. Arch Otolaryngol Head Neck Surg 1984;110: 224–7.

48. Rubin P, Grise J. The differences in response of grafted and normal skin to ionizing irradiation. AJR Am J Roentgenol 1960;84:645.

49. Hom D, Adams G, Monyak D. Irradiated soft tissue and its management. Otolaryngol Clin North Am 1995;28: 1001–19.

50. Tibbles P, Edelsberg J. Hyperbaric oxygen therapy. N Engl J Med 1996;334:1642–8.

51. Boykin JV. Hyperbaric oxygen therapy: a physiological approach to selected problem wound healing. Wounds 1996;8:183–98.

52. Myers RA, Marx RE. Use of hyperbaric oxygen in postradiation head and neck surgery. NCI Monogr 1990;9:151–7.

53. Marx R, et al. Relationship of oxygen dose to angiogenesis induction in irradiated tissue. Am J Surg 1990;160:519–24.

54. Hart GB, Mainous EG. The treatment of radiation necrosis with hyperbaric oxygen. Cancer 1976;37: 2580–6.

55. Marx R. Radiation injury to tissue. In: Kindwall E, editor. Hyperbaric medicine practice. Flagstaff (AZ): Best; 1994. p. 447–503.

56. Knighton DR, Hunt TK, Scheuenstuhl H. Oxygen tension regulates the expression of angiogenesis factor by macrophages. Science 1983;221:1283–5.

57. Perrins DJD. Hyperbaric oxygen and skin coverage. HBO Rev 1983;4:179.

58. Beehner MR, Marx RE. Hyperbaric oxygen induced angiogenesis and fibroplasia in human irradiated tissue. In: Proceedings of the 65th Meeting of the American Association of Oral and Maxillofacial Surgery;1983;78–9.

59. Manson P, et al. Improved capillaries by hyperbaric oxygen in skin flaps. Surg Forum 1980;31:564–6.

60. Marx R, Johnson R, Kline S. Prevention of osteoradionecrosis: a randomized prospective clinical trial of hyperbaric oxygen versus penicillin. J Am Dent Assoc 1985;11:49–54.

61. Neovius E, Lind M, Lind F. Hyperbaric oxygen therapy for wound complications after surgery in the irradiated head and neck: a review of the literature and a report of 15 consecutive patients. Head Neck 1997;19:315–22.

62. Zimmermann JS, Kimmig B. Pharmacological management of acute radiation morbidity. Strahlenther Onkol 1998;3:62–5.

63. Wieman T. Clinical efficacy of becaplermin (rhPDGF-BB) gel. Am J Surg 1998;176 Suppl 2A:74S–9S.

64. Steed D. Modifying the wound healing response with exogenous growth factors. Clin Plast Surg 1998;25:397–405.

65. Jakubowicz DM, Smith RV. Use of becaplermin in the closure of pharyngocutaneous fistulas. Head Neck 2005;27:433–8.

66. Hom DB, Manivel JC. Promoting healing with recombinant human platelet-derived growth factor–BB in a previously irradiated problem wound. Laryngoscope 2003;113:1566–71.

67. Spielberger R, et al. Palifermin for oral mucositis after intensive therapy for hematologic cancers. N Engl J Med 2004;351:2590–8.

68. Robson M, Mustoe T, Hunt T. The future of recombinant growth factors in wound healing. Am J Surg 1998;176 Suppl 2A:80S–2S.

69. Steed D, et al. Effect of extensive debridement and treatment on the healing of diabetic foot ulcers. J Am Coll Surg 1996;183:61–4.

70. Robson M, Smith P. Topical use of growth factors to enhance healing. In: Falanga V, editor. Cutaneous wound healing. London: Martin Dunitz; 2001. p. 379–98.

71. Cooper DM, et al. Determination of endogenous cytokines in chronic wounds. Ann Surg 1994;219:688–91, discussion 691–2.

72. Hom DB, et al. Improving surgical wound healing with basic fibroblast growth factor after radiation. Laryngoscope 2005;115:412–22.

73. Fuks Z, et al. Intravenous basic fibroblast growth factor protects the lung but not mediastinal organs against radiation-induced apoptosis in vivo. Cancer J Sci Am 1995;1:62–72.

74. Haimovitz-Friedman A, Kolesnick RN, Fuks Z. Differential inhibition of radiation-induced apoptosis. Stem Cells 1997;15 Suppl 2:43–7.

75. Houchen C, et al. FGF-2 enhances intestinal stem cell survival and its expression is induced after radiation injury. Am J Physiol 1999;276(1 Pt 1): G249–58.

16

Irradiated Soft Tissue Wounds

George L. Adams, MD, FACS

A CLINICAL PERSPECTIVE

In 1970, Goldman and colleagues published their series of 53 patients treated with preoperative radiation therapy prior to undergoing planned surgical resection for squamous cell carcinoma of the larynx.[1] They felt that by providing 5,500 rads of radiation preoperatively, there was an enhanced survival rate. Surgery was performed 3 to 6 weeks following completion of radiation therapy, and the extent of the surgery was determined by the preoperative original extent of the lesion. They recognized that the addition of radiation therapy may have had an adverse effect on wound healing when surgery was performed. They recommended routinely using a levator scapulae flap to protect the carotid bifurcation in the event of the development of a fistula. They also recommended a meticulous three-layer closure of the pharynx to prevent fistula. Using a much lower dose (2,000 rads of radiation therapy preoperatively), Strong and colleagues in 1978 showed basically no increase in the number of significant complications when surgery was performed a month after radiation therapy.[2] On the other hand, in 1977, Vandenbrouck and colleagues published in 1977 their results showing that postoperative radiation therapy not only had less significant complications, but in their prospective study, there was also a statistically improved survival in patients receiving radiation after surgery.[3] In 1987, the large Radiation Therapy Oncology Group (RTOG) study 7303 led by Kramer and colleagues showed that radiation therapy given pre-operatively versus postoperatively had the same rate of adverse surgical complications (18% in the preoperative group and 14% in the postoperative group), with more severe radiation complications occurring in the postoperative radiation therapy group.[4] Long-term survival was better in the postoperative radiation therapy group.[5]

The rationale behind preoperative radiation therapy was to decrease the size of the malignancy and potentially decrease the implantation of tumor cells at surgery. It was thought that radiation given preoperatively would be more effective given to well-oxygenated tumor cells. Postoperative radiation therapy had the theoretical advantage that the radiation could address the areas of greatest concern and that the surgeon was better able to determine the extent of tumor at resection.[6]

The rate of infection or fistula in patients receiving surgery alone for laryngeal cancer ranges from 10 to 14%. The incidence of fistula and serious complications when radiation and surgery are both employed is as high as 39%, but recent studies report averages closer to 20%.[7] Thus, the prolongation of life and increased survival associated with the combination of treatments leads to the necessity of being prepared to handle the increased incidence of complications, particularly fistula, fibrosis of the larynx, necrosis of wound incisions and flaps, increased difficulty in swallowing, stricture formation, and, most importantly, prolonged wound healing. Although the actual incidence of infection and necrosis in wound complications is no different whether radiation therapy is given pre- or postoperatively, certainly, healing the irradiated wound is more complex and prolonged.[6,8] Planned preoperative radiation therefore should not affect the incidence or type of postoperative complications; whether radiation is delivered pre- or postoperatively, the complication rate and type are the same.

The newer organ preservation protocols (European Organisation for Research and Treatment of Cancer [EORTC], RTOG 9111) administer a full course of radiation therapy with concurrent chemotherapy.[9,10] Although excellent results obtained in organ preservation and reduction of distant metastases have been shown, when surgery is required, the management of wound complications and incidence is much higher than in the previous pre- versus postoperative radiation therapy study.[11]

Surgery is often provided for salvage.[11–13] In the newest prospective randomized combined radiation chemotherapy studies, when there is failure to respond to radiation and chemotherapy, surgery is reserved for salvage. Persistence of cervical adenopathy in some studies and N2 stage cancer in others require a neck dissection.[14,15] Again, even after administration of full-course radiation therapy, when the surgery is limited to the neck, the overall complication rate is acceptably low.[16,17]

The effects of radiation therapy are both acute and long term (Table 16-1).[18–22] The initial effect on the larynx, oral cavity, and oropharyngeal lesions is mucositis, which begins 10 to 12 days after onset of radiation. With continued radiation, this effect becomes less. The effects in patient tolerance when adequate nutrition and general health are satisfactory allow repair of these most rapidly proliferative tissues. The long-term effects on capillaries and even on larger vessels begin several months after completion of therapy.[23] The skin and pharyngeal tissues undergo fibrosis. There is a continued diminution of saliva. There is delayed onset of stricture formation. Surgery performed during this period of time usually requires bringing into the area nonirradiated tissue, whether in the form of a pectoralis myocutaneous or a deltopectoral flap,

Table 16-1 ADVERSE RADIATION EFFECTS ON SOFT TISSUE[18–22]
Increases carotid atherosclerosis
Skin—erythema, fibrosis, pigmentation
Mucositis
Decreased saliva
Perichondritis
Vascular effects
Reduces neovascularization
Increased vascular permeability
Occlusion and thrombosis
Late effects
Atrophy and fibrosis of tissues, less pliable
Effects on wound healing
Affects fibroblast function—reduced collagen
Reduction in wound strength (dose dependent)
Reduced tensile strength
Effects at cellular level
Permanently damages fibroblast
Unable to produce collagen
Affects growth factors and cytokines

but preferably, when possible, free flap reconstruction.

The administration of combined chemotherapy and radiation therapy in organ preservation protocols has not shown a direct increase in the rate of complexity of surgical complications more than radiation therapy followed by surgery alone (Figure 16-1).[24,25] However, healing may be delayed, not from the local effect but from the generally poor nutritional status that has to be dealt with in some patients. Almost all head and neck cancer patients have existing comorbidities, which may include hypothyroidism, anemia, low albumin levels, diabetes, or chronic lung disease, with a long host of other associated problems.[26]

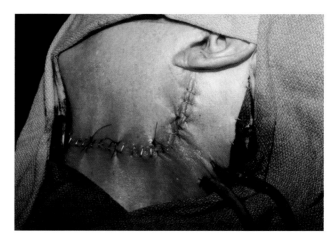

Figure 16-1. Prolene stay sutures remain in place three weeks. Staples are removed in ten days.

Thus, the postoperative complication rate in these patients includes not only the surgical complications but also medical complications.[27] Both have a direct adverse effect on wound healing. Several studies have looked at determining risk factors for patients undergoing either salvage surgery or surgery after planned radiation therapy. Diabetes in some studies has been reported to increase complications, but in others, it is not. A preoperative tracheostomy may or may not affect the incidence of complications.

The general status of the patient, as far as being anemic, or nutritional factors as measured by hypoalbuminemia has an adverse affect on healing. Thus, when feasible, these underlying factors are improved prior to surgery. Factors leading to increased incidence of postoperative wound complications in most studies include intraoperative transfusion, the need for flap reconstruction, the duration of anesthesia, previous chemotherapy, and the operative procedure (Table 16-2).[6,28–31] These factors also correlate with the stage of disease and extent of surgery.

Use of perioperative antibiotics continued for 24 to 48 hours after surgery has been the single largest factor in reducing the incidence of postoperative wound infections (Table 16-3).[32] Patient nutrition has been enhanced by the more aggressive use of percutaneous gastrostomy and even hyperalimentation when required.

Table 16-2 PREDICTORS OF WOUND INFECTIONS

Patient comorbidities
    Poor nutrition (hypoalbuminemia, anemia)[28]
    Diabetes mellitus
    Chronic lung disease and active smoking
    Alcoholism[28]
Previous treatment
    Recidivism—patient who had wound infection with previous head and neck surgery
    Previous radiation
    Not a factor[28–30]
    Is a factor[6,28,31]
    Regardless, increases complexity of managing an infection that does develop
Previous tracheostomy
    Studies disagree
Operation
    Duration of transfusions
    Use of flaps

Table 16-3 SPECIAL CASES FOR PROPHYLACTIC ANTIBIOTICS

Prevention of endocarditis
Orthopedic artificial joints
Cranioplasty
Skull base surgery
Free flap surgery
Mandibular reconstruction bars
Dental extractions (anaerobic infections)

Wound infections in postoperative head and neck patients following radiation and surgery continue to show the same basic group of organisms (Table 16-4).

CLINICAL RECOGNITION OF WOUND INFECTION AFTER SURGERY IN THE IRRADIATED PATIENT

Wound infection is suspected when the patient develops a low-grade fever on the third or fourth day. Pain may have been diminishing but now has increased. The character of the drainage in the suction evacuator changes; it may appear thick, cloudy, or frankly purulent. The volume, which was decreasing, now increases. The neck will start to have a doughy feeling, and some redness develops over the edematous area. Because most wound infections are associated with a leak through the repair of the pharyngeal mucosa, opening and draining the suspected area are indicated immediately. The patient remains fed through the gastrostomy or nasogastric (NG) tube.

If surgery has been a neck dissection only, fistula formation is unlikely, but if the problem begins in the lower neck, a chyle fistula is of potential concern. A salivary fistula developing within 24 to 48 hours of surgery suggests a technical error. If a fistula is demonstrated, these

Table 16-4 MOST COMMON ORGANISMS IN HEAD AND NECK POSTOPERATIVE WOUND INFECTIONS

Staphylococcus aureus
Pseudomonas aeruginosa
Escherichia coli
Enterobacter
Haemophilus sp
Anaerobic organisms

patients can be returned to the operating room and the repair can be made. The tissue at this time is still capable of being repaired primarily or with flap reconstruction if necessary. When there is a question of a fistula formation, and especially if there is concern about NG tube removal, a barium swallow is useful. The presence of a "radiologic fistula" means that the NG tube should remain another week.[33,34]

However, fistulae developing a week or two after surgery are associated with so much inflammation that a primary repair is not possible. The effort is made to adequately drain the wound before further necrosis develops, which can occur rapidly in over 24 to 48 hours. Wound and blood cultures are obtained and systemic antibiotics are started, which would cover *Staphylococcus* and anaerobes until the culture report is returned. This may then require a change in the antibiotic selection.

The mainstay of treatment is adequate drainage of the wound as reliance cannot be made on providing antibiotics alone. Wounds that show obvious copious purulent materials are treated with gauze soaked in a broad-spectrum topical antiseptic microbicide, such as chloroxylenol, particularly in extensive wounds when infection develops that is grossly foul smelling and contains an unacceptably high amount of purulent material. As quickly as possible, usually within 24 hours, the wound is then packed with benzethonium chloride, an antimicrobial non-toxic solution, on 1-inch gauze. Culture results are not yet available, but these chemical solutions are effective against all bacteria. They are also less harmful to the underlying surrounding tissues than preparations such as povidone-iodine, hydrogen peroxide, Dakin's solution, acetic acid, and other topical antiseptics. Within 24 hours, there should no longer be signs of systemic infection. White counts should be decreasing, as well as the patient's fever. If this is not occurring, the wound is not adequately drained. Packing is changed two to three times a day, preferably by a physician or nurse who is used to dealing with such wounds. It should be evident that the purulent nature of the wound is

rapidly decreasing. If this is not occurring or if the fistula is felt to be too large, then the patient should be returned to the operating room, where the wound is better explored.

In this circumstance, a Montgomery salivary bypass tube can be passed (size 12 or larger).[35] This collects and diverts the saliva. By diminishing salivary flow across the wound, the carotid artery is more protected from being exposed.[36] Within 72 hours, this acute purulent wound can be managed by decreasing gauze packing each day. If the fistula is controlled and saliva flow is no longer a major problem, this wound can be converted from the acute purulent phase to a more subacute phase. In the meantime, the skin will have contracted substantially. With time, granulation tissue should start to form. To enhance formation of granulation tissue, new products are available that débride, protect the wound, and are easy to apply. Packing is performed with calcium alginate, with some newer products containing silver. In very large wounds, once granulation tissue is present and purulent material is not present, a pectoralis or deltopectoral flap can be used to close the defect. There is no value in bringing up such a flap prematurely. Placing the flap over a necrotic area or a nondirected fistula will lead to potential flap loss and may even hide latent infection. Primary closure of the underlying pharyngeal tissue is not feasible as these tissues become nonmobile and leathery, and suture placement leads only to the suture being pulling through the tissue as the knot is tied.

ESOPHAGEAL STRICTURE

Increased preference for organ preservation, particularly of the larynx, hypopharynx, or tongue base, has led to combinations of chemotherapy, usually cisplatinum or carboplatinum with or without paclitaxel or 5-fluorouracil administered concomitantly with radiation therapy.[10,37,38] Some protocols include two to three courses of chemotherapy initially, examining for a response, and if there is a 30 to 50% reduction in tumor size, one continues concomitant chemotherapy and radiation therapy.[39-42] Although the protocols seem to be effective in preserving the larynx in 60% of cases, a new series of side effects have been demonstrated. Many patients undergoing this rigorous protocol generally need a percutaneous gastrostomy to maintain adequate nutrition. This dependence on the gastrostomy and lack of swallowing have been considered to aggravate the swallowing problems that are apparent during and immediately after treatment. Simply not using pharyngeal muscles for a period of 6 to 12 weeks may be responsible for the aggravating strictures and difficulty in swallowing that occurs. Patients should be encouraged to swallow during this time, and swallowing exercises may be helpful even if nutritional support relies on tube feedings. A modified barium swallow may demonstrate the lack of an efficient swallowing mechanism, particularly in patients treated for tongue base malignancy, showing that there is limited tongue thrust with limited initiation of the bolus to allow proper swallowing. In others, a stricture develops in the cervical esophagus close to the area of the cricopharyngeus.

In some patients, the stricture becomes progressive and firm and may even become complete. Development of a stricture requires immediate dilatation.[43] This dilatation may require general anesthesia, with the potential of significant risk in nontracheostomized patients when the anesthiologist endeavors to pass the endotracheal tube. The trismus, firmness, and edema of the tongue base tissues make intubation extremely difficult. In fact, in certain cases, if frequent dilatations and trips to the operating room are going to be needed, tracheostomy may be required for this purpose alone if not for control of aspiration and the airway.[44] Fortunately, the majority of patients do respond to careful, repeated gentle dilitation.[45] Those patients who attempt swallowing tend to improve more rapidly. Modified barium swallow may demonstrate a stricture, but at endoscopy, an esophagoscope or a dilator is passed with relative ease. These patients probably have neurogenic loss or paralysis of swallowing muscles.

In a limited number of patients, the stricture progresses to being complete or nearly complete. An NG tube must be kept in position to at least identify the tract. If even this becomes no longer feasible, retrograde dilatation or retrograde assessment of the area through the gastrostomy site is a possible but difficult endoscopic procedure.[46] It must remain carefully stented. Other efforts have been made to resect this and reconstruct the defect with a free flap. Even in the best of hands, this has not always been a satisfactory solution. Some patients will be permanently gastrostomy dependent.

RECONSTRUCTION: REPAIR OF FISTULA AND REPLACEMENT OF CERVICAL SKIN

When the secretions from the fistula are no longer infected and the débrided skin leaves a large defect, with potential exposure of the carotid artery, flap reconstruction is required. At the initial reconstruction for recurrence of tumor or in advanced malignancy, a free flap, usually the forearm, may be the method of choice. If the cervical vasculature is still present (a modified neck dissection) and the tissue is not extremely fibrotic, free flap reconstruction is feasible. It has been effective even in patients who have had full-course radiation.[47,48] However, if there is extensive necrosis, fibrosis, or coexisting morbidities, the pectoralis major myocutaneous muscle is preferred.[49] It not only provides tissue for the reconstruction, it also brings nonirradiated tissue into the field with its own vascular supply and protects the carotid artery. The pectoralis flap derives its blood supply from the pectoral branch of the thoracoacromial artery. The path of this artery lies along a line drawn from the middle third of the clavicle to the xyphoid. The tissue used is generally halfway between the nipple and the midline. After outlining the required skin paddle, stay sutures secure the skin to the underlying fascia. In some patients, there may be excessive soft tissue between the underlying muscle and the skin. The amount of soft tissue that would be brought into the wound would be excessive. In this situation, a myofascial graft is used with a split-thickness skin graft replacing the skin paddle.

If the defect to be repaired is primarily loss of skin with exposed underlying tissues, for example, the carotid artery, then the size of the skin paddle should be substantially larger in each dimension than the cervical defect. More importantly, after cutting and freshening the edges of the defect, it becomes apparent that to suture the flap to vital, healthy tissues will necessitate resection of more cervical skin than was initially planned. Any effort to decrease the size of the defect by mobilizing cervical skin leads to a dead space above the clavicle as the skin stretches across this area. Further, the cervical skin, particularly if a radical neck had been previously performed, is fibrotic, nonmalleable, and adherent to the underlying structures, including the carotid sheath. This skin is best elevated bluntly with the finger in the subplatysmal plane. Even with heavy intensive radiation in the past, this plane may still exist. Doppler ultrasonography is used to identify the carotid artery. The skin tunnel in the lower neck over the clavicle must easily admit four fingers to allow passage of the pectoralis pedicle into the neck. Incisions are designed to preserve the upper chest skin for a potential deltopectoral flap. Large fistulae often require not only repairing the fistula but also replacing overlying cervical skin.

The pectoralis flap is outlined on the chest, and the skin paddle is sutured in place with 3-0 Vicryl, preventing avulsion during the rotation. The myofascial portion is made at least 2 cm wider than the skin paddle. Inferiorly or distally, this should be at least 3 cm. This allows for the shrinkage that will occur at the time of rotation, but, more importantly, it allows for the extra muscle to be tucked in beneath the elevated cervical skin margins, adding an important second layer for closure. The decision on which side to place the skin paddle is made depending on the size of the defect. A large (eg, 6 cm) defect in the pharynx or hypopharynx requires that the skin paddle be used on the internal surface and should be sutured to the underlying mucosa.

Preserve the posterior hypopharyngeal wall as much as possible. Likewise, if the largest portion of the defect is cervical skin, then the skin paddle is used for that purpose and a split-thickness skin graft is applied on the hypopharyngeal side. This split-thickness skin graft in actuality serves only as a temporary biologic dressing when applied on the pharyngeal surface. The cervical skin is trimmed now to fit the paddle rather than vice versa. Relaxing incisions may be required and a skin graft applied if the rotated pedicle is compressed as it crosses the clavicle by the skin bridge. At least two drains are inserted from the chest and brought up into the neck parallel to the newly placed pedicle flap. Care is taken that no drain crosses over or under the flap, with potential obstruction of the venous return. If the patient has had a laryngopharyngectomy, the salivary bypass tube is in place at this time and remains in place for at least 3 weeks (Figures 16-2 to 16-7).

PREVENTION OF ASPIRATION

Patients with large fistulae have the potential for significant aspiration and secondary pneumonia, which can lead to acute respiratory distress syndrome (Figures 16-8 and 16-9). Therefore, it is imperative that when a large fistula develops in

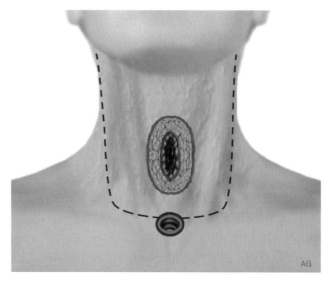

Figure 16-2. Typical area of wound breakdown, often associated with the T-portion of the closure of the laryngopharyngectomy. Saliva must be diverted from the laryngectomy stoma.

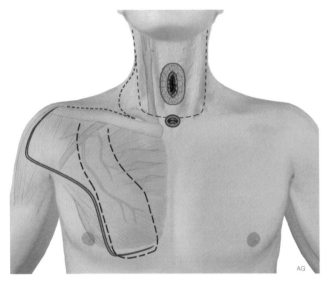

Figure 16-3. Outline of incisions for a pectoralis major myocutaneous flap outlined to preserve a possible deltopectoral flap. Note that the pectoralis flap includes not only the skin paddle, but also a 1–2 cm of additional muscle surrounding the skin paddle.

a previously irradiated patient and immediate repair is not a possibility, a percutaneous gastrostomy should be performed. Leaving an NG tube in place has the potential for vomiting, with immediate aspiration of the secretions through the stoma. Everyone agrees with the goal of salivary diversion to protect the carotid artery, but in severe wound breakdowns, this may not be feasible. Carotid artery exposure is the primary concern, and every effort must be

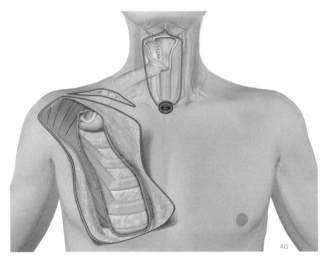

Figure 16-4. The pectoralis flap is tubed to close the defect. In cases where the skin plus subcutaneous fat tissue are so thick that it cannot easily be tubed, the myofascial portion of the flap with a split-thickness skin graft is used.

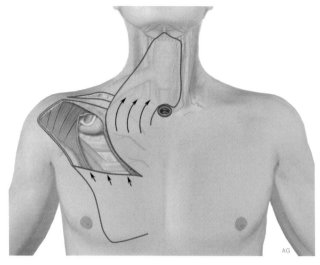

Figure 16-5. The deltapectoral flap completes the closure of the large skin deficit.

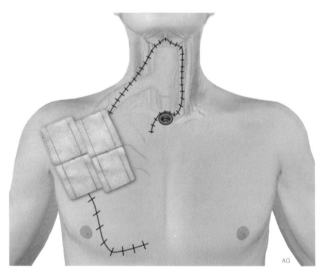

Figure 16-6. A split-thickness skin graft is applied to the exposed area of the shoulder.

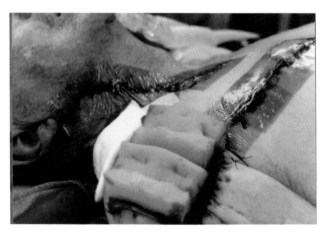

Figure 16-7. The split thickness skin grafts are covered with adaptic gauze and surgical surgical sponges bolster the skin graft in position.

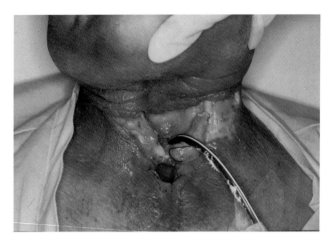

Figure 16-8. A nasogastric tube in the fistula site may promote gross regurgitation with aspiration.

made to protect the artery. The salivary bypass tube is effective in smaller fistulae, but in very large fistulae, moist and repeated careful packing is essential to promote granulation tissue and allow early flap reconstruction.

During this period, an effort is made to prevent salivary contamination of the cervical wound. It is even worse when the fistula opens into the superior portion of the tracheal stoma, where major pulmonary complications can result. It may be necessary to keep an inflated tracheostomy tube cuff in place, even though this does not completely prevent aspiration. The patient is maintained on proton pump inhibitors to neutralize any potential vomitus of gastric juices.

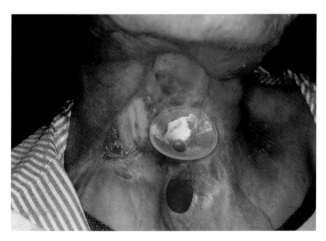

Figure 16-9. Salivary bypass tube collects saliva diverting it from the tracheal stoma.

MANAGEMENT OF THE EXPOSED CAROTID ARTERY

Exposure of the carotid artery with carotid artery "blowout" is the most serious complication of head and neck cancer surgery. Previous radiation therapy combined with fistula and wound breakdown after a composite procedure or laryngopharyngectomy creates this circumstance (Figure 16-10).[50] Preventive measures at the time of surgery include the specific placement of the incision and intraoperative efforts to protect the vessel (Table 16-5). The preferred incision crosses the carotid artery area only once in a transverse direction. For composite resections, this incision crosses the artery in the upper third of the neck

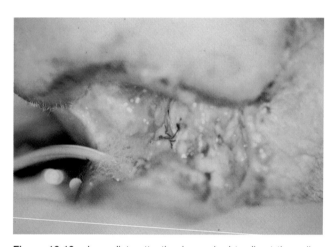

Figure 16-10. Immediate attention is required to divert the saliva from flowing across the carotid artery.

Table 16-5 SURGICAL TECHNIQUES TO PREVENT CAROTID ARTERY EXPOSURE
Begin perioperative antibiotics 1 h before incision
Placement of incision perpendicular to carotid artery
Single, curved transverse incision
Meticulous management of soft tissue, especially mucosa
Watertight pharyngeal closure, adequate size
Use of pedicle flap or free flap if lumen is small
Replace questionably viable skin with rotation flap
Avoid separating pharynx from posterior wall. Avoid separating trachea from esophageal wall (limits blood supply). Eliminate dead space.
Use suction drains carefully placed; soft drains preferred. Observe characteristics of drainage. Keep drains in until < 30 cc/d.
Protect carotid bulb with muscle fascia flap or levator scapulae
If oncologically safe, preserve sternocleidomastoid muscle to protect carotid
Stage neck dissection. If bilateral simultaneous neck dissection, consider tracheostomy.
Use of stay sutures for 3 wk

but not over the bulb. The incision extends posterosuperiorly toward the mastoid to allow for full dissection of the superior cervical lymph nodes toward the jugular foramen. For further exposure, the incision crosses the midline, allowing for a larger flap elevation to be done through a single transverse incision. It is generally not necessary to make a posteroinferior extension from this incision (Figures 16-11 and 16-12).

For laryngopharyngectomy or tumors lying lower in the neck, a broad "smile" incision is useful. The "apron" incision, as originally described along the anterior borders of the sternocleidomastoid muscle and then transversally across the midline, is particularly vulnerable to necrosis in an irradiated patient and directly overlies the carotid artery. By making the incision more transverse and extending across the posterior border of the sternocleidomastoid

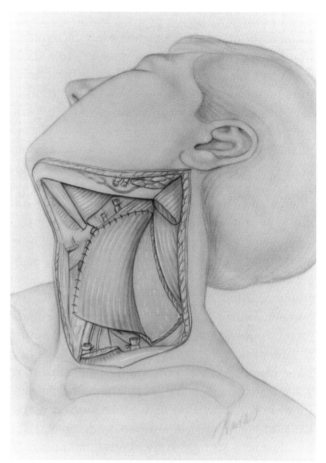

Figure 16-12. A levator scapular flap is outlined. The flap is rotated to cover the carotid artery, but in actuality usually covers only the region of the carotid bulb.

muscle before its upward extension, this large flap has a higher vascular supply and is less likely to necrose, and if that should occur, the carotid artery is less likely to be exposed. Every cervical incision is planned so that it does not cross the carotid artery near the bulb. If, by report, salivary fistulae occur in 30% of patients with ranges up to 50% or higher, then it is imperative that a plan for carotid artery protection is made during surgery.[11,51] The easiest way is to medially rotate a levator scapulae flap. Unfortunately, after rotation, this flap covers only the region of the upper portion of the carotid artery but does cover the carotid bifurcation. In a previously heavily irradiated patient in whom there is substantial fibrosis of the skin, one can predict that this muscle will also be inadequate for this use. In this situation, a pectoralis fasciocutaneous flap can be used to protect the carotid artery.[52]

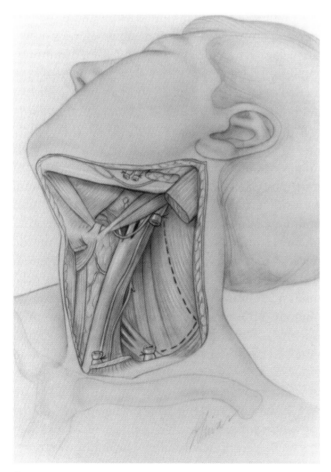

Figure 16-11. A levator scapula flap is rotated to cover the carotid artery. In actuality the flap covers best only the region of the carotid bulb.

A controlled fistula is often discussed in the complications conference, but even recognizing that there is a 50% likelihood that a fistula could occur, creating a controlled fistula in practice is infrequent. Subsequently, each surgeon has his or her own recommendations for pharyngeal closure. Fistulae are more likely to occur in pharyngolaryngectomies because of the amount of mobilization of the underlying mucosa for closure and a more likely tightness of such a closure. In this situation, whenever there is doubt, either a free flap or a pectoralis flap should be considered.[53] Free flap reconstruction, although longer in the operating room, is often accompanied by a shorter overall hospital course, earlier swallowing, and less likely development of a postoperative fistula when primary repair is not possible. A running Connell suture closure of the pharynx is performed, with the first layer being the most important. The sutures are placed sufficiently far from the mucosal and submucosal edges that tearing does not occur as the suture is tightened. If there is adequate tissue for closure, a straight vertical incision appears to be less likely for fistula formation but may lead to some dysphagia. Others prefer the T closure, but it is almost inevitable that the site of fistula is at the T trifurcation. Additional layers of closure include the remaining strap muscles closed as a protective layer. An NG tube is placed for short duration in patients undergoing laryngectomy in a nonirradiated situation. Most authors prefer to leave an NG tube in place for 10 days before feeding a patient after a laryngopharyngectomy when radiation therapy has been administered. Barium swallow has been used as a measure to determine whether it is safe to remove the NG tube and begin feeding.[34] The presence of a "radiologic" fistula, that is, a nonclinically apparent tract leading out into the soft tissues of the neck, is an indication to leave the NG tube for an additional 2 weeks before repeating the radiograph and then allowing swallowing. These radiologic fistulae do not require open surgical drainage unless they become clinically apparent and present as a fistula, as noted earlier in this chapter.

CAROTID ARTERY RUPTURE

Unfortunately, carotid artery rupture may still occur in spite of all efforts to prevent this complication. In at least 50% of cases, sentinel bleeding with up to a few hundred milliliters of blood loss occurs. In other cases, a "ballooning" or "blister" of the artery occurs or the artery becomes soft to palpation, especially in the area of the carotid bulb. This warns that there is an impending blowout of the carotid artery. The patient is admitted to the intensive care unit, and an immediate consultation is made with the interventional radiology team. If the patient is a candidate, a trial internal carotid artery balloon occlusion test performed through the femoral artery is accomplished. Cerebral angiography is performed on both sides to establish the patency of the circle of Willis. A latex balloon is then placed high on the side of the involved artery. The balloon remains inflated while the patient is carefully observed for any signs of neurologic sequelae. After a period of at least 20 minutes, preferably longer, if there are no signs of any neurologic deficit, the balloon can be withdrawn and the internal carotid artery permanently occluded with a series of coils, causing complete obstruction. The preference is to place the coils high in the internal carotid artery to prevent retrograde thrombus formation. The common carotid artery is now occluded in a similar manner. When arteriography demonstrates that the external carotid artery is the sight of the bleeding, it can simply be occluded or ligated. Likewise, when the bleeding is internal into the pharynx, it is usually the superior thyroid or lingual artery, and embolization can be performed. When it is necessary to embolize the internal carotid artery, heparin is delivered for 48 to 72 hours to prevent retrograde thrombus formation with stroke (Figures 16-13 to 16-16). We have adopted this approach because of the postmortem finding in patients who developed delayed cerebral vascular thrombotic stroke, generally 24 hours or later after balloon occlusion and ligation.[54] This occurred gradually and progressively, beginning with a third nerve

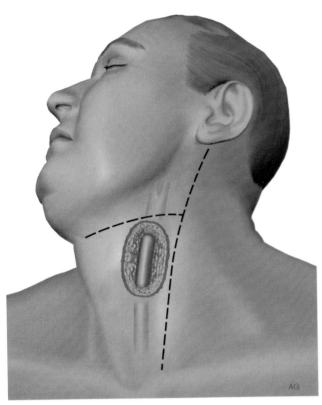

Figure 16-13. Exposed carotid artery and impending carotid artery rupture.

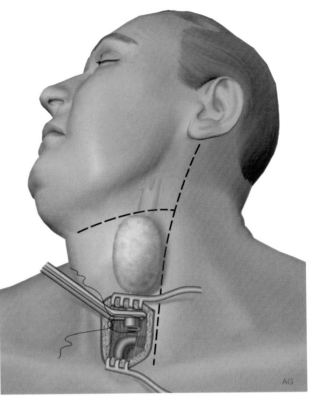

Figure 16-15. Artery ligated through a separate incision after balloon occlusion testing and permanent embolization of internal carotid artery at the skull base by balloon or springs.

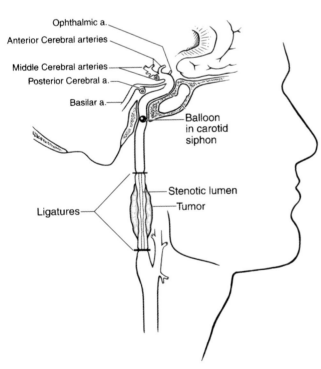

Figure 16-14. Trial balloon occlusion is performed, and if no adverse neurologic events occur, the artery is permanently embolized.

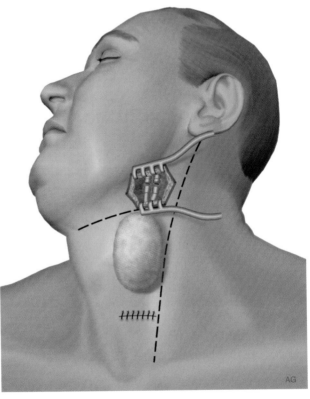

Figure 16-16. Wound packed with calcium alginate and artery ligated.

paralysis followed by progressive loss of consciousness and contralateral paralysis in the preceding 48 hours. This retrograde clot occluded the middle cerebral artery.[54]

If massive bleeding is occurring away from the operating room, the following protocol has been proven effective in at least two-thirds of the patients who were salvaged with this without permanent neurologic sequelae.[55] Manual pressure is maintained on the artery while the patient receives transfusions (Table 16-6). The blood pressure and pulse are maintained, and the patient is then taken to the operating room for ligation. Preferably, the carotid artery is identified and then ligated through a fresh incision distant from the area of necrosis. Both the distal and proximal stumps are suture-ligated and then buried in the surrounding soft tissue to prevent recurrent bleeding. Even in the best of circumstances, thrombotic stroke remains a significant possibility even though this technique reduces the mortality. This protocol is for patients whose carotid artery is exposed with necrosis, infection, and, usually, a fistula. Techniques to reconstruct or bypass the carotid system are obviously preferred but are performed in more ideal circumstances.[56–60]

MANAGEMENT OF THE CHRONIC NONHEALING IRRADIATED WOUND

Once the fistula has been controlled and the carotid artery has been protected, attention turns to the chronic slowly healing or nonhealing wound. Wounds in this phase will not heal unless intervention occurs to bring the wound into an acute phase.[61] This is done by appropriate débridement of the wound and creating the appropriate environment for wound healing. The proper selection of wound dressings creates a moist environment using semiocclusive dressings. Dressings are selected that will promote granulation tissue. This will not occur in the presence of an active infectious process but will occur even if the wound is colonized with specific bacteria. More recent management of such wounds uses technology developed for the management of the chronic diabetic wound. The similarity of the poor vascularity and the need to stimulate wound healing are recognized (Figures 16-17 to 19).

A key point is to maintain the wound in a moist environment. The calcium alginate dressings are kept moist to induce granulation formation and have the advantage that removal is simply by irrigation and therefore is less painful and accepted better by the patient. Also, the dressing changes have to be done only every 2 to 3 days, lessening the requirements for home nursing care. Deeper wounds in cavities require gentle packing soaked in saline. Many compounds commonly used in the infected stage actually can cause tissue damage and delay healing (Table 16-7). The disadvantage of the wet to dry dressing technique is that it reinjures the healing wound as the packing is removed and is painful for the patient. Topical antibiotics are valuable when there is suppuration of the wound.

Table 16-6 PREFERABLE PARAMETERS TO ACHEIVE BEFORE CAROTID LIGATION
Systolic blood pressure > 110 mm Hg
Pulse = 60 to 100 bpm
pO$_2$ > 90 mm Hg
Hemoglobin > 11 g/100 mL
Central venous pressure monitor
Separate skin incision for proximal and distal ligation in healthy tissue

pO$_2$ = oxygen partial pressure.

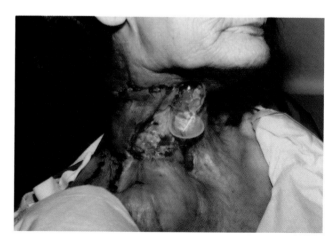

Figure 16-17. The necrotic flap is carefully debrided and the saliva coming from the upper aspect of the wound is collected by the salivary by pass tube.

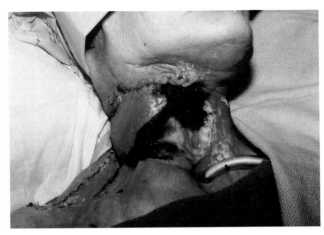

Figure 16-18. When the wound demonstrates in granular surface, a pectoralis major myocutaneous flap can be rotated into position.

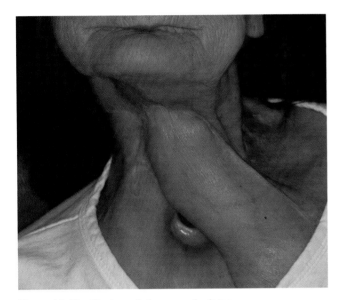

Figure 16-19. Final repair three months later.

Their disadvantage is that they are effective only against certain bacteria and may often lead to colonization with highly resistant organisms.

Table 16-8 LOCAL WOUND CARE
Proper drainage
Débride necrotic tissues
Surgical
Enzymatic
Accuzyme (papain + urea)
Wet to dry
Avoid antiseptics
Povidone-iodine (Betadine) only in grossly purulent wounds
Saline packs as soon as feasible
Topical antibiotics
Silvadene cream 1%
Bacitracin, Neosporin
Dressing
Alginates
Keep wound moist
Change every 2–4 d
Rinse away with water irrigation
Absorbing
Polymem (surfactant + glycerin + superabsorbent polymer)
Duoderm, Hydrogel (hydrophobic polymer)
Hydrogels
Useful for low exudate wounds
Maintain moisture
Hydrocolloids
Useful for medium exudate wounds
Promote autolysis
Promote granulation

Adapted from Hom DB et al.[61]

However, they do have the advantage of keeping the wound moist and are advantageous in a purulent wound (Table 16-8).

Improving the patient's nutritional status is imperative. Anemia and hypothyroidism are two common deterrents to wound healing. Exuberant granulation tissue can be removed by the scalpel. This is usually not highly vascular and appears as clear, edematous tissue overgrowth. The goal is to obtain a nice, granulating bed that has areas with a red (strawberry), healthy-appearing, non-infected granulation. This will now accept a split-

Table 16-7 DRESSING PURPOSE AND PRODUCT CLASSIFICATION	
Wound Goals	**Products Available**
Topically débride devitalized tissue chemically	Enzymatic débridement agents
Mechanically débride devitalized tissue	Wound cleansers, gauze (wet to dry)
Add moisture to the wound	Gauze (impregnated or with saline), hydrogels, wound care systems (2 part)
Maintain a moist wound environment	Ointments, foams, gauze (impregnated or with saline), hydrocolloids, hydrogels, transparent films, wound care systems (2 part)
Fill dead space	Absorption beads, pastes, and powders; alginates; hydrocolloid pastes; powders; foam; gauze
Cover and protect wound	Composites, compression bandages/wraps, foams, gauze dressings (covers/wraps), hydrocolloids, hydrogels (with covers/borders), transparent film dressings
Protect surrounding skin from moisture and trauma	Moisture barrier ointments, foams, hydrocolloids, securement devices, skin sealants, transparent film dressings

thickness skin graft. Assistance from the wound healing team is extremely valuable as it will have access to many of the new dressing compounds that have so enhanced the rapidity with which wounds can be brought to the phase of accepting a skin graft.

PEARLS AND PITFALLS

Recognize the high incidence of postoperative fistula and wound necrosis in patients who have had radiation therapy. Prevention begins pre-operatively with patient nutritional factors and gastrostomy placement if required (Table 16-9). Meticulous management of the repair of the pharynx is required, with elimination of dead space, bringing in nonirradiated tissue, and avoiding overtight closure of the hypopharynx. Early recognition of the development of a fistula and immediate surgical drainage combined with systemic antibiotics and obtaining culture are imperative in treating the wound. The mainstay of treatment is local wound care in conjunction with systemic antibiotics. The wound is packed and the saliva is diverted from the exposed carotid artery and from the stoma or tracheostomy site to avoid aspiration pneumonia. Fistulae will require flap reconstruction. Although free tissue flaps are now preferred, in the contaminated wound in patients with multiple comorbidities, this is not possible. In this situation, the pectoralis myocutaneous flap can be used to close the defect. Neither free flaps nor pectoralis flaps should be brought into the area until the wound infection is brought into control and a healthy granulation tissue bed has been developed.

POTENTIAL FUTURE THERAPY

There are several areas for potential improvement in the healing of an irradiated wound. One is the use of fibroblast growth factor to attempt to improve wound vascularity.[62] The objective of these growth factors would be to improve tissue oxygenation with more rapid and complete wound healing. The potential for improved wound healing with hyperbaric oxygen has also been explored. In anecdotal case reports, the results are promising. However, hyperbaric oxygen alone without careful wound management and proper systemic management will not enhance wound healing. It is unfair to criticize these studies for not being randomized and prospective. It is apparent in reading the reports that patients subjected to hyperbaric oxygen had severe wounds in which no healing process was occurring.[63] A patient with an exposed carotid artery should not be placed in the chamber because this could further increase the risk of rupture. Wound healing is enhanced with new and improved chronic wound dressing products. Some of the newer dressing compounds have both an antibacterial effect and a granulation-promoting effect. Given that complete understanding of healing in the irradiated wound has not been documented, knowledge from chronic stasis ulcers and other chronic wounds has been used to assist irradiated wounds to heal.

The effectiveness of hyperbaric oxygen in the management of chronic osteoradionecrosis of the mandible in head and neck patients is more established. Its use in cartilaginous chronic wound infections and soft tissue wound infections is not as established. However, there is continued enthusiasm about its use and benefits for advanced radionecrosis, particularly of the

---

Table 16-9 POSTOPERATIVE CARE TO DIMINISH LIKELIHOOD OF INFECTION IN THE IRRADIATED PATIENT

Drains remain in place until accumulated drainage < 30 cc over 24 h
Observe drainage for change in character; should go from bloody to serosanguinous to clear
Check for fever, pain, change in appearance of wound twice daily
Have a high suspicion for wound complications in patients in whom pharynx has been entered
Evaluate for nonwound complications, eg, aspiration pneumonia, *Clostridium difficile* infection, deep venous thrombosis
No tight bands across the neck; overly tight tracheostomy ties, elastic band of humidified O_2 dome
Attention to donor sites

larynx.[64] Patients with exposed carotid arteries should not be subjected to hyperbaric oxygen because of the potential adverse affects of inducing carotid artery hemorrhage.

REFERENCES

1. Goldman JR, Gunsberg MJ, Friedman WH, et al. Combined therapy for cancer of the laryngopharynx. Arch Otolaryngol 1970;92:221–5.
2. Strong MS, Vaughan CW, Kayne HL, et al. A randomized trial of preoperative radiotherapy in cancer of the oropharynx and hypopharynx. Am J Surg 1978;136:494–500.
3. Vandenbrouck C, Sancho H, Fur L, et al. Results of a randomized clinical trial of preoperative irradiation versus postoperative in treatment of tumors of the hypopharynx. Cancer 1977;39:1445–9.
4. Kramer S, Gelber RD, Snow JB, et al. Combined radiation therapy and surgery in the management of advanced head and neck cancer: final report of study 73-03 of the Radiation Therapy Oncology Group. Head Neck 1987;10:19–30.
5. Tupchong L, Scott CB, Blitzer PH, et al. Randomized study of preoperative versus postoperative radiation therapy in advanced head and neck carcinoma: long-term follow-up of RTOG study 73-03. Int J Radiat Oncol Biol Phys 1991;20:21–8.
6. Thawley SE. Complications of combined radiation therapy and surgery for carcinoma of the larynx and inferior hypopharynx. Laryngoscope 1981;91:677–700.
7. Genden EM, Rinaldo A, Shaha AR, et al. Pharyngocutaneous fistula following laryngectomy. Acta Otolaryngol (Stockh) 2004;124:117–20.
8. Cummings CW, Johnson J, Chung CK, Sagerman R. Complications of laryngectomy and neck dissection following planned preoperative radiotherapy. Ann Otol Rhinol Laryngol 1977;86:745–50.
9. Denis F, Garaud P, Bardet E, et al. Final results of the 94-01 French Head And Neck Oncology and Radiotherapy Group randomized trial comparing radiotherapy alone with concomitant radiochemotherapy in advanced-stage oropharynx carcinoma. J Clin Oncol 2004;22:69–76.
10. Forastiere AA, Goepfert H, Maor M, et al. Concurrent chemotherapy and radiotherapy for organ preservation in advanced laryngeal cancer. N Engl J Med 2003;349:2091–8.
11. Weber RS, Berkey BA, Forastiere A, et al. Outcome of salvage total laryngectomy following organ preservation therapy: the Radiation Therapy Oncology Group trial 91-11. Arch Otolaryngol Head Neck Surg 2003;129:44–9.
12. Stoeckli SJ, Pawlik AB, Lipp M, et al. Salvage surgery after failure of nonsurgical therapy for carcinoma of the larynx and hypopharynx. Arch Otolaryngol Head Neck Surg 2000;126:1473–7.
13. Agra IMG, Carvalho AL, Pontes E, et al. Postoperative complications after en bloc salvage surgery for head and neck cancer. Arch Otolaryngol Head Neck Surg 2003;129:1317–21.
14. Wolf GT, Fisher SG. Effectiveness of salvage neck dissection for advanced regional metastases when induction chemotherapy and radiation are used for organ preservation. Laryngoscope 1992;102:934–9.
15. Mendenhall WM, Parsons JT, Stringer SP, et al. Radiotherapy alone or combined with neck dissection for T_1-T_2 carcinoma of the pyriform sinus: an alternative to conservation surgery. Int J Radiat Oncol Biol Phys 1993;27:1017–27.
16. Davidson BJ, Newkirk KA, Harter KW, et al. Complications from planned, posttreatment neck dissections. Arch Otolaryngol Head Neck Surg 1999;125:401–5.
17. Dagum P, Pinto HA, Newman JP, et al. Management of the clinically positive neck in organ preservation for advanced head and neck cancer. Am J Surg 1998;176:448–52.
18. Feehs RS, McGuirt WF, Bond MG, et al. Irradiation: a significant risk factor for carotid atherosclerosis. Arch Otolaryngol Head Neck Surg 1991;117:1135–7.
19. Muzaffar K, Collins SL, Labropoulos N, Baker WH. A prospective study of the effects of irradiation on the carotid artery. Laryngoscope 2000;110:1811–4.
20. Bernstein EF, Sullivan FJ, Mitchell JB, et al. Biology of chronic radiation effect on tissues and wound healing. Clin Plast Surg 1993;20:435–53.
21. Tokarek R, Bernstein EF, Sullivan F, et al. Effect of therapeutic radiation on wound healing. Clin Dermatol 1994;12:57–70.
22. Porock D. Factors influencing the severity of radiation skin and oral mucosal reactions: development of a conceptual framework. Eur J Cancer Care 2002;11:33–43.
23. Chandler JR. Radiation fibrosis and necrosis of the larynx. Ann Otol Rhinol Laryngol 1979;88:509–14.
24. Sassler AM, Esclamado RM, Wolf GT. Surgery after organ preservation therapy: analysis of wound complications. Arch Otolaryngol Head Neck Surg 1995;121:162–5.
25. Panje WR, Namon AJ, Vokes E, et al. Surgical management of the head and neck cancer patient following concomitant multimodality therapy. Laryngoscope 1995;105:97–101.
26. Piccirillo JF. Importance of comorbidity in head and neck cancer. Laryngoscope 2000;110:593–602.
27. Robbins KT, Favrot S, Hanna D, Cole R. Risk of wound infection in patients with head and neck cancer. Head Neck 1990;12:143–8.
28. Schwartz SR, Yueh B, Maynard C, et al. Predictors of wound complications after laryngectomy: a study of over 2000 patients. Otolaryngol Head Neck Surg 2004;131:61–8.
29. Johnson JT, Bloomer WD. Effect of prior radiotherapy on postsurgical wound infection. Head Neck 1989;11:132–6.

30. Penel N, Lefebvre D, Fournier C, et al. Risk factors for wound infection in head and neck cancer surgery: a prospective study. Head Neck 2001;23:447–55.

31. Coskin H, Erisen L, Basut O. Factors affecting wound infection rates in head and neck surgery. Otolaryngol Head Neck Surg 2000;123:328–33.

32. Weber RS. Wound infection in head and neck surgery: implications for perioperative antibiotic treatment. Ear Nose Throat J 1997;76:790–8.

33. Krouse JH, Metson R. Barium swallow is a predictor of salivary fistula following laryngectomy. Otolaryngol Head Neck Surg 1992;106:254–7.

34. Giordano AM Jr, Cohen J, Adams GL. Pharyngocutaneous fistula after laryngeal surgery: the role of the barium swallow. Otolaryngol Head Neck Surg 1984;92:19–23.

35. León X, Quer M, Burgués J. Montgomery® salivary bypass tube in the reconstruction of the hypopharynx: cost-benefit study. Ann Otol Rhinol Laryngol 1999;108:864–8.

36. Zaki HS, Kharchaf M, Carrau RL. Prosthetic management of pharyngocutaneous fistula by means of a salivary conduit. Laryngoscope 2001;111:548–51.

37. Tishler RB, Busse PM, Norris CM Jr, et al. An initial experience using concurrent paclitaxel and radiation in the treatment of head and neck malignancies. Int J Radiat Oncol Biol Phys 1999;43:1001–8.

38. Jacobs C, Lyman G, Velez-Garcia E, et al. A phase III randomized study comparing cisplatin and fluorouracil as single agents and in combination for advanced squamous cell carcinoma of the head and neck. J Clin Oncol 1992;10:257–63.

39. Demard F, Chauvel P, Santini J, et al. Response to chemotherapy as justification for modification of the therapeutic strategy for pharyngolaryngeal carcinomas. Head Neck 1990;12:225–31.

40. Shirinian MH, Weber RS, Lippman SM, et al. Laryngeal preservation by induction chemotherapy plus radiotherapy in locally advanced head and neck cancer: the M.D. Anderson Cancer Center experience. Head Neck 1994;16:39–44.

41. Urba SG, Wolf GT, Bradford CR, et al. Neoadjuvant therapy for organ preservation in head and neck cancer. Laryngoscope 2000;110:2074–80.

42. Clayman GL, Weber RS, Guillamondegui O, et al. Laryngeal preservation for advanced laryngeal and hypopharyngeal cancers. Arch Otolaryngol Head Neck Surg 1995;121:219–23.

43. Laurell G, Kraepelien T, Mavroidis P, et al. Stricture of the proximal esophagus in head and neck carcinoma patients after radiotherapy. Cancer 2003;97:1693–700.

44. Eisbruch A, Lyden T, Bradford CR, et al. Objective assessment of swallowing dysfunction and aspiration after radiation concurrent with chemotherapy for head-and-neck cancer. Int J Radiat Oncol Biol Phys 2002;53:23–8.

45. Sullivan CA, Jaklitsch MT, Haddad R, et al. Endoscopic management of hypopharyngeal stenosis after organ sparing therapy for head and neck cancer. Laryngoscope 2004;114:1924–31.

46. Lew RJ, Shah JN, Chalian A, et al. Technique of endoscopic retrograde puncture and dilatation of total esophageal stenosis in patients with radiation-induced strictures. Head Neck 2004;26:179–83.

47. Chepeha DB, Annich G, Pynnonen MA, et al. Pectoralis major myocutaneous flap vs revascularized free tissue transfer. Arch Otolaryngol Head Neck Surg 2004;130:181–6.

48. Choi S, Schwartz DL, Farwell DG, et al. Radiation therapy does not impact local complication rates after free flap reconstruction for head and neck cancer. Arch Otolaryngol Head Neck Surg 2004;130:1308–12.

49. Suh JD, Sercarz JA, Abemayor E, et al. Analysis of outcomes and complications in 400 cases of microvascular head and neck reconstruction. Arch Otolaryngol Head Neck Surg 2004;130:962–6.

50. Hom DB, Adams G, Koreis M, Maisel R. Choosing the optimal wound dressing for irradiated soft tissue wounds. Otolaryngol Head Neck Surg 1999;121:591–8.

51. Joseph DL, Shumrick DL. Risks of head and neck surgery in previously irradiated patients. Arch Otolaryngol 1973;97:381–4.

52. McCrory AL, Magnuson JS. Free tissue transfer versus pedicled flap in head and neck reconstruction. Laryngoscope 2002;112:2161–5.

53. Adams GL, Madison M, Remley K, Gapany M. Preoperative permanent balloon occlusion of internal carotid artery in patients with advanced head and neck squamous cell carcinoma. Laryngoscope 1999;109:460–6.

54. Smith TJ, Burrage KJ, Ganguly P, et al. Prevention of postlaryngectomy pharyngocutaneous fistula: the Memorial University experience. J Otol 2003;32:222–5.

55. Porto DP, Adams GL, Foster C. Emergency management of carotid artery rupture. Am J Otolaryngol 1986;7:213–7.

56. Chazono H, Okamoto Y, Matsuzaki Z, et al. Extracranial-intracranial bypass for reconstruction of internal carotid artery in the management of head and neck cancer. Ann Vasc Surg 2003;17:260–5.

57. Freeman SB, Hamaker RC, Borrowdale RB, Huntley TC. Management of neck metastasis with carotid artery involvement. Laryngoscope 2004;114:20–4.

58. Gavilán J, Ferlito A, Silver CE, et al. Status of carotid resection in head and neck cancer. Acta Otolaryngol (Stockh) 2002;122:453–5.

59. Muhm M, Grasl MC, Burian M, et al. Carotid resection and reconstruction for locally advanced head and neck tumors. Acta Otolaryngol (Stockh) 2002;122:561–4.

60. Aslan I, Hafiz G, Baserer N, et al. Management of carotid artery invasion in advanced malignancies of head and neck: comparison of techniques. Ann Otol Rhinol Laryngol 2002;111:772–7.

61. Hom DB, Adams GL, Monyak D. Irradiated soft tissue and its management. Otolaryngol Clin North Am 1995; 28:1003–19.

62. Hom DB, Simplot TC, Pernell KJ, et al. Vascular and epidermal effects of fibroblast growth factor on irradiated and nonirradiated skin flaps. Ann Otol Rhinol Laryngol 2000;109:667–75.

63. Wang C, Schwaitzberg S, Berliner E, et al. Hyperbaric oxygen for treating wounds: a systematic review of the literature. Arch Surg 2003;138:272–9.

64. Filntisis GA, Moon RE, Kraft KL, et al. Laryngeal radionecrosis and hyperbaric oxygen therapy: report of 18 cases and review of the literature. Ann Otol Rhinol Laryngol 2000;109:554–62.

17

Nonunion of the Mandible and Irradiated Mandible

Stephen P.R. MacLeod, BDS, MB ChB, FDS RCS (Ed and Eng), FRCS (Ed)

The mandible is commonly subjected to trauma. Healing usually proceeds uneventfully. Delayed union, or even nonunion, does occur, however. The cause for this is usually apparent and can be corrected to allow healing to progress. Inadequate fixation, infection, and microvascular inadequacy are the most common causes and may coexist in a given case. This chapter summarizes the management of nonunion of mandibular fractures and nonhealing of mandibular wounds, with reference to the irradiated mandible. Adjuvant therapies and possible future therapies are discussed.

HEALING OF THE MANDIBLE

The mandible and the maxilla are unique bones characterized by structures projecting from them, the teeth. The teeth project into the oral cavity, a potentially hostile environment, which possesses a diverse microbial ecosystem. The periodontal ligaments around the teeth provide a potential source of communication between the cancellous space of the mandible and the oral cavity. This potential space is realized whenever a tooth is extracted or the mandible is fractured through a tooth socket. In spite of this, infection of the mandible is a surprisingly unusual event. This is because of the robust host defense system present. The excellent blood supply to the head and neck is the cornerstone of the host defense system. The bone of the mandible is the site of many muscular insertions, which, along with the periosteum, provide a valuable contribution to the blood supply of the mandible with increasing age. The involution of the inferior alveolar artery with age leads the centrifugal supply from the periosteum and muscles to assume a dominant role in the blood supply to the mandible.[1,2] Disruption of this blood supply can result in the mandible having a diminished ability to respond to trauma. This can lead to problems with healing of mandibular injuries, whether they are fracture sites or surgical wounds (most commonly extraction sites). Irradiation of the mandible leads to endarteritis obliterans of the periosteal vessels of the mandible. Marx and Johnson reviewed the effects of irradiation to the mandible and described the mandible after irradiation to be hypovascular, hypocellular, and hypoxic.[3,4] In such an environment, any trauma may lead to the development of osteoradionecrosis (ORN). This is seen much more commonly in the mandible than in the maxilla, presumably because of the greater dependence on the periosteal blood supply in the mandible and the thicker cortical plate in the mandible.

Radiation is not the only cause of impairment of the periosteal microvascular circulation. It was recently recognized that chronic bisphosphonate use has been associated with necrosis of the jaws. The mechanism of this is not fully elucidated and may differ from ORN in a number of ways, with the role of osteoclasts being reevaluated. Intrinsic bone diseases, such as Paget's disease and fibrous dysplasia may predispose patients to impaired healing.

Rarely, apparently spontaneous ulceration and sequestration may occur.[5] This usually occurs on the lingual aspect of the posterior mandible in the region of the mylohyoid line. It is thought that disruption of the periosteal microcirculation by minor trauma in a region of cortical bone predisposes to this sequestration.

A number of conditions can impair host defenses and lead to infections with impaired healing of bone. The causes of immunocompromise are discussed elsewhere but can be viewed as falling into one of four groups: systemic, congenital defects, iatrogenic, or social.

In addition to the host factors and anatomic features of the mandible, the biomechanics of the fixation of mandibular fixation are important. Excessive movement has been shown to have a deleterious effect on fracture healing. This led to the concept of rigid internal fixation to allow bone healing by primary bone healing. The desirability of primary bone healing was questioned recently, and there is an increasing acceptance of the concept of functionally stable fixation, which allows for a small amount of healing via callus formation. Central to the use of functionally stable fixation is the understanding of the concepts of load sharing and load bearing. Put simply, load-sharing osteosynthesis depends on the ability of the bone to share some of the functional load during the period of healing, whereas load-bearing osteosynthesis requires that the full functional load be borne by the fixation. Recognition of the concept of load sharing has allowed for the use of resorbable fixation systems and smaller metal fixation systems in certain cases. In contrast, many cases of malunion and nonunion can be traced to not recognizing a situation in which load-bearing osteosynthesis was required (Figure 1).

DELAYED UNION, MALUNION, AND NONUNION

In ideal circumstances, adequate reduction and fixation of a mandibular fracture in an otherwise

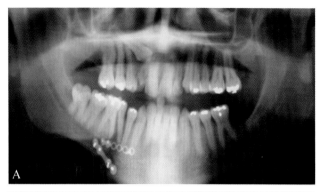

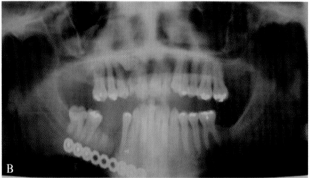

Figure 1.   *A*, Panorex radiograph showing nonunion of the mandible secondary to inadequate fixation. *B*, Panorex radiograph showing postoperative reduction and rigid internal fixation using a 2.4 mm locking reconstruction plate.

healthy adult will allow healing in 4 to 6 weeks and in 2 to 4 weeks for a child. In the dentate patient, the occlusion should be restored to the premorbid state. Healing extended beyond this period represents delayed union.[6] It is possible that such healing represents a variation of normal and complete healing may ultimately occur. In the mandible, healing that has not occurred within 4 months is delayed. If healing has not occurred within 6 to 8 months of treatment, nonunion of the fracture is present. In some cases, a fibrous union may be present. In rare instances, this may be functionally adequate. Inadequate reduction or loss of reduction leads to malunion. In such cases, the bone may have fully healed but is functionally impaired. In the mandible, this most commonly manifests as a post-treatment malocclusion. If the fracture was in the condylar region, altered mandibular movement may be seen. Inadequate fixation allows movement of the bone ends. This can lead to eburnation of the bone ends, deposition of fibrous tissue, and, if communication with the oral cavity persists (eg, via the periodontal ligament), the introduction of infection. An appreciation of the difference between the types of impaired bony union is important in the planning and timing of treatment.

Mathog and colleagues reviewed 900 patients with mandibular fractures seen over a 5-year period and found a 2.8% incidence of nonunion.[7] They concluded that the incidence of nonunion appears to be unchanged over time, regardless of the varied and presumably advanced methods of fixation and reduction. They found that the body region of the mandible was most commonly affected. This is consistent with other reports.[6]

MY APPROACH TO MANAGEMENT

When dealing with a mandibular injury that has not healed as planned, it is important to have a systematic approach to formulating treatment goals. The goals I lay out are as follows:

1. Optimizing host healing potential
2. Eradication of any infection
3. Restoration of bony continuity
4. Restoration of occlusion or preparation for occlusal reconstruction
5. Pain-free movement of the mandible with normal range

A careful history and examination will help identify any factors that need to be corrected to optimize healing potential. Review of notes and imaging from any previous treatment can be helpful in identifying factors that may have compromised healing (eg, reliance on load-bearing osteosynthesis in a complex fracture, poor patient compliance with treatment). Correction of these is an essential first step.

Infection is typically a consequence of excessive mobility at the fracture site as a result of delayed treatment or inadequate fixation. Osteomyelitis of the mandible, although often stated as a concern in cases of infected nonunion, is, fortunately, rare. The infections seen are more frequently an osteitis and resolve quickly with adequate stable fixation of the mandible, débridement, and antibiotics. Adequate rigid fixation

will help with healing and should not be delayed to allow solely medical management of any infection present. Recent work by Benson and colleagues showed that primary bone grafting can be carried out in such circumstances with predictable results.[8]

Restoration of bony continuity may be possible by adequate rigid internal fixation alone as this will provide an optimal environment for healing. If a gap defect is present, then bone grafting may be required. There are a variety of possible sources for cancellous grafts, cortico-cancellous grafts, or osseous flaps. In the absence of massive tissue loss as seen with gunshot injuries, most cases will not require microvascular reconstruction. As mentioned above, primary grafting, even in the presence of purulence, is a viable treatment option if there is an adequate vascular bed, host factors have been optimized, and the fracture is rigidly fixed. The use of platelet-rich plasma (PRP) has been advocated by some as an adjunct to bone grafting. I find that the main value of PRP with cancellous bone grafting is that it improves the handling of the graft and helps it stay where it is placed.

In most cases, it will be necessary to place the fixation via a transcutaneous approach. This must be discussed with the patient in advance. Placement of adequate rigid fixation via a transoral approach is complicated by an inability to get the screws at the correct angle to the plate to allow bicortical fixation without compromising the tooth roots or inferior alveolar canal.

My preferred fixation device is the locking reconstruction plate. This provides good rigidity and the ability for bicortical fixation. The locking of the screw into the plate allows the plate to act as an "internal" external fixator and allows for slight latitude in the contouring of the plate to the bone. This minimizes torquing forces on the bone and loosening of the screws, with subsequent hardware failure. The locking reconstruction plate has an important application in the management of the atrophic edentulous mandible, which is particularly prone to nonunion and malunion. The saddle area of the mandible is a common site of fracture as it is the site of greatest resorption in the edentulous mandible. It is an area that is frequently brittle and prone to fragmentation if screw placement is attempted. The locking reconstruction plate allows spanning of the fracture site and the placement of the screw in the region of the symphysis and angles, where bone thickness is better preserved and screw placement is more predictable (Figure 2).

Restoration of the occlusion may be challenging. Many patients present with a premorbid occlusion that is not optimal. Sufficient teeth may not be present to determine the occlusion. This may be due to previous tooth loss, loss of teeth at the time of the injury, or subsequent tooth loss as a result of infection after injury. Not infrequently, patients are unable to explain what the problem with their occlusion is; they complain only that their "bite" is not right. In such cases, study models, in addition to clinical examination and radiographs, may be helpful.

The study models can be observed for clues to help determine the occlusion, such as wear facets. In cases in which there is an element of union of the fracture, "model surgery" can be carried out to cut the models in the region of the previous fractures and allow movement of the tooth-bearing segments into a position that allows more optimal occlusion. Splint fabrication to facilitate the postioning of the jaws in an optimal occlusion is also possible on the study models. In cases in which there has been malunion of condylar fractures, the study models may show how an optimal occlusion may be obtained by repositioning of the maxilla, a more stable and technically straightforward procedure than reosteotomy of the condylar fracture.

In some cases, such as as a result of tooth loss or extensive comminution, it may not be possible to restore the occlusion. In such cases, thought must be given to secondary restoration of the

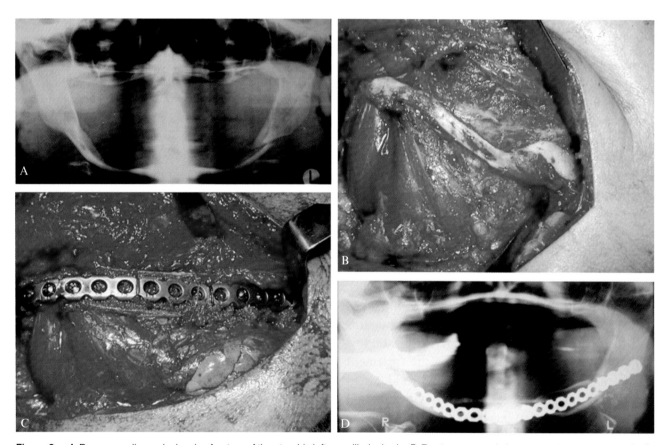

Figure 2. *A*, Panorex radiograph showing fracture of the atrophic left mandibular body. *B*, Fracture exposed via a transcutaneous approach. *C*, Fracture rigidly fixed and bone graft placed. *D*, Postoperative Panorex radiograph showing rigid fixation and bone graft in place. Note placement of the bone graft on non fractured atrophic right side to facilitate subsequent implant placement.

occlusion. It may be possible to carry out ancillary procedures at the time of correction of the nonunion or malunion to help optimize later rehabilitation of the occlusion. An example of this would be the placement of bone grafts to augment the alveolus and allow subsequent implant placement.

For restoration of the occlusion to be successful at the time of surgery, adequate control of the occlusion is vital. If used, arch bars must be accurately contoured and securely fixed to the teeth. The teeth must be firmly held in occlusion at the time of rigid fixation. It is vital that the surgeon is happy with the occlusion at the time of the rigid fixation. If the occlusion is wrong, the rigid fixation "rigidly fixes" the mistake in place. I occasionally run some cold-cure acrylic across the intermaxillary fixation to help secure the occlusion at the time of the rigid fixation. It is easily removed with the wires at the end of the case.

The last of the treatment goals, pain-free movement with normal range, depends on optimal operative and postoperative management. Adequate rigid internal fixation allows restoration of mandibular continuity and an early return to functional movement. Patients must be followed in the postoperative period and trained to practice range of motion exercises to help stretch shortened muscles, reduce edema, and break down any adhesions present. This phase of treatment is frequently overlooked by both the surgeon and patients. A number of aids are available. Tongue spatulas, stacked on top of each other and placed between the incisors, are as effective as the new devices, such as the Therabite (Atos Medical Inc, 11390 West Theodore Trecker Way, West Allis, WI 53214), if used diligently. Poor compliance with follow-up is an unfortunate reality among this group of patients. It is important to emphasize this phase of therapy when agreeing on the treatment plan with patients. A realistic goal would be an interincisal opening of 35 to 40 mm with minimal deviation. If treatment has been delayed, it may be necessary to carry out a manipulation under anesthesia (brisement force) to break down any adhesion present.

To summarize my approach to the nonunited mandibular fracture:

1. Identify and optimize host factors
2. Treat any associated infection
3. Determine occlusion and plan for perioperative control
4. Expose fractures
5. Débride the fracture site as needed. Mobilize the fracture site.
6. Control the occlusion
7. Apply rigid fixation
8. Bone graft if required
9. Careful soft tissue closure externally and intraorally
10. Early temporomandibular joint mobilization of the mandible postoperatively
11. Physical therapy with rehabilitation

OSTEORADIONECROSIS

As mentioned earlier, radiation to the mandible can result in changes to the bone and its microcirculation, diminishing the potential of the bone to heal after trauma or surgery. If the bone is sufficiently devitalized, healing may not occur. The devitalized bone may persist unhealed and become exposed transcutaneously and/or transorally. If this situation persists for more than 3 months, it is known as ORN, although there has been no agreement on strict diagnostic criteria. It is distinct from tumor recurrence. Store and Boysen suggested the following definition of ORN: radiologic evidence of bone necrosis in the radiation field where tumor recurrence has been excluded.[9] This definition recognizes the fact that the radiographic changes may precede any overt clinical symptoms. The severity of the condition may vary from a small amount of painless exposed bone (Figure 3) to pathologically fractured bone with multiple orocutaneous fistulae and intractable pain (Figure 4). Schwartz and Kagan proposed a classification system that is based on clinical findings.[10] They also identify several facts about ORN:

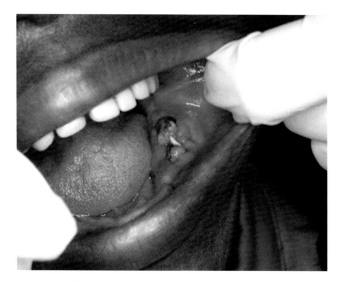

Figure 3. Early osteoradionecrosis of the left mandible.

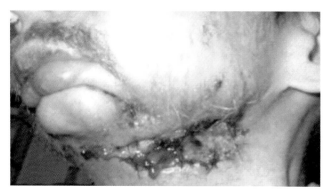

Figure 4. Florid osteoradionecrosis and soft tissue radiation injury. Multiple local recurrences precluded hyperbaric oxygen therapy.

1. It is more common in the mandible than in the maxilla.
2. It is more likely to occur if the mandible is in a treatment field of greater than 6,000 cGy.
3. It frequently follows some form of trauma to the bone, often dental extraction (Figure 5).

4. It is primarily a wound healing and not an infective problem, although infection, particularly with *Actinomyces* spp, may complicate it.[11]

Although host factors, similar to those implicated in nonunion of the mandible, are implicated in the onset of ORN, the radiation to the bone predisposes the bone to necrosis. The mechanism for this is disputed. Marx and Johnson suggested that radiation to the jawbones renders the bone hypocellular, hypoxic, and hypovascular.[3] This was used as the rationale for the utility of hyperbaric oxygen (HBO) therapy in the management and prevention of ORN. This mechanism was challenged recently.[12] Osteoclasia secondary to radiation damage to the osteoclasts has been suggested as the basis of ORN. This view has been supported by those who contend that ORN shares its pathogenesis with the recently noted entity of bisphosphonate-related osteonecrosis. A third mechanism suggests that fibroatrophic changes may be significant.[12] The incidence of ORN has been estimated between 4 and 35% after irradiation.[11] The interval between radiation and the development of ORN may be several years. Indeed, it has been suggested that the risk of developing ORN increases with time after radiation. The introduction of megavoltage radiation techniques may lead to a decreased incidence.

Classification of ORN is controversial. Marx was, apparently, the first to classify ORN.[4] His system was based on the response to HBO therapy and did not directly address the under-

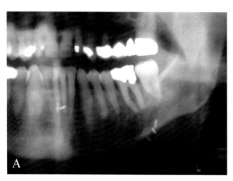
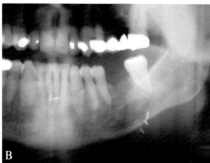
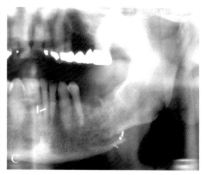

Figure 5. *A*, Panorex radiograph showing apical radiolucency associated with tooth number 19. *B*, Panorex radiograph following extraction showing progression of radiolucency consistent with stage II osteoradionecrosis (ORN). *C*, Panorex radiograph showing progression of ORN with pathologic fracture.

lying disease. More recently, Schwartz and Kagan proposed a clinical staging of the condition.[10] In stage I, there is exposed cortical bone with minimal soft tissue ulceration. In stage II, there is localized necrosis of the cortical and medullary bone. It is subdivided into two groups depending on the amount of soft tissue ulceration. Stage III shows diffuse involvement of the bone, including the lower border. As with stage II ORN, there is subdivision into two groups.

Clinical findings in ORN include pain, swelling, and soft tissue ulceration, including orocutaneous fistulae. Malocclusion may occur following pathologic fracture, but as many patients with ORN are edentulous, the fracture may represent an incidental radiographic finding (Figure 6).

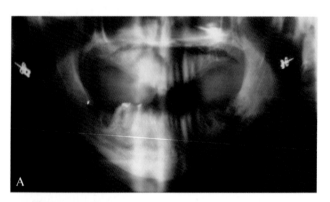

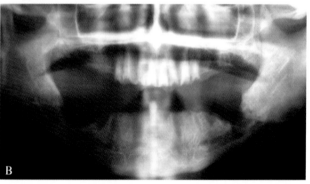

Figure 6. *A*, Panorex radiograph showing bilateral osteoradionecrosis (ORN). The right side was entirely symptomless. Note the multiple retained roots. *B*, Panorex radiograph showing pathologic fracture of the left mandible. This occurred approximately 3 months after 40 dives of hyperbaric oxygen, débridement of areas of ORN bilterally, and removal of retained, carious mandibular roots (the maxillary roots were retained at the patient's request to help retain an overdenture). The patient was unaware of the fracture of the left mandible.

TREATMENT

Prevention of ORN is the first consideration. Preoperative dental evaluation for patients with a head and neck malignancy for whom radiotherapy (and or chemotherapy) is considered should be routine practice. If teeth with a poor prognosis in the proposed field of radiation are identified, early removal should be considered. It has been suggested that 2 to 3 weeks of healing should be allowed prior to starting radiotherapy. This is frequently not possible, and in such cases, radiotherapy should not be delayed. If subsequent extraction is required, prophylactic HBO may be helpful in the prevention of ORN. The use of HBO prophylactically is not universally accepted as there have been no randomized trials demonstrating its value.[13] A number of case reviews do, however, suggest that HBO is of value in preventing ORN.[14] Prophylactic antibiotics are typically given regardless of HBO use, but the basis for this is empiric.

Established ORN can be a significant management challenge. Treatment not infrequently fails to prevent the progression of ORN. Conservative treatment of early ORN (exposed bone with no radiographic changes) includes optimizing host factors, refraining from smoking, and good oral hygiene, including the use of antiseptic mouthrinses. Antibiotics are commonly prescribed.

The use of HBO for the treatment of ORN has been suggested by many authors for decades.[3,12] HBO is thought to reverse the hypoxia, hypovascularity, and hypoxia of irradiated bone by improving the oxygen gradient and stimulating a number of growth factors, leading to fibroblast proliferation, increased collagen synthesis, and angiogenesis. The production of oxygen free radicals is thought to be antibacterial and may help eradicate any associated infection. HBO has been used extensively as an adjunct to conservative and surgical management of ORN. There are, however, few controlled trials showing a clear benefit. This, coupled with the prolonged treatment time, a limited number of hyperbaric facilities, and cost, has led to difficulties in insurance coverage for HBO therapy, making the establishment of good-quality trials difficult.

Regardless of the use of HBO, ORN that fails to respond to conservative measures needs to be débrided. In the absence of radiographic changes in the lower border or pathologic fracture, transoral débridement should be attempted where possible with minimal disruption to the oral soft tissues. Débridement to bleeding bone should be carried out. Soft tissue closure over the bone may be difficult owing to scarring and fibrosis. An antiseptic impregnated pack (eg, gauze soaked in Whitehead's varnish) may be placed over a small mucosal defect to protect forming granulation tissue from trauma. If a large mucosal defect is present, fresh soft tissue needs to be brought into the area. This can be done with regional flaps or free tissue transfer.

In advanced cases of ORN (pathologic fracture, orocutaneous fistula), resection of the involved bone with rigid fixation is required. This is similar to the management of the mandibular nonunion. However, in cases of ORN, the segmental defect is typically significantly larger. A decision needs to be made whether to carry out a primary reconstruction using free tissue transfer or an interval reconstruction. Free tissue transfer has been suggested to represent the standard of care (Figure 7),[12] but many patients with ORN are high-risk patients for major reconstructive surgery. For high-risk patients, resection of the necrotic bone and rigid fixation using a reconstruction plate may provide good medium-term symptom relief.

MY APPROACH TO MANAGEMENT

To summarize my approach to ORN of the mandible:

1. Identify and optimize host factors; assess the patient's fitness for reconstruction
2. Treat any associated infection; exclude the recurrence of neoplasia
3. Determine the extent of ORN
4. HBO therapy, if possible

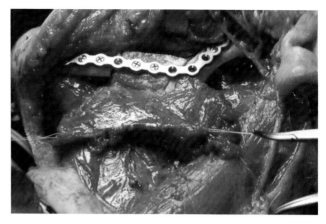

Figure 7. Deep circumflex iliac artery free flap in situ to reconstruct a defect after segmental resection. Note the abundant soft tissue recruited with the flap. Courtesy of Mr. D.A. Mitchell, Leeds, England.

5. Assess the response to HBO
6. Débride as needed if the response is inadequate
7. If there is a segmental defect and the patient is a candidate for definitive reconstruction free tissue transfer, ensure that adequate fresh soft tissue is brought in
8. If unable to definitively reconstruct, rigidly fix the mandible with a reconstruction plate and a locoregional flap to recruit soft tissue
9. Careful soft tissue closure externally and intraorally
10. Postoperative HBO therapy

NEW THERAPIES

An improved understanding of the importance of stable rigid fixation of mandibular fractures has reduced but not eliminated the problem of nonunion. Further advances in bone biotechnology might help identify those growth factors, bone morphogenetic proteins, etc., that can help accelerate poor healing and perhaps obviate the need for autogenous bone grafting, which is currently the most effective adjunct. The true role of PRP in assisting healing has not been determined.

The rethinking of the underlying pathophysiology of ORN has led to possible alternative management therapies. The fibroatrophic model for ORN has opened opportunities for the use of antioxidants and antifibrotic drugs.

Pentoxifylline and vitamin E were recently investigated.[16] The need for controlled trials of HBO to determine its role in the management of ORN remains. The recognition of bisphosphonate-related osteonecrosis has highlighted the need for a better understanding of the role of the osteoclast.[17] Therapies used for other osteoclast-related diseases, such as topical phenytoin in osteopetrosis, may have a role.[18] A more complete understanding of the underlying pathology will direct future therapies.

REFERENCES

1. Bradley JC. Age changes in the vascular supply of the mandible. Br Dent J 1972;132:142–4.
2. Bradley JC. The clinical significance of age changes in the vascular supply to the mandible. Int J Oral Surg 1981; 10 Suppl 1:71–6.
3. Marx RE, Johnson RP. Problem wounds in oral and maxillofacial surgery: the role of hyperbaric oxygen. In: Davis JC, Hunt TK, editors. Problem wounds: the role of oxygen. New York: Elsevier; 1988. p. 65–123.
4. Marx R. A new concept in the treatment of osteoradionecrosis. J Oral Maxillofac Surg 1983;41:168–71.
5. Peters E, Lovas GL, Wysocki GP. Lingual mandibular sequestration and ulceration. Oral Surg Oral Med Oral Pathol 1993;75:740–3.
6. Mathog RH, Boies LR. Nonunion of the mandible. Laryngoscope 1976;86:908–20.
7. Mathog RH, Toma V, Clayman L, Wolf S. Nonunion of the mandible: an analysis of contributing factors. J Oral Maxillofac Surg 2000;58:746–52.
8. Benson PD, Marshall MK, Engelstad ME, et al. The use of immediate bone grafting in reconstruction of clinically infected mandibular fractures: bonegrafts in the presence of pus. J Oral Maxillofac Surg 2006;64:122–6.
9. Store G, Boysen M. Mandibular osteoradionecrosis: clinical behaviour and diagnostic aspects. Clin Otolaryngol 2000;25:378–84.
10. Schwartz HC, Kagan AR. Osteoradionecrosis of the mandible: scientific basis for clinical staging. Am J Clin Oncol 2002;25:168–71.
11. Hansen T, Kunkel M, Kirkpatrick CJ, Weber A. *Actinomyces* in infected osteoradionecrosis—underestimated? Hum Pathol 2006;37:61–7.
12. Teng MS, Futran ND. Osteoradionecrosis of the mandible. Curr Opin Otolaryngol Head Neck Surg 2005;13:217–21.
13. Sulaiman F, Huryn JM, Zlotolow IM. Dental extractions in the irradiated head and neck patient: a retrospective analysis of Memorial Sloan-Kettering Cancer Center protocols, criteria, and end results. J Oral Maxillofac Surg 2003;61:1123–31.
14. Chavez JA, Adkinson CD. Adjunctive hyperbaric oxygen therapy in irradiated patients requiring dental extractions: outcomes and complications. J Oral Maxillofac Surg 2001;59:518–22.
15. Peleg M, Lopez EA. The treatment of osteoradionecrosis of the mandible: the case for hyperbaric oxygen and bone graft reconstruction. J Oral Maxillofac Surg 2006; 64:956–60.
16. Delanian S, Depondt J, Lefaix JL. Major healing of refractory mandible osteoradionecrosis after treatment combining pentoxifylline and tocopherol: a phase II trial. Head Neck 2005;27:114–23.
17. Hellstein JW, Marek CL. Bisphosphonate osteochemonecrosis (bis-phossy jaw): is this phossy jaw of the 21st century? J Oral Maxillofac Surg 2005;63:682–9.
18. Topical phenytoin treatment in bimaxillary osteomyelitis secondary to infantile osteopetrosis: report of a case. Nuray Er, Oğuzcan Kasaboğlu, Aytuğ Atabek, Kerem Öktemer, Murat Akkocaoðlu. J Oral Maxillofac Surg 2006;64:1160–4.

18

Irradiated Temporal Bone

Yoav Hahn, MD; Hilary A. Brodie, MD, PhD

Treatment of tumors of the head and neck and brain malignancies often includes radiation therapy. Radiation therapy is used both as primary treatment and adjunctive therapy postoperatively in relatively high doses. Radiation used alone or in combination with surgery has significantly impacted survival rates in the treatment of head and neck cancer. In addition, suffering has been reduced by palliation. However, the effects of radiation therapy on surrounding structures are at times profound, often introducing a new set of problems. This chapter focuses on the effects of radiation on the temporal bone and in particular on the complication of osteoradionecrosis of the temporal bone.

Radiation therapy to tissue produces hypoxia, hypovascularity, and hypocellularity and impairs normal collagen synthesis and cell production. This series of effects can lead to tissue breakdown and a chronic, nonhealing wound. Osteoradionecrosis has been defined as exposed irradiated bone that fails to heal over a period of 3 months.[1] Exposure of nontarget organs during radiotherapy of the head and neck is unavoidable. Numerous animal and human studies have examined the deleterious effects of radiation. However, clear-cut data on the incidence, type, and severity of radiation-induced ear toxicity are scarce.

HISTORY

Historically, radiotherapy was involved in the management of numerous benign and malignant human disorders, including chronic ear infections, hearing loss, and otitis media.[2] A technique called "nasopharyngeal radium therapy" was developed in the 1920s to treat children with hearing loss caused by repeated ear infections. Insertion of an applicator with a capsule of radium through each nostril with placement of the radium near the eustachian tube orifice for 8 to 12 minutes was the method of treatment. In addition to otitis media, this treatment was used for tonsillitis, sinusitis, bronchitis, asthma, and repeated viral and bacterial infections. Five hundred thousand to 2 million civilians, mostly children, received these treatments, as estimated by the US Veterans Affairs Office. Also, between 8,000 and 20,000 military personnel received them during World War II and up until about 1960.[3]

These treatments were abandoned because of a significantly increased risk of the development of head and neck cancers.[4-6] The effect of radiation on the inner ear was soon recognized and intensively studied in human and animal studies.[7] Animal models have been used to study the effects of radiation since 1905 when Ewald placed beads containing radium in the area of the middle ear in pigeons and noted labyrinthine symptoms.[8] In 1962, the first human study on the effects of radiation therapy on the ear was published and included audiologic tests in 14 head and neck cancer patients.[9]

ETIOLOGY AND FINDINGS

Radiation damage can occur from the external ear to the central auditory pathways and may cause significant damage to the osseous temporal bone. It may result in conductive, sensorineural, or mixed hearing loss, and the bony damage may involve a localized area or be a diffuse process with severe ramifications.

External Ear

The effects of radiation to the external ear may involve the pinna, external auditory canal, and periauricular region. These effects may be broken down into acute and late reactions. Acute events include erythema, dry and moist desquamation, or ulceration of the skin of the auricle and external auditory canal (Figure 1). These acute changes are often associated with otalgia and otorrhea. Late skin changes include atrophy, ulceration, external auditory canal stenosis, otitis externa, and cholesteatoma formation.[10] In 1962, Borsanyi reported a series of 100 consecutive patients who received radiation to the head and neck. Breakdown of the external canal skin occurred in 10% of patients. Destruction of the apocrine and sebaceous glands and epithelial damage decreased wax secretion.[11] Skin necrosis has been observed in up to 13% of patients treated with hypofractionated orthovoltage x-rays or electron irradiation for tumors of the pinna[12,13] and seems to be lower in cases of brachytherapy[14] or irradiation for skin cancer at other sites. Two studies reviewing 313 and 138 patients treated with orthovoltage or electrons

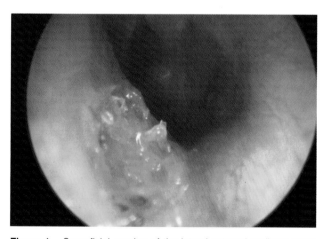

Figure 1. Superficial erosion of the lateral external auditory canal secondary to radiation damage.

showed that the risk of late skin necrosis was higher with a high daily fraction size (> 4 Gy) and a large field size (> 5 cm^2).[13] There is no demonstrated impact of the patient's age, histology, tumor location, radiation modality, and beam energy, whereas the impact of the total dose remains controversial.

Middle Ear

The effects of radiation on the middle ear are well known. The term *radiation otitis media* has been used to describe the syndrome of hyperemia of the tympanic membrane, serous middle ear effusion, mucosal edema, and, occasionally, suppurative otitis media.[15] Patients are known to develop a sterile transudate within the middle ear, contributing to a conductive hearing loss. Otitis media can be induced by transient edema and dysfunction of the eustachian tube. Blockage of the eustachian tube occurs in the cartilaginous segment or at the pharyngeal opening of the tube. The eustachian tube normally functions to equilibrate the pressure within the middle ear to atmospheric pressure. Equilibration occurs when swallowing, which transiently opens the eustachian tube. At rest, the eustachian tube remains closed to minimize resonance of sound while speaking and to avoid reflux into the middle ear. Compromise of normal eustachian tube function, along with resorption of gas by the middle ear mucosa, leads to negative pressure within the middle ear, retraction of the tympanic membrane, and increased tension in the ossicular chain. This combination of events often leads to increased impedance of sound and a resultant conductive hearing loss. The tympanic membrane is observed to be thickened in some cases several months after radiation.[16] In addition, radiation has been known to cause ossicular fixation, ossicular erosion, middle ear adhesions, and tympanic membrane perforations.[17,18] A study by Leach examined the changes in the temporal bone following radiation therapy.[19] The middle ear and mastoid cells were filled with exudates, and marked bony resorption was noted. In addition, the organ of Corti was destroyed.

The conductive hearing loss that may result from radiation to the temporal bone may be transient or permanent based on the etiology. If the hearing loss is due to an effusion within the middle ear, this may be transient in nature as long as the effusion resolves. On the other hand, if changes to the ossicular chain occur, the resultant hearing loss may be permanent in nature. Also, radiation damage to the eustachian tube may result in a persistently patent or patulous eustachian tube. In this condition, the patient will complain of autophony, hearing the resonance of his or her own breathing and voice in the affected ear.

Eustachian tube dysfunction, together with resorption of oxygen by middle ear mucosa, leads to the creation of a vacuum in the middle ear. This, in turn, leads to retraction of the tympanic membrane into the middle ear and superior aspect of the middle ear, the epitympanum. Pockets can form as the tympanic membrane retracts inward. The most common locations for retraction pocket formation are the posterosuperior quadrant of the middle ear (Figure 2) and into the epitympanum (Figure 3). As the depth of the pocket progresses, desquamating keratin

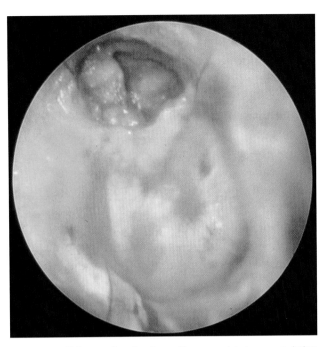

Figure 3. Epitympanic retraction with some debris accumulating within the pocket.

often collects within the pocket, forming a cholesteatoma. The collection of keratin debris results in further expansion of the pocket and erosion of bone, which the newly forming cholesteatoma encounters. The contents of the sac often become infected, leading to chronic or recurrent otorrhea. Cholesteatomas form over months to years and are often insidious in nature. As they expand, cholesteatomas can erode through the ossicles, labyrinth, and facial nerve and even intracranially. Figure 4 demonstrates

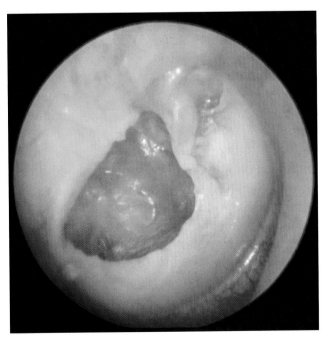

Figure 2. Large broad based retraction pocket into the posterosuperior quadrant of the middle ear. There is no buildup of skin or debris within the pocket.

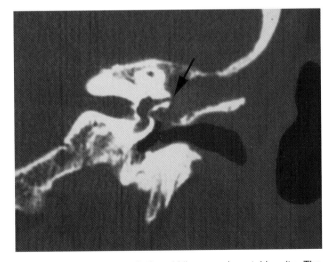

Figure 4. Cholesteatoma in the middle ear and mastoid cavity. The horizontal semicircular canal has been eroded by the cholesteatoma.

erosion of the horizontal semicircular canal on a coronal computed tomographic (CT) scan of the temporal bone by a cholesteatoma. Eventually, these skin cysts can lead to intracranial complications of meningitis, brain abscess, lateral sinus thrombosis, and otitic hydrocephalus. Given that these result from eustachian tube dysfunction, they can be prevented by bypassing the eustachian tube with insertion of a pressure equalization tube into the tympanic membrane. The pressure equalization tube allows for continuous equilibration of middle ear pressure with atmospheric pressure, thereby preventing the negative pressure from developing in the middle ear.

Inner Ear

Sensorineural hearing loss is a serious radiation-induced complication to the inner ear. This hearing loss may occur in the acute setting but more commonly affects the hearing months to years after the completion of radiation therapy. Sensorineural hearing loss may develop either as a primary toxic effect of radiation therapy on the cochlea or as a secondary effect of arterial occlusion or chronic infection. Progressive degeneration and atrophy of the inner ear sensory structures, fibrosis, and ossification of the inner ear fluid spaces are seen. Hemorrhage in the inner ear spaces and edema of the membranous labyrinth have been demonstrated, along with loss of cells in inner and outer hair cells, atrophy and degeneration of the stria vascularis, a reduced number of capillaries, degeneration of endothelial cells in vessels, and atrophy of the spiral ganglion cells and the cochlear nerve.[20]

Radiation-induced sensorineural hearing loss occurs in about one-third of patients treated with definitive radiation with fields including the inner ear.[21–23] Borsanyi observed temporary perceptive hearing loss with recruitment in 6 of 40 patients, which he attributed to transient radiation vasculitis.[15] Leach reported a 36% incidence of sensorineural loss, with early and late sequelae developing in a non-dose-dependent fashion.[19] Delayed sensorineural hearing loss often has a

chronic, progressive, and irreversible pattern.[24] It typically develops 6 to 24 months after irradiation and may progress to complete deafness over weeks and months. Impairment may also affect the vestibular system in a similar fashion; toxicity to neuroepithelial cells or the secondary effects of ischemia or infection may cause vertigo and abnormalities on electronystagmography (ENG). Changes on ENG have been seen in as many as 44% of patients who underwent radiation that involved the ear.[25] Many of these patients, however, remain asymptomatic because of the gradual loss of vestibular function and compensation that occurs.

PATHOGENESIS

Tissues have a unique response to the effects of radiation. Some tissues, such as lymphatics and skin, are more radiosensitive, whereas others, such as bone and nerve tissue, are generally more radioresistant. Healthy bone may withstand radiation very well. However, the incidence of osteoradionecrosis of the mandible is found to be between 5 and 10% when treating an intraoral malignancy. This has been described as an "acceptable incidence" of osteoradionecrosis after radiation to the oral cavity.[26] The mandible is certainly at risk because of its close proximity to oral secretions, infected teeth, a relatively poor blood supply, and superficial location. Historically, chronic damage to normal tissue irradiated with high-dose radiation was thought to be caused by trauma and infection.[27] In the 1980s, Marx suggested a new pathogenesis for radiation-induced tissue breakdown: the hypoxic-hypocellular-hypovascular ("three H") principle, tissue breakdown, and a nonhealing chronic wound.[28] Marx postulated that the body relies on cellular turnover to maintain healthy function. The hypoxic-hypocellular-hypovascular tissue that is created by the radiation damage has retarded cellular turnover, and fibrosis and spontaneous tissue breakdown ensue.

Whereas direct cellular injury results from radiation, an indirect effect secondary to obliterative endarteritis results in permanent epithelial thickening and subepithelial fibrosis. Fine blood vessel density is reduced by the edema of the vascular endothelium in bone and leads to aseptic vascular necrosis. Osteoblastic activity ceases, whereas osteoclastic cells continue breaking down bone. This causes a relative inequality in these cells, with a shift toward increased bone porosity and bone regeneration below normal. Histopathologically, empty lacunae and a preponderance of osteoclasts with spicules of dead bone surrounded by connective tissue are seen.[29] The end result is an aseptic necrosis followed by reparative fibrosis, with the affected bone prone to injury, fracture, and infection. Similar to the mandible, the temporal bone's susceptibility to radiation damage appears to be related to such factors as its superficial location, close proximity to infection, a relatively poor blood supply, and histologically compact architecture.[30]

RISK FACTORS

It is not entirely clear why some patients develop osteoradionecrosis but others do not. Certain factors that have been shown to be associated with the development of osteoradionecrosis include the dosage of radiation given, underlying medical conditions that may impair the patient's immune system and healing process (diabetes and immunosuppression), or preexisting or concomitant infection of the middle ear and temporal bone. Patients with a preexisting hearing impairment, autoimmune disease, recurrent otitis media, Meniere's disease, otosclerosis, acoustic nerve tumors, paraneoplastic syndromes, mastoiditis, surgical damage, microvascular disease, otologic insults with delayed effects (eg, previous irradiation, syphilis), and genetic anomalies (eg, Cogan's syndrome, Usher's syndrome) or with idiopathic sudden sensorineural hearing loss are at high risk.[31] The type of radiation that is used may also have a factor in the development of osteoradionecrosis. When megavoltage is used, the absorption of energy by bone and soft tissue is equal as opposed to orthovoltage, which causes

an increased absorption by bone. However, clinical studies have not shown a difference in severity or a decreased incidence of disease with megavoltage.[32,33]

Assessing the risk of postirradiation ear damage related to the site of disease reveals that nasopharyngeal carcinoma, which has as its primary treatment combination chemotherapy and radiotherapy, places otologic structures most at risk. Even with CT- guided treatment plans for radiotherapy of the nasopharynx, the cochlea may actually receive a greater calculated radiation dose than the primary tumor site.[34] In addition, for primary cancers of the nasopharynx, it is unavoidable that the eustachian tubes always receive essentially the full tumor dose. Consequently, audiograms show significant hearing loss in up to 50% of patients treated with radiotherapy for tumors of the nasopharynx.[35] Radiation for nasopharyngeal carcinoma has also been associated with tinnitus, with up to 30% of patients reporting intermittent tinnitus at 12 months after treatment.[36] In addition, a patulous eustachian tube is commonly seen in patients after radiation for nasopharynx tumors. There has been no correlation shown between the dose of radiation and the late effect of a patulous eustachian tube (Table 1).[21,37,38]

SCORING SYSTEMS

Radiation-induced changes in the temporal bone have been studied extensively from the pathologic aspect. Only more recently, however, have

Table 1 FACTORS ASSOCIATED WITH THE HIGH RISK OF POSTIRRADIATION HEARING IMPAIRMENT
Total radiotherapy dose
Cisplatin-based chemotherapy
Fraction dose > 2 Gy
Number of isocenters used
Conventional RT vs IMRT
Neurofibromatosis 2
Hearing deficit before RT
Secretory otitis media after RT
Site of tumor
Involvement of the upper cervical lymph nodes
Tumor size

IMRT = intensity-modulated radiation therapy; RT = radiation therapy.

various scoring systems been developed to assess the damage secondary to radiation. The Radiation Therapy Oncology Group (RTOG) criteria include acute but not late ear morbidity and can be applied in a retrospective analysis (Table 2). The late effects of radiation-induced ear toxicity can be better scored by the Late Effects of Normal Tissue/Somatic Objective Management Analytic (LENT/SOMA) scoring system (Table 3). This system categorizes patients into different grades based on subjective and objective findings and recommends management based on the extent of injury. This system has not yet been validated in clinical practice, however.[32]

DOSING AND TECHNIQUE

Data on the dose-response relationship for ear morbidity are not great despite the numerous reports on radiation-induced hearing loss. The general policy of avoiding unnecessary irradiation of normal tissue should always be attempted. Studies have established general tolerance doses (TDs) for ear morbidity; the TD for acute radiation otitis has been set at 40 Gy and for chronic otitis at 65 to 70 Gy.[39] In addition, this same source found a TD of 60 Gy for sensorineural hearing loss and a TD of 70 Gy for vestibular damage. A review of multiple studies demonstrated that at least one-third of patients who received 70 Gy near the inner ear developed hearing impairment of 10 dB or more in the 4 kHz region.[40] In addition, the risk of otomastoiditis secondary to radiation is higher if the dose exceeds 50 Gy and if the portals include a field that is both anterior and posterior to the clival line.[41] These data listed above have been confirmed by several authors; some studies, however, do not show a relationship between radiation dose and ear damage.[25,42] Further large-scale, prospective studies are needed to evaluate this issue. Still unknown is precisely how much radiation of the inner ear occurs with standard protocols. Further studies are necessary

Table 2 ACUTE RADIATION EAR MORBIDITY ACCORDING TO THE RTOG SCORING CRITERIA	
Score	Ear Morbidity
0	No change over baseline
1	Mild external otitis with erythema, pruritus, secondary to dry desquamation not requiring medication. Audiogram unchanged from baseline.
2	Moderate external otitis requiring topical medication, serous otitis media, hypoacusis on testing only
3	Severe external otitis with discharge or moist desquamation, symptomatic hypoacusis, tinnitus; not drug related
4	Deafness

RTOG = Radiation Therapy Oncology Group.

Table 3 LATE RADIATION EAR MORBIDITY ACCORDING TO THE LENT/SOMA SCALE			
	Grade 1	Grade 2	Grade 3	Grade 4
Subjective				
Pain	Occasional and minimal	Intermittent and tolerable	Persistent and intense	Refractory and excruciating
Tinnitus	Occasional	Intermittent	Persistent	Refractory
Hearing	Minor loss	Frequent difficulties with faint speech	Frequent difficulties with loud speech	Complete deafness
Objective				
Skin	Dry desquamation	Otitis externa	Superficial ulceration	Deep ulceration, necrosis
5Hearing	< 10 dB loss in one or more frequencies	10–15 dB loss	15–20 dB loss	> 20 dB loss
Management				
Pain	Occasional non-narcotic	Regular non-narcotic	Regular narcotic	Parenteral narcotics
Skin	Occasional lubrication	Regular eardrops	Eardrums	Surgical intervention
Hearing loss			Hearing aid	Hearing aid

LENT/SOMA = Late Effects of Normal Tissue/Somatic Objective Management Analytic.

to quantify radiation scatter to the inner ear structures.

DIAGNOSIS

All patients who are to undergo radiation with fields that include the nasopharynx and temporal bone should have a baseline audiogram, including tympanometry and pure-tone audiometry, prior to initiation of therapy. In addition, patients should have a careful examination of the external auditory canal and tympanic membrane. Pure-tone audiometry tests the patient's subjective hearing thresholds and differentiates conductive, sensorineural, and mixed hearing loss. Tympanometry serves to objectively detect middle ear acoustic impedance and details middle ear aeration, ossicular chain mobility, and eustachian tube function. These tests should be performed on all patients with risk of damage to their hearing organ. The data should be used as baseline studies, and comparison should be made after the treatment course is complete. Should any of the findings be abnormal, a full otologic examination and workup should be initiated.

Ear complications following radiation therapy require débridement of the external auditory canal and careful inspection of the ear canal and tympanic membrane using an operating microscope. A follow-up audiogram assesses hearing and differentiates conductive from sensorineural hearing loss. A purely conductive hearing loss is associated with a disease process affecting the middle ear or external auditory canal. A sensorineural hearing loss component on an audiogram signifies damage proximal to the middle ear (ie, cochlear or retrocochlear lesions). These patients should be followed to monitor for progression of hearing loss, and further studies may need to be added to identify the cause of hearing loss.

Imaging of the temporal bone and brain is used to identify certain pathologies and to guide treatment options. CT demonstrates the condition of the temporal bone and middle ear. It is useful in assessing the size and extent of damage from cholesteatomas and the condition of the middle ear and mastoid mucosa. This preopera-

tive information guides the surgeon in the approach and provides warnings for potential complications. The CT scan in Figure 18-4 reveals erosion of the lateral semicircular canal by a cholesteatoma. Preoperative identification will reduce the likelihood of removing the matrix covering the fistula and thereby avoid severely damaging the inner ear. The management of osteoradionecrosis of the temporal bone can be guided with CT scans, which can demonstrate areas of necrotic bone and sequestra. CT scans can also detect fibrosis and neo-ossification within the lumen of the cochlea and labyrinth (Figure 5). Magnetic resonance imaging (MRI) can demonstrate postradiation injuries, such as labyrinthitis, ossification of the cochlea, hemorrhage into the inner ear spaces, neuronitis, and white matter lesions. In patients who develop very delayed ear disease or hearing loss, radiation-induced malignancies must be considered. These lesions are generally readily identified with MRI.

In addition to CT scans, bone scan and positron emission tomography (PET) can also be useful in accurate imaging of the bony structures and be helpful in evaluation of the extent of osteoradionecrosis.[43] However, bone and PET scans are rarely required in the management of radiation-induced injuries of the temporal bone. ENG can play a role in the assessment and management of vestibular injuries.

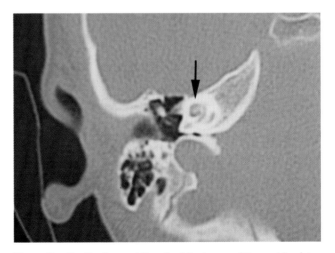

Figure 5. Ossification and fibrosis of the lumen of the cochlea from osteoradionecrosis can be visualized on CT scan imaging.

MANAGEMENT

External Ear

Patients who have undergone radiation to the region of the ear require counseling and guidance regarding care for the ear. Instrumenting the ear canal with any object, including cotton swabs, may result in otitis externa and lead to breakdown of external auditory canal skin. This may be the sentinel event in the development of osteoradionecrosis of the temporal bone. Patients are prone to manipulation of their ear canals because of the pruritis of the canal that frequently accompanies radiation therapy. When the pruritis is associated with dry canal skin, a drop of mineral oil in the ear canal, once a day, is often helpful.

In general, osteoradionecrosis nearly always starts with a nonhealing cutaneous defect. Initial treatment of temporal bone osteoradionecrosis consists of local therapy with débridement of squamous and purulent debris and maintenance of a dry, healthy environment. Removal of bony sequestra is required when these fragments of dead bone are expelled from the canal. Topical antibiotic otic drops and systemic antibiotics play a limited role in the management of this disease. This is a chronic, unresolving condition, and otic drops merely predispose the patient to otomycosis. Oral antibiotics are generally ineffective for the reason that the disease began in the first place: poor blood supply. Oral antibiotics are used, however, if adjacent cellulitis develops. Treatment of early otitis externa infections needs to be aggressive to decrease the chance that the infection may spread or incite a more diffuse inflammatory reaction. Cases of localized osteoradionecrosis may be treated with conservative measures. Ramsden and colleagues used conservative management (as described above) successfully for localized cases of osteoradionecrosis, with healing occurring from several months to 4 years after the initiation of therapy.[45] The more diffuse, aggressive case requires surgical intervention with complete removal of necrotic tissue wherever it is present.

Reconstruction with vascularized regional flaps and obliteration of the mastoid cavity may be necessary.

The disease process may involve a wider area than is clinically evident. Thus, minimal surgical débridement may not be adequate. It may be difficult to determine when all diseased tissue has been removed. All areas of frank necrosis need to be exenterated until healthy, viable bone or a vital structure is encountered. Often a repeat exploration of the area is required to débride devitalized bone and soft tissue further. In Ramsden and colleagues' study, five of nine patients requiring surgical treatment for diffuse osteoradionecrosis of the temporal bone required reexploration. Further studies have also found that multiple visits to the operating room are required to débride all devitalized bone. Inadequate treatment of osteoradionecrosis can lead to progressive involvement of adjacent structures, such as the facial nerve, sigmoid sinus, labyrinth, temporal lobe, and cerebellum, and other cranial nerves via the skull base.

Middle Ear

A reduction in middle ear pressure may ensue after radiation to the surrounding areas secondary to dysfunction of the eustachian tube. Radiation damage to the eustachian tube may hinder its ability to function in the manner described. Vasoconstricting medications, including nasal sprays and oral decongestants, rarely provide much assistance in reestablishing eustachian tube function. Nasal steroid sprays have been somewhat successful in reducing nasopharyngeal edema and improving eustachian tube function. If conservative measures fail, insertion of a ventilating tube into the tympanic membrane can function to relieve pain and improve hearing. Ventilating tubes are required when retraction pocket formation is identified. Early intervention can prevent cholesteatoma formation. Late intervention with ventilation tubes will not prevent further development of cholesteatomas once initiated. In one randomized trial, hearing improvement and a lower risk of sensorineural hearing loss were found in patients treated with ventilation tubes.[46] If negative pressure secondary to eustachian tube dysfunction is not the only problem and it is felt that there are middle ear mucosal changes, such as productive mucosa and granulation tissue, grommet tube insertion may not be indicated. In such cases, placement of tubes has actually been shown to initiate and sustain inflammatory processes and pain, resulting in persistent otorrhea and hearing deterioration.[47] Repeated myringotomies with aspiration of effusion from the middle ear rather than grommet insertion may be employed in these cases.[48]

One significant problem encountered by patients with hearing loss secondary to radiation therapy is the complications associated with hearing aids. By their nature, hearing aids predispose patients to recurrent and chronic otitis externa. They can traumatize the canal wall, trap debris in the canal, and maintain a humid environment conducive to bacterial and fungal growth. One solution to this problem of amplification is a bone conduction hearing aid, which avoids the use of an ear mold. There are two varieties. One attaches over the head and places an ossilator onto the mastoid cortex. These aids are cumbersome and mildly uncomfortable. If the skin under the ossilator is also compromised, these are problematic. A bone-anchored hearing aid is the second option. This aid involves an osseointegrated screw placed into the skull to which a vibratory hearing aid is attached. The advantage of this device is that acoustic signal is transformed into vibration and transferred via the skull to directly stimulate the inner ear, bypassing the external and middle ears. Although ideal for most patients with conductive or moderate sensorineural hearing loss who cannot wear a traditional hearing aid because of chronic otitis externa, this aid is potentially problematic postradiation. Although the site for the screw implantation may be out of the field of radiation, the vessels supplying the skin around the implant may have passed through the radiation field and are potentially compromised.

Thus, the patient may experience significant wound complications.

Inner Ear

The auditory and vestibular organs may be negatively impacted by radiation therapy to the temporal bone. Studies have shown that radiation-induced sensorineural hearing loss and vestibular system impairment may be caused by primary neuroepithelial toxicity or by the secondary effects of ischemia or infection.[49] Generally, postirradiation sensorineural hearing loss should be treated as idiopathic sensorineural hearing loss. Although there is no standard treatment for these conditions, some treatments are being considered. Corticosteroid treatment may reduce edema and inflammation in the inner ear after radiation, but the clinical results have been disappointing.[50,51] Several factors have been shown to be correlated with better recuperation of hearing acuity. These include younger age, a good preirradiation hearing level, and a short time between the onset of the hearing loss and radiotherapy.[52]

There may be some benefit from the use of hyperbaric oxygen (HBO) therapy on the recovery of hearing. The benefits of this treatment have been shown in some studies, although its value has not been confirmed by other groups.[53] The best management of moderate sensorineural hearling loss after radiation therapy is standard air conduction hearing aids. Cochlear implants may be considered in patients with profound bilateral hearing loss. Cochlear implants, however, are contraindicated in the face of osteoradionecrosis of the temporal bone and are relatively contraindicated if the patient has developed labyrinthitis ossificans (neo-ossification of the cochlea).

Hyperbaric Oxygen Therapy

HBO therapy can elevate the oxygen tension within the tissue and may stimulate collagen synthesis and fibroblastic proliferation, thus facilitating wound healing.[54] HBO therapy should be an adjunct to aggressive management of osteoradionecrosis. Devitalized bone or soft tissue cannot be treated with HBO therapy; this sequestrum must be aggressively removed. Prevention of osteoradionecrosis is the key, and at the earliest signs of this process, intensive local treatments need to be initiated. HBO therapy may serve a role under these circumstances in limiting the extent of the osteoradionecrosis. Once severe soft tissue necrosis, sequestrum, or massive infection has developed, HBO therapy without surgical intervention is unlikely to help. However, HBO treatment can be used as an adjunct to a planned surgical procedure.

The use of HBO therapy as an adjunct to healing in the treatment of osteoradionecrosis has been well described. In a review by Davis and colleagues, the use of HBO therapy in conjunction with adequate surgical débridement and appropriate antibiotic therapy resulted in healing of 20 of 23 cases of osteoradionecrosis of the mandible and 15 of 16 patients with soft tissue osteoradionecrosis of the head and neck.[55] Hart and Mainous have also reported impressive results with the use of HBO therapy in the treatment of osteoradionecrosis of various sites in 68 patients.[56] Marx demonstrated that HBO therapy is valuable in both the treatment and prevention of osteoradionecrosis.[57] Marx and Ames demonstrated that bone previously irradiated showed increased fibroblastic stroma and new vessel proliferation when exposed to HBO.[58] It has been shown that maximal fibroplasia and neovascularization occur after 30 treatment dives, using 100% oxygen through a hood for 90 minutes while pressurized to 2.4 atmospheres absolute. Marx's studies on tissue oxygen tension have shown that oxygen-induced angiogenesis becomes measurable after 8 treatments, plateaus at 80 to 85% of nonirradiated tissue vascularity after 20 treatments, and remains at this level whether or not HBO is continued.[59]

There are no prospective, controlled, randomized, double-blinded trials to prove the efficacy of HBO therapy for osteoradionecrosis of the temporal bone. These studies are difficult to perform because of the relatively low frequency of the disease, together with the multiple variables related to the disease process and management of the wounds.

CONCLUSION

Osteoradionecrosis is a well-known complication of radiation therapy. The temporal bone's superficial location, close proximity to infection, relatively poor blood supply, and histologically compact architecture make it susceptible. The effects of radiation may damage all components of the temporal bone from the ear and external canal to the inner ear structures. Early and aggressive therapy of osteoradionecrosis is critical to prevent extension and decrease the morbidity associated with this disease process.

REFERENCES

1. Mark RE. Osteoradionecrosis: a new concept of its pathophysiology. J Oral Maxillofac Surg 1983;41:283–99.
2. Kang HK, Bullman TA, Mahan CM. A mortality follow-up study of WWII submarines who received nasopharyngeal radium irradiation treatment. Am J Ind Med 200, 38:441–6.
3. VA Office of Public Affairs News Service. Veterans Affairs fact sheet. Nasopharyngeal radium therapy. Available at: www.va.gov (accessed Dec 2005).
4. Hempelmann LH, Hall WJ, Phillips M, et al. Neoplasms in persons treated with x-rays in infancy: 4th survey in 20 years. J Natl Cancer Inst 1975;55:519–30.
5. Sandler DP, Comstock GW, Matanoski GM. Neoplasms following childhood radium irradiation of the nasopharynx. J Natl Cancer Inst 1982;68:3–8.
6. Verduijn PG, Hayes RB, Looman C, et al. Mortality after nasopharyngeal radium irradiation for eustachian tube dysfunction. Ann Otol Rhinol Laryngol 1989;98:839–44.
7. Sataloff RT, Rosen DC. Effects of cranial irradiation on hearing acuity: a review of the literature. Am J Otol 1994;15:772–80.
8. Ewald CA. Die Wirkung des Radium auf das Labyrinth. Zentralbl Physiol 1905;10:298–9.
9. Borsanyi S, Blanchyard C. Ionizing radiation and the ear. JAMA 1962;181:958–61.
10. Jereczek-Fossa BA, Zarowski A, Milani F, Orecchia R. Radiotherapy-induced ear toxicity. Cancer Treat Rev 2003;29:417–30.
11. Van Hasselt CA, Gibb AG. Related ear problems. In: van Hasselt CA, Gibb AG, editors. Nasopharyngeal carcinoma. 2nd ed. Hong Kong: The Chinese University Press; 1998. p. 297–308.

12. Ashamalla HL, Thom SR, Goldwein JW. Hyperbaric oxygen therapy for the treatment of radiation-induced sequelae in children. The University of Pennsylvania experience. Cancer 1996;77:2407–12.

13. Silva JJ, Tsang RW, Panzarella T, et al. Results of radiotherapy for epithelial skin cancer of the pinna: the Princess Margaret Hospital Experience, 1982-1993. Int J Radiat Oncol Biol Phys 2000;47:451–9.

14. Mazeron JJ, Ghalie R, Zeller J, et al. Radiation therapy for carcinoma of the pinna using iridium 192 wires: a series of 70 patients. Int J Radiat Oncol Biol Phys 1986;12:1757–63.

15. Borsanyi SJ. The effects of radiation therapy on the ear: with particular reference to radiation otitis media. South Med J 1962;55:740–93.

16. Elwany S. Delayed ultrastructural radiation induced changes in the human mesotympanic middle ear mucosa. J Laryngol Otol 1985;99:343–53.

17. Kristensen H. Irradiation and otosclerosis. Acta Otolaryngol (Stockh) 1967;63:114–20.

18. Gyorkev I, Pollock FJ. Radiation necrosis of the ossicles. Arch Otolaryngol 1960;71:793.

19. Leach W. Irradiation of the ear. J Laryngol Otol 1965;79:870–80.

20. Bohne BA, Marks JE, Glasgow GP. Delayed effects of ionizing radiation on the ear. Laryngoscope 1985;95:818–28.

21. Ho Wk, Wei WI, Kwong DL, et al. Long-term sensorineural hearing deficit following radiotherapy in patients suffering from nasopharyngeal carcinoma: a prospective study. Head Neck 1999;21:547–53.

22. Chen WC, Liao CT, Tsai HC, et al. Radiation-induced hearing impairment in patients treated for malignant parotid tumour. Ann Otol Rhinol Laryngol 1999;108:1159–64.

23. Johannesen TB, Rasmussen K, Winther FO, et al. Late radiation effects on hearing, vestibular function, and taste in brain tumour patients. Int J Radiat Oncol Biol Phys 2002;53:86–90.

24. Grau C, Overgaard J. Postirradiation sensorineural hearing loss: a common but ignored late radiation complication. Int J Radiat Oncol Biol Phys 1996;36:515–7.

25. Gabriele P, Orecchia R, Magnano M, et al. Vestibular apparatus disorders after external radiation therapy for head and neck cancers. Radiat Oncol 1992;25:25–30.

26. Rankow RM, Weissman B. Osteoradionecrosis of the mandible. Ann Otol 1971;8:603–11.

27. Meyer I. Infectious diseases of the jaws. J Oral Surg 1970;28:17–27.

28. Marx RE. Osteoradionecrosis: a new concept of its pathophysiology. J Oral Maxillofac Surg 1983;41:283–8.

29. Schuknecht H, Karmody C. Radionecrosis of the temporal bone. Laryngoscope 1966;76:1416–28.

30. Thornley GD, Gullane PJ, Ruby RRF, et al. Osteoradionecrosis of the temporal bone. J Otolaryngol 1979;8:396–400.

31. Shotland LI, Ondrey FG, Mayo KA, et al. Recommendations for cancer prevention trials using potentially ototoxic agents. J Clin Oncol 2001;19:1658–63.

32. Ramsden RT, Bulman CH, Lorigan BP. Osteoradionecrosis of the temporal bone. J Laryngol Otol 1975;89:941–55.

33. Rankow RM, Weissman B. Osteoradionecrosis of the mandible. Ann Otol 1971;8:603–11.

34. Ondrey FG, Greig JR, Herscher L. Radiation dose to otologic structures during head and neck cancer radiation therapy. Laryngoscope 2000;110:217–21.

35. Raaijmakers E, Engelen AM. Is sensori-neural hearing loss a possible side effect of nasopharyngeal and parotid irradiation? A systematic review of the literature. Radiother Oncol 2002;65:1–7.

36. Lau Sk, Wei WI, Sham JST, et al. Early changes of auditory brain stem evoked response after radiotherapy for nasopharyngeal carcinoma: a prospective study. J Laryngol Otol 1992;106:887–92.

37. Cheng PW, Young YH, Lou PJ. Patulous eustachian tube in long-term survivors of nasopharyngeal carcinoma. Ann Otol Rhinol Laryngol 1999;108:201–4.

38. Andrews DW, Suarez O, Godman HW, et al. Stereotactic radiosurgery and fractionated stereotactic radiotherapy for the treatment of acoustic schwannomas: comparative observations of 125 patients treated at one institution. Int J Radiat Oncol Biol Phys 2001;50:1265–78.

39. Sataloff RT, Rosen DC. Effects of cranial irradiation on hearing acuity: a review of the literature. Am J Otol 1994;15:772–80.

40. Raaijmakers E, Engelen AM. Is sensori-neural hearing-loss a possible side effect of nasopharyngeal and parotid irradiation? A systematic review of the literature. Radiother Oncol 2002;65:1–7.

41. Nishimura R, Baba Y, Murakami R, et al. MR evaluation of radiation otomastoiditis. Int J Radiat Oncol Biol Phys 1997;39:155–66.

42. Young YH, Cheng PW, Ko JY. A 10-year longitudinal study of tubal function in patients with nasopharyngeal carcinoma after irradiation. Arch Otolaryngol Head Neck Surg 1997;123:945–8.

43. Jereczek-Fossa BA, Orecchia R. Radiotherapy-induced mandibular bone complications. Cancer Treat Rev 2002;28:65–74.

44. Ramsden RT, Bulman CH, Lorigan BP. Osteoradionecrosis of the temporal bone. J Laryngol Otol 1975;89:941–55.

45. Guida RA, Finn DG, Buchalter IH, et al. Radiation injury to the temporal bone. Am J Otol 1990;11:6–11.

46. Chowdhury CR, Ho JH, Wright A, et al. Prospective study of the effects of ventilation tubes on hearing after radiotherapy for carcinoma of the nasopharynx. Ann Otol Rhinol Laryngol 1988;97:142–5.

47. Morton RP, Woolons AC, McIvor NP. Nasopharyngeal carcinoma and middle ear effusion: natural history and the effect of ventilation tubes. Clin Otolaryngol 1994;19:529–31.

48. Chen CY, Young YH, Hsu WC. Failure of grommet insertion in post-irradiation otitis media with effusion. Ann Otol Rhinol Laryngol 2001;110:746–8.

49. Winther FO. X-ray irradiation of the ear of the guinea pig: an electron microscopic study of the degenerating vestibular sensory cell. Acta Otolaryngol (Stockh) 1970;69:307–19.

50. Sakamoto T, Shirato H, Takeichi N, et al. Medication for hearing loss after fractionated stereotactic radiotherapy for vestibular schwannoma. Int J Radiat Oncol Biol Phys 2001;50:1295–8.

51. Minoda R, Masuyama K, Habu K, et al. Initial steroid hormone dose in the treatment of idiopathic sudden deafness. Am J Otol 2000;21:819–25.

52. Sakamoto T, Shirato H, Satoh N, et al. Audiological assessment before and after fractionated stereotactic irradiation STI for acoustic neuroma. Radiother Oncol 1998;49:185–90.

53. Fattori B, Berrettini S, Casani A, et al. Sudden hypoacusis treated with hyperbaric oxygen therapy: a controlled study. Ear Nose Throat J 2001;80:655–60.

54. Rudge FW. Osteoradionecrosis of the temporal bone: treatment of hyperbaric oxygen therapy. Mil Med 1993; 158:196–8.

55. Davis JC, Dunn JM, Gates GA, et al. Hyperbaric oxygen; a new adjunct in the management of radiation necrosis. Arch Otolaryngol Head Neck Surg 1979;105:58–61.

56. Hart GB, Mainous EG. The treatment of radiation necrosis with hyperbaric oxygen. Cancer 1976;37: 2580–5.

57. Marx RE. Osteoradionecrosis: a new concept of its pathophysiology. J Oral Maxillofac Surg 1983;41:283–8.

58. Marx RE, Ames JR. The use of hyperbaric oxygen therapy in bony reconstruction of the irradiated and tissue-deficient patient. J Oral Maxillofac Surg 1982;40:412.

59. Marx RE, Johnson RP, Kline SN. Prevention of osteoradionecrosis: a randomized prospective clinical trial of hyperbaric oxygen versus penicillin. J Am Dent Assoc 1985;111:49–54.

19

Cranial Suture Biology and Craniosynostosis

Randall P. Nacamuli, MD; Derrick C. Wan, MD; Michael T. Longaker, MD, MBA

Craniosynostosis, or premature fusion of the cranial sutures, is a relatively common birth defect, with an estimated incidence of around 1 in 2,500 live births.[1] The functional and aesthetic sequelae of craniosynostosis include hydrocephalus, elevated intracranial pressure, blindness, deafness, compromised airway, and dysmorphic facies.[2] Since its first formal identification by a German surgeon in the early 1800s, physicians and investigators have put forth several theories attempting to explain the etiology and physiology of craniosynostosis.[3–5] In 1851, Virchow hypothesized that craniosynostosis arose as a consequence of cretinism or meningeal inflammation.[4] He also described the phenomenon of compensatory calvarial growth parallel to the axis of the fused suture (ie, anteroposterior growth with sagittal craniosynostosis, medial-lateral with coronal craniosynostosis), now known as Virchow's law. In the late 1950s, Moss proposed that the derangements of suture morphogenesis that lead to craniosynostosis arise owing to abnormalities in the development of the skull base, with transmission of abnormal mechanical forces to the developing cranial suture via the dura mater.[5] This theory was based on the observation that resection of the synostosed suture alone did not correct the observed problems with cranial vault expansion. Although today we know that skull base deformities may not be the cause of craniosynostosis, the fundamental observation that surgical treatment of the suture alone is insufficient to restore normal craniofacial development has led to the development of modern surgical treatments for craniosynostosis.[6]

Exactly what the etiology of premature suture fusion is remains unknown, although much insight has been gained in recent years, owing in large part to data obtained from clinical genetics studies and rodent models of cranial suture fusion. To facilitate the development of novel therapeutic strategies with which to treat craniosynostosis, a more complete understanding of cranial suture biology must be obtained. In this chapter, we review the clinical genetics data that have provided a major foothold for laboratory research into craniosynostosis and the animal models and studies that have advanced our understanding of the molecular and cellular biology of cranial sutures.

GENETICS OF CRANIOSYNOSTOSIS

Crouzon was perhaps the first to realize that there may be a heritable component to premature suture fusion when he identified a familial form of craniosynostosis.[7] Although sporadic, non-syndromal craniosynostosis accounts for the majority of cases, approximately 15 to 25% of all cases of craniosynostosis are syndromic and are associated with mutations in a few different genes, specifically the fibroblast growth factor receptors (*FGFRs*), the transcription factors *TWIST* and *MSX2*, and, most recently, the epidermal-like growth factor *NELL1*.[8–12]

In the early 1990s, investigators such as Wilkie, Reardon, Jabs, and Meunke, among others, determined that mutations in *FGFRs* 1, 2, and 3 were associated with Apert's, Crouzon's, Jackson-Weiss, and Pfeiffer's craniosynostotic syndromes.[13–16] Overall, the most common of the genetic mutations encountered in patients with syndromic craniosynostoses are heterozygous *FGFR* mutations, which alter the ligand binding domain, thus changing the affinity of the receptor for the target molecule. For example, the vast majority of patients with Apert's syndrome have an activating mutation in *FGFR2*, thus leading to gain of function in the fibroblast growth factor (FGF) signaling pathway. At a similar point in time, genetic linkages were made for several other craniosynostotic syndromes, leading to the association of gain-of-function mutations in *MSX2* with Boston-type craniosynostosis.[8,17,18] Interestingly, defects in calvarial ossification, such as parietal foramina, have been linked to loss-of-function mutations in *MSX2*.[19] In 1997, two investigative groups simultaneously detected numerous mutations leading to loss of function for the gene *TWIST* in patients with craniosynostotic Saethre-Chotzen syndrome.[12,20] Interestingly, subsequent screening of patients has indicated that mutations in *FGFR2* and *FGFR3* may also be associated with Saethre-Chotzen syndrome.[21] The most recent addition to the relatively short list of mutations associated with craniosynostosis is *NELL1*.[10] In 1999, Ting and colleagues used differential-display polymerase chain reaction to search for novel genes being expressed in specimens from patients with unilateral coronal synostosis and identified Nell1, a protein with multiple epidermal-like growth factor domains.[10]

Although the above clinical genetics studies have been invaluable in identifying the mutations associated with craniosynostotic syndromes and have provided a solid basis for further laboratory investigation, analysis of clinical samples derived from patients with craniosynostosis has been less informative. This is in large part due to the fact that specimens of synostosed sutures represent only the physiologic state of the suture after fusion has already occurred. Thus, longitudinal analysis of the dynamic process of suture fusion starting in utero is not feasible, and only limited glimpses into in vivo human suture biology are possible. Another limitation is the inability to obtain samples of the dura mater underlying the suture, a key regulator of calvarial development and craniofacial ossification.[22,23] These restrictions have led to the development of multiple animal models of craniosynostosis, with the rodent model proving most useful for the study of suture fusion.[24,25]

MURINE MODELS OF SUTURE FUSION AND PATENCY

Rats and mice provide an ideal model with which to study cranial suture biology given the numerous similarities between rodent and human calvaria. Although the calvaria are obviously different in shape, the main cranial sutures found in humans are also found in rats and mice, namely, the coronal, sagittal, and frontal (metopic) sutures. Furthermore, as described initially by Moss in the 1950s, the murine posterior frontal suture (equivalent to the metopic suture in man) fuses in a predictable fashion, from anterior to posterior, early in life, whereas the other sutures remain patent, just as in humans.[26,27] This allows for samples to be obtained from sutures before, during, and after fusion, with readily available control tissue from patent coronal or sagittal sutures. Coupled with the high degree of conservation between the genetic code of humans and mice, murine suture fusion provides an ideal model with which to investigate the complex molecular, cellular, and tissue interactions that regulate suture fusion and patency.[28]

Anatomically, the cranial suture can be simplified to four components: the osteogenic fronts of the calvaria, intervening suture mesenchyme, underlying dura mater, and overlying periosteum. Opperman and colleagues demonstrated that the periosteum is not an integral mediator of suture fate and that fetal rat coronal sutures remain patent regardless of the presence or absence of periosteum.[29] These data are consistent with other studies examining calvarial healing, in which the periosteum was not found to be an important mediator of reossification.[23,30,31] Subsequent studies by Opperman and colleagues examined the role of the dura mater in the maintenance of embryonic and neonatal rat coronal suture patency.[25,32] In these experiments, coronal sutures cultured in vivo or in vitro without the underlying dura mater went on to fuse, whereas control sutures cultured with the attached dura mater remained patent. Similar results have been obtained with embryonic mouse sagittal sutures.[33]

The importance of the dura mater in the regulation of postnatal cranial suture fate was demonstrated in another series of studies involving anatomic rearrangement of cranial sutures and their associated dura mater. Physiologic posterior frontal suture fusion was shown to be delayed in vivo when the proximity of the underlying dura mater is disrupted, either by surgical manipulation or interposition of a nonpermeable membrane.[34] Interestingly, Levine and colleagues were able to reverse suture fate by performing strip craniectomies on rats and rotating the posterior frontal and sagittal sutures 180°, such that the dura-suture interactions were reversed.[24] This orientation led to abnormal fusion of the sagittal suture (localized over the posterior frontal dura mater after rotation) and patency of the posterior frontal suture (over the sagittal dura mater after rotation).

All of the above studies demonstrate that the interaction between suture-associated dura mater and the overlying suture is integral for determining suture fate and further suggest that soluble factors are mediating this event. The importance of these as yet unidentified soluble factors was demonstrated in mouse fetal coronal sutures that had been stripped of their dura mater (and thus should have fused) by adding conditioned media from intact coronal sutures. This approach prevented the expected obliteration of the suture. Further analysis of the conditioned media revealed that the soluble factors responsible were

heparan binding factors, such as FGF2 or transforming growth factor β (TGF-β).[35]

FGF SIGNALING

Given the association of gain-of-function *FGFR* mutations with syndromic premature suture fusion and data from the studies discussed above, several investigators have concentrated on FGF ligands as candidate factors regulating suture fate. *FGF2* is specifically known to be involved with calvarial osteogenesis.[36] Histologic studies have demonstrated that there is both messenger ribonucleic acid (mRNA) and protein for *FGF2* in the dura mater underlying rat cranial sutures and that increased levels are detected in the dura mater associated with the posterior frontal suture.[37,38] A more detailed analysis of the regional, suture-associated dura mater further demonstrated that the dura mater underlying the fusing posterior frontal suture had a more osteogenic profile than the dura underlying the sagittal suture, as determined by mRNA levels of bone extracellular matrix molecules (collagen I, alkaline phosphatase, osteocalcin).[39] Coculture of primary dura mater cells isolated from the posterior frontal suture or sagittal suture with primary calvarial osteoblasts also confirmed the more osteogenic nature of the posterior frontal dura mater.[40]

The relevance of the *FGF2* ligand to postnatal cranial suture fate was elegantly demonstrated by using adenoviruses to overexpress *FGF2* or block FGF signaling in vivo. Rat fetuses were injected in utero with adenovirus either overexpressing *FGF2* or expressing a truncated dominant negative *FGFR*. Coronal sutures exposed to viruses overexpressing *FGF2* went on to fuse, whereas posterior frontal sutures in which FGF signaling was blocked remained patent.[41] Thus, manipulation of FGF signaling was capable of directly altering and "reversing" the fate of patent and fusing cranial sutures.

Recently, new insight into how FGF signaling may regulate cranial suture fusion has been provided and implicates a novel regulator of a skeletally ubiquitous signaling pathway, bone morphogenic proteins (BMPs). *BMPs* are the most osteogenic growth factors known and are capable of inducing ectopic bone formation.[42] Based on the observations that, despite remaining patent, transcripts for *BMP2* and *BMP4* are found in embryonic sagittal suture complexes and that *BMP4* protein is detected in postnatal sagittal and coronal suture mesenchyme,[43] Warren and colleagues hypothesized that there must be an antagonistic factor opposing the osteogenic capacity of *BMPs* and thus allowing for maintenance of suture patency.[44] BMP antagonists function by binding to BMPs and preventing them from interacting with their cell surface receptors, thus decreasing BMP biologic activity, and have been implicated in diverse developmental processes, such as mandibular outgrowth, proximal-distal patterning in the lung, and joint formation.[45–49] In situ hybridization studies have suggested that the BMP antagonist *Noggin* is expressed in coronal, sagittal, and posterior frontal sutures perinatally but is down-regulated in the posterior frontal suture during the process of suture fusion; histologic assessment of staining in transgenic Noggin-LacZ knock-in mice has confirmed these observations. Noggin directly binds to BMP2, BMP4, and BMP7, thus preventing ligand-receptor interaction.[50] Although primary calvarial osteoblast cultures produce Noggin and up-regulate its production in response to BMP stimulation, FGF signaling was found to block Noggin translation in a dose-dependant fashion in vitro either by direct application of recombinant growth factor or by transfecting osteoblasts with *FGFR2* gain-of-function mutations. Overexpression of Noggin in postnatal posterior frontal sutures of mice altered suture fate with abnormal maintenance of suture patency, suggesting that BMP signaling is required for suture fusion.[44] Finally, overexpression of FGF2 in postnatal coronal sutures led to diminished Noggin transcription and coronal craniosynostosis. This study thus suggests that increased signaling via the FGF pathway (such as in the gain-of-function mutations seen in syndromic

craniosynostosis) decreases sutural expression of the BMP antagonist Noggin, allowing increased suture osteogenesis and eventual craniosynostosis.[44] Another antagonist of BMP activity, *BMP3*, has also been detected in association with patent and fusing sutures, with higher expression in the sagittal suture relative to the posterior frontal, and has been shown to be down-regulated in calvarial osteoblasts by FGF2.[51] Interestingly, *BMP3* null mice have been described but have not yet yielded any further insight into suture development.[52]

One of the most powerful investigative tools available to researchers is transgenic mice. By using transgenic mice, mutations in genes associated with craniosynostosis can be introduced into the mouse model, allowing precise, detailed histologic and molecular analysis of the effects of the mutation on suture fusion. Introduction of an *FGFR1* gain-of-function mutation orthologous to the mutation associated with Pfeiffer's syndrome (Pro252Arg) into mice led to the increased expression of the osteoblast transcription factor Cbfa1 and development of premature sagittal and coronal synostosis, as well as other abnormalities associated with Pfeiffer's syndrome.[49] Other researchers have used slightly different techniques to reproduce this *FGFR1* mutation in mice, with consistent histologic findings.[53] An *FGFR2* gain-of-function mutation representative of the mutation associated with Pfeiffer's and Crouzon's syndromes (Cys342Tyr) has also been studied.[54] Mice carrying this mutation demonstrated premature coronal suture fusion in association with up-regulation of markers of osteoblast differentiation, including Cbfa1. The transgenic system has also been used to replicate the Ser252Trp *FGFR2* mutation causing some forms of Apert's syndrome, with affected mice developing coronal craniosynostosis.[55] Conditional *FGFR2* knockout mice have also been generated, leading to loss of *FGFR2* function in skeletal tissues.[56] These mice were noted to have persistent patency of the normally fusing posterior frontal suture, further emphasizing the role of FGFR signaling in cranial suture fusion and patency.

TRANSFORMING GROWTH FACTOR β

Although *TGF-β* is ubiquitously associated with bone and skeletal biology, clinical genetics has yet to uncover a form of craniosynostosis associated with mutations in the TGF-β signaling pathway. Despite this observation, numerous studies in both humans and rodents have suggested that TGF-β signaling is an important part of suture development and patency.[57] Altered levels of *TGF-β* isoforms have been noted in fused coronal sutures—when compared with the patent contralateral side—from individuals with unilateral coronal craniosynostosis. Similarly, increased *TGF-β* has also been demonstrated in lambdoid suture tissue samples from children with persistent plagiocephaly.[58] Studies conducted in rodent models have been consistent with human clinical data. Opperman and colleagues' initial experiments with embryonic rat coronal sutures (as discussed above) suggested that *TGF-β* family members were candidate growth factors regulating suture fusion and patency.[35] Subsequent in vitro investigation manipulating the levels of various *TGF-β* isoforms demonstrated that individual *TGF-β* isoforms had specific roles in embryonic suture biology, with *TGF-β3* maintaining suture patency and *TGF-β2* modulating fusion.[58–60]

Research into the function of *TGF-β* in postnatal rodent suture fusion and patency has focused on the posterior frontal and sagittal sutures and associated dura mater. During posterior frontal suture fusion in the rat, elevated mRNA and/or protein for TGF-β1 and TGF-β2 have been described, as well as histologic localization of TGF-β receptors to the dura mater and osteogenic fronts of posterior frontal sutures in comparison with the patent sagittal suture at identical time points.[38,39,61,62] Dura mater as a source of TGF-β ligand has been further demonstrated by analyzing either the dura mater alone or the suture complex with the dura mater removed in mice and rats.[63–65] These studies again suggest that the greatest source of *TGF-β* is the dura mater underlying the fusing posterior frontal suture as higher levels of *TGF-β1* were found in the posterior frontal suture–associated dura when compared with sagittal suture–associated dura. Similarly, low levels of ligand were detected in the nondura components of the suture.[63] More recently, functional validation of an active role for *TGF-β* in the regulation of suture fate has been described. Using an in vitro mouse system, Mehrara and colleagues and Song and colleagues demonstrated that adenovirus-mediated blocking of TGF-β signaling using the dominant-negative approach prevented posterior frontal suture fusion.[66,67] This result may be due to alterations in the regulation of *MSX2* as osteoblasts cocultured with dura mater in the context of TGF-β signaling blockade have elevated levels of *MSX2*, as well as increased expression of osteopontin.[67] This would be internally consistent with the *MSX2* gain-of-function mutation associated with Boston-type craniosynostosis.[17,18]

TWIST AND *MSX2*

The transcription factor *TWIST* is a basic helix-loop-helix transcription factor that regulates osteoblast differentiation.[68] Haploinsufficiency is found in patients with Saethre-Chotzen syndrome, and mice that are haploinsufficient for *twist* likewise develop coronal synostosis (homozygous null mice are embryonic lethal).[69] Studies in vitro have demonstrated that high levels of *TWIST* maintain osteoprogenitors in a proliferative state, whereas low levels of *TWIST* permit osteoblastic differentiation.[68] This mechanism appears to be, at least in part, due to the ability of the "*TWIST* Box," a novel deoxyribonucleic acid (DNA) binding domain, to bind Runx2 target sequences and prevent Runx2 function.[70] Interestingly, haploinsufficient *twist* mutant mice have been demonstrated to express FGFR2 aberrantly in the suture mesenchyme.[71] Thus, in addition to directly preventing Runx2-mediated differentiation of osteoprogenitors cells, *TWIST* may negatively regulate *FGFR2*, such that *TWIST* loss-of-function mutations lead to increased osteogenesis via up-regulation of *FGFRs* and increased Runx2 activity.

MSX2 is a transcription factor thought to regulate osteoblast proliferation and differentiation, and gain-of-function mutations that confer enhanced DNA binding activity are associated with Boston-type craniosynostosis.[8,17] In humans, loss-of-function mutations in *MSX2* are associated with deficiencies in calvarial ossification, and human calvarial phenotypes observed with both gain- and loss-of-function mutations have been replicated using transgenic mice.[19,72,73] Studies by Ishii and colleagues performed in *MSX2* mutant mice have demonstrated that defects in calvarial ossification arise secondary to attenuation in the number and proliferation of skeletogenic mesenchymal cells.[74] Similar to *TWIST*, *MSX2* has been shown to interfere with the function of Runx2 by binding to it and preventing transcription of target genes.[75] It is interesting to note that although both *MSX2* and *TWIST* are negative regulators of differentiation and act to maintain osteoprogenitors in a proliferative state, opposite types of mutations (gain vs loss of function) lead to pathologic bone formation and craniosynostosis. One proposed explanation is that *TWIST* and *MSX2* regulate mesenchymal cell differentiation at different stages of development. Thus, overexpression of *MSX2* during early suture morphogenesis may lead to elevated mesenchymal cell proliferation and an enlarged pool of osteogenic cells, which, in turn, gives rise to excess bone and suture fusion.[73] Conversely, *TWIST* may be a late inhibitor of differentiation, such that *TWIST* insufficiency results in unrestricted differentiation of a normal size population of precursor cells. These interactions further underscore the complexity of the signaling cascades regulating suture fate.

NELL1

Illustrating yet again the advantages of transgenic animals, researchers have been able to create mice that overexpress *nell1*. *NELL1* was initially identified and isolated from patients with nonsyndromic, unilateral coronal synostosis by Ting and colleagues.[10] Mice that overexpressed *nell1* suffered from craniosynostosis and increased calvarial differentiation.[76] Interestingly, despite generalized tissue expression, abnormal findings were noted only in calvarial bone. Additional studies demonstrated that osteoblasts transfected with *NELL1* viral expression constructs undergo elevated apoptosis.[77] These findings suggest that *NELL1* may have important roles in both cranial suture development and calvarial osteoblast differentiation.

SUMMARY

Although craniosynostosis has been recognized as a clinical entity for over 150 years, it is only in the past 15 years that investigators have started to make pioneering discoveries about the cellular and molecular biology that orchestrates normal suture physiology and the derangements that lead to pathologic fusion. With data gathered from clinical genetics, rodent models, and transgenic animals, a clearer picture of the myriad and complicated interactions between growth factors such as *FGF* and *TGF-β*, transcription factors such as *TWIST* and *MSX2*, and novel molecules such as *Noggin* and *Nell1* has developed. Clearly, the most exciting tools available to researchers today are transgenic mice and the ability to create tissue-restricted and conditional mutations in genes of interest.

Despite these huge advances in our understanding of cranial suture biology, current primary therapy for premature suture fusion is still surgical intervention. It is hoped that as research progresses, biologic therapies can be designed to prevent the development of craniosynostosis. Perhaps delivery of Noggin or other osteogenic antagonists to the mesenchyme of fusing sutures could halt progression of synostosis and allow enough time for normal calvarial vault expansion. The development of novel therapeutic strategies may some day allow early postnatal or even in utero treatment of affected fetuses and avoid the morbidity associated with skull vault remodeling.

REFERENCES

1. Lajeunie E, Le Merrer M, Bonaiti-Pellie C, et al. Genetic study of nonsyndromic coronal craniosynostosis. Am J Med Genet 1995;55:500–4.
2. Posnick JC. Craniofacial syndromes and anomalies. In: Posnick JC, editor. Craniofacial and maxillofacial surgery in children and young adults. Vol 1. Philadelphia: WB Saunders; 2000. p. 391–527.
3. Otto AW. Lehrbuch der Pathologischen Anatomie. Berlin: Rücher; 1830.
4. Virchow R. Ueber den Cretinismus, namentlich in Franken, und ueber pathologische Schaedelformen. Verh Phys Med Gesellsch Wuerzburg 1851;2:231–71.
5. Moss ML. The pathogenesis of premature cranial synostosis in man. Acta Anat 1959;37:351–70.
6. Tessier P. [Total facial osteotomy. Crouzon's syndrome, Apert's syndrome: oxycephaly, scaphocephaly, turricephaly]. Ann Chir Plast 1967;12:273–86.
7. Crouzon O. Dysostose cranio-faciale héréditaire. Bull Mem Soc Med Hop Paris 1912;33:545–55.
8. Jabs EW, Muller U, Li X, et al. A mutation in the homeodomain of the human MSX2 gene in a family affected with autosomal dominant craniosynostosis. Cell 1993;75:443–50.
9. Twigg SR, Kan R, Babbs C, et al. Mutations of ephrin-B1 (EFNB1), a marker of tissue boundary formation, cause craniofrontonasal syndrome. Proc Natl Acad Sci U S A 2004;101:8652–7.
10. Ting K, Vastardis H, Mulliken JB, et al. Human NELL-1 expressed in unilateral coronal synostosis. J Bone Miner Res 1999;14:80–9.
11. Bellus GA, Gaudenz K, Zackai EH, et al. Identical mutations in three different fibroblast growth factor receptor genes in autosomal dominant craniosynostosis syndromes. Nat Genet 1996;14:174–6.
12. el Ghouzzi V, Le Merrer M, Perrin-Schmitt F, et al. Mutations of the TWIST gene in the Saethre-Chotzen syndrome. Nat Genet 1997;15:42–6.
13. Reardon W, Winter RM, Rutland P, et al. Mutations in the fibroblast growth factor receptor 2 gene cause Crouzon syndrome. Nat Genet 1994;8:98–103.
14. Jabs EW, Li X, Scott AF, et al. Jackson-Weiss and Crouzon syndromes are allelic with mutations in fibroblast growth factor receptor 2. Nat Genet 1994;8:275–9.
15. Wilkie AOM, Slaney SF, Oldridge M, et al. Apert syndrome results from localized mutations of FGFR2 and is allelic with Crouzon syndrome. Nat Genet 1995;9:165–71.
16. Muenke M, Schell U, Hehr A, et al. A common mutation in the fibroblast growth factor receptor 1 gene in Pfeiffer syndrome. Nat Genet 1994;8:269–74.
17. Ma L, Golden S, Wu L, Maxson R. The molecular basis of Boston-type craniosynostosis: the Pro148→His mutation in the N-terminal arm of the MSX2 homeodomain stabilizes DNA binding without altering nucleotide sequence preferences. Hum Mol Genet 1996;5:1915–20.
18. Warman ML, Mulliken JB, Hayward PG, Muller U. Newly recognized autosomal dominant disorder with craniosynostosis. Am J Med Genet 1993;46:444–9.
19. Wilkie AOM, Tang Z, Elanko N, et al. Functional haploinsufficiency of the human homeobox gene MSX2 causes defects in skull ossification. Nat Genet 2000;24:387–90.
20. Howard TD, Paznekas WA, Green ED, et al. Mutations in TWIST, a basic helix-loop-helix transcription factor, in Saethre-Chotzen syndrome. Nat Genet 1997;15:36–41.
21. Paznekas WA, Cunningham ML, Howard TD, et al. Genetic heterogeneity of Saethre-Chotzen syndrome, due to TWIST and FGFR mutations. Am J Hum Genet 1998;62:1370–80.
22. Hobar PC, Schreiber JS, McCarthy JG, Thomas PA. The role of the dura in cranial bone regeneration in the immature animal. Plast Reconstr Surg 1993;92:405–10.
23. Hobar PC, Masson JA, Wilson R, Zerwekh J. The importance of the dura in craniofacial surgery. Plast Reconstr Surg 1996;98:217–25.
24. Levine JP, Bradley JP, Roth DA, et al. Studies in cranial suture biology: regional dura mater determines overlying suture biology. Plast Reconstr Surg 1998;101:1441–7.
25. Opperman LA, Sweeney TM, Redmon J, et al. Tissue interactions with underlying dura mater inhibit osseous obliteration of developing cranial sutures. Dev Dyn 1993;198:312–22.
26. Sahar DE, Longaker MT, Quarto N. Sox9 neural crest determinant gene controls patterning and closure of the posterior frontal cranial suture. Dev Biol 2005;280:344–61.
27. Moss ML. Fusion of the frontal suture in the rat. Am J Anat 1958;102:141–66.
28. Waterston RH, Lindblad-Toh K, Birney E, et al. Initial sequencing and comparative analysis of the mouse genome. Nature 2002;420:520–62.
29. Opperman LA, Persing JA, Sheen R, Ogle RC. In the absence of periosteum, transplanted fetal and neonatal rat coronal sutures resist osseous obliteration. J Craniofac Surg 1994;5:327–32.
30. Uddstromer L, Ritsila V. Osteogenic capacity of periosteal grafts. A qualitative and quantitative study of membranous and tubular bone periosteum in young rabbits. Scand J Plast Reconstr Surg 1978;12:207–14.
31. Ozerdem O, Anlaici R, Bahar T. Roles of periosteum, dura and adjacent bone on healing of cranial osteonecrosis. J Craniofac Surg 2003;14:371–9.
32. Opperman LA, Passarelli RW, Morgan EP, et al. Cranial sutures require tissue interactions with dura mater to resist osseous obliteration in vitro. J Bone Miner Res 1995;10:1978–87.
33. Kim HJ, Rice DP, Kettunen PJ, Thesleff I. FGF-, BMP- and Shh-mediated signalling pathways in the regulation of cranial suture morphogenesis and calvarial bone development. Development 1998;125:1241–51.
34. Roth DA, Bradley JP, Levine JP, et al. Studies in cranial suture biology: part II. Role of the dura in cranial suture fusion. Plast Reconstr Surg 1996;97:693–9.

35. Opperman L, Passarelli R, Nolen A, et al. Dura mater secretes soluble heparin-binding factors required for cranial suture morphogenesis. In Vitro Cell Dev Biol 1996;32:627–32.

36. Moore R, Ferretti P, Copp A, Thorogood P. Blocking endogenous FGF-2 activity prevents cranial osteogenesis. Dev Biol 2002;243:99–114.

37. Mehrara BJ, Mackool RJ, McCarthy JG, et al. Immunolocalization of basic fibroblast growth factor and fibroblast growth factor receptor-1 and receptor-2 in rat cranial sutures. Plast Reconstr Surg 1998;102:1805–17; discussion 1818–20.

38. Most D, Levine JP, Chang J, et al. Studies in cranial suture biology: up-regulation of transforming growth factor-beta1 and basic fibroblast growth factor mRNA correlates with posterior frontal cranial suture fusion in the rat. Plast Reconstr Surg 1998;101:1431–40.

39. Greenwald JA, Mehrara BJ, Spector JA, et al. Regional differentiation of cranial suture-associated dura mater in vivo and in vitro: implications for suture fusion and patency. J Bone Miner Res 2000;15:2413–30.

40. Warren SM, Greenwald JA, Nacamuli RP, et al. Regional dura mater differentially regulates osteoblast gene expression. J Craniofac Surg 2003;14:363–70.

41. Greenwald JA, Mehrara BJ, Spector JA, et al. In vivo modulation of FGF biological activity alters cranial suture fate. Am J Pathol 2001;158:441–52.

42. Wozney JM, Rosen V, Celeste AJ, et al. Novel regulators of bone formation: molecular clones and activities. Science 1988;242:1528–34.

43. Kim H, Rice D, Kettunen P, Thesleff I. FGF, BMP, and Shh mediated signaling pathways in the regulation of cranial suture morphogenesis and calvarial bone development. Development 1998;125:1241–51.

44. Warren SM, Brunet LJ, Harland RM, et al. The BMP antagonist noggin regulates cranial suture fusion. Nature 2003;422:625–9.

45. Stottmann RW, Anderson RM, Klingensmith J. The BMP antagonists Chordin and Noggin have essential but redundant roles in mouse mandibular outgrowth. Dev Biol 2001;240:457–73.

46. Lu MM, Yang H, Zhang L, et al. The bone morphogenic protein antagonist gremlin regulates proximal-distal patterning of the lung. Dev Dyn 2001;222:667–80.

47. Brunet LJ, McMahon JA, McMahon AP, Harland RM. Noggin, cartilage morphogenesis, and joint formation in the mammalian skeleton. Science 1998;280:1455–7.

48. Massague J, Chen YG. Controlling TGF-beta signaling. Genes Dev 2000;14:627–44.

49. Zhou YX, Xu X, Chen L, et al. A Pro250Arg substitution in mouse Fgfr1 causes increased expression of Cbfa1 and premature fusion of calvarial sutures. Hum Mol Genet 2000;9:2001–8.

50. Groppe J, Greenwald J, Wiater E, et al. Structural basis of BMP signaling inhibition by Noggin, a novel twelve-membered cystine knot protein. J Bone Joint Surg Am 2003;85-A Suppl 3:52–8.

51. Nacamuli RP, Fong KD, Lenton KA, et al. Expression and possible mechanisms of regulation of BMP3 in rat cranial sutures. Plast Reconstr Surg 2005;116:1353–62.

52. Daluiski A, Engstrand T, Bahamonde ME, et al. Bone morphogenetic protein-3 is a negative regulator of bone density. Nat Genet 2001;27:84–8.

53. Hajihosseini MK, Lalioti MD, Arthaud S, et al. Skeletal development is regulated by fibroblast growth factor receptor 1 signalling dynamics. Development 2004;131:325–35.

54. Eswarakumar VP, Horowitz MC, Locklin R, et al. A gain-of-function mutation of Fgfr2c demonstrates the roles of this receptor variant in osteogenesis. Proc Natl Acad Sci U S A 2004;101:12555–60.

55. Chen L, Li D, Li C, et al. A Ser250Trp substitution in mouse fibroblast growth factor receptor 2 (Fgfr2) results in craniosynostosis. Bone 2003;33:169–78.

56. Yu K, Xu J, Liu Z, et al. Conditional inactivation of FGF receptor 2 reveals an essential role for FGF signaling in the regulation of osteoblast function and bone growth. Development 2003;130:3063–74.

57. Roth DA, Gold LI, Han VK, et al. Immunolocalization of transforming growth factor beta 1, beta 2, and beta 3 and insulin-like growth factor I in premature cranial suture fusion. Plast Reconstr Surg 1997;99:300–9.

58. Lin K, Nolen A, Gampper T, et al. Elevated levels of transforming growth factors beta 2 and beta 3 in lambdoid sutures from children with persistent plagiocephaly. Cleft Palate Craniofac J 1997;34:331–7.

59. Opperman LA, Chhabra A, Cho RW, Ogle RC. Cranial suture obliteration is induced by removal of transforming growth factor (TGF)-beta 3 activity and prevented by removal of TGF- beta 2 activity from fetal rat calvaria in vitro. J Craniofac Genet Dev Biol 1999;19:164–73.

60. Opperman LA. Cranial sutures as intramembranous bone growth sites. Dev Dyn 2000;219:472–85.

61. Roth DA, Longaker MT, McCarthy JG, et al. Studies in cranial suture biology: Part I. Increased immunoreactivity for transforming growth factor-beta (β1, β2, β3) during rat cranial suture fusion. J Bone Miner Res 1997;12:311–21.

62. Mehrara BJ, Most D, Chang J, et al. Basic fibroblast growth factor and transforming growth factor beta-1 expression in the developing dura mater correlates with calvarial bone formation. Plast Reconstr Surg 1999;104:435–44.

63. Spector JA, Mehrara BJ, Greenwald JA, et al. A molecular analysis of the isolated rat posterior frontal and sagittal sutures: differences in gene expression. Plast Reconstr Surg 2000;106:852–61.

64. Sagiroglu JS, Mehrara BJ, Chau D, et al. Analysis of TGF-beta production by fusing and nonfusing mouse cranial sutures in vitro. Ann Plast Surg 1999;42:496–501.

65. Gosain AK, Recinos RF, Agresti M, Khanna AK. TGF-beta1, FGF-2, and receptor mRNA expression in suture mesenchyme and dura versus underlying brain

in fusing and nonfusing mouse cranial sutures. Plast Reconstr Surg 2004;113:1675–84.

66. Mehrara BJ, Spector JA, Greenwald JA, et al. Adenovirus-mediated transmission of a dominant negative transforming growth factor-beta receptor inhibits in vitro mouse cranial suture fusion. Plast Reconstr Surg 2002; 110:506–14.

67. Song HM, Fong KD, Nacamuli RP, et al. Mechanisms of murine cranial suture patency mediated by a dominant negative transforming growth factor-beta receptor adenovirus. Plast Reconstr Surg 2004;113: 1685–97.

68. Lee MS, Lowe GN, Strong DD, et al. TWIST, a basic helix-loop-helix transcription factor, can regulate the human osteogenic lineage. J Cell Biochem 1999;75:566–77.

69. Carver EA, Oram KF, Gridley T. Craniosynostosis in Twist heterozygous mice: a model for Saethre-Chotzen syndrome. Anat Rec 2002;268:90–2.

70. Bialek P, Kern B, Yang X, et al. A twist code determines the onset of osteoblast differentiation. Dev Cell 2004;6: 423–35.

71. O'Rourke MP, Tam PP. Twist functions in mouse development. Int J Dev Biol 2002;46:401–13.

72. Satokata I, Ma L, Ohshima H, et al. Msx2 deficiency in mice causes pleiotropic defects in bone growth and ectodermal organ formation. Nat Genet 2000;24:391–5.

73. Liu YH, Tang Z, Kundu RK, et al. Msx2 gene dosage influences the number of proliferative osteogenic cells in growth centers of the developing murine skull: a possible mechanism for MSX2-mediated craniosynostosis in humans. Dev Biol 1999;205:260–74.

74. Ishii M, Merrill AE, Chan YS, et al. Msx2 and Twist cooperatively control the development of the neural crest-derived skeletogenic mesenchyme of the murine skull vault. Development 2003;130:6131–42.

75. Shirakabe K, Terasawa K, Miyama K, et al. Regulation of the activity of the transcription factor Runx2 by two homeobox proteins, Msx2 and Dlx5. Genes Cells 2001; 6:851–6.

76. Zhang X, Kuroda S, Carpenter D, et al. Craniosynostosis in transgenic mice overexpressing Nell-1. J Clin Invest 2002;110:861–70.

77. Zhang X, Carpenter D, Bokui N, et al. Overexpression of Nell-1, a craniosynostosis-associated gene, induces apoptosis in osteoblasts during craniofacial development. J Bone Miner Res 2003;18:2126–34.

20

Vocal Fold Scar

Robert Thayer Sataloff, MD, DMA

A vocal fold scar poses great diagnostic and therapeutic challenges. Normal phonation requires not only adequate neuromotor function as supplied by the vagus nerve but also sufficient pliability of vocal fold soft tissues to permit complex mucosal wave motion. The layered structure of the vocal fold (Figure 1) is essential to normal phonation. Functionally, the epithelium and superficial layer of lamina propria constitute the cover of the vocal fold. The medial belly of the thyroarytenoid (vocalis) muscle functions as the body; and the intermediate and deep layers of lamina propria, which together constitute the vocal ligament, are a transition layer. There are few fibroblasts in the epithelium and superficial layer; but the vocal ligament and body are rich in fibroblasts. If fibroblasts proliferate and cause scar involving the superficial layer of lamina propria, the mucosal wave is impaired, and dysphonia usually results. The complex processes involved in vocal fold wound healing and scar formation are reviewed in Chapter 7, "Wound Healing of the Larynx."

There are many causes of vocal fold scarring. Phonotrauma from voice abuse or misuse, vocal fold hemorrhage, neoplasm, radiation, sulcus vocalis, and any other condition that causes vocal fold tissue injury may result in scar formation. Unfortunately, laryngologists encounter scar most frequently among patients who have remained or become dysphonic after laryngeal surgery.

Occasionally, a cause unrelated to scarring, such as arytenoid dislocation or vocal fold paresis, can be found and treated. More often, however, the problem is scar producing an adynamic segment, decreased bulk of one vocal fold following a stripping, or some other serious structural abnormality in a mobile vocal fold. None of the surgical procedures available for these conditions are consistently effective. If surgery is considered at all in such patients, it should be discussed realistically and somewhat pessimistically. The patient should be aware that the chances of returning the voice to normal or professional quality are slight, and there is a chance of making it worse. However, advances in the management of vocal fold scar have increased our therapeutic options.

Symptomatic vocal fold scarring alters phonation by interfering with the mucosal wave. This may be due to the obliteration of the layered structure of the vibratory margin, as seen commonly after vocal fold stripping or, to a limited extent, after other vocal fold surgery or trauma. Similar disruption of the layered structure and mucosal wave function also may occur congenitally, as in some cases of sulcus vocalis. Scarring may cause dysphonia by mechanical restriction of vibration or glottic closure, as seen in some cases of dense vocal fold web, or fibrotic masses on the membranous vocal fold, such as those that may form subsequent to vocal fold hemorrhage.

It is also necessary to distinguish a raised scar that causes failure of glottic closure by mass effect from the more common scar that effectively thins the vocal fold edge and causes failure of glottic closure by adhering the epithelium to the vocal ligament or muscle. In the former case,

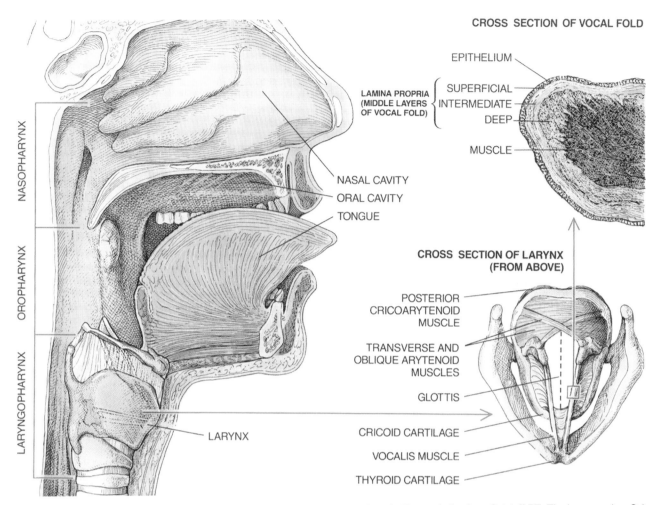

CROSS SECTION OF VOCAL FOLD

EPITHELIUM

LAMINA PROPRIA
(MIDDLE LAYERS
OF VOCAL FOLD)
SUPERFICIAL
INTERMEDIATE
DEEP

MUSCLE

NASAL CAVITY
ORAL CAVITY
TONGUE

NASOPHARYNX

OROPHARYNX

LARYNGOPHARYNX

CROSS SECTION OF LARYNX
(FROM ABOVE)

POSTERIOR
CRICOARYTENOID
MUSCLE

TRANSVERSE AND
OBLIQUE ARYTENOID
MUSCLES

GLOTTIS

LARYNX

CRICOID CARTILAGE

VOCALIS MUSCLE

THYROID CARTILAGE

Figure 1. Cross section of the vocal fold showing its layered structure. Reproduced with permission from Sataloff RT. The human voice. Sci Am 1992;267:108–15.

treatment usually includes resection of the scar tissue mass to reestablish a straight vocal fold edge. However, most of this chapter discusses the even more challenging problem of a vocal fold scar that has obliterated the layered structure and mucosal wave. Scar involving the posterior, subglottic, and arytenoid regions may also be troublesome, but this discussion is limited to scarring involving the membranous portion of the vocal folds.

Reliable, valid, objective voice assessment is essential in diagnosing a vocal fold scar, as well as in the assessment of other voice disorders. It is also important for measuring treatment outcomes. Accurate assessment of vibration is critical, and strobovideolaryngoscopy is virtually indispensable to proper diagnosis and management of a vocal fold scar.[1,2] Under continuous light, the vocal folds vibrate approximately 250 times per second while phonating at middle C. The human eye cannot discern necessary details during such rapid motion. Assessment of the vibratory margin may be performed through high-speed photography, strobovideolaryngo-scopy, high-speed video, videokymography, elec-troglottography, or photoglottography. Only strobovideolaryngoscopy provides the necessary clinical information in a practical fashion. For example, in a patient with a poor voice following laryngeal surgery and a normal-appearing larynx during indirect laryngoscopy, stroboscopic light reveals adynamic segments (scar) that explain the problem even to an untrained observer (such as a patient). In most instances, stroboscopy provides all of the clinical information necessary to assess vibration. However, objective voice analysis, particularly aerodynamic and acoustic assessment, is extremely valuable for diagnosis, therapy, and evaluation of treatment efficacy.

THERAPY FOR VOCAL FOLD SCAR

Therapy for a vocal fold scar depends on the size, location, and severity of the scar; the vocal needs of the individual patient; patient motivation; and the skill of the voice team. In general, once the vibratory margin of the vocal fold has been scarred (the layered structure obliterated), it is not possible to return the voice to normal. However, several options are available to improve voice quality.

Voice therapy is essential for anyone interested in obtaining optimal results. Most patients do not use their vocal mechanisms optimally even prior to vocal injury, and they develop even greater strain as they struggle to compensate for dysphonia. Consequently, even in the presence of a vocal fold scar, teaching the individual to make effective use of the support and resonator systems generally improves vocal intensity and ease and helps diminish fatigue. Nearly everyone with significant vocal fold injury develops compensatory behaviors in an effort to decrease breathiness and hoarseness. These gestures are usually hyperfunctional, counterproductive, and, in some cases, dangerous, potentially causing vocal fold injury through increased adductory forces. Such unconscious adjustments are seen even in the most skilled voice professionals after sustaining a vocal fold injury and scar. Expert voice therapy eliminates this compensatory muscular tension dysphonia, further decreasing fatigue and allowing a more accurate assessment of vibratory margin function. After the voice technique has been optimized and the vocal fold scar has matured (usually about 6 to 12 months), judgments can be made about the acceptability of the final voice result. If voice function is not satisfactory to the patient, then surgery may be considered. However, it is essential for the laryngologist to be sure that the patient's expectations are reasonable. These do not include restoration to normalcy. However, in some cases, it is possible to decrease hoarseness and breathiness substantially.

SURGERY FOR VOCAL FOLD SCAR

A vocal fold scar causes dysphonia by disrupting or obliterating the mucosal wave and by interfering with glottic closure. Clear understanding of these facts is necessary if one is to design rational surgical intervention. At present, there is no generally accepted or routinely successful surgical treatment for vocal fold scar. Numerous procedures have been tried, and some techniques are useful in selected cases. Very little information has been published on older attempts at surgical procedures to correct a vocal fold scar; anecdotally, many experienced voice surgeons admit to having attempted such surgery. Procedures to restore the mucosal wave have included injection of steroids into the vibratory margin, elevation of a microflap to lysis of adhesions followed by simply replacing the microflap, elevation of a microflap with the placement of steroids under the flap, and other procedures. Although none of these procedures produce consistently excellent results, they may help somewhat. Microflap elevation with steroids is still used (M. Bouchayer, personal communication, April 1995), but the results are not consistent. Pontes and Behlau suggested a unique approach to the treatment of sulcus vocalis that essentially involves multiple releasing incisions.[3]

The voice results have been surprisingly good, considering the limited success achieved by previous procedures for this condition. These principles have been applied to an iatrogenic vocal fold scar and appear to have some merit in severe, extensive scarring (P. Pontes, personal communication, April 1995). However, before addressing the difficult problem of trying to restore the mucosal wave, it is important to consider the role of glottic insufficiency. In most cases, correcting glottic insufficiency decreases vocal effort and increases volume. Given that effortful phonation is more troublesome to many patients than their hoarseness and that medialization procedures are common and straightforward and rarely cause dysphonia to worsen, it is often prudent to correct glottic insufficiency before addressing mucosal wave abnormalities. In addition, sometimes once good vocal fold contact has been established, spontaneous compensation renders the mucosal wave dysfunction much less symptomatic, and the risks of vibratory margin surgery may be avoided.

The problem of glottic incompetence is addressed through medialization surgery. Most medialization procedures in past decades have involved injection of Teflon. Because this implant material can itself cause significant scarring, otolaryngologists have abandoned its use in most cases since the mid- to late 1980s. At present, the medialization techniques of choice are thyroplasty with or without arytenoid repositioning or injection of a substance other than Teflon. For extensive failure of glottic closure, I have found type I thyroplasty to be most effective. Arytenoid repositioning surgery is not appropriate in most scar patients who have mobile vocal folds. For limited medialization, a lateral injection of autologous fat (in the same place where Teflon used to be injected) has proven successful.[4] Approximately 30 to 40% overinjection is necessary to account for resorption.[5] Other materials may be used for injection medialization, including autologous fascia, calcium hydroxylapatite, collagen, Gelfoam, and other substances. Each has specific advantages and disadvantages, and I still find all of them useful in the management armamentarium. In patients with a scar, special consideration must be given to the end point in surgical medialization. In patients with a bilateral vocal fold scar, a good surgical result may cause worsening dysphonia. If a bilateral vocal fold scar is approximated firmly, this may result in increased resistence to airflow, increased phonation threshold pressures, and increased vocal effort and fatigue. Although the examination result looks good becuase of complete glottal closure on stroboscopy, such patients generally consider themselves worse than they were preoperatively. They do better with near-closure (a slight glottal gap) unless and until mucosal wave function can

be restored. Such problems can be predicted preoperatively in many cases by testing phonation while performing external laryngeal compression. They can also be avoided intraoperatively by performing medialization procedures (particularly thyroplasty) under local anesthesia so that phonatory results can be monitored.

Collagen injection has been investigated extensively and reported by Ford and colleagues.[6–9] Long-term results from skin injections of collagen have shown a reduction in scar tissue in the treated areas. Collagen injectables come as a viscous form that can be injected easily in small quantities. Consequently, collagen injections are ideally suited for small adynamic segments. The ease and accuracy of injection allow for attempts at augmentation in areas of scar, as well as for managing difficult problems such as persistent posterior glottic incompetence and combined recurrent and superior laryngeal nerve paralysis. Concerns regarding the efficacy and safety of this material[9] seem to be less warranted, and experience using collagen has been encouraging, especially since autologous and allogenic human collagen products have been available to replace bovine collagen. Collagen can be injected into the region of the vocal ligament for treating limited vocal fold scarring. Such cases are common, for example, after laser resection of vocal nodules. For more extensive scarring, as may be seen following stripping of an entire vocal fold, collagen appears to be less effective.

In 1995, I introduced a technique for autologous fat implantation into the vibratory margin of the vocal fold as a treatment for vocal fold scarring.[5] The technique involves fat implantation into the vibratory margin, not injection.

To recreate a mobile vibratory margin, a mucosal pocket is created and filled with fat to prevent readherence of the mucosa to the vocal ligament and vocalis muscle. An incision is made on the superior surface (Figure 2A), and a small access tunnel is elevated toward the vibratory margin. The superior incision is placed in a position that will permit angled instruments to be passed through the tunnel to reach the anterior and posterior limits of the vocal fold scar.

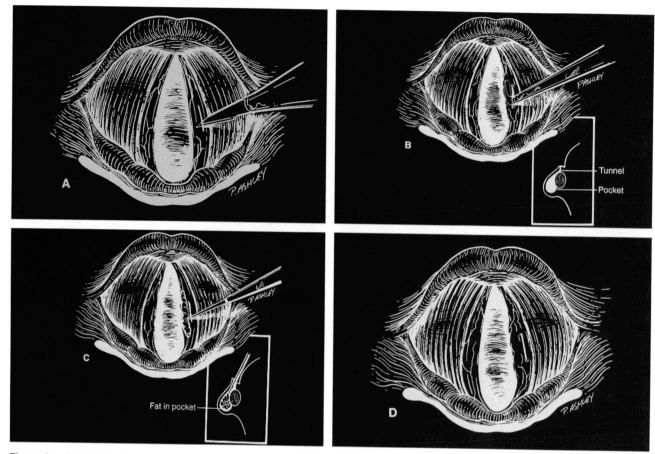

Figure 2. *A*, A small incision is made on the superior surface of the scarred vocal fold, and a narrow access tunnel is excavated to provide access to the medial edge. *B*, Through the access tunnel, an angled instrument is used to elevate a pocket. It is essential that the mucosa along the medial and inferior margins be kept intact. *C*, A Brünings syringe with the largest needle is passed through the tunnel and used to deposit fat in the pocket. *D*, When the needle is removed, the small access tunnel closes spontaneously, preventing extrusion of the fat. Fat should not extrude even when pressure is placed against the medial margin. If fat extrusion occurs, a suture can be placed. Reproduced with permission from Sataloff RT. Professional voice: the science and art of clinical care. 2nd ed. San Diego (CA): Singular Publishing Group; 1997.

Although working through a small access tunnel is technically more difficult than elevating a large flap, this technique is advantageous because it closes spontaneously without sutures on removal of instruments and prevents fat extrusion from the surgically created pocket. If a larger incision is made along the superior surface, sutures are necessary to prevent fat extrusion, and even small sutures create additional tissue trauma.[10] A pocket is created along the medial margin using a right-angled dissector and an angled knife or scissors, as needed (Figure 2B). The pocket extends to the superior aspect of the vibratory margin and inferiorly for at least 3 to 5 mm to encompass all of the vertical extent of the medial surface ordinarily involved in creating the mucosal wave vertical phase difference during

phonation. Fat harvested at the beginning of the surgery is then used to fill the tunnel (Figure 2C). Instruments are then withdrawn, and the access tunnel closes and provides sufficient resistance against fat extrusion (Figure 2D). The procedure may be performed under local or general anesthesia; I prefer general anesthesia. At the conclusion of the procedure, under local anesthesia, the patient is asked to phonate briefly and to cough to be certain that the implant is secure. Under general anesthesia, the medial margin is palpated firmly with the side of a suction to be sure that the implant is secure. Although no problems that have prevented closure of the mucosal flap have occurred to date, if extrusion occurred, fibrin adhesive would be tried or a suture closure would be placed.

Experience with lipoinjection has provided convincing evidence that it is important to avoid extensive manipulation or trauma to the fat. The fat is harvested in large globules either by resecting a small amount of fat (usually from the abdomen) with traditional instruments or by harvesting it with the largest available liposuction cannula (8–10 mm). The fat is rinsed gently with saline, but it is not morselized. Packing the fat through the access tunnel with microinstruments has been attempted, but it is technically difficult to pack the fat tightly and evenly, and this method appears to cause more trauma to the access tunnel, flap, and fat than delivering the fat through a Brünings syringe. At present, the fat is loaded into the Brünings syringe, and the largest Brünings needle (18 gauge) is used to deliver the fat into the preformed vibratory margin pocket. Gross examination with a microscope indicates that passing the fat through the Brünings syringe can elongate the fat globules and traumatize them to some degree, but they appear to be largely intact and survival is noted.

Occasionally, surgeons are faced with extreme cases of vibratory margin scarring. These are especially common after major trauma or extensive cancer surgery. When a nonvibrating, scarred vocal fold is lateralized so that glottic closure is impossible, and when the involved hemilarynx is so densely scarred that the vocal fold cannot be medialized adequately, even with thyroplasty, occasionally more extensive surgery for a vocal fold scar may be appropriate. For example, some cases may be improved through resection of the scarred hemilarynx and creation of a pseudo–vocal fold using modifications of strap muscle techniques employed routinely for cordectomy or vertical hemilaryngectomy.[11] This is a rare and aggresssive option for the treatment of vocal fold scarring.

Familiarity with the latest concepts in vocal fold anatomy and physiology is essential in understanding the consequences of vocal fold scar and current paradigms for diagnosis and treatment. The vocal folds constitute only one part of the voice. If the surgeon does not pay adequate attention to the function of the power source and resonator, working with a skilled voice team, diagnostic judgments, and surgical outcome will not be optimal. However, substantial advances have been made in team-based care of patients with a vocal fold scar over the last two decades.[12,13] Even more advances are anticipated in the coming years through techniques that modify wound healing; enhance substances such as hyaluronic acid, decorin, and fibromodulin, control substances such as fibronectin; and provide other techniques that help prevent adverse vocal fold scarring. In addition, it may be possible to increase our ability to prevent vocal fold scarring through genetic screening that identifies the patients who are most prone to adverse healing processes. Hyaluronidase inhibitors and hyaluronic acid are already available, although more experience will be required to determine their clinical value. It is hoped that it will be possible to eliminate surgery for vocal fold scarring altogether when genetic engineering makes it possible to recreate a superficial lamina propria. At present, although clinicians continue to help patients through voice therapy, surgical medialization, and vibratory margin surgery, it is important for all of us to recognize that no good solution to this challenging problem exists and to devote conscientious attention to further research.

Acknowledgments

Modified from Sataloff RT. Vocal Fold Scar. In: Sataloff RT: Professional Voice: The Science and Art of Clinical Care, 3rd ed. San Diego (CA): Plural Publishing; 2005.

REFERENCES

1. Sataloff RT, Spiegel JR, Carroll LM, et al. Strobovideolaryngoscopy in professional voice users: results and clinical value. J Voice 1988;1:359–364.
2. Sataloff RT, Speigel JR, Hawkshaw MJ. Strobovideolaryngoscopy: results and clinical value. Ann Otol Rhinol Laryngol 1991;100:725–757.
3. Pontes P, Behlau M. Treatment of sulcus vocalis: auditory perceptual and acoustic analysis of the slicing mucosa surgical technique. J Voice 1993;7(4):365–376.
4. Mikaelian D, Lowry LD, Staaloff RT. Lipoinjection for unilateral vocal fold paresis. Laryngoscope 1991;101:465–468.

5. Sataloff RT, Spiegel JR, Hawkshaw M, et al. Autologous fat implantation for vocal fold scar: a preliminary report. J Voice 1997;11(2):238–246.

6. Ford CN, Bless DM, Loftus JM. The role of injectable collagen in the treatment of glottic insufficiency: a study of 119 patients. Ann Otol Rhinol Laryngol 1973;101(3):23–247.

7. Ford CN, Bless DM. Collagen injected in the scarred vocal fold. J Voice 1988;1:116–118.

8. Ford CN, Bless DM. Selected problems treated by vocal fold injections of collagen. Am J Otolaryngol 1993; 14(4):257–261.

9. Spiegel JR, Sataloff RT, Gould WJ. The treatment of vocal fold paresis with injectable collagen. J Voice 1987;1: 119–121.

10. Feldman MD, Sataloff RT, Epstein G, Ballas SK. Autologous fibrin tissue adhesive for peripheral nerve anastomosis. Arch Otolaryngol Head Neck Surg 1987; 113:963–967.

11. Spiegel JR, Sataloff RT. Surgery for carcinoma of the larynx. In: Gould WJ, Sataloff RT, Spiegel JR, editors. *Voice Surgery*. St. Louis, Mo: CV Mosby Co; 1993. p. 307–338.

12. Neuenschwander MC, Sataloff RT, Abaza M, et al. Management of fold scar with autologous fat implantation: perceptual results. J Voice 2001;15(2):295–304.

13. Benninger MS, Alessi D, Archer S, et al. Vocal fold scarring: current concepts and management. Otolaryngol Head Neck Surg 1996;115(5):474–482.

Clinical Considerations of Wound Healing in the Subglottis and Trachea

Todd D. Otteson, MD; Aron Parekh, PhD; Joseph E. Dohar, MD, MS

Concerns with wound healing in other anatomic locations, including the head and neck, primarily involve a delay or an inability to heal. By contrast, the clinical problem facing surgeons of the subglottis and trachea is overly exuberant scar formation leading to subglottic and/or tracheal stenosis. Any surgical manipulation of the subglottis or trachea is performed while always being conscious of the possibility of scar formation with attendant stenosis. Any degree of stenosis for any reason may significantly compromise airway lumen patency and induce a potentially life-threatening airway obstruction. Knowledge of the basic science of mucosal and cartilaginous wound healing in the subglottis and trachea influences clinical and surgical decision making and directs potential therapies to inhibit such exuberant scar formation.

CLINICAL HEALING PROBLEM: SCAR FORMATION IN THE SUBGLOTTIS AND TRACHEA LEADING TO AIRWAY STENOSIS

Although several systemic processes may cause subglottic stenosis, injury to the subglottis sustained from endotracheal intubation is the most common cause of acquired airway stenosis, particularly in neonates and infants. In fact, subglottic stenosis resulting from endotracheal intubation injury has become standard for airway mucosal wound healing studies. Wounds resulting from intubation present the full spectrum of injury, ranging from mild edema to complete deformation of the mucosa and cartilaginous framework of the airway, ultimately leading to fibrosis and stenosis.[1]

Estimates of the incidence of subglottic stenosis in the neonatal population secondary to endotracheal intubation are reported to be as high as 8.3%.[2] More recently, improved intensive care has markedly decreased the incidence of clinically significant injury. A report of 281 intubated neonates found none who developed subglottic stenosis.[2] The authors cited greatly enhanced understanding and techniques of caring for infants requiring ventilatory support and a trend toward fewer days of ventilation and intubation as reasons for this significant decrease in the incidence of neonatal subglottic stenosis.

Predisposing Factors

A number of predisposing factors may allow one to predict which patient and in which circumstances an infant may develop subglottic stenosis. Elegant postmortem histologic studies demonstrate a relationship between the duration of intubation and the corresponding glottic and subglottic injury causing subglottic stenosis.[3,4] The longer the child is intubated, the more likely it is that he or she will develop subglottic stenosis.

Albert and colleagues prospectively studied 30 infants by performing endoscopic laryngeal and subglottic examination at the time of extubation and analyzed the severity of the laryngeal injury to several presumed predisposing factors.[5] The age of the infant correlated, implying that younger neonates were more prone to subglottic stenosis. The activity of the infant and the resultant instability of the endotracheal tube correlated with an increased incidence of laryngeal and subglottic injury.

Gastroesophageal reflux has also been implicated as a factor contributing to subglottic injury in intubated patients.[6] A study using the rabbit model irrigated the larynx and trachea of intubated animals with normal saline or acid solutions of varying pH. At the time of sacrifice, control animals intubated and irrigated with only normal saline showed minimal trauma. Animals irrigated with a solution of pH 4.0 showed an inflammatory response involving the submucosa and muscle. The degree of damage was greater with longer periods of irrigation. At pH 1.4, there was severe mucosal ulceration, deep submucosal hemorrhage with a marked inflammatory response, and necrosis. These results occurred after only a few hours of continuous irrigation. The clinical corollary is that any injury sustained at the time of endotracheal intubation is severely exacerbated by untreated gastroesophageal reflux.

Histopathology of Subglottic Stenosis

The postmortem histopathology of subglottic stenosis in infants and children after endotracheal intubation has been well studied.[7–9] Ulceration was common. The depth of the ulceration ranged from superficial to full thickness, involving the perichondrium and even the cartilage.[7–10] When the epithelium regenerated, it was primarily as squamous metaplasia.[9] Fibrous scar formation caused a clinically narrowed airway. Goldstein and colleagues induced a subglottic mucosal wound and obtained histologic sections at varying time intervals.[11] At day 7, the animals exhibited mucosal reepithelialization and mucosal hypertrophy with much less squamous metaplasia than encountered in other studies. At day 21, there was an intact mucosa.

A unique study examining the resected, stenotic portion of the airway removed by partial cricotracheal resection demonstrated some key histopathologic findings with particular clinical relevance.[10] Twenty-five specimens consisting of the resected area of stenosis were stained to visualize basic histopathology and elastin, and were immunohistochemically stained for the presence of macrophages. Occasionally, the luminal surface of the stenotic ring had islands of normal epithelium. The vast majority, however, had squamous metaplasia. This abnormal squamous metaplastic surface exhibits diminished mucociliary function and is thought to become more vulnerable to repetitive injury, such as would be caused by reintubation. Lesions confined to the soft tissue eventually form a membranous stenosis, more superficial in location. If the injury is deeper to the level of the perichondrium, there is compact, abundant hypertrophic scar formation. Injured or absent perichondrium seems to play an active role in the aberrant wound healing of the subglottis and trachea. Surgical decision making must take into account the paramount importance of perichondrial preservation to prevent subglottic scar formation.

The rabbit animal model confirms these general principles. The structure of the rabbit larynx is remarkably similar to that of the human larynx. It includes the organization of the cartilaginous components of the larynx, as well as the character of the respiratory epithelium and the components of the subepithelial layer,[12] making the rabbit the ideal small animal model for subglottic stenosis. Endolaryngeal injuries involving only the mucosal and submucosal layers caused disorderly regeneration of the epithelium and a marked thickening of the subepithelial layer, primarily composed of a loose fibrous netting.[13] When the injury extends to the perichondrium and cartilage, the cartilage is deformed, with inconsistent thickness, dense scar tissue, and marked luminal narrowing and collapse.[13] Animals sacrificed because of respiratory distress prior to the end of the study showed severe subglottic stenosis composed of dense fibrosis and cartilage thickening, with a pinpoint lumen.[12]

Dohar and colleagues serendipitously confirmed the notion that the development of subglottic stenosis is directly related to the depth of injury, independent of circumferential extent.[14] Animals with injury reaching the perichondrium experienced respiratory obstruction resulting from edema and granulation tissue. A histologic section showed chronic inflammatory cellular infiltrates and fibroplasia, resulting in a reparative process, not a regenerative process. Injury to the connective tissue is a critical component of the development of subglottic stenosis.

APPROACH TO THE CLINICAL HEALING PROBLEM: SURGICAL MANIPULATION OF THE AIRWAY; MAXIMIZING THE LUMEN WHILE MINIMIZING THE SCAR

It cannot be emphasized enough that the best treatment for subglottic and tracheal stenosis is prevention at the outset. Atraumatic intubation with an appropriately sized endotracheal tube depending on the age and size of the child is important. Minimizing trauma from endotracheal tube mobility and avoiding frequent reintubations also diminish the risk of subglottic stenosis. Prophylaxis with antireflux therapy and the judicious administration of antibiotics to prevent iatrogenic pulmonary infection may also modulate scar formation in the subglottis and trachea. Unfortunately, randomized, controlled, and double-blinded clinical trials have not been done. Thus, in pediatric intensive care, there is no well-established standard of care guiding the use of these two classes of drugs for this particular clinical outcome. Unlike adult critical care practice, in which anti-reflux medications are often routinely employed for stress ulcer prophylaxis, no such routine practice exists in children.

More conservative surgical interventions to treat subglottic and tracheal stenosis have generally proven less than satisfactory with regard to long-term outcomes of airway lumen patency. Several studies have reported the use of carbon dioxide laser treatment, either as a sole treatment modality or as an adjunct to other therapeutic approaches, in the treatment of subglottic stenosis of variable severity with mediocre results. General principles include the need for multiple procedures[15] and the avoidance of circumferential laser treatment, which may cause further airway stenosis. Studies on the laser resection of subglottic hemangiomas emphasize some overlying principles of laser treatment of the subglottis.[16] Laser treatment should be conservative, treating only a third of the lumen circumference at one procedure, and should avoid underlying cartilage.[17] Partial cricotracheal resection specimens that included a luminal surface treated with the carbon dioxide laser reveal a much more intense scar formation than patients with stenosis from intubation alone. Cartilage injury was also pronounced, including the loss of large segments of the cricoid ring and replacement by fibrous tissue with resultant airway stenosis. Conservative use of the laser in the subglottis, as long as no perichondrial or cartilaginous injury is induced, may have some merit in the treatment of mild subglottic stenosis or as an adjunct with other treatment modalities. Again, comparative clinical trials are lacking.

The use of microdébridement to treat recurrent respiratory papillomatosis was first reported in 1999 and has gained popularity.[18] A recent article extolled the virtues of the microdébrider and its expanding role in pediatric endoscopic airway surgery, including its use to resect portions of airway stenosis.[19] Nine patients with airway stenosis underwent endoscopic escharectomy. Long-term airway patency results were not reported. Histologic studies detailing the natural history of subglottic and tracheal wound healing resulting from microdébridement are necessary. If long-term results demonstrate success with airway lumen patency, the microdébrider may become the method of choice for the airway surgeon. As is true for medicine in general, this swinging pendulum between "cold" steel and "hot" cautery and laser techniques is still seeking its optimal point between the extremes.

The mainstay of the treatment of subglottic stenosis is expansion of the laryngotracheal framework, including anterior cartilage graft placement, anterior and posterior graft placement, and anterior cricoid split, among others. Success of laryngeal expansion procedures in general is excellent, with a decannulation rate near 90%.[20] The specific technique of laryngotracheal reconstruction (LTR) has been well reported in the literature and is not the focus of this chapter. Rather, a review of the aspects of wound healing relative to the LTR procedure, an analysis of certain patients who fail LTR, and the benefits of meticulous perioperative management are discussed.

TECHNIQUES TO TREAT THE CLINICAL HEALING PROBLEM: LTR

Cotton and colleagues described the five stages of LTR as (1) characterization of the subglottic stenosis, (2) expansion of the lumen, (3) stabilization of the enlarged lumen framework, (4) healing of the surgical site, and (5) decannulation.[21]

Characterization of subglottic stenosis is performed endoscopically and is classified depending on the size of the endotracheal tube that will pass comfortably through the narrowest point of the stenosis and allow a leak at a pressure of between 10 and 25 cm H_2O. Comparison is then made with the expected normal size for age, and the percentage of stenosis is assessed. The stenosis is then graded by the Myer-Cotton grading scale (Table 1). The decision for surgical intervention and the type of surgery best suited to treat the type and severity of stenosis depends on the Myer-Cotton grade of

the stenosis and the length of the stenotic segment.

Expansion of the airway lumen may be accomplished with or without cartilage grafting. If anterior cartilage grafting is necessary, expansion of the lumen may be accomplished by suturing an appropriately shaped graft to the incised portion of the cricoid cartilage and the proximal trachea (Figures 1 to 4), carefully preserving the perichondrial layer of the cartilage graft, which will face the airway lumen and which will provide a matrix for regenerated epithelialization with respiratory epithelium (pseudostratified, columnar, and ciliated). The cartilage graft is typically harvested from the rib.[22] Some surgeons have recommended auricular or thyroid alar cartilage, touting the benefits of reduced morbidity and surgical accessibility of these alternative donor sites. If the posterior subglottis is involved or if the stenosis is severe, a cartilage graft may be secured within a vertical split in the posterior cricoid plate. Recent literature suggests that endoscopic placement of a posterior cartilage graft holds some promise for less invasive luminal expansion.[23]

The final three stages of LTR ensue over a span of months in the case of an indwelling tracheostomy and airway stenting. Alternatively,

Table 1. MYER-COTTON SUBGLOTTIC STENOSIS CLASSIFICATION	
Classification	Degree of Obstruction
Grade I	No obstruction to 50% obstruction
Grade II	51–70% obstruction
Grade III	71–99% obstruction
Grade IV	No detectable lumen

Adapted from Myer, Charles M, O'conner David M, and Cotton, RT. Proposed grading system for subglottic stenosis based on endotracheal tube sizes. Ann Otol Rhinol Laryngol 1994;103:319–23.

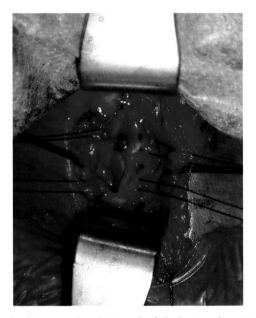

Figure 1. Intraoperative photograph of single-stage larygotracheal reconstruction for a grade II subglottic stenosis showing the incision through inferior thyroid cartilage, cricoid, and superior tracheal rings. The endotracheal tube is visible through the incision.

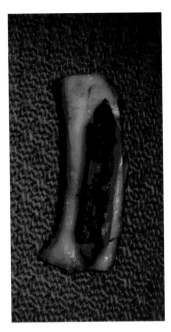

Figure 2. Rib graft carved for placement in the incision present in Figure 22-1. Note preservation of the perichondrium, which will face the airway lumen.

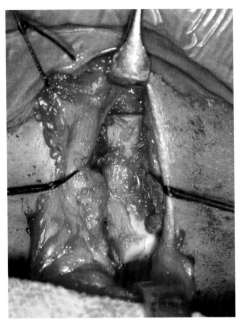

Figure 4. Rib graft sutured in place with the perichondrial surface facing the airway lumen. The wound was subsequently closed with a drain in place.

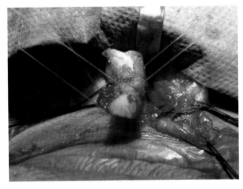

Figure 3. Rib graft now positioned in situ with sutures placed but not tied.

this may be compressed into a shorter period of weeks when the patient is intubated. These techniques are known as two-stage LTR and single-stage LTR, respectively. Cotton and colleagues reported in 1995 that 30% of a series of LTR patients had the single-stage technique.[21] Each has its own operative indications and postoperative healing considerations. Many authors have emphasized the importance of capable anesthesia, nursing, and intensive care unit staff[21,24] to ensure successful extubation after single-stage LTR. Single-stage LTR requires sedation or paralysis for at least 1 week postoperatively to allow mucosal healing to take

place. Airway endoscopy with removal of any airway granulation tissue typically occurs between 7 and 14 days postoperatively, prior to extubation. Additional details regarding a successful single-stage LTR follow in the section on pearls and pitfalls.

The two-stage procedures employ the same techniques of airway expansion, but rather than endotracheal intubation, the patient is not decannulated and an endolaryngeal stent is placed until mucosal healing is complete, on average, 6 weeks. This technique has the advantage of a short intensive care unit hospitalization and no paralysis, obviating potential adverse sequelae. The length of time from surgery to successful decannulation is much longer than the single-stage counterpart, at times lasting several months and necessitating serial airway endoscopy procedures to ensure lumen patency and resect granulation tissue (on average, 6.2 airway endoscopic procedures prior to decannulation).[25]

Stent Placement

Airway stents are recommended for lumen patency during all or part of the healing process.

Maintenance with metal alloy airway stents has been in use since the 1950s. Montgomery introduced the T tube in 1965, and the Aboulker stent was introduced in the 1960s for the treatment of subglottic stenosis in both children and adults.[26] Evans introduced the use of a Silastic sheet that was rolled as a lumen keeper, taking advantage of the mechanical tendency to unroll to maintain lumen patency, obliterate airway dead space, and allow mucosal regeneration.[27] The use of silicone stents was first reported in 1990[28] and was later reported again by Temes and colleagues for the treatment of subglottic stenosis.[29]

Zalzal identified the ideal stent as available in many sizes and appropriate for all situations.[26] The stent should exist in many shapes to fit reconstructed areas. The ideal shape would be that of the reconstructed lumen and have the capability of molding to fit the exact size of the lumen. This is of particular concern if the stent passes through the glottis because the shape of the laryngeal inlet is vastly different from that of the tracheal lumen. The stent should be safe, without any risk of airway obstruction. The stent should not induce a foreign body reaction, inflammation, or infection. A stent should be hard enough to keep reconstructed structures and grafts in place but soft enough not to cause discomfort or pressure necrosis in other areas. The stent should allow voice production while allowing safe intake of food without aspiration.[26] This is a challenge at times because if a stent has a hole in the proximal end to allow passage of air through the glottis with voice production, the patient is automatically at risk of aspiration through the hole. The key is the superior or inferior positioning of the stent relative to the arytenoids. If the stent is placed higher than the level of the arytenoids, aspiration is inevitable; if the stent is placed lower than the level of the aryentoids, there is an increased risk of glottic and subglottic granulation tissue.[26]

Although stents may be employed in a variety of clinical scenarios, the focus of the current chapter is the reaction of the mucosa and deeper soft tissues to an indwelling airway stent. This finds application in the postoperative LTR patient with a stent in place. The stents most commonly used after pediatric airway reconstruction are the Aboulker stent and the Montgomery T tube. These stents are similar in terms of the mucosal response to the stent as a foreign body, but there are distinct differences.

The Aboulker stent is made of highly polished Teflon. After a few days or weeks, the stent-tracheostomy complex causes mucosal irritation and secondary infection, which causes granulation tissue to form at the superior or inferior ends of the stent or at the tracheostomy site. If the stent projects throught the glottis, the stent may cause erosion of the base of the epiglottis, with resultant granulation tissue. When a short stent is used, granulation tissue forms at the lower end of the stent in the area above the tracheostomy, with stasis of secretions and mucosal irritation strongly contributing. The granulation tissue is circumferential and will eventually lead to a severe circumferential tracheal stenosis with suprastomal collapse.[26] All of these sequelae may be avoided if the Aboulker stent is used for a period not to exceed 5 weeks.[26] Granulation tissue at the distal end of a long stent is rare but has been noted in patients with tracheomalacia, perhaps secondary to mucosal erosion from irritation of the lower tip of the stent. The stent surface should be polished in an effort to minimize granulation tissue formation. Patients with long stents should be flexibly scoped to assess the presence and degree of granulation tissue at the distal tip of the stent.[26]

The Montgomery T tube is made of silicone, which is biologically inert (Figure 5). In one study in which long-term Montgomery T-tube stents were placed without concurrent LTR in an effort to gradually dilate the area of stenosis and eventually allow closure of the tracheostomy site, 25% of the patients developed severe granulation tissue obstruction at the distal stent site, requiring urgent removal of the stent at some point during the stenting process.[30] The Montgomery T-tube stent, because of its composition, can remain in situ for many months without inciting

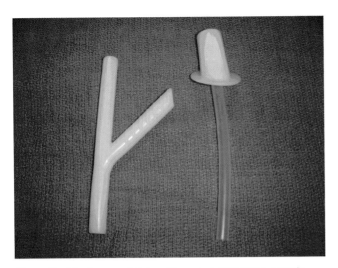

Figure 5. Montgomery T tube with a removable inner cannula.

the same degree of inflammatory response typically seen with Aboulker stents for the same time period.

Stenting is an important adjunct to LTR. It prevents both restenosis and collapse of the airway lumen. The stents in use today have their pros and cons, but no one stent is ideal. There is a large body of research in various animal models investigating both the indications for stenting and the materials used. One study involving LTR in 42 rabbits placed polyvinyl endotracheal stents in half of the animals and no stent in the other half of the animals. There was a trend toward increased mucosal edema and granulation tissue formation, particularly in the animals stented for a longer period of time.[31] Another study advocated placement of a long-term subglottic stent at the time of tracheostomy or extubation as a means of preventing subglottic stenosis. They used two different stent materials Portex (Smiths Medical, St. Paul, MN) and Vygon (Vygon Corp., Norristown, PA) and then sacrificed the animals with stents in place in one group and 1 week after removing the stent in the other group. All of the inflammatory changes induced by the stents were confined to the mucosa, with no evidence of underlying injury to the laryngeal framework. This was already diminishing at 1 week after stent removal.[32] Other studies have used stents constructed of silicone[33] and Medpor (Porex Corp., Newnan, GA).[34]

In addition to the obvious granulation tissue response that occurs even with the most inert stents, there is a risk of secondary infection induced by the stent, causing additional inflammation and greater degrees of stenosis. Pathogens contaminating the surgical incision may exacerbate the inflammatory response, more so if there is active infection. A study emphasizing the type and frequency of organisms that colonized the stents placed during LTR yielded interesting results. The biofilm of 23 stents was cultured and grew between two and seven organisms, most commonly *Streptococcus viridans*, *Pseudomonas aeruginosa*, *Neisseria* species, *Haemophilus influenzae*, and *Candida* species.[35] These data have implications in the practical use of antibiotics while an airway stent is in place and guide empiric prophylactic antibiotic choices.

PEARLS AND PITFALLS: MAXIMIZING HEALING AFTER LTR

When considering aspects of LTR that make the most difference in postoperative success, some are independent of whether the procedure is single stage or two stage. Meticulous handling of the rib graft with attention to maintaining the vitality of the perichondrial layer, which will face the airway lumen, is paramount. Planning for endoscopic procedures prior to extubation or stent removal or decannulation is important, particularly if excision of airway granulation tissue must be performed.

Single-Stage LTR

Yellon and colleagues described their protocol for decreasing morbidity following LTR. Clindamycin and antipseudomonal antibiotics were prophylactically administered in patients while intubated, and there was a significant decrease in the number of infectious complications in patients receiving these antibiotics (8%) compared with those receiving alternative regimens (50%).[24] The use of intravenous steroids has been controversial. Some advocate their use to help diminish edema and inflammation, but Yellon and colleagues advocate avoidance of administering both corticosteroids and neuro-muscular blockers, reporting decreased compli-cations with postextubation muscle weakness when avoiding this combination. Antireflux therapy was also strongly recommended.[24]

Cotton and colleagues agreed that it is "imperative" that any gastroesophageal reflux be controlled either medically or surgically before any reconstruction.[21] They also suggested that pulmonary function is an important factor in the timing of single-stage LTR and that the patient must be free of supplementary oxygen for at least 3 months before single-stage LTR.

Two-Stage LTR

The postoperative course of a two-stage LTR requires vigilant monitoring of the distal tip of the stent with flexible endoscopy.[26] Meticulous tracheostomy tube suctioning must be reinforced to caregivers because the potential for obstruc-tion of the tube with secretions or granulation tissue may be life-threatening. Stents have been previously discussed, but the choice of stent depending on the airway lesion and surgeon preference deserves mention. Most surgeons advocate painstaking control of gastroesopha-geal reflux before, during, and after airway reconstruction in an effort to diminish airway inflammation that may predispose the patient to granulation tissue formation and additional stenosis. Perioperative antibiotics are also routi-nely administered with a variable length of treatment.

Mitomycin-C: Pearl or Pitfall?

Mitomycin-C is an antibiotic that is metabolized to an alkylating agent, inhibiting deoxyribonu-cleic acid (DNA) synthesis and inhibiting cell division and fibroblast proliferation. Its use in the pediatric airway has been somewhat con-troversial for two reasons: (1) Does its topical use in the airway have any effect on preventing subglottic and tracheal scar formation and

stenosis? (Does the benefit outweigh the risk?) and (2) What are the potential short- and long-term side effects (including a theoretical risk of carcinogenesis) that would preclude its use in children?

Both animal and human studies examining the efficacy of mitomycin-C in an airway model exist. Correa and colleagues elicited subglottic stenosis in a canine model with the carbon dioxide laser and then carried out radial incisions and dilations of the subglottic airway.[36] Animals were randomly assigned to receive either a 1% topical solution of mitomycin-C to the subglottic area for 5 minutes or no other treatment. Weekly microlaryngoscopy and photodocumentation of the airway were performed for 6 weeks. Eighty percent of the control animals developed sub-glottic stenosis so severe that they had to be sacrificed early. All treatment group animals survived the study. Morphometric analysis of the subglottic photographs confirmed a greater than 100% increase in the percentage of the relative airway. There was a corresponding decrease in collagen formation in the subglottic wounds of the animals treated with mitomycin-C. Rahbar and colleagues treated 15 patients with mitomy-cin-C as an adjuvant to the endoscopic laser management of laryngotracheal stenosis and found that 93% of patients had an improvement in their airway and resolution of preoperative symptoms.[37] A mean follow-up of 18 months revealed no complications from treatment with mitomycin-C.[37]

A pig model evaluating the efficacy of topical mitomycin-C after performing single-stage LTR with stenting showed that mitomycin-C did not affect the acute inflammatory response, reepithe-lialization of the graft site, or formation of the subepithelial fibroproliferative response. Those treated with mitomycin-C did show better graft incorporation, less necrosis of the graft, and neochondrification of the graft.[38] These findings suggest an equivocal efficacy at best. A human study by Hartnick and colleagues treated patients who underwent LTR with mitomycin-C or placebo at the time of extubation or stent removal and found nearly identical results between the two groups, suggesting that no effect was gained by treatment with mitomycin-C.[39] One wonders if the results may have been more favorable if the treatment with mitomycin-C was performed at the time of LTR rather than at the time of stent removal.

Although short-term complication rates for the topical use of mitomycin-C in the airway have proven favorable, its systemic use has known toxicities. Pulmonary toxicity consisting of dyspnea and cough occurs with an incidence of 2.8 to 12%.[40] Approximately 40% of patients who develop pulmonary toxicity will die of progressive pulmonary disease.[40] A syndrome of renal failure has been described in 10% of patients, usually appearing after 6 months of therapy.[40] Mitomycin-C has been shown to be carcinogenic and teratogenic in animal studies.[40] Caution should be exercised and patients should be carefully monitored if several doses of mitomycin-C are planned or if therapy is administered in a manner other than topically.

POTENTIAL FUTURE THERAPIES

Modulation of Growth Factors

The success of LTR as measured by tracheostomy decannulation approaches 90%.[20,24] Future therapies for the treatment of subglottic stenosis depend on an accurate investigation and understanding of the remaining 10% of patients who fail LTR. Why do these patients fail, and can intrinsic factors for each patient be studied to determine the risk factors for failure? Once elucidated, may these risk factors be mitigated to allow for greater postoperative success?

Walner and colleagues approached this exact question by histologically examining the area of resected stenosis, testing for various growth factors and extracellular matrix components.[41] They found that the patients they deemed "adequate wound healers" had a positive correlation with vasculature fibronectin, vasculature tenascin, and stromal fibronectin. Those "poor wound healers" in the study had a positive correlation with stromal vascular endothelial

growth factor. Animal studies by the same group suggested a role for platelet-derived growth factor (PDGF) in laryngotracheal wound healing.[42] Some animals had an increased inflammatory response but did not have granulation tissue severe enough to cause life-threatening airway obstruction.

Scioscia and colleagues biopsied the subglottis of various patients with subglottic stenosis and stained these specimens for various growth factors.[43] They demonstrated fibrogenic growth factors deposited in the upper airway tissues of patients with subglottic stenosis, in particular transforming growth factor β_2 (TGF-β_2) and PDGF. There were differences between patients with idiopathic subglottic stenosis and post-traumatic or postintubation subglottic stenosis, suggesting a distinct pathogenic mechanism. They surmised that PDGF and TGF-β_2 may act in concert to produce the pathologic fibrotic process of subglottic stenosis. Dillard and colleagues also suggested that TGF-β may play a role in the pathogenesis of subglottic stenosis.[44] Clearly, this is an area in which much more research, especially regarding individual growth factors and their role in the formation of subglottic stenosis and in an appropriate postoperative healing response after LTR, needs to be performed.

The primary goal of LTR is to provide an adequate airway to allow tracheostomy decannulation. A patient may be one considered a success because of the ability to decannulate but often at the expense of functional phonation and a competent swallowing mechanism. Many authors have described the high incidence of abnormal vocal quality after LTR. Zalzal and colleagues found 15 of 16 patients with an aberrant voice subsequent to LTR and decannulation.[45] Bailey and colleagues found that 75% of children with a Cotton grade I stenosis had an acceptable voice postoperatively, but for grades II, III, and IV, the percentage of patients with acceptable voices fell to between 40 and 50%.[46] Similar results in vocal function were observed by Sell and MacCurtain., MacArthur and colleagues, and Smith and colleagues.[47–49]

Dysphonia after LTR occurs for a variety of reasons, including blunting of the anterior commissure (especially after laryngofissure), vocal cord dysfunction after stent placement, and arytenoid abnormalities.[45,46] Evaluation of the voice is currently performed by flexible laryngoscopy to assess vocal cord function, vocal acoustic analysis, usually showing a decreased fundamental frequency of phonation, diminished frequency range, and decreased vocal intensity.[49] Smith and colleagues reported the utility of stroboscopy to aid in the diagnosis of the vocal abnormality in these patients.[49] In summary, the future of LTR is to effectively decannulate patients while allowing a maximally functional voice.

Lathyrogens

Beta-aminopropionitrile (β-APN) is a lathyrogen, a compound that interferes with collagen and elastin cross-linking. Studies investigating the mechanism of lathyrogens in superficial skin wound healing demonstrate some efficacy of these compounds for inhibiting wound contracture when injected subcutaneously.[50] Interference of the collagen cross-linking process keeps a larger portion of the synthesized collagen soluble, ultimately reducing the amount of collagen available for wound contraction. This effect is due to a defect in the maturation of a newly formed scar; mature collagen already present in tissue is unaffected.[51] Lathyrogens have been shown to reduce the effect of the scar in esophageal stricture.[51] Doolin and colleagues, in an elaborate animal study, tracheostomized dogs and then induced a circumferential subglottic injury through the tracheostomy.[51] They had a control group, a group treated with oral steroid, and a group given β-APN. They found that subglottic stenosis owing to inflammation and scar was qualitatively less in the animals treated with lathyrogen. Quantitative immunohistochemical staining for collagen III was significantly reduced by β-APN. The administration of lathyrogens may hold promise in the prevention and treatment of "soft" or immature subglottic stenosis owing to airway inflammation. No studies investigating the efficacy of lathyrogens in the human airway have been published.

Secretion Analysis as a Predictor of Healing

Branski and colleagues suggested a novel approach to assist in the management of patients following intubation injury through an animal study collecting subglottic secretions for analysis.[52] The secretions were collected at various time intervals after inducing a subglottic mucosal injury with the carbon dioxide laser and were subjected to an enzyme-linked immunoassay for interleukin-1β (IL-1β) and prostaglandin E_2 (PGE$_2$). They found measurable amounts of both inflammatory mediators with a distinct temporal pattern post-trauma. The IL-1β levels were increased on days 4 to 18, and the PGE$_2$ levels were increased on days 7 to 18. Analysis of airway secretions in the future may be helpful in determining the natural wound healing process in the subglottis and provide a marker for treatment efficacy.

Tissue Engineering of Subglottic and Tracheal Tissue

Previous attempts at solving the issue of surgical airway reconstruction in patients in whom sufficient tissue for surgery is absent have included prostheses, nonviable tissue grafts, and airway transplantation but have failed because of graft failure, tissue necrosis, and eventual restenosis, all owing to a lack of revascularization.[53] The emerging field of tissue engineering holds promise for solving these problems, with its ability to replace worn, damaged, or poorly functioning tissue and restore cellular functions by creating new tissue. Of all of the strategies employed for this goal, a synthetic polymer scaffold that mimics extracellular matrix seeded with autologous cells grown in culture shows the highest likelihood for tissue incorporation and healing. A discussion of the general principles of tissue engineering follows elsewhere in this text;

the principles of tissue engineering specifically pertaining to the trachea deserve discussion.

Tissue engineering of the trachea involves replacement of the epithelium and cartilage. The challenges associated with maintenance of functional respiratory epithelium without loss of ciliated cells have been overcome by basing resorbable scaffolds on nonwoven collagen to grow human respiratory epithelial cells, and these constructs have been shown to maintain ciliated cells over time.[54] Ciliogenesis has also been demonstrated. Collagen scaffolds have been shown to promote differentiation of stem cells into fully differentiated airway epithelium that exhibits structural features and mucus secretion akin to native respiratory epithelium.[55]

To create a full tissue equivalent of the trachea, tissue-engineered respiratory epithelium must be supported by long segments of cartilage. Collagen-coated mesh tubes implanted in an animal model to promote regeneration of tracheal cartilage were found to provide good airway framework support but also caused the formation of granulation tissue.[56] Various scaffolds seeded with chondrocytes or bone marrow stromal cells were allowed to mature in vitro and were then implanted, maintaining the cartilaginous phenotype.[57] Polyglycolic acid scaffolds have been used with ovine chondrocytes for fetal tracheal repair, resulting in successful engraftment and reepithelialization, and with histological features comparable to those of native trachea.[58]

A tissue-engineered cartilage composed of pig chondrocytes seeded on a copolymer scaffold was allowed to develop in a subcutaneous pocket prior to implantation as an anterior cartilage graft for LTR.[59] These implants incorporated into the cricoid area and mucosalized, and a patent airway was maintained. A similar tissue-engineered LTR study was performed in rabbits with a different scaffold material, but a high mortality resulted owing to airway obstruction.[60] As research continues on appropriate scaffold materials and maintenance of functional respiratory epithelium in vitro, the ideal LTR graft and even the ideal neotrachea may be realized.

CONCLUSION

The challenge for any surgeon working in the subglottis and trachea is the development of subglottic stenosis. An understanding of the fundamental aspects of mucosal and cartilaginous wound healing, as well as factors that predispose the patient to stenosis, has direct clinical application after LTR surgery. The future of subglottic and tracheal surgery is the development of an ideal graft, minimally invasive surveillance of predictive markers for stenosis, and an understanding of why the patients who cannot be decannulated after LTR fail.

REFERENCES

1. Dohar JE, Stool SE. Respiratory mucosa wound healing and its management: an overview. Otolaryngol Clin North Am 1995;28:897–912.
2. Walner DL, Loewen MS, Kimura RE. Neonatal subglottic stenosis—incidence and trends. Laryngoscope 2001; 111:48–51.
3. Gau GS, Ryder TA, Mobberley MA. Iatrogenic epithelial change caused by endotracheal intubation of neonates. Early Hum Dev 1987;15:221–9.
4. Gould SJ, Howard S. The histopathology of the larynx in the neonate following endotracheal intubation. J Pathol 1985;146:301–11.
5. Albert DM, Mills RP, Fysh J, et al. Endoscopic examination of the neonatal larynx at extubation: a prospective study of variables associated with laryngeal damage. Int J Pediatr Otorhinolaryngol 1990;20:203–12.
6. Gaynor EB. Gastroesophageal reflux as an etiologic factor in laryngeal complications of intubation. Laryngoscope 1988;98:972–9.
7. Dankle SK, Schuller DE, McClead RE. Prolonged intubation of neonates. Arch Otolaryngol Head Neck Surg 1987;113:841–3.
8. Dankle SK, Schuller DE, McClead RE. Risk factors for neonatal acquired subglottic stenosis. Ann Otol Rhinol Laryngol 1986;95:626–30.
9. Chen JC, Holinger LD. Acquired laryngeal lesions. Pathologic study using serial macrosections. Arch Otolaryngol Head Neck Surg 1995;121:537–43.
10. Duynstee MLG, de Krijger RR, Monnier P, et al. Subglottic stenosis after endotracheal intubation in infants and children: result of wound healing processes. Int J Pediatr Otorhinolaryngol 2002;62:1–9.
11. Goldstein NA, Hebda PA, Klein EC, Dohar JE. Wound management of the airway mucosa: comparison with

skin in a rabbit model. Int J Pediatr Otorhinolaryngol 1998;45:223–5.

12. Bean JK, Verwoerd-Verhoef HL, Verwoerd CDA. Injury and age-linked differences in wound healing and stenosis formation in the subglottis. Acta Otolaryngol (Stockh) 1995;115:317–21.

13. Verwoerd-Verhoef HL, Bean JK, Adriaansen FCPM, Verwoerd CDA. Wound healing of laryngeal trauma and the development of subglottic stenosis. Int J Pediatr Otorhinolaryngol 1995;32(Suppl):S103–5.

14. Dohar JE, Klein EC, Betsch JL, Hebda PA. Acquired subglottic stenosis—depth and not extent of the insult is key. Int J Pediatr Otorhinolaryngol 1998;46:159–70.

15. Koufman JA, Thompson JN, Kohut RI. Endoscopic management of subglottic stenosis with the CO_2 surgical laser. Otolaryngol Head Neck Surg 1981;89:215–20.

16. Azizkhan RG. Laser surgery: new applications for pediatric skin and airway lesions. Curr Opin Pediatr 2003;15:243–7.

17. Benjamin B, Jacobson I, Eckstein R. Idiopathic subglottic stenosis: diagnosis and endoscopic laser treatment. Ann Otol Rhinol Laryngol 1997;106:770–4.

18. Myer CM, Willging PJ, McMurray S, et al. Use of the laryngeal microresector system. Laryngoscope 1999;109:1165–6.

19. Rees CJ, Tridico TI, Kirse DJ. Expanding applications for the microdebrider in pediatric endoscopic airway surgery. Otolaryngol Head Neck Surg 2005;133:509–13.

20. Cotton RT, O'Connor DM. Pediatric laryngotracheal reconstruction: 20 years' experience. Acta Otol Rhinol Laryngol Belg 1995;49:367–72.

21. Cotton RT, Myer CM, O'Connor DM, Smith ME. Pediatric laryngotracheal reconstruction with cartilage grafts and endotracheal tube stenting: the single-stage approach. Laryngoscope 1995;105:818–21.

22. Cotton RT. Management of subglottic stenosis in infancy and childhood: review of a consecutive series of cases managed by surgical reconstruction. Ann Otol Rhinol Laryngol 1978;87:649–57.

23. Inglis AF, Perkins JA, Manning SC, Mouzakes J. Endoscopic posterior cricoid split and rib grafting in 10 children. Laryngoscope 2003;113:2004–9.

24. Yellon RF, Parameswaran M, Brandom BW. Decreasing morbidity following laryngotracheal reconstruction in children. Int J Pediatr Otorhinolaryngol 1997;41:145–54.

25. Saunders MW, Thirlwall A, Jacob A, Albert DM. Single- or two-stage laryngotracheal reconstruction; comparison of outcomes. Int J Pediatr Otorhinolaryngol 1999;50:51–4.

26. Zalzal GH. Stenting for pediatric laryngotracheal stenosis. Ann Otol Rhinol Laryngol 1992;101:651–5.

27. Evans JNG. Laryngotracheoplasty. Otolaryngol Clin North Am 1977;10:119–23.

28. Dumon JF. A dedicated tracheobronchial stent. Chest 1990;97:328–32.

29. Temes RT, Wernly JA, Cooper JD, et al. Internal fixation of high tracheal stents. Ann Thorac Surg 1995;59:1023–4.

30. Froehlich P, Truy E, Stamm D, et al. Role of long-term stenting in treatment of pediatric subglottic stenosis. Int J Pediatr Otorhinolaryngol 1993;27:273–80.

31. Jewett BS, Cook RD, Johnson KL, et al. Effect of stenting after laryngotracheal reconstruction in a subglottic stenosis model. Otolaryngol Head Neck Surg 2000;122:488–94.

32. Albert DM, Cotton RT, Conn P. Effect of laryngeal stenting in a rabbit model. Ann Otol Rhinol Laryngol 1990;99:108–11.

33. Liu HC, Lee KS, Huang CJ, et al. Silicone T-tube for complex laryngotracheal problems. Eur J Card Thorac Surg 2002;21:326–30.

34. Hashem FK, Homsi MA, Mahasin ZZ, Gammas MA. Laryngotracheoplasty using the Medpor implant: an animal model. J Otolaryngol 2001;30:334–9.

35. Simoni P, Wiatrak BJ. Microbiology of stents in laryngotracheal reconstruction. Laryngoscope 2004;114:364–7.

36. Correa AJ, Reinisch L, Sanders DL, et al. Inhibition of subglottic stenosis with mitomycin-C in the canine model. Ann Otol Rhinol Laryngol 1999;108:1053–60.

37. Rahbar R, Shapshay SM, Healy GB. Mitomycin: effects on laryngeal and tracheal stenosis, benefits and complications. Ann Otol Rhinol Laryngol 2001;110:1–6.

38. Coppit G, Perkins J, Munaretto J, et al. The effects of mitomycin-C and stenting on airway wound healing after laryngotracheal reconstruction in a pig model. Int J Pediatr Otorhinolaryngol 2000;53:125–35.

39. Hartnick CJ, Hartley BEJ, Lacy PD, et al. Topical mitomycin application after laryngotracheal reconstruction. Arch Otolaryngol Head Neck Surg 2001;127:1260–4.

40. Compendium of Pharmaceuticals and Specialties. Mutamycin. Toronto, CA: Canadian Pharmacists Association, Toronto, Canada; 2004.

41. Walner DL, Heffelfinger SC, Stern Y, et al. Potential role of growth factors and extracellular matrix in wound healing after laryngotracheal reconstruction. Otolaryngol Head Neck Surg 2000;122:363–6.

42. Walner DL, Cotton RT, Willging JP, et al. Model for evaluating the effect of growth factors on the larynx. Otolaryngol Head Neck Surg 1999;120:78–83.

43. Scioscia KA, April MM, Miller F, Gruber BL. Growth factors in subglottic stenosis. Ann Otol Rhinol Laryngol 1996;105:936–43.

44. Dillard DG, Gal AA, Roman-Rodriguez J, et al. Transforming growth factor and neutralizing antibodies in subglottic stenosis. Ann Otol Rhinol Laryngol 2001;110:393–400.

45. Zalzal GH, Loomis SR, Derkay CS, et al. Vocal quality of decannulated children following laryngotracheal reconstruction. Laryngoscope 1991;101:425–9.

46. Bailey CM, Clary RA, Pengilly A, Albert DM. Voice quality following laryngotracheal reconstruction. Int J Pediatr Otorhinolaryngol 1995;32(Suppl):S93–5.

47. Sell D, MacCurtain F. Speech and language development in children with acquired subglottic stenosis. J Laryngol Otol Suppl 1988;17:35–8.

48. MacArthur CJ, Kearns GH, Healy GB. Voice quality after laryngotracheal reconstruction. Arch Otolaryngol Head Neck Surg 1994;120:641–7.

49. Smith ME, Mortelliti AJ, Cotton RT, Myer CM. Phonation and swallowing considerations in pediatric laryngotracheal reconstruction. Ann Otol Rhinol Laryngol 1992;101:731–8.

50. Joseph HL, Roisen FJ, Anderson GL, et al. Inhibition of wound contraction with locally injected lathyrogenic drugs. Am J Surg 1997;174:347–50.

51. Doolin EJ, Strande LF, Tsuno K, Santos MC. Pharmacologic inhibition of collagen in an experimental model of subglottic stenosis. Ann Otol Rhinol Laryngol 1998;107:275–9.

52. Branski RC, Sandulache VC, Dohar JE, Hebda PA. Mucosal wound healing in a rabbit model of subglottic stenosis: biochemical analysis of secretions. Arch Otolaryngol Head Neck Surg 2005;131:153–7.

53. Grillo HC. Tracheal replacement: a critical review. Ann Thorac Surg 2002;73:1995–2004.

54. Ziegelaar BW, Aigner J, Staudenmaier R, et al. The characterization of human respiratory epithelial cells cultured on resorbable scaffolds: first steps toward a tissue engineered tracheal replacement. Biomaterials 2002;23:1425–38.

55. Coraux C, Nawrocki-Raby B, Hinnrasky J, et al. Embryonic stem cells generate airway epithelial tissue. Am J Respir Cell Mol Biol 2005;32:87–92.

56. Omori K, Nakamura T, Kanemaru S, et al. Cricoid regeneration using in situ tissue engineering in canine larynx for the treatment of subglottic stenosis. Ann Otol Rhinol Laryngol 2004;113:623–7.

57. Kojima K, Ignotz RA, Kushibiki T, et al. Tissue-engineered trachea from sheep marrow stromal cells with transforming growth factor $\beta 2$ released from biodegradable microspheres in a nude rat recipient. J Thorac Cardiovasc Surg 2004;128:147–53.

58. Fuchs JR, Terada S, Ochoa ER, et al. Fetal tissue engineering: in utero tracheal augmentation in an ovine model. J Pediatr Surg 2002;37:1000–6.

59. Kamil SH, Eavey RD, Vacanti MP, et al. Tissue-engineered cartilage as a graft source for laryngotracheal reconstruction. Arch Otolaryngol Head Neck Surg 2004;130:1048–51.

60. Grimmer JF, Gunnlaugsson CB, Alsberg E, et al. Tracheal reconstruction using tissue-engineered cartilage. Arch Otolaryngol Head Neck Surg 2004;130:1191–6.

22

The Facial Nerve after Injury

Kofi D.O. Boahene, MD; Mark May, MD

Injury to the facial nerve is a common clinical problem. Common causes include Bell's palsy, surgical trauma, and involvement with benign and malignant neoplasms. Evidence of faulty regeneration is the rule following spontaneous regeneration or nerve repair. Aberrant facial nerve regeneration results in motor dysfunction and is characterized by a combination of facial muscle hypokinesis (weakness) and hyperkinesis (hypertonus, synkinesis, spasm, and hemifacial contracture). Faulty facial nerve recovery may result in significant functional, aesthetic, and emotional disability. This chapter focuses on the theoretical and practical clinical aspects of motor dysfunction following facial nerve injury.

ANATOMY

The facial nerve is a mixed motor and sensory nerve composed of approximately 10,000 neurons. Seventy percent of the neurons are myelinated and innervate the muscles of facial expression. The motor fibers originate from the precentral and postcentral gyri of the frontal lobe (motor face area). These fibers project to the facial nucleus in the lower pons via the corticobulbar tract and internal capsule and through the upper and midbrainstem. The facial nucleus contains a musculotopic arrangement of four major nuclei subgroups: dorsomedial, ventromedial, intermediate, and lateral. Each subnucleus innervates a small group of facial muscles. For example, cells in the intermediate group inner-

vate the frontalis, orbicularis oculi, corrugator supercilli, and zygomaticus. The subnuclei innervating the sphincteric muscles of the eye and mouth are extensive, reflecting the greater need for complex movements in this area for speech, oral continence, eye protection, and facial expression. In contrast, nuclei representation for less used facial muscles, such as the depressor septi nasi or auricular muscles, is rudimentary. The delicate musculotopic arrangement of the facial nucleus is disrupted following facial nerve injury.[1]

Once the facial nerve exits the brainstem, the musculotopic arrangement is lost.[2] Within the parotid gland, the nerve divides into superior (temporofacial) and inferior (cervicofacial) divisions, which are interconnected by a rich network of fibers, each programmed during embryogenesis to reach a specific muscle target.

After facial nerve injury, characteristic changes occur in the cell body, proximal and distal axonal segments, and myoneural junction, disrupting the delicate nerve-muscle network. These changes influence the degree of recovery after spontaneous regeneration or nerve repair. Seddon and Sunderlund classified the fundamental types of nerve injury based on axonal integrity and the status of the endoneurium and perineurium.[3,4] However, in clinical situations, injuries to the facial nerve may not cause an all-or-nothing injury that fits perfectly into one of Seddon's or Sunderlund's injury classification. Rather, a mixed pattern of injury is often observed. The degree of regeneration is closely related to the level of injury. One can expect some level of faulty regeneration as long as nerve degeneration occurs (Figure 1).

CLINICAL MANIFESTATION OF FACIAL NERVE INJURY

Within days to weeks of facial nerve injury, symptoms of facial hypotonus or hypokinesis are seen. Depending on the location and severity of injury, these may include brow ptosis, lagophthalmos, drooping of the corner of the mouth, collapse of the nasal alae, and an asymmetric smile. The severity of these findings depends on the intrinsic facial muscle tone and skin turgor. Children who have excellent skin turgor as opposed to the elderly are spared the early signs of hypotonus, with the exception of asymmetric facial movement. Most often, the signs of facial nerve injury are not apparent before 10 days because it takes that long to affect the facial muscles.

In cases in which axonal disruption has occurred, nerve regeneration begins and becomes clinically apparent between 2 and 4 months. Axonal regeneration results in varying degrees of motor dysfunction even under optimal nerve repair conditions using advanced microsurgical techniques. A continuum of symptoms from chronic hypokinetic to chronic hyperkinetic disorders can be used to describe the long-standing changes that may result for facial nerve injury. With no recovery, complete facial hypotonus is observed. With partial recovery, symptoms of hypokinesis are present. With increasing recovery, hyperkinesis (hypertonus, synkinesis, spasm, and hemifacial contracture) becomes a problem.

Chronic Hypokinetic Disorders

Chronic hypokinetic problems resulting from faulty facial nerve regeneration are those that reflect inadequate motor input and hypotonus. In the forehead, the horizontal rhytids are lost and the brow becomes ptotic. Lagophthalmos, reduced blink reflex, and lower eyelid ectropion

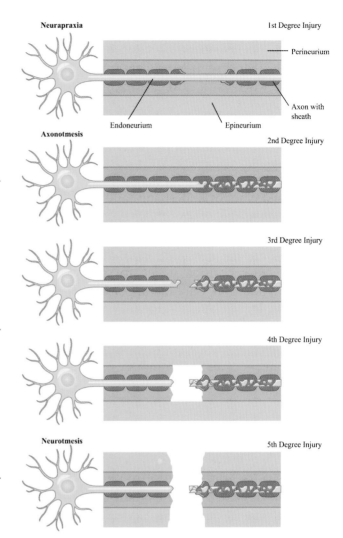

Figure 1. Sunderland nerve injury classification.[4]

cause chronic corneal exposure. In addition, loss of tone in the orbicularis oculi results in an apparent lengthening of the lower eyelid and pseudofat herniation, giving the patient an aged and chronically tired look. When the dilator nasalis muscles are affected, the alar and nasal valves collapse, resulting in nasal obstruction. Drooping of the mouth and oral incontinence may also be seen.

Chronic Hyperkinetic Disorders

The clinical signs and symptoms of hyperkinesis depend on the muscle group involved and the extent of regeneration. Hypertonicity of the orbicularis oculi muscle may give rise to narrowing of the palpebral fissure. This appearance may be made worse with eating, drinking, talking, or blowing out the cheek, reflecting the presence of synkinesis from faulty regeneration. This palpebral fissure narrowing should be distinguished from true ptosis resulting from levator muscle dysfunction.[5] A careful history usually reveals additional clues of underlying faulty facial nerve regeneration, such as crocodile tears and synkinesis. The supratarsal crease in facial paralysis patients remains unchanged, in contrast to the higher crease position in levator muscle dehiscence. In addition, only the upper lid is involved in true ptosis, whereas both the upper and the lower eyelid position contributes to narrowing of the palperbral fissure seen in orbicularis oculi hypertonicity. Lagophthalmos is usually absent. It will be an error to attempt to correct this palpebral fissure asymmetry with levator muscle repair because this may result in lagophthalmos and corneal exposure. Hypertonicity of the zygomaticus major and other perioral levator muscles causes deepening of the nasolabial fold and exaggerated elevation of the corner of the mouth. Involvement of the chin musculature causes dimpling with peau d'orange changes. With involvement of the platysma, contracture and banding in the neck become apparent and painful.

Hyperkinesis of the affected side can also present as facial spasm varying from isolated blepharospasm to severe painful hemifacial mass contracture. These short-lived spasms may be triggered by voluntary or emotional facial expression, such as smiling and kissing, which creates a situation of significant psychosocial disability. Blepharospasm and hemifacial spasm resulting from aberrant facial nerve regeneration may mimic that seen in essential blepharospasm and essential hemifacial spasm. However, careful history, a clinical examination, and electrophysiologic evaluation permit the separation of the two entities. Unlike spasms resulting from aberrant facial nerve regeneration, voluntary facial movement does not necessarily trigger

essential hemifacial spasms. In essential hemifacial spasm, facial contraction is usually paroxysmal and consists of irregular, rapid, clonic bursts of electromyographic (EMG) activity simultaneously involving the upper and lower facial musculature.[6] In contrast, the EMG firing rate in aberrant regeneration is slower. Essential hemifacial spasm is believed to result from vascular compression at the facial nerve root exit zone and usually responds to posterior fossa decompression. Nerve decompression will have no effect on spasms arising from faulty facial nerve regeneration.

Another common manifestation of faulty facial nerve regeneration is facial synkinesis. Synkinesis is the abnormal synchronization of movement accompanying voluntary and reflex activity of muscles that normally do not contract together. Three prevalent theories proposed as responsible for synkinesis are (1) aberrant regeneration of facial nerve fibers, (2) peripheral ephaptic transmission of impulses between regenerating axons, and (3) somatotopic reorganization within the facial nerve nucleus. Clinically, mild forms of synkinesis following facial nerve injury may consist of a hardly detectible chin twitch that accompanies a blink. In extreme cases, there is mass movement on the affected side and loss of the ability to carry out fine mimetic movement without gross facial contraction. In one study, the incidence of clinical synkinesis following facial paralysis was reported to be as high as 55%.[7] Using electrophysiologic criteria, synkinetic movement can be detected in nearly all patients with proximal facial nerve injury.[8] Synkinetic movement can be observed in the early postinjury period but becomes more overt as regeneration proceeds during the first year postinjury. The commonly observed clinical patterns of synkinesis are predictable rather than random.[9] The most common pattern is mouth movement with voluntary eye closure. The zygomaticus muscle is also commonly involved. These abnormal movements are limited to the side of injury and may progress to a tonic type of contracture involving all of the mimetic muscles.

TREATMENT OF CLINICAL SEQUELAE OF FACIAL NERVE INJURY

Current approaches to treating clinical sequelae of facial nerve injury include noninvasive, semi-invasive, and invasive strategies. Treatment strategies can be targeted toward chonic hypokinetic and chronic hyperkinetic problems.

Chronic Hypokinetic Problems

The current treatment of chronic hypokinetic disorders includes surgical reanimation with nerve grafting, free neuromuscular transfer or pedicled musculofascial transposition, and a spectrum of static techniques (Table 1). For a detailed description of the various techniques by the coauthor, see May.[10] Primary neurorrhaphy, whenever feasible, is the mainstay of reanimation of the hypokinetic face. Presently, advances in microsurgery have allowed precision in anatomic alignment of the severed nerves aided by visual magnification. At best, one can expect improved voluntary movement and symmetry at rest, but the execution of fine mimetic movement without signs of aberrancy remains elusive. When primary neurorrhaphy is not possible, nerve grafting with a bridging donor graft is the recommended procedure. In clinical situations in which the proximal nerve stump is unavailable, nerve substitution techniques with other cranial nerves, particularly the hypoglossal

nerve, assume a prominent role. The single most important factor influencing the clinical outcome of nerve repair is the timing of repair. The most optimal results occur when repair is done within 30 days of the nerve injury. Beyond this period, somatotopic alterations in the facial nerve nucleus and collagenization along the nerve axon remarkably diminish the degree of functional recovery. Two technical principles are key. First, neurorrhaphy should be tensionless. It is preferred to place an interposition graft whenever the two nerves do not passively align. Second, the endoneural surfaces should be matched. Neural matching ensures the suturing of proximal and distal nerve segments with comparable axonal concentration. Neural matching is particularly important when interposition grafts are used and in cranial nerve substitution procedures. It is important to note that the gross diameter of a nerve graft does not necessarily reflect the axonal concentration but rather the ratio of connective tissue to axons. Hence, time must be spent preparing the nerve segments by trimming back and stripping epineurium at both ends to uncover healthy endoneurim to determine an axonal surface match.

Chronic Hyperkinetic Problems

Several medical and surgical approaches have been used to either prevent or treat hyperkinetic

Table 1. PROBLEM-ORIENTED TREATMENT OF CHRONIC HYPOKINESIS		
Anatomic Site	**Clinical Problem**	**Treatment**
Brow	Ptosis	Brow-lift
Upper eyelid	Lagophthalmos	Gold weight implant, tarsorrhaphy
Lower eyelid	Ectropion	Medial canthoplasty, lateral canthoplasty
		Lower lid fascial sling, cartilage graft
Nose	Valve collapse	Suspension slings, cartilage grafts
Mouth	Drooping	Neuromuscular retraining
		Static sling (fascial lata, palmaris longus tendon, AlloDerm, Gore-Tex), suspension sutures
		Temporalis suspension, masseter suspension, SMAS suspension
		Free neuromuscular transfer (gracilis, latissimus, serratus)
		Lateral lip-lift
	Incontinence	Commissuroplasty, wedge resection
	Lower lip palsy	Digastric transposition

SMAS = superficial muscular aponeurotic system.

disorders of facial nerve regeneration. Presently, there is no single treatment modality effective in restoring normal facial nerve function once aberrant regeneration has occurred. Preventive measures, including high-dose steroids, early nerve decompression, and selective neurectomy, have all yielded inconsistent results. Table 2 provides a problem-oriented approach to treating chronic hyperkinetic disorders resulting from faulty facial nerve regeneration.

Prior to initiating any treatment, a complete history and thorough clinical examination should be performed. It is important to clearly establish the etiology of the facial paralysis, with particular attention to excluding occult neoplasms masquerading as Bell's palsy.[11] The nature of the aberrant movement disorder should be defined, differentiating hypokinetic disorders from hyperkinetic ones. Clinical findings should be properly documented using video and photodocumentation. A comprehensive treatment plan can then be formulated, which may include (1) noninvasive, (2) semi-invasive, and (3) invasive modalities.

Noninvasive Therapy: Neuromuscular Retraining

Neuromuscular retraining uses selective motor training enhanced by visual and surface EMG feedback to facilitate symmetric facial movement, optimize muscle tone, and control unde-

sired motor hyperkinesis.[12] The best candidates are highly motivated patients with realistic expectations. Neuromuscular retraining unlinks undesired motions from the desired ones using slow, small-amplitude, desired motions while consciously suppressing the undesired ones. As the undesired activity is suppressed, the range of the primary movement gradually extends, increasing excursion, strength, and motor control. Surface EMG biofeedback is an essential complementary tool that helps bring the normally unconscious control of specific muscles under conscious control. Surface EMG feedback provides the patient with information regarding the rate and strength of the muscle contraction in real time. In the properly selected patient, neuromuscular training is an effective, relatively inexpensive, and noninvasive means of treating motor dysfunction arising from faulty regeneration (Figure 2).

Semi-Invasive Therapy

Botulinum toxin (Botox) offers a minimally invasive and effective treatment of facial hyperkinesis, such as blepharospasm, ptosis, facial contracture, and synkinesis. Botulinum toxin is a potent neurotoxin produced by *Clostridium botulinum*. The toxin blocks acetylcholine release at the neuromuscular junction, causing a chemical denervation. Botulinum toxin temporarily weakens targeted muscles, with effects lasting 3

Table 2. PROBLEM-ORIENTED TREATMENT OF CHRONIC HYPERKINESIS		
Anatomic Site	Clinical Problem	Treatment
Eye	Ptosis	NMR, botulinum toxin, levator resection, brow pexy
	Blepharospasm	NMR, botulinum toxin
	Synkinesis	NMR, botulinum toxin
Cheek-mouth	Deep nasolabial fold	NMR, Botulinum toxin into zygomaticus
		Zygomaticus myolysis
Mouth	Synkinesis, contracture	NMR, botulinum toxin
Chin	Dimpling, synkinesis	NMR, botulinum toxin, mentalis myolysis
Neck	Synkinesis, contracture	Platysmal myectomy,
		Botulinum toxin

NMR = neuromuscular retraining.

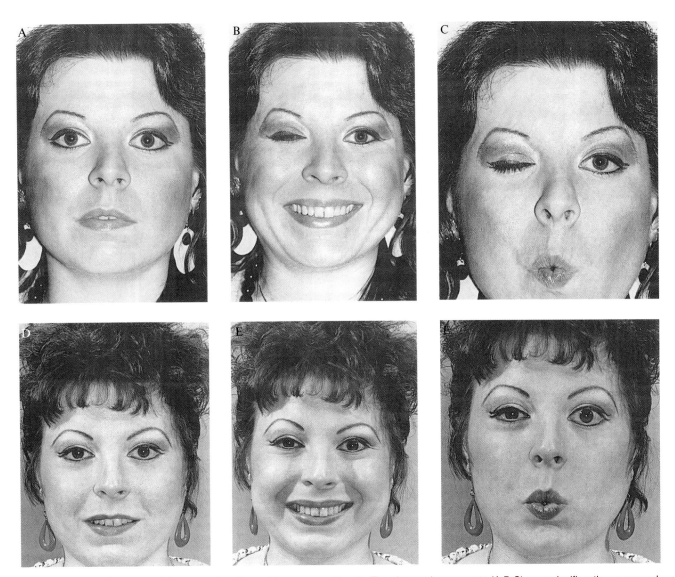

Figure 2.   Patient 2 years post-herpes zoster oticus with severe synkinesis. The abnormal movements (A,B,C) were significantly suppressed following surface EMG feedback therapy (D,E,F).

to 6 months. When combined with neuromuscular retraining, botulinum toxin provides chemical suppression of undesired muscle movement during which the patient can practice more normal movement patterns without synkinetic interference.

Prior to initiating botulinum toxin treatment, patients should be prescreened for potential contraindications. The toxin should be avoided in pregnant or lactating women and in patients with known neuromuscular diseases, such as myasthenia gravis, Eaton-Lambert syndrome, and motoneuron disease. It should be used with caution in patients taking aminoglycosides, which may potentiate the effect of the toxin by interfering with neuromuscular transmission. Next, the offending target muscles should be identified and mapped out. Selection of the appropriate dose depends on the target muscles, severity of symptoms, and individual differences. In general, it is safer to administer incremental doses spaced 2 weeks apart until the optimal response is achieved.

Blepharospasm and narrowed palpebral fissures resulting from synkinetic facial nerve regeneration can be managed with botulinum

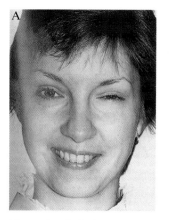
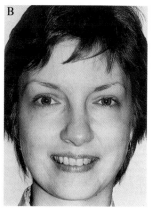

Figure 3. *A*, Patient with aberrant regeneration following Bell's palsy with involuntary eye closure with an effort smile. *B*, Note relief of spasm one week following upper and lower lid injection with botulinum toxin.

toxin injection. The rationale of this approach is to weaken the hypertonic and spastic effects of the protagonist (orbicularis oculi) while enhancing the dynamic range of the antagonists (Müller's muscle and levator muscle).[13] The net effect is a reduction in spasticity, widening of the palpebral aperture, and improvement in eye symmetry. Mild cases of periorbital muscle spasm can be treated with 0.5 to 1.0 units of botulinum toxin injected subdermally at the medial and lateral aspects of the pretarsal orbicularis oculi muscle (Figure 3). Higher doses may be used in severe and long-standing cases in which the orbicularis oculi has

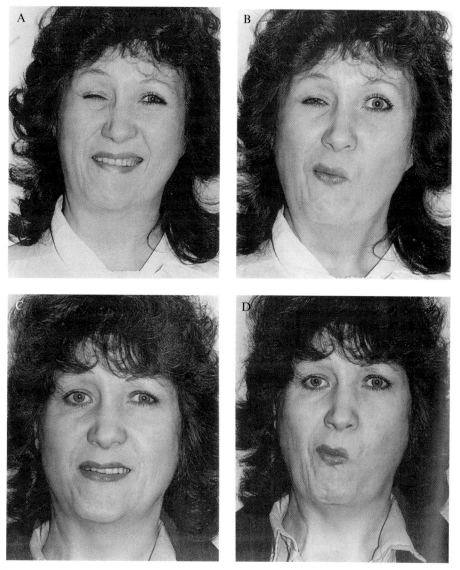

Figure 4. Patient with aberrant regeneration following Bell's palsy. *A* Demonstrates smile with effort. *B*, Involuntary eye closure when the lip is pursed. *C* and *D*, Note improvement after botulinum toxin injection.

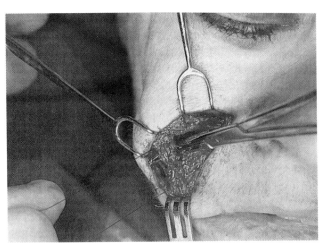

Figure 5. Selective resection for hypertonic zygomatic major muscle.

become hypertrophic. In severe cases of blepharospasm, injection is directed to the midpretarsal region of both lids and the lateral raphe region.

Patients with spasm of the perioral elevators resulting in an exaggerated pull of the corner of the mouth and a deepened nasolabial crease can be injected in the submalar area and the nasolabial crease (Figure 4). Similarly, chronic spasm of the mentalis and platysma can be relieved with direct injection into the offending muscles.

Invasive Therapy

In patients who have not responded to less invasive therapy, selective myectomy of offending hyperkinetic muscles provides an effective and permanent alternative to treating hyperkinetic dysfunction of faulty regeneration. Two approaches to myolysis, chemical and surgical, have been described. Chemical myectomy relies on the myotoxic properties of the chemotherapy agent doxorubi-

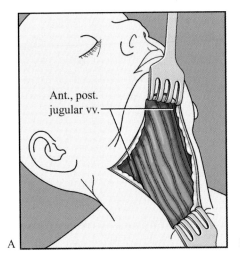

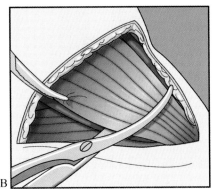

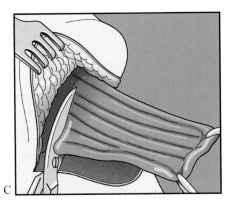

Figure 6. Technique of platysma resection.

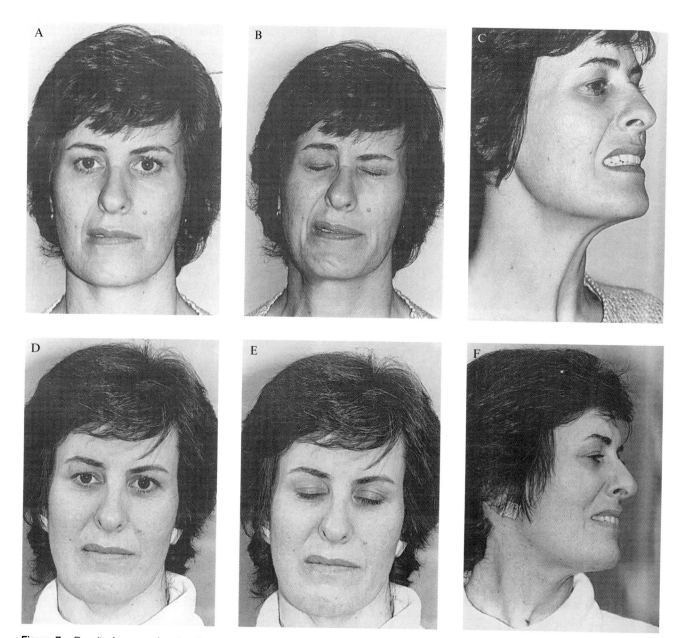

Figure 7. Result of surgery for chronic hyperkinesis following Bell's palsy. *A,B,C,* Preoperative appearance at rest, with eye closure and smiling. *D,E,F* Post operative appearance following resection of frontalis attachment to brow, zygomatic major, levator labii superioris, mentalis, and platysma muscles. Note that the right eyebrow does not elevate with eye closure. Also note the improvement in nasolabial fold, chin dimpling and platysmal spasm noted preoperatively.

cin.[14] Early clinical studies in blepharospasm and hemifacial spasm showed promising results, but complications of skin injury have limited its widespread use. The senior author prefers selective myectomy to other forms of myolysis. Prior to proceeding with myectomy, a thorough clinical evaluation should map out the involved muscle groups. An accurate determination of the degree of hyperkinesia should be made. Orbicularis oculi myectomy can be approached through standard upper and lower eyelid blepharoplasty incisions. The preseptal, preorbital, and pretarsal orbicularis oculi is dissected off the skin and resected. In mild cases of blepharospasm, a strip of pretarsal orbicularis oculi may be preserved. The levator muscle should be reattached.

Deep nasolabial creases arising from hyperkinesis of the zygomaticus muscle can be treated with partial resection of the muscle (Figure 5). An incision directly in the nasolabial groove provides exposure to the zygomaticus muscle and other levator muscles of the mouth. Prominent chin dimpling responds well to resection of the mentalis muscle through a submental approach. Depression and asymmetry of the lower lip secondary to hyperactivity of the depressor labii inferioris muscle can be improved by resecting this muscle. Resection of the platysma for unsightly banding and painful contracture is by far the most effective and rewarding of the surgical myectomies performed for chronic hyperkinetic disorders (Figure 6). This is because the platysma muscle is large, lending itself to a relatively easy identification and resection. Platysma resection can be accomplished through a horizontal incision in a natural skin rhytid in the neck. Subcutaneous dissection between the anterior and posterior jugular veins followed by separation of the platysma from the underlying fascia isolates the muscle (Figure 7). The muscle can then be divided along the mandibular border and its inferior aspect.

Most cases of selective surgical myectomy can be performed under local anesthesia with minimal discomfort to the patient. Selective myectomy produces immediate and long-lasting symptomatic improvement.

Selective Neurolysis

Prior to myectomy, peripheral facial neurectomy was considered the only effective surgical treatment for hyperkinesis of aberrant facial nerve regeneration. Selective nerve injury can be carried out by various methods, including alcohol injection, percutaneous thermolysis, or selective nerve avulsion. The senior author found selective neurolysis unpredictable because of the aberrant nature of the regenerating nerves, potential injury to intact adjacent nerves, and regeneration of the lysed nerve.

FUTURE APPROACHES TO TREATING SEQUELAE OF FACIAL NERVE INJURY

Many unanswered questions in the field of peripheral nerve repair remain. Current basic science investigations and the explosion in tissue engineering techniques may provide the basis for novel treatment approaches that may enhance clinical outcome following facial nerve injury. The primary areas that are being explored include the role of axonal guidance channels and neurotrophic factors in nerve repair

SUMMARY

The sequelae of faulty facial nerve regeneration, regardless of cause, are characterized by facial muscle hypokinesis or hyperkinesis. Although there are no effective preventive measures, these motor dysfunctions can be adequately controlled with a combination of invasive and less invasive techniques. Successful treatment depends on correctly defining the motor dysfunction, identifying the muscle groups involved, and selecting the appropriate intervention.

REFERENCES

1. Bratzlavsky M, Eecken H. Altered synaptic organization in facial nucleus following facial nerve regeneration: an electrophysiological study in man. Ann Neurol 1977;2: 71–3.
2. Gacek RR, Radpour S. Fiber orientation of the facial nerve, with special reference to peripheral facial palsy. Acta Med Acad Sci Hung 1957;10:249–59.
3. Seddon HJ. Three types of nerve injury. Brain 1943;66: 237–88.
4. Sunderland S. Nerve and nerve injuries. 2nd ed. London: Churchill Livingstone; 1978.
5. Chen C, Malhotra R, Muecke J, et al. Aberrant facial nerve regeneration: an underrecognized cause of ptosis. Eye 2004;18:158–62.
6. Valls-Sole J, Montero J. Movement disorders in patients with peripheral facial palsy. Mov Disord 2003;18: 1424–35.
7. Yamamoto E, Nishimura H, Hirono Y. Occurrence of sequelae in Bell's palsy. Acta Otolaryngol Suppl (Stockh) 1988;446:93–6.

8. Kimura J, Rodnitzky RL, Okawara SH. Electro-physiologic analysis of aberrant regeneration after facial nerve paralysis. Neurology 1975;25:989–93.

9. Moran CJ, Neely JG. Patterns of facial nerve synkinesis. Laryngoscope 1996;106:1491–6.

10. May M. Surgical rehabilitation of facial paralysis. In: May M, editor. The facial nerve. New York: Thieme; 1986. p. 695–781.

11. Boahene DO, Driscol C, Olsen KD, McDonald TJ. Facial nerve paralysis secondary to occult malignant neoplasms. Otolaryngol Head Neck Surg 2004;130:459–65.

12. Diels HJ. New concepts in nonsurgical facial nerve rehabilitation. Adv Otolaryngol Head Neck Surg 1995;9:289.

13. Fagien S. Botox for the treatment of dynamic and hyperkineti facial lines and furrows: adjunctive use in facial aesthetic surgery. Plast Reconstr Surg 2004; 114(7):1892–1902.

14. Wirtschafter JD. Clinical doxorubicin chemomyectomy. An experimental treatment for benign essential blepharospasm and hemifacial spasm. Ophthalmology 1991;98: 357–66.

23

General Approach to a Poorly Healing Problem Wound: Practical and Clinical Overview

David B. Hom, MD, FACS; Harley Dresner, MD

Acute wounds of the face and neck are known to heal faster compared with acute wounds of the rest of the body owing to their improved blood supply and blood perfusion. However, when poor healing occurs, severe compromise in the airway, swallowing, speaking, smell, taste, and hearing can occur, which significantly reduces quality of life. In addition, poor healing of the face and neck can be devastating to patients and their relatives owing to their increased visible disfigurement in public and society. Poor healing to the face and neck can also be life-threatening owing to airway obstruction or exsanguination from a ruptured major vessel.

The causes of poor tissue healing in the face and neck region are different from those in the rest of the body. The face and neck region is unique in that it has better vascularity and improved blood perfusion and is not in a dependent position in relation to the heart compared with the rest of the body. Vasodilation may also occur more often in the face and neck region (ie, emotional response causing facial blushing). Furthermore, less repetitive trauma occurs to the face and neck region compared with the extremities.

In the face and neck area, poor healing is most likely secondary to nonhealing surgical wounds (from previous radiation, chemotherapy, steroids, diabetes, ischemia, or revision surgery),

trauma, and burns. In addition, retained foreign bodies and adverse reactions to various implant material can cause a prolonged inflammatory process, resulting in poor healing. These causes are in contrast to etiologies for chronic wounds below the neck, which are due to venous insufficiency, arterial disease, diabetes, vasculitis, and trauma.[1]

Normal wound healing must occur in an orderly fashion, consisting of four overlapping phases: hemostatic phase, inflammatory phase, proliferative phase, and maturing phase (Figure 1). Delays of healing in any phase interfere with all subsequent phases, resulting in a chronic, nonhealing wound.[2] Therefore, treatment objectives strive to transform the state of a poorly healing wound into an acute healing state by removing the healing barriers contributing to it (Figure 2).[3]

During healing, all wounds require close scrutiny and monitoring for signs of impaired healing. If healing does not progress to what is expected, recognizing wound deterioration is the first step. The following clinical signs are indicative of signs of poor healing in a wound: persistent inflammation over 7 days, increased odor, increased exudate, delayed epithelialization, surrounding skin maceration, incision dehiscence, and necrotic tissue. These signs indicate that the normal acute healing state has

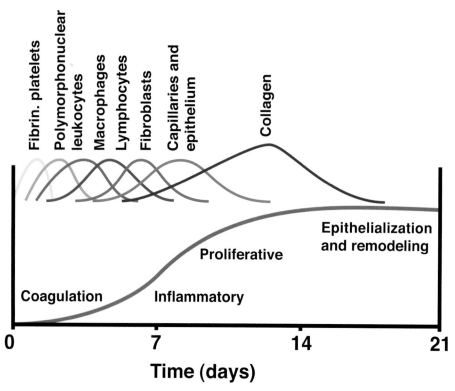

Figure 1. The wound healing process over time.

transformed into a chronic one. A chronic wound can be either in a deteriorating state (further destruction is ongoing) or a static state (no change is occurring).

CLASSIFYING A WOUND

In classifying a wound, it is important to determine if it is in the acute versus chronic state and if it should be treated surgically or non-surgically. A chronic wound is defined as a wound that has failed to heal in an orderly and timely fashion. Next, the wound needs to be classified by depth, either being defined as superficial (blister), partial thickness, full thickness (over muscle, fascia, perichondrium, or periosteum), or deep full thickness (down to bare bone, bare cartilage, nerve, large vessel, joint cavity) or as a fistula communicating with the upper airway or upper alimentary tract. Wounds

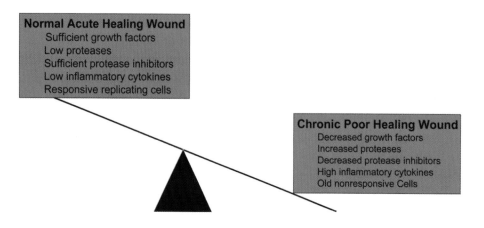

Figure 2. Microenvironment differences between a normal acute wound versus a chronic poorly healing wound (Adapted from Mast B and Schultz G, *Interactions of cytokines, growth factors and proteases in acute and chronic wounds.* Wound Rep Reg, 1996;4:411–420).

that need to be treated surgically are those that require débridement and/or skin coverage (skin flap, skin graft, free flap).

APPROACHING A CHRONIC PROBLEM WOUND

In evaluating a chronic wound, several levels of comprehensive assessments must be made to plan for the most appropriate wound management goals for the patient. These three stages of assessment are at the environmental, systemic, and wound levels (Figure 3).

At the environmental level, realistic goals of the patient's circumstances and situation should be addressed. Is the patient severely compromised, or does he or she have a terminal illness? In such instances, the optimal goal is to maximize quality of life and minimize pain.[4] On the other hand, in a healthy patient, conversion of a deteriorating wound into a healed wound is the ultimate goal.[5]

At the systemic level, the medical condition should be evaluated with a thorough medical history and physical examination. The influence of systemic disorders that impede wound healing should be considered, including diabetes, renal failure, immunodeficiency states such as human immunodeficiency virus (HIV) and malignancy, and malnutrition. Table 1 lists the extrinsic, intrinsic, and psychosocial factors that contribute to a poorly healing wound. Administration of immunosuppressant, anticoagulant, and glucocorticoid medications may also delay healing.[6] Table 2 shows medications that delay healing.

At the wound level, wound assessment involves documenting the wound location, wound dimensions, depth, exposure of underlying structures (ie, vessel, nerves, bone, cartilage), and proximity to important anatomic structures (great vessels, nerves, eyes, joints) (Table 3). The state of the wound bed can be necrotic, exudative, granulating, or epithelializing (Figure 4). When evaluating a wound bed, the characteristics of healthy granulation tissue are as follows: a bright red color, moist, shiny, and does not bleed easy. The characteristics of unhealthy granulation tissue are as follows: a

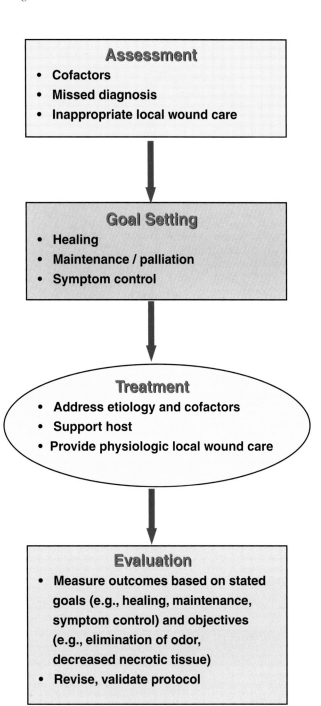

Figure 3. Hierarchy in treatment goals of wound assessment. Permission Granted From Rolstad, B. S. and Nix. D (2001). Management of Wound Recalcitrance and Deterioration. *Chronic Wound Care: A Clinical Source book for Healthcare Professionals.* D. K. Krasner, G. T. Rodeheaver and S. R.G. Wayne, PA, HMP Communications: 731–742.

dark red bluish color, dry, friable, and bleeds easily. Exudate in the wound can be described as serous (clear), sanguinous (red), serosanguineous (light red), seropurulent (cloudy yellow), and purulent (pus). Heavy exudate formation indi-

Table 1. FACTORS THAT IMPAIR HEALING
Intrinsic
Infection
Foreign bodies
Ischemia
Cigarette smoking
Metabolic disorders (diabetes, renal failure)
Circulatory disorders (congestive heart failure, anemia)
Respiratory disorders (COPD)
Immune deficiency (HIV, rheumatoid arthritis)
Malignancy
Old age
Extrinsic
Mechanical forces (shear, pressure)
Nutritional deficiencies
Radiation
Chemotherapeutic agents
Alcoholism
Distant malignancies
Hereditary healing disorders
Uremia
Medications (described in more detail in Table 24-2)
Psychosocial
Patient/family poor compliance, negative perceptions
Poor health care–patient relationships
Decreased access to state-of-the-art wound care (wound specialist, technology, products)
Fictitious injury

COPD = chronic obstructive pulmonary disease; HIV = human immunodeficiency virus.

Table 2. MEDICATIONS THAT CAN IMPAIR HEALING
Steroids
Anticoagulants
Antiplatelet agents (ie, aspirin, aspirin-related products)
Penicillamine
Cyclosporine
Colchicine
Phenylbutazone

Table 3. DEFINING A WOUND TO DETERMINE THE BEST FORM OF TREATMENT
Location
Wound depth (partial or full thickness, underlying structures exposed)
Dimensions and volume (ie, cavitary, fistula)
Wound bed state (clean, necrotic, granulating)
Exudate (type and amount)
Wound margin state (undefined, distinct)
Presence of infection

cates that either uncontrolled edema or an increased bacterial burden has occurred. Chronic exudate slows the proliferation of keratinocytes, fibroblasts, and endothelial cells.[7] Metalloproteinases present in exudate break down essential matrix material and trap growth factors, rendering them unavailable for healing.[8] Prolonged exposure to exudate can macerate the skin at the wound margin either through excessive water content or an insufficient absorptive capacity of the wound dressing. The application of skin sealants can reduce the extent of surrounding skin maceration.[9] Erythema, edema, or pain at the wound margin may indicate inflammation, infection, unrelieved pressure, or allergy to treatment products.

The status of the wound perimeter is evaluated by checking for erythema, warmth, maceration, induration, and chronicity of the wound edge. If the wound edge has a distinct thick, rolled, transitional border, it demonstrates that a chronic wound has been formed because the epithelial cells have migrated down into the deeper wound edge, for some time being unable to cross the wound bed.[10] If a fistula is present, it is important to describe where is it connected and where the salivary flow is being directed.

After this comprehensive evaluation, an interview with the patient, caregiver, and, if possible, the family should be made to discuss the ultimate wound healing goals and the wound care procedures planned. Specifically, the topics to be discussed are daily wound maintenance, symptom control, and short-term goals. By not including this information to the caregiver and family, a good wound care plan can lead to failure owing to poor compliance or unrealistic expectations. At times, a social worker may be important to help coordinate these outpatient plans with the family.[11] Complete healing is the preferred ultimate outcome; however, in severely compromised patients, wound maintenance or symptom control may be a more realistic goal.

For complex wounds, an interdisciplinary team may be required consisting of a surgeon, a wound care specialist, a clinic nurse, a nutritionist, and a primary medical physician. For finding a wound care specialist, many hospitals have a wound, ostomy, and continence clinical nurse specialist who is proficient in addressing proper wound dressings and care for chronic wounds. If swallowing or speaking is compromised, a speech pathologist is also helpful in assisting the patient.

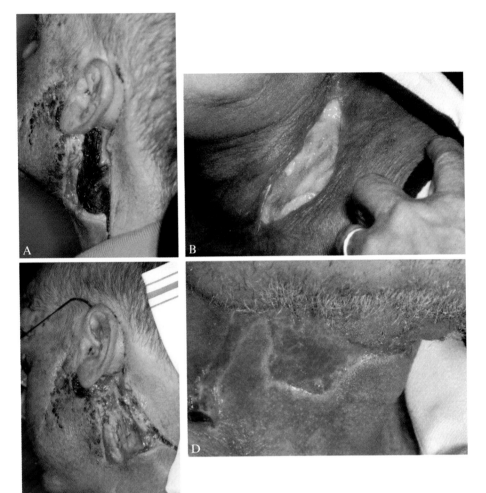

Figure 4. Wound types. *A*, Necrotic. Wound cavity with dark eschar and excessive yellow exudates. The treatment goal in this case is to promote débridement and absorb wound exudates. Possible dressings are calcium alginate rope, hypertonic saline gauze, and hypertonic gel. *B*, Exudative. Wound cavity with excessive yellow exudates. The treatment goal in this case is to absorb wound exudates. The wound may be dressed with calcium alginate rope. *C*, Granular. This is a granulating wound with minimal or moderate exudates. The treatment goal here is to promote wound granulation. Dressings may be in the form of hydrogel-impregnated gauze calcium alginate. *D*, Requires reepithelialization. This type of wound shows red granulation tissue in the wound bed. The treatment goal in this case is to maintain moisture, promote epithelial resurfacing, and protect new epithelium. The wound may be dressed with a hydrogen sheet, hydrocolloid, or foam when the wound is moist.

If the infection status is of concern, an infectious disease physician may be helpful.

In approaching a wound for optimal wound healing, several principles need to be pursued (Table 4).[12] With sound physiologic wound care, a chronic wound ideally should begin to show signs of healing within 2 to 4 weeks.[10] If treatment does not occur by this time, the patient must be reevaluated to ensure (1) proper nutri-tion, (2) adequate blood supply, (3) proper wound care and dressing, (4) protection from injury, and (5) control of wound bacterial contamination. During wound healing, the daily allowance of protein should be increased up to 1.8 g/kg/d in comparison with the daily recommendation in healthy individuals of 0.8 g/kg/d.[13] Wound healing can also be delayed when transcutaneous oxygen partial pressure measurements are less than 30 mm Hg.[14] In addition, in all nonhealing wounds, recurrence of neoplasia needs to be ruled out with a biopsy. Table 5 lists the order of treatment in approaching a poorly healing wound of the head and neck.

Table 4. MAJOR TENETS FOR OPTIMAL LOCAL WOUND CARE
Débride necrotic tissue
Identify and treat infection
Pack dead spaces lightly
Absorb excess exudates
Maintain a moist wound surface.
Maintain open fresh wound edges
Protect the wound from trauma and infection
Insulate the wound
Divert salivary drainage

LABORATORY EVALUATION

Routine diagnostic laboratory values should include albumin, glucose, hemoglobin, blood urea

Table 5. ORDER OF TREATMENT IN APPROACHING A POORLY HEALING WOUND OF THE HEAD AND NECK
Remove necrotic tissue and foreign bodies
Divert salivary flow and secretions
Control and prevent infection
Optimize exudate control
Promote granulation tissue
Promote reepithelialization or consider skin flap or skin graft coverage

nitrogen, creatinine, and a complete white cell count. An albumin concentration below 3.0 g/L can delay wound healing.[13] The erythrocyte sedimentation rate, rheumatoid factor, and antinuclear factor can be considered. A patient with a history of radiation to the head and neck region should have thyroid-stimulating hormone levels checked to rule out hypothyroidism. For any persistent nonhealing wound over several months, a biopsy should be considered to rule out malignancy. In addition, if any previous trauma or surgery had been performed at the site, a retained foreign body should be ruled out. Other laboratory values to consider in evaluating a poorly healing wound are VDRL, HIV, hepatitis screen, purified protein derivative, antinuclear antibodies, and peripheral antineutrophil cytoplasmic antibody to rule out systemic disorders.

Wound swab cultures are helpful when an infection is suspected and identification of the microorganism is needed to determine the optimal antibiotics. However, routine swab cultures are not needed when an infection is not present and the open wound is colonized.[15]

If any simultaneous infectious process exists in another body location, it will be a bioburden for the healing of the wound at the face and neck region.[16] In this instance, both sites need to be addressed properly to achieve optimal healing.

Given that scarring is an important cosmetic and functional issue to the face and neck, full-thickness wounds, once infection has been controlled, can be addressed by using local, regional, or distant skin flaps or skin grafts for wound coverage (Figure 5). Skin grafts are frequently considered a second choice for coverage owing to their color mismatch, different texture, and increased contraction. In some partial-thickness wounds, certain sites of the face will scar minimally when allowed to heal by secondary intention with the assistance of moist

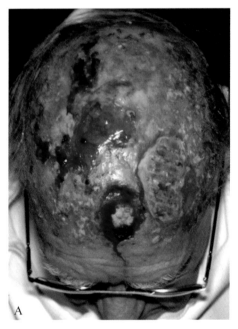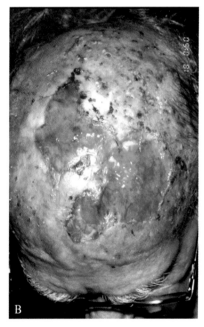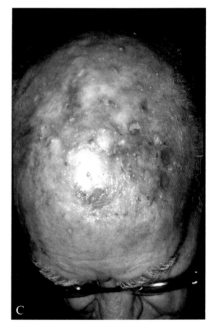

Figure 5. A) An 82-year-old male presenting with a 2-year history of a persistent, nonhealing, full-thickness ulcer on his scalp. Ten years previously, he received radiation to the scalp. Two years before presentation, he had excision of a squamous cell cancer from the scalp with no evidence of recurrence by multiple biopsies. Poor granulation tissue formation was evident. B) By burring down additional outer calvarial bone and keeping the scalp moist, sufficient granulation tissue developed for later split-thickness skin grafting. C) The chronic wound transformed into an acute wound. A free flap was not required.

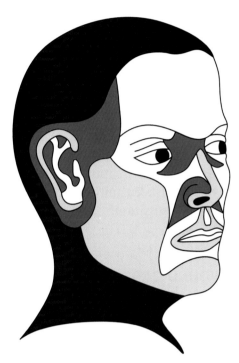

Healing by Secondary Intention

Facial: Concave surfaces heal with less scarring (dark blue)
NEET - nose, ears, eyes, temple

Facial: Convex surfaces heal with more scarring (light blue)
NOCH - nose, oral lip, cheeks, helix

Other facial: Surfaces (white) heal fair

Figure 6. Facial aesthetic appearance of facial areas when healed by second intention. Dark Blue Color (NEET Area, concave surfaces of the nose, eye, ear, and temple)—give good to excellent results in appearance. White Color (FAIR Area, forehead, antihelix, eyelids and rest of the nose, lips and cheeks)—give satisfactory results in appearance, it could result in hypopigmented scars. Light Blue Color (NOCH Area, convex surfaces of the nose, oral lips, cheeks, chin and helix)—give variable results in appearance. Superficial wounds are acceptable to some patients; however, deeper wounds heal with depression, contraction, or potential for hypertrophic scars. Permission Granted From Zitelli JA. Wound healing by secondary intention: a cosmetic appraisal. *Am Acad Dermatol* 1983;9:407–15.

dressings.[17] Figure 6 depicts the aesthetic results of healing by secondary intention of partial-thickness wound sites on the face. The disadvantages of healing by secondary intention are (1) more contraction of the surrounding soft tissue perimeter, (2) increased risk of hypopigmentation of the reepithelialized scars, and (3) a longer period of healing.

REFRACTORY WOUND

If a wound fails to heal despite instituting these measures, reevaluation of the current management and identification of the contributing causes of poor healing need to be undertaken. At the systemic level, the metabolic states, such as undiagnosed diabetes, anemia, or malignancy, need to be ruled out. At times, concurrent factors play a role in poor healing, such as in an insulin-dependent diabetic who is chronically on steroids for asthma.

As the healing wound changes over time, its management also needs to be modified accord-

ingly. The major question during each periodic assessment should be "Is the wound healing?" Clinical studies have demonstrated that a reduction in the ulcer area greater than 20% after 2 to 4 weeks of treatment indicates favorable healing progression.[10] If wound improvement does not occur after 2 to 4 weeks of treatment, the wound needs to be further reevaluated.

Clinical evidence signifying a decline in wound healing status is increased odor, increased pain, increased exudate, dehiscence, tissue necrosis, and breakdown of the perimeter around the wound. If the wound is not healing, the following questions should be asked:

1. Is there a misdiagnosis of the cause of the poor healing?
2. What are the extrinsic or intrinsic factors contributing to the poor healing?
3. Is inappropriate wound care being given?

If the goal is full healing, the patient should be treated more aggressively both surgically and medically. Adjuvant medical therapies, such as hyperbaric oxygen, negative pressure vacuum devices, growth factors, and biosynthetic dressings, are now available for the clinician.[18] These modalities of treatment are described in Section 3 of this book. Recently, growth factor therapy has been reported to have potential to improve the healing of previously irradiated chronic surgical wounds to the head and neck.[19,20] However, the off-label use of growth factor treatment to head and neck wounds has not been fully established and requires further investigation.

WOUND CARE

A common question is "What should I put on the wound?" The answer is based on the assessment goals for that patient on three levels (environmental level, patient level, and wound level), as previously discussed. The overall goal is to minimize local, systemic, and environmental factors that contribute to poor healing and maintain an optimal local wound milieu. It should be emphasized that local wound care and dressing selection are only two of the important components of optimal wound care. The other factors are nutritional support, adequate pain palliation, infection control, protecting the wound from trauma, and ensuring sufficient vascular perfusion to the wound site.

WOUND BED PREPARATION

Recent principles of wound bed preparation have been proposed to help improve the healing of chronic wounds. The acronym TIME (which stands for tissue, infection, moisture, and epidermal treatment) has been used to serve as a practical guide for clinicians in chronic wound management (Table 6).[2] These principles of wound bed preparation incorporate essential healing concepts to encourage chronic wounds to heal. This clinical approach is a very helpful and feasible protocol for clinicians.

Necrotic tissue promotes bacterial growth, prolongs inflammation, inhibits phagocytosis, limits the effectiveness of antimicrobial therapy, inhibits epithelialization, and causes suboptimal cosmesis. Therefore, necrotic tissue and eschar must be removed in a chronic wound. This

Time acronym	Clinical observations	Proposed pathophysiology	WBP clinical actions	Effect of WBP actions	Clinical outcomes
Table 6. WOUND BED PREPARATION USING THE TIME PRINCIPLE					
T	Tissue non-viable or deficient	Defective matrix and cell debris impair healing	Debridement (episodic or continuous) • autolytic, sharp surgical, enzymatic, mechanical or biological • biological agents	Restoration of wound base and functional extra-cellular matrix proteins	Viable wound base
I	Infection or inflammation	High bacterial counts or prolonged inflammation ↑ inflammatory cytokines ↑ protease activity ↓ growth factor activity	• remove infected foci topical/systemic • antimicrobials • anti-inflammatories • protease inhibition	Low bacterial counts or controlled inflammation: ↓ inflammatory cytokines ↓ protease activity ↑ growth factor activity	Bacterial balance and reduced inflammation
M	Moisture imbalance	Desiccation slows epithelial cell migration Excessive fluid causes maceration of wound margin	Apply moisture balancing dressings Compression, negative pressure or other methods of removing fluid or surgical skin coverage	Restored epithelial cell migration, desiccation avoided oedema, excessive fluid controlled, maceration avoided	Moisture balance
E	Edge of wound-non advancing or undermined	Non migrating keratinocytes Non responsive wound cells and abnormalities in extracellular matrix or abnormal protease activity	Re-assess cause or consider corrective therapies • debridement • skin grafts, skin flaps • biological agents • adjunctive therapies	Migrating keratinocytes and responsive wound cells Restoration of appropriate protease profile	Advancing edge of wound

WBP = Wound Bed Preparation.
Permission From Schultz, G. S., R. G. Sibbald, Falanga et al. (2003). *Wound Repair Regen* 11:S1–S28.

objective is accomplished by a variety of débridement techniques. Surgical débridement physically excises devitalized tissue and nonfunctional cells. This method is preferred in wounds with widespread infection, infected bone, and large amounts of necrosis.[16] Autolytic débridement is the most conservative type that allows for endogenous proteolytic enzymes to liquefy and spontaneously separate eschar from healthy tissue. Maintaining a moist wound surface promotes the rehydration of slough and necrotic tissue while allowing leukocytes and enzymes present in exudate to break down avascular tissue.[21]

Wound cleaning is another important factor for effective wound bed preparation management. A quotation regarding wound cleaning is "Don't put in a wound what you wouldn't put in your own eye." This statement is based on the fact that the strength of wound cleaning solutions is directly proportional to their cellular toxicity. Thus, a solution's cleaning capacity must be weighed against the potential cellular toxicity to the wound. Cleaning solutions are classified as either wound cleansers or skin cleansers. Skin cleansers (ie, Hibiclens, Betadine, Dakin solution, hydrogen peroxide) can be used intermittently in wounds, but when used in a repetitive fashion, a potential for toxicity to normal cells exists.[22] Normal saline and commercial wound cleansers are more acceptable options to chronically clean wounds.

Following cleaning, moisture balance and exudate management, need to be addressed. Achieving moisture balance at the wound-dressing interface accelerates granulation tissue formation and reepithelialization by increasing the speed of epithelial cell migration and allows for a shorter distance for epithelial cells to travel. In contrast, migrating epidermal cells in dry wounds need to take a more circuitous route beneath the physical barriers of scab, crusts, and devitalized dermis to reach their destination.[23] Effective exudate management can use highly absorbent dressings or, more recently, the vacuum-based mechanical systems.[21] These methods are described in more detail in Section 3 of this book.

Enzymatic débridement uses exogenous enzymes to dissolve necrotic tissue and liquefy slough. Commonly used preparations include papain-urea, papain-urea chlorophyllin, and collagenase. Collagenase products degrade collagen fibers that anchor necrotic tissue to the underlying wound bed. Urea unfolds proteins, and papain helps denature proteins.[21]

Mechanical débridement physically removes debris from the wound bed by wet-to-dry dressings, wound irrigation, or whirlpool therapy. Wet-to-dry dressings loosen eschar and induce nonselective mechanical separation of debris on dressing removal. However, wet-to-dry dressing removal causes pain and bleeding, and may damage the newly formed granulation tissue during dressing change. High-pressure irrigation and whirlpool therapy effectively remove bacteria, particulate matter, and necrotic debris from wounds. However, these modalities may not be appropriate for granulating wounds with fragile endothelial and epithelial cells. Lastly, biologic débridement uses maggots to digest necrotic tissue, slough, and bacteria. Larval therapy can quickly eradicate infection and rapidly stimulate growth of granulation tissue. In the head and neck region, one needs to protect orifices (ear canal, nose, mouth, and tracheostomy) to prevent the larvae from entering. Despite the disadvantages of poor aesthetics, local discomfort, itching, and application problems, maggots are beginning to assume a larger role in chronic wound management as antibiotic resistance increases.

ADDRESSING INFECTION

Although all chronic wounds contain bacteria, bacterial presence may represent either colonization or infection. A colonized wound does not have bacterial invasion into viable tissue and thus elicits a minimal host immune response.[15] A wound infection implicates bacterial invasion and replication within host tissue and results in a strong host immune response. Infection delays wound healing, but colonization usually does not.[15] Clinical criteria for identifying a chronic wound infection include increased exudate, surface discoloration, increased odor, superficial pocketing or bridging of the wound base, dehiscence, cellulitis, friable granulation tissue that bleeds easily, abscess formation, fever, and increased pain.[9]

Local factors that increase the likelihood of wound infection include reduced wound perfusion, a large wound area or depth, chronicity, necrosis, foreign bodies, metabolic disorders (eg, diabetes mellitus), alcohol abuse, smoking, and corticosteroid medication use. An increased bacterial load delays wound healing; substantial impairment occurs when there is greater than 10^5 organisms per gram of tissue. However, the number of organisms present may not be as important as the type and pathogenicity of the organism. For example, β-hemolytic streptococci are pathologic at much lower bacteria loads. In addition, if a foreign body or implant is present in the region, much less bacterial inoculum is needed to begin a wound infection.[16,24]

Removal of devitalized material and excess exudate most effectively reduces the level of bacterial contamination in chronic wound infection. Systemic antibiotics should be used when active infection cannot be managed with local measures and when there are signs of fever, an underlying deep structure infection, and spreading cellulitis. As bacterial antibiotic resistance increases, the selective use of topical antiseptics has gained renewed interest. For example, some iodine and silver preparations have bacteriocidal effects even against multidrug-resistant organ-isms such as methicillin-resistant *Staphylococcus aureus*. Antiseptic agents act across three target areas: the cell membrane, cytoplasmic organelles, and the bacteria's nucleic acids. This multitarget effect suggests that bacterial resistance to topical antiseptics may be less likely to emerge.[21]

WOUND DRESSINGS

Wound dressings are selected according to the initial characteristics of the chronic wound (Table 7).[11] Dressing modifications are instituted as the wound progresses through subsequent stages of healing. The ideal dressing maintains a moist wound environment, absorbs excess exudate, and keeps the surrounding skin dry. Additionally, the ideal dressing is nonadherent, hypoallergenic, comfortable, capable of being sterilized, and cost-effective. Unfortunately, no single dressing fulfills all of these characteristics.[9] Six major moisture-retentive dressing categories exist: gauzes, transparent films, hydrocolloids, hydrogels, alginates, and foams. Chapter 31 of this book describes the dressing materials in more detail. The following is an overall summary of the dressing classifications.

Gauzes

Gauzes are inexpensive dressings suitable for low-exudate wounds. Moist gauzes commonly treat full-thickness, open, necrotic, cavitary wounds. Used in a wet-to-dry fashion, the moist

	Appearance of wound bed				Appearance of granulation tissue		
Dressing	Black (necrotic)	Yellow (dry)	Sloughy (moist)	Red (infected)	Bed (wet)	Red (bleeding)	Pink/purple (healthy granulation/ reepithellalization)
Foam			++	++	+++		
Hydrofiber			+++	++	+++	+	
Crystalline NaCl gauze			+++	+++	++		
Calcium alginate			+	+++	+++	+++	
Hydrocolloid	+	++	++		++		++
Hydrogel	++	+++		+		+	+++
Adhesive film							+++
Non-adhesive film			++				
Enzymes	+++	+++					++

Table from Sibbald et al 2000 with permission.

gauze adheres to the wound bed as it dries. During wound dressing changes, the dry adhered dressing removes the nonviable tissue. To maintain sufficient moisture, gauzes should be rewetted at least three times a day. This protocol hastens débridement, promotes granulation, and prevents excessive desiccation.[25] When used as secondary dressings, gauzes provide padding and protection. The disadvantages in using gauze include limited absorbency, frequent dressing changes, and nonselective adherence and removal of healthy granulation tissue. In addition, dressing change removal induces pain, bleeding, and repeated epidermal trauma. New saline or hydrogel-impregnated gauzes may reduce these deleterious effects by being more gentle to healthy granulation tissue on dressing removal.[9]

Hydrogels

Hydrogels are water- or glycerine-based dressings that add moisture to the wound. They are available as amorphous gels, sheets, and impregnated gauzes. The gels are moisture retentive, nonadherent, and nonocclusive. These highly comfortable dressings afford a cool, soothing sensation. Hydrogels promote débridement, granulation, and reepithelialization.[25] They are used on granular and necrotic wounds of all depths. The sheets are used on partial-thickness wounds; amorphous gels and impregnated gauzes are used for full-thickness wounds and cavitary wounds. Hydrogels require daily dressing changes and may require a secondary dressing to keep it in place. Hydrogels may leak if wound exudate production is heavy.

Calcium Alginates

Calcium alginate dressings, derived from seaweed, are nonocclusive, nonadhesive, moisture-retentive dressings applied once or twice daily to partial- and full-thickness wounds. They are available in ropes, ribbons, and sheets. Alginates absorb moderate to heavy wound exudate and are used to fill wound dead space which produce exudate.[25] As the

exudate is absorbed, the alginate forms into a viscous hydrogel at the wound interface. Alginates are not used on dry or low-exudate wounds. They should also be avoided in blind sinus or fistula tracts. Secondary dressings are usually necessary to secure alginates in the proper position.

Foams

Foams are composed of polyurethanes with variable conformability, permeability, and absorbency.[25] Foams are generally nonadherent, moisture-retentive dressings that support autolytic débridement. Most foams require changing every 1 to 5 days depending on the amount of drainage. Typically, they are secured with tape, wrap bandages, or stretch netting. Foams are used as primary dressings and as wound fillers. They are appropriate choices for partial- and full-thickness wounds with moderate to heavy exudate and moist, necrotic slough. Similar to alginates, foams are contraindicated in dry wounds and may require secondary dressings for fixation. They are useful at tracheostomy sites for cushioning the side flange of the tracheostomy tube from traumatizing the skin.

Hydrocolloids

Low exudate, sloughy, and necrotic wounds may be treated with hydrocolloids or hydrogels.[9] Hydrocolloids have a water-impermeable polyurethane outer layer and a nonadherent hydrocolloid inner layer. Opaque and transparent wafer, paste, and powder forms are available. Most hydrocolloids are occlusive, providing excellent microbial barriers. They maintain a moist wound environment, promote autolysis, and insulate the wound bed. However, hydrocolloids may produce excessive granulation tissue and malodor. Dressing changes are typically performed every 3 to 5 days based on the occurrence of loosening, wrinkling, and leakage of exudate.[9]

Hydrocolloids are indicated for partial-thickness wounds and shallow full-thickness wounds with clean bases. For cavitary wounds, they should be used with a filler such as calcium alginate to obliterate the dead space.[25] The wafers work well on areas of moist desquamation and are also used to secure other types of dressings. Hydrocolloids require low maintenance and provide a high degree of comfort. These dressings should not be used on heavy-exudate or infected wounds.[9]

Transparent Films

Transparent films are thin, semipermeable dressings fabricated from polyurethane. Films are conformable, water resistant, and impervious to bacterial penetration.[25] Additionally, films resist shearing forces and permit wound inspection without dressing removal. Films have limited absorbency and will therefore leak if exudate production underneath the membrane becomes heavy. These factors dictate the frequency of dressing changes, which may be challenging. Films are thus used on superficial and partial-thickness wounds with little or no exudate. Placement of films over dry, necrotic eschar supports autolytic débridement. These dressings are also applied secondarily over gauze or alginate packing. Films are contraindicated in heavy-exudate or infected wounds and must be used cautiously on thin, fragile skin.[9]

CONCLUSION

Chronic wounds are different from acute wounds in that they require strategic wound bed preparation to achieve successful wound healing. More recent, comprehensive wound management strategy includes (1) accurate and systematic wound assessment, (2) adequate débridement and cleaning; (3) effective exudate management, (4) restoration of proper moisture and bacterial balance, (5) promotion of granulation tissue formation and reepithelialization, (6) selection of the appropriate dressing, and (7) periodic reassessment with dressing modification as indicated.[9] Chronic wound management has advanced rapidly over the last 25 years through the collaborative efforts of many specialists and researchers to optimize the wound tissue environment. The next generation of wound healing advancements may involve directing selected cells to replicate and migrate within a wound to optimize tissue repair.

REFERENCES

1. Banerjee D, Jones V, Harding K. The overall clinical approach to chronic wounds. In: Falanga V, editor. Cutaneous wound healing. London: Martin Dunitz; 2001. p. 165–85.
2. Schultz GS, Sibbald RG, Falanga V, et al. Wound bed preparation: a systematic approach to wound management. Wound Repair Regen 2003;11 Suppl 1:S1–28.
3. Mast B, Schultz G. Interactions of cytokines, growth factors and proteases in acute and chronic wounds. Wound Repair Regen 1996;4:411–20.
4. Rolstad BS, Nix D. Management of wound recalcitrance and deterioration. In: Krasner DK, Rodeheaver GT, Sibbald RG, editors. Chronic wound care: a clinical source book for healthcare professionals. Wayne (PA): HMP Communications; 2001. p. 731–42.
5. Orsted H, Sibbald RG. A coordinated approach to chronic wound care. Ostomy Wound Manage 2001;47:68.
6. Flanagan M. A practical framework for wound assessment. Br J Nurs 1997;6:68–11.
7. Keast DH, et al. MEASURE: a proposed assessment framework for developing best practice recommendations for wound assessment. Wound Repair Regen 2004;12(3 Suppl):S1–17.
8. Falanga V. Classifications for wound bed preparation and stimulation of chronic wounds. Wound Repair Regen 2000;8:347–52.
9. Flanagan M. Wound bed preparation: a guide to advanced wound management. Largo (FL): Smith & Nephew; 2003.
10. Rijswijk LV. Wound assessment and documentation. In: Krasner DK, Rodeheaver GT, Sibbald RG, editors. Chronic wound care: a clinical source book for healthcare professionals. Wayne (PA): HMP Communications; 2001. p. 101–15.
11. Sibbald RG, et al. Preparing the wound bed—debridement, bacterial balance, and moisture balance. Ostomy Wound Manage 2000;46:14–22, 24–8, 30–5.
12. Hom DB, et al. Choosing the optimal wound dressing for irradiated soft tissue wounds. Otolaryngol Head Neck Surg 1999;121:591–8.
13. Mazzotta MY. Nutrition and wound healing. J Am Podiatr Med Assoc 1994;84:456–62.
14. Hunt TK, Pai MP. The effect of varying ambient oxygen tensions on wound metabolism and collagen synthesis. Surg Gynecol Obstet 1972;135:561–7.
15. Crow S, Thompson P. Infection control perspective. In: Krasner DK, Rodeheaver GT, Sibbald RG, editors. Chronic wound care: a clinical source book for healthcare professionals. Wayne (PA): HMP Communications; 2001. p. 357–67.

16. Dow G. Infection in chronic wounds. In: Krasner DK, Rodeheaver GT, Sibbald RG, editors. Chronic wound care: a clinical source book for healthcare professionals. Wayne (PA): HMP Communications; 2001. p. 343–56.

17. Zitelli JA. Wound healing by secondary intention: a cosmetic appraisal. J Am Acad Dermatol 1983;9:407–15.

18. Li V, Kung E, Li W. Molecular therapy for wounds: modalities for stimulating angiogenesis and granulation. In: Lee B, editor. The wound mangagement manual. New York: McGraw-Hill; 2005. p. 17–43.

19. Jakubowicz DM, Smith RV. Use of becaplermin in the closure of pharyngocutaneous fistulas. Head Neck 2005;27:433–8.

20. Hom DB, Manivel JC. Promoting healing with recombinant human platelet-derived growth factor--BB in a previously irradiated problem wound. Laryngoscope 2003;113:1566–71.

21. Lionelli G, Lawrence W. Wound dressings. Surg Clin North Am 2003;83:617–38.

22. Rodeheaver GT. Wound cleansing, wound irrigation, wound disinfection. In: Krasner DK, Rodeheaver GT, Sibbald RG, editors. Chronic wound care: a clinical source book for healthcare professionals. Wayne (PA): HMP Communications; 2001. p. 369–83.

23. Winter G. Formation of the scab and the rate of epithelialization of superficial wounds in the skin of the young domestic pig. Nature 1962;193:293–4.

24. Sibbald RG, et al. Preparing the wound bed 2003: focus on infection and inflammation. Ostomy Wound Manage 2003;49:23–51.

25. Turner T. The development of wound management products. In: Krasner DK, Rodeheaver GT, Sibbald RG, editors. Chronic wound care: a clinical source book for healthcare professionals. Wayne (PA): HMP Communications; 2001. p. 293–310.

24

Nutrition and Wound Healing

Ryan Katz, MD; Adrian Barbul, MD, FACS

SPECIFIC THERAPY IN ITS CURRENT STATE

Although the importance of adequate nutrition for the healing wound has long been understood, the science of wound healing is still in its infancy. As such, our current nutritional therapies consisting of enteral or parenteral nutritional supplementation in surgical patients are often imprecise. We now understand that optimizing nutrition is more than just optimizing calories; it is also meeting the specific and complex nutritional requirements of the patient given the pathology, with the unique proteins, lipids, vitamins, and trace elements at our disposal.

SHORTCOMINGS

Unfortunately, given our limited understanding of the wound healing process, a specific mechanism and effect of each nutritional supplement are often difficult to clarify. Thus, we are often severely limited in our ability to precisely identify and adequately correct complex nutritional deficits to ensure adequate wound healing in our surgical patients.

FUTURE PROMISES

With early and appropriate identification of those patients at risk of wound healing problems, specific diets tailor-made to promote, speed, initiate, or resume the wound healing process can be instituted preoperatively or postoperatively as needed.

It has been known since biblical times that there is a close link between adequate nutrition and wound healing. Since then, clinical experience and rigorous scientific studies have confirmed the importance of nutrition to the healing wound.

The wound healing process is a complex series of events that is initiated with organ or tissue damage. Under ideal circumstances, this process results in wound closure and allows for continued organ function. The elusive goal has been to more clearly define these circumstances. It is well accepted that there are certain tenets to optimize the wound healing process, including careful approximation of wound edges, gentle tissue handling, elimination of dead space, keeping wounds clean and moist, and minimizing bacterial load. Some of these time-honored technical teachings are centuries old, and further progress needs to be made if the incidence of wound infection and failure is to be minimized. The internal wound environment—specifically, the availability of protein, nutrients, vitamins, cofactors, and caloric energy necessary to synthesize matrix and to build, break down, and remodel healing wounds—has proven to be just as essential for successful healing.

This chapter discusses the concept of nutritional supplementation in the surgical patient and reviews the importance of a baseline nutritional assessment. A brief evaluation of enteral and parenteral nutrition is followed by a review of the literature evaluating the role of nutritional supplementation in the wound healing process. The chapter specifically focuses on nutritional supplementation with protein and lipids, the amino acids arginine and glutamine, vitamins C and A, and the trace element zinc.

NUTRITION IN SURGICAL PATIENTS

Trauma, surgical or accidental, causes significant metabolic perturbations characterized by mobilization of amino acids from muscle and other organs, gluconeogenesis, and hypermetabolic responses. Many of these metabolic responses are mediated by the wound itself via afferent nerve fibers, which perceive pain, inflammation, and changes in pH.[1]

For wounds to heal appropriately, the requisite building blocks and energy stores must be available. In addition, an adequate blood supply is required to ensure the delivery of nutrients and reparative cells to the wound bed. Compared with other locations in the human body, the blood supply to the head and neck is often not in question. However, in patients who have had previous surgery or in those with a clinical history of diabetes, trauma, or radiation, compromised macro- or microvascular circulation may impair the wound healing process. For these patients, optimization of nutritional status is imperative and nutritional assessment and planning should begin at the preoperative consultation.

NUTRITIONAL ASSESSMENT

Prior to implementing nutritional therapy, the physician must first determine if a patient requires such intervention and, if so, to what extent. Malnutrition is well recognized as a risk factor for healing and needs to be determined and possibly treated preoperatively. On the other hand, most operations in well-nourished patients are successful with uncomplicated healing responses, even if nutritional intake is absent or curtailed for 7 to 10 days. Evaluation of preoperative nutritional status is an important consideration because improper administration or implementation of nutritional therapies can

result in increased patient morbidity and unnecessary health care costs.

A complete history and physical examination should be performed on each patient. This alone has been found to be 80 to 90% accurate in evaluating patient nutritional status; the addition of multiple or complex biochemical, immune, or anthropometric measurements does not greatly increase the accuracy of nutritional assessment.[2] Malnutrition may be expected if the history reveals unintentional weight loss (20% weight loss is indicative of severe malnutrition), if the patient appears cachectic with obvious muscle wasting, or if the patient has a history of or reason for alimentary malabsorption. These factors, along with any comorbidities, such as diabetes, other endocrinopathies, or renal or liver failure, must be noted because they will guide nutritional management. Some biochemical markers that have been used as aids in diagnosing malnutrition include measurement of serum proteins (albumin < 3.5 mg/dL, prealbumin < 15 mg/dL, transferrin < 200 mg/dL), nitrogen balance, total cholesterol, and creatinine. Baseline assessment documenting the status of these markers should be obtained prior to implementing any nutritional therapy, and optimization of nutritional status should be tailored to each patient's unique history, pathology, and expected therapy.

Malnutrition contributes to increased morbidity and mortality in both the hospital and the community. Specifically, malnutrition (which can be as prevalent as 50% in hospitalized patients) predisposes patients to increased septic complications, prolonged ventilator dependence, pneumonia, and impaired or failed wound healing.[3–5] Determining who would truly benefit from nutritional supplementation is still a matter of some debate, but there is evidence that preoperative nutritional support reduces infectious complications and anastomotic breakdown in severely malnourished patients undergoing major elective surgery.[6] Postoperative nutritional support should be considered in patients expected to be unable to eat for a period of at least 2 weeks, although it may not be beneficial in patients who are able to eat within 2 weeks after surgery.[7]

ENTERAL VERSUS PARENTERAL NUTRITION

In malnourished preoperative patients or in postoperative patients unable to tolerate a diet (or unable to meet nutritional and caloric needs) for a protracted period of time, enteral or parenteral feeds should be started or resumed as early as possible. There have been multiple prospective studies to demonstrate that enteral feeding is superior to parenteral feeding in reducing morbidity from septic complications (pneumonia, abdominal abscesses, line sepsis) in those patients requiring nutritional supplementation.[7–10] Further studies reveal that enteral nutrition stimulates gut luminal brush border hydrolase, increases microvillus height, and decreases mucosal permeability.[4,11] These findings suggest that enteral feeding reduces septic complications by preventing bacterial translocation across the gut mucosa.

Unfortunately, the enteral route is not always available or well tolerated by patients. In these circumstances, parenteral nutrition should be used as a means of maximizing the intake of proteins and calories necessary for satisfactory wound healing. However, parenteral nutrition does not afford the patient the apparent immunologic benefits of enteral feeding and should therefore be either replaced by enteral feeding when possible or augmented with enteral feeding as tolerated. Furthermore, it should be noted that parenteral nutrition carries the potential for intravenous line complications, including the morbidity associated with line insertion and the ever-present risk of line sepsis.

PROTEIN AND LIPID SUPPLEMENTATION

Both proteins and lipids are important sources of calories, and having deficiencies in either could result in significant morbidity and disturbances in the wound healing process. However, isolated protein deficiency is actually very rare.

Inadequate protein stores are instead most commonly seen in the setting of chronic malnutrition. Historically, evaluation of a patient's albumin level has served as a bellwether for protein stores, nutritional status, and subsequent healing ability. In early studies of patients and animals with hypoalbuminemia, wound healing was compromised by delayed fibroplasia, decreased wound strength, and an increased incidence of wound dehiscence.[12,13] Interestingly, this impaired wound healing response may be more a result of global malnutrition than actual deficiencies in protein stores.[14] Today, there is no doubt that adequate energy stores are necessary for successful wound healing, and it has been repeatedly demonstrated that, in malnourished patients, the healing of wounds will be slower and more prone to infectious complications and will overall be weaker than in those patients with adequate energy stores.[12–14]

Although it may not play a direct role in contributing to the ultimate wound strength or collagen content, protein does provide both energy and amino acids necessary for the proper functioning of the wound healing process. Thus, protein plays an important role in the overall diet and must be supplemented to overcome daily losses and meet each patient's differing protein-energy requirements. For example, most postoperative patients have protein requirements in the range of 1.2 to 2 g/kg/d, whereas patients with extensive burns may require greater than 2 g/kg/d. Furthermore, patients with renal failure and those with gastrointestinal malabsorption (seen in inflammatory bowel disease) or excessive gastrointestinal losses (associated with diarrhea or fistulae) will also have increased protein requirements. When in doubt, a nitrogen balance can be calculated to determine the patient's nitrogen status and hence protein requirements. For adequate and timely wound healing, protein supplementation should be such that the patient has a net positive nitrogen balance and meets daily protein-energy requirements. Protein supplementation can be achieved enterally or parenterally; there are a number of protein-rich "shakes" and total parenteral nutrition formulations to meet this end. The optimal form of protein supplementation for wound repair has yet to be elucidated but most likely involves a combination of intact proteins and specific amino acids (see below).

Lipids, the primary components of all cell membranes, play an integral role in the wound healing process. As a source of calories other than glucose and protein, a diet replete in lipids may theoretically limit protein catabolism in the stressed or wounded state. In young rats, healing of skin, the stability of sutures in gut anastomoses, and reepithelialization of partial-thickness burns have all been shown to be compromised in the setting of essential fatty acid deficiency.[15] Impaired wound healing has also been documented in humans with essential fatty acid deficiencies.[16] Most often these deficiencies arise in the hospital setting when a patient is placed on parenteral nutrition. Thus, it is important in the postsurgical, burn, trauma, or severely stressed patient to supplement parenteral formulas with lipids. In practice, it has become common, especially in a critical care setting, to see parenteral formulas containing up to 30 to 50% of nonprotein calories in the form of lipid emulsions. In theory, this may be of benefit to selected patient populations by decreasing the respiratory quotient (amount of endogenous carbon dioxide produced relative to oxygen consumed). Tailoring the amount of lipid supplementation should be done carefully, taking into consideration the potential risk of infectious complications, hyperlipidemia, and a higher postoperative mortality rate with increased fat administration.[17]

ARGININE

Endogenously, arginine is synthesized from ornithine via a citrulline intermediate. Like glutamine, arginine is a nonessential amino acid that, in the setting of severe injury, major surgery, or critical illness, becomes conditionally essential.[18,19] The physiologic role of this amino acid is varied and includes nitrogen scavenging, protein metabolism, the creation of high-energy creatine phosphate bonds, and polyamine biosynthesis. In addition, as the only known substrate for the enzyme nitric oxide synthase (NOS), arginine appears to be indispensable for formation of the biologic effector molecule nitric oxide (NO) (Figure 1).[19] NO released through the activity of NOS regulates collagen formation, cell proliferation, and wound contraction in distinct ways during the course of wound healing.

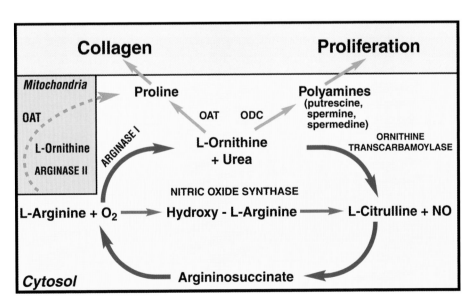

Figure 1. Arginine is a substrate for nitric oxide synthase (NOS) and contributes to cell proliferation and collagen synthesis. Adapted from Witte MB and Barbul A.[19]

OAT = ornithine decarboxylase
ODC = ornithine aminotransferase

Early studies examining animals with arginine-deficient diets clearly demonstrate the importance of this amino acid to the healing wound. In the 1970s, one such experiment examined the morbidity and mortality of rats fed an arginine-deficient diet and subjected to dorsal incision and closure. When compared with rats fed a normal diet, those with dietary arginine restrictions were found to have decreased perioperative weight gain, increased perioperative mortality, and overall weaker scars with less collagen.[19] Subsequent studies demonstrated that injured rats whose diets were supplemented with arginine developed scars with higher breaking strengths and more collagen than the control rats fed normal diets.[20,21] These experiments, coupled with the knowledge that local wound environments are marked by very low arginine levels, suggest that arginine is being actively used during the wound healing process and that its supplementation may aid in developing stronger scars with more collagen. Indeed, this concept has been studied in human volunteers subjected to wounding. When compared with placebo controls, those individuals with arginine-supplemented diets demonstrated healing wounds with significantly higher levels of hydroxyproline—an indirect marker of collagen deposition.[22,23]

Although these results are noteworthy and encouraging, dietary arginine supplementation has not yet become a widely implemented measure to augment the process of wound healing. Perhaps this is because the exact role played by arginine within the healing wound is uncertain. It does seem apparent that arginine supplementation boosts initial collagen production and subsequent deposition. Yet even without arginine supplementation, most wounds go on to heal with functionally strong scars. Of important exception are the fragile and often chronic wounds of diabetics, in whom many of the wound healing problems are attributed to NO dysregulation and local deficiencies of arginine.[24,25] In wounds of diabetic rodents, dietary arginine supplementation appears to restore order to the dysregulated NO pathway and increase wound breaking strength and collagen content.[24] In humans, topical administration of arginine to chronic diabetic ulcers appears to result in more rapid and complete wound closure.[26] Although arginine supplementation may not be recommended for all patients with wounds, it should be considered for diabetic patients with chronic wounds or a history of complicated wound healing. Furthermore, arginine supplementation should be recommended to patients in whom malnutrition is suspected.

GLUTAMINE

In a physiologic state, glutamine is the most abundant amino acid in blood and tissue.[27] This is a testament to the multiple roles it plays in the human body as an ammonia scavenger, nitrogen donor during protein metabolism, and precursor of nucleotides and nucleic acids.[28] The cyclization of glutamate, the acid form of glutamine, produces proline, which is necessary for collagen formation and connective tissue stability. In addition, glutamine appears to play an important role in the growth of rapidly dividing cells such as fibroblasts, enterocytes, and lymphocytes and also has an immunologic function, enhancing or enabling macrophage phagocytosis and cytotoxity.[27,28]

The pool of glutamine, an otherwise nonessential amino acid, becomes depleted and may contribute to a relative immunosuppressive state in the setting of trauma, sepsis, critical injury, burns or severe wounds, bone marrow transplantation, intense chemotherapy, or radiotherapy.[29–33] Given that the formation of a well-healed wound requires a properly functioning immune system, fibroblast division, and protein and nucleic acid metabolism, it would be fair to ask whether glutamine supplementation could enhance the wound healing process. To date, no convincing data have been obtained to support a role for glutamine in wound healing. There is, however, some evidence that enteral glutamine supplementation in elective surgical patients and burn victims may lead to decreased hospital stay and infectious complications.[34,35] Furthermore, in critically ill patients in whom glutamine depletion is thought to contribute to immunosuppression and increased hospital morbidity, glutamine supplementation may be of benefit.[35]

Before initiating glutamine supplementation, it is important to assess the patient's hepatic, renal, and central nervous system (CNS) function, and the benefits of supplementation must be weighed against the accumulation of ammonia (a degradation product of glutamine) and the potential deleterious effects on the CNS. Similarly, since glutamine is a fuel of rapidly dividing cells, some physicians would withhold supplementation in patients with known tumors.

VITAMIN SUPPLEMENTATION

Specific vitamin deficiencies can greatly impair the wound healing process and can often be identified through careful assessment of the patient's diet, clinical history, and social history. Although rarely seen in Western civilizations, vitamin C deficiency must be considered in severely malnourished patients, alcoholics, patients with chronic illness, the elderly, and patients on special restrictive diets. In that it is essential for proline hydroxylation and, ultimately, collagen cross-linking, vitamin C is of utmost importance for ultimate wound healing and strength. Initial manifestations of vitamin C deficiency may not be recognized as they mainly present as lethargy and weakness. However, chronic vitamin C deficiency will ultimately result in signs and symptoms consistent with vascular fragility (petechia, easy bruising, purpura, hemarthrosis) and tissue instability (bleeding gums, impaired wound healing, the breakdown of scars, and reopening of wounds). Fortunately, such extremes are not common and can be prevented and often reversed with the proper and timely administration of enteral or parenteral vitamin C.[36] Of note, the recommended daily allowance of vitamin C is 40 mg/d for adults. For those patients with chronic illness or those undergoing surgery, elevated doses of 150 mg/d are recommended. In the severely burned patient with massive tissue damage, levels as high as 500 mg/d to 2 g/d should be administered while tissue turnover and repair are ongoing. Because it is water soluble, there is no known true vitamin C toxicity.[27,37] However, excessive doses of vitamin C can lead to renal stones or diarrhea.

A fat-soluble vitamin, vitamin A is absorbed with the other fat-soluble vitamins in the terminal ileum. As such, vitamin A deficiency should be considered in anyone who is malnourished (impoverished, alcoholic, vegan, elderly, or chronically ill patients) or has a history of inflammatory bowel disease or previous bowel surgery. Unlike the other fat-soluble vitamins, vitamin A—specifically, its derivative, retinoic acid—plays a direct and multifaceted role in the wound healing process.

Clinically, the manifestations of vitamin A deficiency are myriad and include ophthalmologic symptoms (night blindness, scleral Bitot's spots, corneal dryness and ulceration, and, in extreme cases, blindness), dermatologic symptoms (dry skin, dry or brittle hair and fingernails, phrynoderma, excessive keratinization of epithelial tissues), and hematologic symptoms (anemia, leukopenia). Of these, all but excessive keratinization can be reversed with appropriate supplementation.[36] In practice, doses of 25,000 to 30,000 IU/d are recommended for treatment of mild clinical symptoms, with higher doses being reserved for more severe clinical pathology. Although vitamin A toxicity can occur with chronic use and high doses, regimens as high as 100,000 IU/d have been used safely in cancer patients.[27] Clinical signs of toxicity include arthralgias, nausea, vomiting, CNS changes, and even elevated intracranial pressure.

From a wound healing perspective, retinoic acid plays a role in promoting fibroblast proliferation and cell differentiation. Retinoic acid can restore wound tensile strength and collagen content in diabetics, patients on chronic steroids, and those with wounds in irradiated tissue beds.[27,38,39] Thus, in these patient populations, vitamin A supplementation is likely to be beneficial. However, controversy remains as to whether retinoids can be of benefit to those patients with unimpaired wound healing. One trial designed to test the effect of oral vitamin A supplementation on wound healing in rats with a mild vitamin A deficiency demonstrated a significant increase in wound tensile strength at 5 days but no significant increase when measured at 2 weeks.[40] A more recent study in mice examining the use of a topical retinoid on incisional wounds demonstrated a temporary but significantly decreased initial wound breaking strength.[41] Compared with controls, the group treated with retinoic acid displayed a prolonged inflammatory phase that seemed to impair the early deposition of collagen; at 1 week, this resulted in markedly weaker scars. However, this effect was transient, and wound strength among treatment and control groups equilibrated by 3 weeks. Another study examining pretreatment of full-thickness wounds in photodamaged human skin with topical retinoic acid demonstrated more rapid epithelialization in the treatment group.[42] Taken together, these results are difficult to interpret and do not make a strong case for either topical or enteral vitamin A supplementation in patients without chronic wounds or impaired wound healing.

TRACE ELEMENTS: ZINC

Trace elements should be considered mandatory for adequate nutrition. These molecules act as enzymatic cofactors and play a variety of roles in regulating the body's metabolic processes. Of the seven known trace elements, zinc is perhaps the most well known for its effects on the wound healing process.

An essential element, zinc has long been recognized to have a beneficial effect on wound healing. It is mostly absorbed enterally through the jejunum. Thus, impaired zinc absorption should be considered in any patient with chronic diarrhea, malabsorption, or a history of small bowel resection. Given that it is a cofactor in many enzymatic reactions, it is not surprising to find that there are multiple manifestations of zinc deficiency. Hallmarks of the deficient state include dermatitis, alopecia, immunocompromise, growth retardation, skin lesions, diarrhea, and impaired wound healing.[43,44] The exact mechanism by which zinc deficiency impairs the wound healing process is unknown but may be due to a delayed inflammatory response.[43,45] Deprived of sufficient zinc, healing wounds have been shown to exhibit an increased time to wound closure, delayed fibroblast proliferation, decreased collagen deposition, and decreased wound tensile strength.

Treatment of the zinc-deficient state can be achieved by either parenteral (2 mg/d) or enteral (15 mg/d) supplementation. Requirements may be increased in patients with large wounds (as in burns), impaired absorption, or pathologic losses. For patients who are not zinc deficient, however, there are no known benefits to zinc supplementation.[27]

REFERENCES

1. Bessey PQ. Metabolic response to critical illness. In: Souba WW, editor. ACS surgery: principles and practice. New York: WebMD Inc.; 2004. p. 1417–43.
2. Jeejeebhoy KN, Detsky AS, Baker JP. Assessment of nutritional status. JPEN J Parenter Enteral Nutr 1990; 14(5 Suppl):193S–6S.
3. Bistrian BR, Blackburn GL, Vitale J, et al. Prevalence of malnutrition in general medical patients. JAMA 1976; 235:1567–70.
4. Kudsk KA. Early enteral nutrition in surgical patients. Nutrition 1998;14:541–4.
5. Kudsk KA. Enteral versus parenteral feeding. Effects on septic morbidity after blunt and penetrating abdominal trauma. Ann Surg 1992;215:503–11; discussion 511–3.
6. Veterans Affairs Total Parenteral Nutrition Cooperative Study Group. Perioperative total parenteral nutrition in surgical patients. N Engl J Med 1991;325:525–32.
7. Souba WW. Nutritional support. N Engl J Med 1997;336: 41–8.
8. Kudsk KA. Effect of enteral and parenteral feeding in malnourished rats with E. coli-hemoglobin adjuvant peritonitis. J Surg Res 1981;31:105.
9. Saluja SS. Enteral nutrition in surgical patients. Surg Today 2002;32:672–8.
10. Moore FA, Moore EE, Jones TN, et al. TEN versus TPN following major abdominal trauma-reduced septic morbidity. J Trauma 1989;29:916–22.
11. DeWitt RC, Kudsk KA. The gut's role in metabolism, mucosal barrier function, and gut immunology. Infect Dis Clin North Am 1999;13:465–81.
12. Lindstedt E, Sandblom P. Wound healing in man: tensile strength of healing wounds in some patient groups. Ann Surg 1975;181:842–6.

13. Thompson WD, Ravdin IS, Frank IL. Effect of hypoproteinemia on wound disruption. Arch Surg 1938;36:500–8.

14. Felcher A, Schwartz J, Shechter C, et al. Wound healing in normal and analbuminemic (NAR) rats. J Surg Res 1987;43:546–9.

15. Hulsey TK, O'Neill JA, Neblett WR, Meng HC. Experimental wound healing in essential fatty acid deficiency. J Pediatr Surg 1980;15:505–8.

16. O'Neill JA Jr, Caldwell MD, Meng HC. Essential fatty acid deficiency in surgical patients. Ann Surg 1977;185:535–42.

17. Hart DW, Wolf SE, Zhang XJ, et al. Efficacy of a high-carbohydrate diet in catabolic illness. Crit Care Med 2001;29:1318–24.

18. Williams JZ, Barbul A. Nutrition and wound healing. Surg Clin North Am 2003;83:571–96.

19. Witte MB, Barbul A. Arginine physiology and its implication for wound healing. Wound Repair Regen 2003;11:419–23.

20. Seifter E, Rettura G, Barbul A, Levenson SM. Arginine: an essential amino acid for injured rats. Surgery 1978;84:224–30.

21. Barbul A, Fishel RS, Shimazu S, et al. Intravenous hyperalimentation with high arginine levels improves wound healing and immune function. J Surg Res 1985;38:32834.

22. Barbul A, Lazarou SA, Efron DT, et al. Arginine enhances wound healing and lymphocyte immune responses in humans. Surgery 1990;108:3317.

23. Kirk SJ, Hurson M, Regan MC, et al. Arginine stimulates wound healing and immune function in elderly human beings. Surgery 1993;114:155–9.

24. Witte MB, Thornton FJ, Tantry U, Barbul A. L-Arginine supplementation enhances diabetic wound healing: involvement of the nitric oxide synthase and arginase pathways. Metabolism 2002;51:1269–73.

25. Jude EB, Boulton AJ, Ferguson MW, Appleton I. The role of nitric oxide synthase isoforms and arginase in the pathogenesis of diabetic foot ulcers: possible modulatory effects by transforming growth factor beta 1. Diabetologia 1999;42:748–57.

26. Arana V, Paz Y, Gonzalez A, et al. Healing of diabetic foot ulcers in L-arginine-treated patients. Biomed Pharmacother 2004;58:588–97.

27. Barbul A, Purtill WA. Nutrition in wound healing. Clin Dermatol 1994;12:133–40.

28. Baudouin SV, Evans TW. Nutritional support in critical care. Clin Chest Med 2003;24:633–44.

29. Askanazi J, Michelsen CB, Carpentier YA, et al. Sequential changes in muscle and plasma amino acids during injury, infection, and convalescence. Surg Forum 1979;30:90–2.

30. Parry-Billings M, Evans J, Calder PC, Newsholme EA. Does glutamine contribute to immunosuppression after major burns? Lancet 1990;336:523–5.

31. Parry-Billings M, Baigrie RJ, Lamont PM, et al. Effects of major and minor surgery on plasma glutamine and cytokine levels. Arch Surg 1992;127:1237–40.

32. Novak F, Heyland DK, Avenell A, et al. Glutamine supplementation in serious illness: a systematic review of the evidence. Crit Care Med 2002;30:2022–9.

33. Coeffier M, Dechelotte P. The role of glutamine in intensive care unit patients: mechanisms of action and clinical outcome. Nutr Rev 2005;63:65–9.

34. Peng X, Yan H, You Z, et al. Clinical and protein metabolic efficacy of glutamine granules-supplemented enteral nutrition in severely burned patients. Burns 2005;31:342–6.

35. Wernerman J, Hammarqvist F. Glutamine: a necessary nutrient for the intensive care patient. Int J Colorectal Dis 1999;14:137–42.

36. Zaloga GP. Vitamins. In: Zaloga GP, editor. Nutrition in critical care. 1st ed. St. Louis: Mosby-Year Book; 1994. p. 217–42.

37. Hathcock JN, Azzi A, Blumberg J, et al. Vitamins E and C are safe across a broad range of intakes. Am J Clin Nutr 2005;81:736–45.

38. Ehrlich HP, Hunt TK. Effects of cortisone and vitamin A on wound healing. Ann Surg 1968;167:324–8.

39. Ehrenpreis ED, Jani A, Levitsky J, et al. A prospective, randomized, double-blind, placebo-controlled trial of retinol palmitate (vitamin A) for symptomatic chronic radiation proctopathy. Dis Colon Rectum 2005;48:1–8.

40. Gerber LE, Erdman JW Jr. Effect of dietary retinyl acetate, beta-carotene and retinoic acid on wound healing in rats. J Nutr 1982;112:1555–64.

41. Muehlberger T, Moresi JM, Schwarze H, et al. The effect of topical tretinoin on tissue strength and skin components in a murine incisional wound model. J Am Acad Dermatol 2005;52:583–8.

42. Hung VC, Lee JY, Zitelli JA, Hebda PA. Topical tretinoin and epithelial wound healing. Arch Dermatol 1989;125:65–9.

43. Gray M. Does oral zinc supplementation promote healing of chronic wounds? J Wound Ostomy Continence Nurs 2003;30:295–9.

44. Sandstead HH, Lanier VC Jr, Shephard GH, Gillespie DD. Zinc and wound healing. Effects of zinc deficiency and zinc supplementation. Am J Clin Nutr 1970;23:514–9.

45. Lim Y, Levy M, Bray TM. Dietary zinc alters early inflammatory responses during cutaneous wound healing in weanling CD-1 mice. J Nutr 2004;134:811–6.

25

Controlling Infection

Rebecca E. Fraioli, MD; Jonas T. Johnson, MD

OVERVIEW

Specific Therapy in Its Current State

Prevention of perioperative surgical site infection is critical to ensure normal wound healing. Perioperative antibiotic prophylaxis begun prior to the surgical incision and continued for a period of 24 hours has been demonstrated to decrease rates of wound infection for clean-contaminated surgeries of the head and neck. No benefit has been shown from the use of perioperative antibiotics for clean (uncontaminate) surgery or for a duration longer than 24 hours. Many antibiotic agents are effective, but when the wound is contaminated by oropharyngeal flora, the antibiotic chosen should cover both anaerobes and gram-positive aerobes.

Shortcomings

Perioperative antibiotic prophylaxis decreases the incidence of wound infection by decreasing the level of bacterial contamination of the wound at the time of surgery. Antibiotics are not able to compensate for technical failure, such as closure of the wound under tension or poor blood supply to skin flaps. It is important to recognize the limitations of perioperative antimicrobial prophylaxis because prolonging the duration of antibiotic coverage past 24 hours will not further decrease the risk of wound infection but will place the patient at risk of antibiotic-associated complications.

Future Promise

The targeted use of perioperative antimicrobial prophylaxis can minimize surgical site infection and thereby prevent delays in wound healing. The risk of antibiotic-associated complications can be minimized if antibiotic agents are routinely given for only 24 hours in duration.

INTRODUCTION

Wound healing is a complex process that depends on the coordinated interaction of a number of cell types and their products. Normal wound healing consists of orderly progression through the well-defined stages of inflammation, proliferation, and maturation, ultimately resulting in a healed wound (see Chapter 1).[1] Bacteria are omnipresent in our environment; therefore, it is evident that wound healing may progress even in the presence of some degree of bacterial contamination. However, it has long been recognized that wound healing is impaired in the presence of frank infection.[1,2]

Carrel and Hartmann reported in 1916 that wound healing stopped progressing when a surgical wound became infected.[3] The importance of this observation is clear if one considers that perioperative surgical wound infection is the most common nosocomial infection in surgical patients.[4] Wound infection rates have been estimated to occur in 3 to 4% of all surgical procedures.[4,5]

The precise mechanism by which infection impairs wound healing is unknown; however, it is believed that inflammatory mediators released during infection prolong the inflammatory phase and thereby interrupt the normal progression of wound healing. The inflammatory phase of wound healing is stimulated directly by tissue injury. Injury causes liberation of phospholipase A from the cell membrane, causing arachidonic acid to be broken down into inflammatory mediators, including prostaglandins and leukotrienes. The clotting cascade is also activated by the injury, as are components of complement. This initial inflammatory response to tissue injury causes extensive inflammatory mediator release, with the subsequent migration of inflammatory cells to the wound within the next 48 to 72 hours.[2] The polymorphonuclear leukocyte (PMN) is the predominant inflammatory cell type for the first 48 hours. These cells begin to infiltrate the wound within hours after injury.[1]

Normally, the PMN is replaced by the macrophage as the predominant inflammatory cell type in the wound within 72 hours after injury.[2] Macrophages appear to play a critical role in wound healing owing to their ability to phagocytose necrotic debris and to secrete proangiogenic and profibroblastic growth factors. Secretion of these factors appears to initiate the transition from the inflammatory to the proliferative stage of wound healing.[1] In contrast, the PMN does not appear to be critical for normal wound healing. In fact, the continued presence of PMNs at high levels in the infected wound likely contributes to the deleterious effects of infection on wound healing. PMN granules contain hydrolytic enzymes, and the continued release of these, as well as oxygen free radicals, in the wound causes ongoing tissue damage. High concentrations of bacteria in a wound thus cause tissue damage, not only by their direct production of toxins but also by the continued recruitment of PMNs and prolongation of the inflammatory phase.[2]

Recent studies have demonstrated that even in the absence of frank infection, high bacterial counts in a wound may delay healing. Bendy and colleagues demonstrated that epithelialization of decubitus ulcers will occur only if the bacterial count is below 10^6 bacteria/mL^3 of tissue.[6] Stenberg and colleagues showed that full-thickness 1.5 cm^2 experimental wounds on a rat's back contract in 22 days in control rats but take longer to contract after the experimental addition of 10^5 colony-forming units (cfu) of *Escherichia coli.*[7] Finally, a number of experiments examining skin graft take revealed a 94% graft survival when bacterial counts were below 10^5 cfu bacteria/g tissue but only a 19% graft survival when bacterial counts in the recipient site were $> 10^6$ cfu.[2] The critical concentration above which bacterial contamination interferes with wound healing appears to be a bacterial count of 10^5 to 10^6 cfu/g tissue.[6,8] To maintain wound healing on its normal course, then, the goal should be to maintain the concentration of bacteria contaminating the wound below this concentration.

Because it has been demonstrated that bacterial concentrations below 10^5 cfu bacteria/g tissue do not generally cause wound infection or impair wound healing, efforts to reduce the level of bacterial contamination in a wound to or below this level are warranted.[8] Evidence demonstrates that the main source of bacterial contamination of a wound is from endogenous sources. For example, in patients developing wound abscess following cholecystectomy, 8 of 10 had positive intraoperative cultures of the biliary tract.[9] In the head and neck, contamination of the wound by oropharyngeal flora is a major risk factor for postoperative wound infection. It has been estimated that the normal salivary bacterial count is in the range of 10^8 to 10^9 cfu/mL, consisting of 50 to 100 different bacterial types at any one location.[10] When surgery is undertaken in this area, the normally sterile underlying tissues are exposed to these bacterial contaminants. In fact, bacteriologic analysis of wound infection has demonstrated that organisms cultured from the wound are typically oropharyngeal flora that would likely be contaminants at the time of surgery.[11,12]

ANTIBIOTIC PROPHYLAXIS

The use of antibiotics as prophylaxis for prevention of wound infection following head and neck surgery has been studied extensively. As expected by the high concentration of bacteria in normal oropharyngeal secretions, postoperative wound infection rates following head and neck surgery are high.[13-15] Infection rates as high as 87% have been reported for contaminated procedures when no antibiotic prophylaxis is used.[16]

The degree of contamination of the wound with oral and respiratory secretions varies according to the type and duration of the procedure. Therefore, different surgical procedures have varying risks of postoperative wound infection and, as such, have different requirements for antibiotic prophylaxis. In the United States, the Centers for Disease Control and Prevention (CDC) established guidelines aimed at preventing surgical site infection (SSI). The CDC guidelines include a classification system based on the level of contamination of a wound.[17,18] Surgeons can use the guidelines preoperatively to help predict the risk of SSI for any procedure and should base the decision of whether to give antimicrobial prophylaxis on these as well as procedure- and specialty-specific guidelines. A summary of these class descriptions and the associated risk of infection is shown in Table 1.[18]

Clean (Class I)

According to the CDC guidelines, a "clean" wound is one in which no infection exists preoperatively and no gross contamination occurs during surgery. This latter criterion is satisfied if, during surgery, no entry is made into the respiratory or alimentary tracts, sterile techniques are maintained, and the wound is closed primarily. Examples of surgical procedures of the head and neck that fall into this category are thyroidectomy, parotidectomy, and

Table 1. RISK OF INFECTION BY WOUND CATEGORY		
Class	Description	Risk of Infection
I	Clean	Low (< 3–5%)
II	Clean-contaminated	Intermediate (10–80%)
III	Contaminated	High (over 80%)
IV	Dirty	Already infected

submandibular gland excision. Johnson and Wagner demonstrated that infection rates without antimicrobial prophylaxis following clean procedures are extremely low (< 5%).[19] Antimicrobial prophylaxis is not necessary for clean surgery of the head and neck.

Clean-Contaminated (Class II)

This class of wound results when a tissue is clean prior to the procedure but the alimentary, respiratory, genital, or urinary tract is entered as part of the procedure, under controlled conditions, and without gross spillage of secretions into the wound. A large proportion of head and neck. Examples include composite resection of oropharyngeal tumors and laryngectomy. Prospective randomized placebo-controlled trials clearly demonstrate the benefit of antimicrobial prophylaxis for reducing postoperative wound infection in clean-contaminated procedures.[13,15,16,20] These studies clearly demonstrate both the efficacy of and the necessity for antimicrobial prophylaxis in clean-contaminated surgery of the head and neck. A meta-analysis of this data demonstrated a 43.7% reduction in infection rates with use of antibiotic prophylaxis compared with placebo.[21] With appropriate prophylaxis, postoperative wound infection occurs in less than 10% of clean-contaminated cases.[18] Unusual spillage of secretions or other gross contamination during the procedure will upgrade the procedure to class III.[22] It is worth mentioning that there are certain common procedures that come under the definition of clean-contaminated surgery but do not carry the same high risk of postoperative wound infection. Intranasal surgery is one such example. Forty to 50% of patients have colonization of the nose by *Staphylococcus aureus*, and there have been reports of bacteremia following intranasal surgery such as septoplasty.[23,24] However, Silk and colleagues demonstrated that the rate of bacteremia following septoplasty is low and that antimicrobial prophylaxis for nasal septoplasty is not indicated.[23]

Contaminated (Class III)

Contaminated wounds include traumatic wounds, wounds from procedures in which there was a major violation of sterile technique, and wounds that have been exposed to gross spillage from the upper aerodigestive or gastrointestinal tract. Antimicrobial prophylaxis with various agents and regimens has been able to significantly reduce the postoperative SSI rates to approximately 10–17%.

Infected or "Dirty" (Class IV)

Dirty wounds are those in which known contamination exists prior to the initiation of surgery. Examples include traumatic wounds grossly contaminated with environmental debris and surgical wounds clinically infected at the time of surgery. It is important to note that class IV wounds are considered infected prior to the time of surgery. This consideration is due either to the presence of gross infection within the surgical site or to the fact that wounding occurred accidentally and without the benefit of sterile conditions or antimicrobial prophylaxis. Postoperative infection rates in these cases are greater than 27%, even with appropriate antimicrobial therapy.[18] Antibiotics are therefore mandatory in such cases. Again, class IV wounds are those in which the critical period for prophylaxis has lapsed. Antimicrobial therapy should be administered as treatment, not as prophylaxis, and should be dosed accordingly.[25]

Special Cases: Neck Dissection

Neck dissection is a clean case, without direct contamination of the wound intraoperatively. Nevertheless, as pointed out by Carrau and colleagues, neck dissection is a prolonged operation, with the need for wide wound exposure and intraoperative changes in neck positioning.[26] All of these factors may predispose the patient to postoperative wound infection. A retrospective analysis of the incidence of postoperative wound infection following uncontaminated neck dissec-

tion with or without antimicrobial prophylaxis failed to demonstrate a statistically significant decrease in wound infection with the use of prophylaxis. However, a trend suggesting a benefit of prophylaxis was identified.[26] Prospective randomized trials will be needed to definitively answer this question. In the meantime, a single preoperative dose of antibiotic prophylaxis for uncontaminated neck dissection is reasonable.

SPECTRUM OF ANTIMICROBIAL PROPHYLAXIS

The most common sources of wound contamination and postoperative wound infection following surgery of the head and neck are skin flora and oropharyngeal flora. The predominant skin contaminant is *S. aureus*. Oropharyngeal flora normally consists of 90% anaerobic bacteria and 10% gram-positive aerobes. Gram-negative aerobic bacteria are not normal colonizers of the oropharnyx, although conditions such as the presence of a tracheostomy, a long hospital stay, and the presence of a necrotic oral tumor are risk factors that increase the likelihood of gram-negative aerobes colonizing the oropharnyx and thus, potentially, the wound.[27]

Bacteriology of postoperative wound infections after clean-contaminated surgery of the head and neck has demonstrated that these infections are virtually always polymicrobial. Organisms commonly cultured from wounds include gram-positive (*Staphylococcus* and *Streptococcus*) and gram-negative (eg, *E. coli*, *Klebsiella*, *Serratia*, *Proteus*, *Pseudomonas*) aerobic bacteria, anaerobic bacteria (gram-negative bacilli, including *Bacteroides*, *Lactobacillus*, and *Propionibacerium*), and fungi.[11,15,28,29] However, the pathogenicity of each class of organism is not equally well established.

Gram-Positive Aerobes

These bacteria are present both on the skin and in the oropharynx, which are the two most common sites from which the surgical site may become contaminated. Most studies demonstrating the efficacy of preoperative prophylactic antibiotics at decreasing the incidence of postoperative wound infection have used antibiotics covering these organisms. Gram-positive aerobes are among the most important bacteria to cover with perioperative antibiotic prophylaxis.

Gram-Negative Aerobes

The pathogenicity of aerobic gram-negative organisms in postoperative wound infection following head and neck surgery is not definitively established. Most studies have failed to demonstrate a reduction in the incidence of wound infection when antibiotic prophylaxis was extended to include coverage of gram-negative bacteria.[29–32] Therefore, coverage of aerobic gram-negative organisms is not recommended as a routine component of prophylaxis for contaminated surgery of the head and neck. Nevertheless, as discussed above, certain "special cases" in which gram-negative bacteria are more likely to colonize the oropharynx have been identified. In these cases, inclusion of gram-negative coverage in the antibiotic prophylaxis may be warranted. Such cases include hospitalized patients with tracheostomies and patients who have received preoperative radiation therapy.[28]

Anaerobes

Anaerobic bacteria (most of which are gram negative) from the oropharyngeal cavity appear to play a pathogenic role in the development of postoperative wound infection. Several studies have demonstrated that adding anaerobic coverage to antibiotic prophylaxis reduces the incidence of wound infection when compared with antibiotic prophylaxis regimens without anaerobic coverage.[28,33–35] In addition, in one experimental trial, three patients developed postoperative bacteremia. In each case, the same anaerobic pathogen was isolated from both the blood and the wound of the patient.[15] Antibiotic

prophylaxis for clean-contaminated surgery of the head and neck should therefore include coverage of anaerobic bacteria.

Fungi

Fungi are common isolates from wound infection cultures. However, evidence suggests that fungi grown from wound cultures represent contaminants and not true pathogens. Rubin and colleagues isolated fungi (all *Candida* species) in 48% of postoperative wound infection culture specimens.[11] No antifungal therapy was given, and all of the infections in the series resolved. Antifungal therapy is not recommended as prophylaxis for head and neck surgery.

SELECTION OF AGENT FOR ANTIMICROBIAL PROPHYLAXIS

Prospective randomized trials have demonstrated the efficacy of a variety of antibiotics in preventing postoperative wound infection following contaminated surgery of the head and neck (Table 2). Although it is difficult to compare the results of different antibiotics between trials owing to methodologic differences, within each study, various antibiotic agents providing coverage for anaerobes and gram-positive aerobes were found to have equivalent efficacy between antibiotic agents covering anaerobes and gram-positive aerobes. The dosage of the antibiotic must be higher than the minimal inhibitory concentration (MIC). This is illustrated by the findings of two separate studies at the University of Pittsburgh examining the ability of prophylactic cefazolin to prevent postoperative wound infection. An initial study using cefazolin dosed at 500 mg IV every 8 hours for 24 hours only 500 mg resulted in a wound infection rate of 33%, whereas a later study examining cefazolin at a concentration of 2 g given every 8 hours for 4 doses had a wound infection rate of only 8.5%.[33,36]

Table 2. RATES OF WOUND INFECTION WITH 24 HOURS OF PERIOPERATIVE ANTIBIOTIC PROPHYLAXIS

Antibiotic (Dose)	Rate of Wound Infection (%)	Reference
Amoxicillin-clavulanate (2g IV q8° X 4 doses)	/57 (22.8)	Rodrigo et al.[32]
Ampicillin-sulbactam (1.5 g IV q6° X 4 doses)	11/81(14)	Johnson et al.[30]
Cefazolin (500 mg IV q8° X 24°)	7/21 (33)	Johnson et al.[33]
Cefazolin (1g IV q6-8° X 4 doses)	4/25 (16)	Seagle et al.[62]
Cefazolin (1g IM or IV then 0.5 g IM/IV q6° X 3 doses)	12/32 (38)	Becker and Parell[16]
Cefazolin (2g IV q8° X 4 doses)	5/59 (8.5)	Johnson et al. [36]
Cefazolin (2g IV X 1 then 1g IV q8° X 3 doses)	/50 (26)	Rodrigo et al. [32]
Carbenicillin (10g IV q8° X 24°)	10/72 (14)	Piccart et al. [63]
Moxalactam (30 mg/kg IV q8° X 3 doses)	1/16 (6.2)	Fee et al. [41]
Moxalactam (2g IV q8° X 4 doses)	2/59 (3.4)	Johnson et al. [36]
Clindamycin (600 mg IV q8° X 4 doses)	2/52 (3.4)	Johnson et al. [31]
Clindamycin (600 mg IV q6° X 5 doses)	12/88 (14)	Johnson et al. [30]
Clindamycin+gentamicin (300 mg + 1.7 mg/kg both IV q8° X 4 doses)	2/29 (7.0)	Johnson et al. [33]
Clindamycin+gentamicin (600 mg + 1.7 mg/kg both IV q8° X 4 doses)	2/52 (3.4)	Johnson et al. [31]
Clindamycin+gentamicin (600 mg + 80 mg both IV q8° X 4 doses)	/52 (21.2)	Rodrigo et al. [32]
Cefoperazone (2g IV q8° X 4 doses)	4/39 (10)	Johnson et al. [15]
Cefotaxime (2g IV q8° X 4 doses)	3/32 (9.4)	Johnson et al. [15]
Cefotaxime (1g IM q12° X 2 doses)	4/30 (13.3)	Mustafa et al.[42]

Adapted from Grandis J and Johnson J.[12]

TIMING OF ANTIBIOTIC PROPHYLAXIS

A landmark study by Burke used experimental lesions in an animal model of wound infection to demonstrate that there is a limited "effective period" during which antibiotic prophylaxis can reduce the incidence of wound infection.[37] This critical period begins the moment that the surgical incision is made and bacteria contaminate the tissue; strikingly, it lasts for only 3 hours after the contamination occurs. Antibiotic administration is most effective when given just prior to the surgical incision, thereby ensuring that an effective tissue concentration will be present the moment the bacterial contamination occurs. The effective period lasts only up to 3 hours following bacterial inoculation. Initiation of prophylactic antibiotics greater than 3 hours after bacterial contamination is not effective. Human studies have since corroborated these earlier findings.[38]

DURATION OF ANTIBIOTIC PROPHYLAXIS

Several large, prospective, randomized clinical trials have established the efficacy of antibiotic prophylaxis of 24-hour duration in clean-contaminated head and neck surgery. Overwhelmingly, these studies have failed to demonstrate a decrease in infection rates with increased duration of prophylaxis.[39-42] With the exception of certain special cases, perioperative prophylactic antibiotics should not be given for a period longer than 24 hours.

Special Cases

Skull Base Surgery
There still may be special cases for which a longer course of antibiotic prophylaxis may be justified. These are cases such as skull base surgery, in which contamination of the intracranial contents with nasal and oral bacteria is common. Carrau demonstrated a statistical benefit from extending the duration of prophylaxis to 48 hours from 24 hours but no further benefit when prophylaxis was extended beyond 48 hours.[43]

Flaps
Despite the fact that prolonged antibiotic prophylaxis is commonly used following flap reconstructions, prospective randomized trials do not support this practice. Prolongation of antimicrobial prophylaxis from 1 day to 5 days did not reduce wound infection rates following either pedicled flap or free flap reconstruction.[39,44] Despite common belief, flap reconstruction does not appear to be a special case for antibiotic prophylaxis.

COST OF ANTIMICROBIAL PROPHYLAXIS

It has been estimated that 30% of the entire cost of hospitalization is due to antibiotic prophylaxis.[45] In the current environment of escalating health care costs, the importance of limiting antibiotic prophylaxis to cases in which it is truly needed is obvious. Nevertheless, the expense of wound infection, including that resulting from delayed wound healing, is of such great magnitude that, from a dollar-cost perspective, the savings of even a few wound infections may justify the cost of antibiotic prophylaxis.[36,46,47]

COMPLICATIONS OF ANTIMICROBIAL PROPHYLAXIS

As Burke pointed out as far back as 1977, prophylactic use of antibiotics is useful only if its potential benefit outweighs the risk of side effects or complications from the drug.[48] In the determination of whether and how to give adequate prophylaxis, one must consider many variables, including cost, toxicity, the emergence of antibiotic-resistant organisms, and antibiotic-associated illness (eg, *Clostridium difficile* colitis).

Antimicrobial drugs may have significant toxicity, as in the ototoxicity and nephrotoxicity associated with the aminoglycoside group of antibiotics. In addition to the direct toxicity of some antimicrobials, some patients may have allergic or other adverse drug reactions. Indiscriminate antibiotic use may hasten the emergence of resistant strains of bacteria.[49] Finally, although *C. difficile* colitis is more frequent after long-term administration of antibiotics, it has been documented even after an appropriate, short prophylactic regimen of antibiotics.[50] *C. difficile* colitis has the potential for grave complications and is increasingly becoming a real issue for patients undergoing surgery of the head and neck.

LIMITATIONS OF ANTIBIOTIC PROPHYLAXIS

Surgical Technique

Johnson and colleagues pointed out nearly two decades ago that antibiotics do not prevent the development of postoperative wound infection in cases in which there is technical failure.[15] In another study, Brown and colleagues attributed 59% of postoperative wound infections to a "probable flaw in surgical technique or judgment," such as tissue trauma or wound closure under tension.[51]

Most patients who develop postoperative wound infection do so despite having received antibiotic prophylaxis. As discussed above, extending the duration of antibiotic prophylaxis does not further decrease the incidence of wound infection. This suggests that wound infections occurring despite antibiotic prophylaxis are not due to an inadequacy or failure of prophylaxis but to some other cause.[5] Factors such as poor surgical technique, patient smoking, low intraoperative patient temperature, and wound ischemia appear to predispose the patient to postoperative wound infection.[52–57] Failure to address these factors cannot be compensated for by antimicrobial prophylaxis. In terms of surgical technique, exacting attention must be paid to hemostasis prior to wound closure. Postoperative hematoma may compromise tissue perfusion and also directly predispose the patient to wound infection by providing a culture medium for bacterial growth. Irrigation of the wound and placement of suction drains in dependent portions of the neck are crucial to remove debris and prevent its reaccumulation.[25]

Avoidance of wound closure under tension and devascularization of skin flaps is also crucial. This is illustrated by the fact that infection rates in surgical defects reconstructed with a pedicled myocutaneous flap are higher than those closed primarily or reconstructed with free tissue transfer with microvascular anastomosis.[44,58] Wound infection rates following closure with a pedicled flap have been reported in the range of 20 to

36%.[33,39,51,50] With a 24-hour course of adequate antimicrobial prophylaxis, wound infection rates for nonirradiated tissue following free flap reconstructions of the head and neck appear to be at or below 11%, which is comparable to infection rates in wounds closed primarily.[44,58,59]

TREATMENT OF POSTOPERATIVE WOUND INFECTION

Early recognition of developing wound infection and prompt initiation of therapy is crucial to limit patient and wound morbidity. Early treatment limits the exposure of tissue to salivary enzymes and bacterial toxins, both of which contribute to flap autolysis and, if unchecked, may result in exposure of critical structures.[5] Diagnosis of postoperative wound infection after surgery of the head and neck is not always straightforward. Many of the classic signs of inflammation, such as erythema, edema, and induration, are normal sequelae of head and neck surgical procedures.[5] In addition, low-grade fever and mild leukocytosis (10,000 white blood cell/mm^3) are common in the immediate postoperative period, limiting the predictive value of these signs for the diagnosis of wound infection.[60]

To objectively assess a surgical wound for the presence of infection, a wound grading system such as that employed by Johnson and colleagues is useful (Table 3).[33] Figures 1 to 4 show examples of visual assessment. Wounds with erythema and induration that do not progress to drain purulent material are not felt to represent true wound infection, and the administration of therapeutic antibiotics for such a wound exposes

	Table 3. Wound Grading Scale
Grade	**Wound Description**
0	Normal healing
1	Erythema around suture line < 1 cm
2	1–5 cm erythema
3	Greater than 5 cm erythema and induration
4	Purulent drainage either spontaneously or by incision and drainage
5	Orocutaneous fistula

Adapted from Johnson et al.[33]

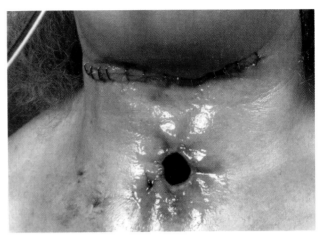

Figure 1. This patient underwent total laryngectomy 9 days previously. There is no erythema or induration. This wound is scored 0.

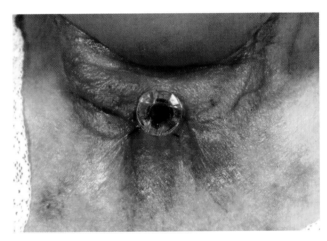

Figure 2. This photograph demonstrates a wound 10 days following laryngectomy. There is persistent erythema and edema extending > 2 cm from the incision. This is graded 2+.

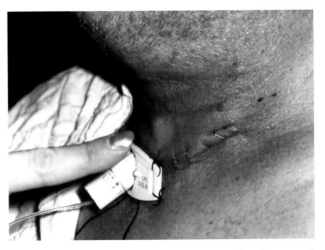

Figure 3. This patient underwent major head and neck surgery 6 days previously. Notice the 2+ erythema and induration. The erythema blanches with digital pressure.

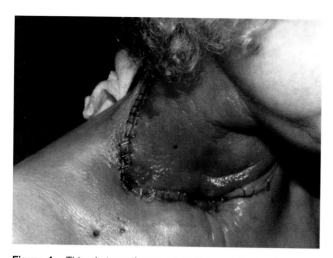

Figure 4. This photograph was taken 7 days following laryngectomy and neck dissection. There is diffuse erythema and edema of the flap. We grade this 3+. Note that the distribution of the wound changes correspond with the interruption of the venous and lymphatic drainage secondary to the design of the superiorly based flap.

the patient to the risks of antibiotic administration, which in this case exceed the benefits.

Postoperative wound infections, as with all soft tissue infections, benefit from débridement of devitalized tissue and drainage of purulent debris (see Chapter 26). Pathogenic aerobic bacteria that thrive in the low-oxygen environment of devitalized tissue and necrotic debris are best eradicated by surgical débridement and drainage. Opening the wound exposes it to ambient oxygen pressures and eliminates the anaerobic environment. In most cases, this is best accomplished in the operating room, where the extent of tissue destruction can best be evaluated, the wound can be well irrigated, and drainage can be established in the most optimal locations.[5]

In some cases, purulent secretions noted in the patient's suction drains are the first sign of developing infection. In such cases, every effort should be made to maintain the patency of these drains. Adequate drainage of purulent debris prevents the formation of an abscess cavity and is necessary for resolution of the infection. Drains should be maintained for 10 to 14 days after purulence is noted to allow time for the wound cavity to heal and close.[61] For patients with cellulitis or sepsis, antibiotic use is appropriate.

Selection of antibiotics should be based on the findings of Gram's stain and wound culture and sensitivity reports.

Empiric therapy while awaiting sensitivity reports should provide coverage for anaerobes and gram-positive and gram-negative aerobic bacteria. The antibiotic used for prophylaxis at the time of surgery should not be used for empiric therapy. Suitable choices include ticarcillin with clavulanic acid or ampicillin-sulbactam. In a penicillin-allergic patient, a combination of clindamycin with an aminoglycoside is suitable. The addition of vancomycin for coverage of methicillin-resistant *S. aureus* should be considered in institutional settings in which the rate of infection with this organism is high. The duration of antimicrobial treatment should be based on clinical findings.

GUIDELINES FOR ANTIBIOTIC PROPHYLAXIS

In summary, prophylactic antibiotics covering gram-positive aerobic bacteria and anaerobes are recommended for clean-contaminated surgery of the head and neck. This includes any surgery in which there is expected to be gross contamination of the wound with secretions from the upper aerodigestive tract. Clean and selected clean-contaminated surgeries, such as nasal septoplasty, generally do not necessitate antimicrobial prophylaxis. In general, antimicrobial prophylaxis should be continued for only 24 hours postoperatively. Increased duration of prophylaxis has not been shown to further reduce postoperative wound infection rates and may increase the risk of antibiotic-related complications. Many different antibiotic agents have been used for prophylaxis of wound infection with comparable results. However, it is crucial that the concentration of the antibacterial agent in the blood be above the MIC for the bacteria and that the trough between doses during the operation not fall below this MIC.

REFERENCES

1. Krizek T. Biology of Tissue Injury and Repair. In: Georgiade G, Georgiade N, Riefkohl R, Barwick W, editors. Textbook of Plastic, Maxillofacial, and Reconstructive Surgery. Philadelphia: Williams & Wilkins; 1992. p. 3–8.

2. Robson MC, Stenberg BD, Heggers JP. Wound healing alterations caused by infection. Clin Plast Surg 1990;17: 485–492.

3. Carrel A, Hartmann A. Cicatrization of wounds: The relation between the size of the wound and the rate of its cicatrization. J Exp Med 1916;24:429.

4. Malone DL, Genuit T, Tracy JK, et al. Surgical site infections: reanalysis of risk factors. J Surg Res 2002; 103:89–95.

5. Johnson JT, Weber RS. Management of Postoperative Head and Neck Wound Infections. In: Johnson JT, Yu VL, editors. Infectious Diseases and Antimicrobial Therapy of the Ears, Nose, and Throat. Philadelphia: W.B. Saunders; 1996. p. 563–565.

6. Bendy RH Jr, Nuccio PA, Wolfe E, et al. Relationship of Quantitative Wound Bacterial Counts to Healing of Decubiti: Effect of Topical Gentamicin. Antimicrobial Agents Chemother 1964;10:147–155.

7. Stenberg BD, Phillips LG, Hokanson JA, et al. Effect of bFGF on the inhibition of contraction caused by bacteria. J Surg Res 1991;50:47–50.

8. Robson MC, Mannari RJ, Smith PD, et al. Maintenance of wound bacterial balance. Am J Surg 1999;178:399–402.

9. Robson MC. Wound infection. A failure of wound healing caused by an imbalance of bacteria. Surg Clin North Am 1997;77:637–650.

10. Bartlett JG, Gorbach SL. Anaerobic infections of the head and neck. Otolaryngol Clin North Am 1976;9: 655–678.

11. Rubin J, Johnson JT, Wagner RL, et al. Bacteriologic analysis of wound infection following major head and neck surgery. Arch Otolaryngol Head Neck Surg 1988; 114:969–972.

12. Grandis J, Johnson J. The Use of Antibiotics in Head and Neck Surgery. In: Myers E, Suen J, editors. Cancer of the Head and Neck. Philadephia: W.B. Saunders Company; 1996. p. 97–104.

13. Dor P, Klastersky J. Prophylactic antibiotics in oral, pharyngeal and laryngeal surgery for cancer: (a double-blind study). Laryngoscope 1973;83:1992–1998.

14. Goode RL, Abramson N, Fee WE, et al. Effect of prophylactic antibiotics in radical head and neck surgery. Laryngoscope 1979;89:601–608.

15. Johnson JT, Yu VL, Myers EN, et al. Efficacy of two third-generation cephalosporins in prophylaxis for head and neck surgery. Arch Otolaryngol 1984;110:224–227.

16. Becker GD, Parell GJ. Cefazolin prophylaxis in head and neck cancer surgery. Ann Otol Rhinol Laryngol 1979; 88:183–186.

17. Mangram AJ, Horan TC, Pearson ML, et al. Guideline for Prevention of Surgical Site Infection, 1999. Centers for Disease Control and Prevention (CDC) Hospital Infection Control Practices Advisory Committee. Am J Infect Control 1999;27:97–132; quiz 133-134; discussion 196.

18. Garner J, Hughes J, Davis B. CDC Guideline for Prevention of Surgical Wound Infections, 1985. Infect Control Hosp Epidemiol 1986;7:193–200.

19. Johnson JT, Wagner RL. Infection following uncontaminated head and neck surgery. Arch Otolaryngol Head Neck Surg 1987;113:368–369.

20. Becker GD. Identification and management of the patient at high risk for wound infection. Head Neck Surg 1986; 8:205–210.

21. Velanovich V. A meta-analysis of prophylactic antibiotics in head and neck surgery. Plast Reconstr Surg 1991;87: 429–434; discussion 435.

22. McGuckin M, Goldman R, Bolton L, et al. The clinical relevance of microbiology in acute and chronic wounds. Adv Skin Wound Care 2003;16:12–23; quiz 24-15.

23. Silk KL, Ali MB, Cohen BJ, et al. Absence of bacteremia during nasal septoplasty. Arch Otolaryngol Head Neck Surg 1991;117:54–55.

24. Slavin SA, Rees TD, Guy CL, et al. An investigation of bacteremia during rhinoplasty. Plast Reconstr Surg 1983;71:196–198.

25. Johnson JT. Principles of Antibiotic Prophylaxis. In: Johnson JT, Yu VL, editors. Infectious Diseases and Antimicrobial Therapy of the Ears, Nose, and Throat. Philadelphia: W.B. Saunders; 1996. p. 589–593.

26. Carrau RL, Byzakis J, Wagner RL, et al. Role of prophylactic antibiotics in uncontaminated neck dissections. Arch Otolaryngol Head Neck Surg 1991;117: 194–195.

27. Johnson JT, Weber RS. Prophylaxis for Contaminated Head and Neck and Cranial Base Surgery. In: Johnson JT, Yu VL, editors. Infectious Diseases and Antimicrobial Therapy of the Ears, Nose, and Throat. Philadelphia: W.B. Saunders; 1996. p. 594–598.

28. Johnson JT, Yu VL. Role of aerobic gram-negative rods, anaerobes, and fungi in wound infection after head and neck surgery: implications for antibiotic prophylaxis. Head Neck 1989;11:27–29.

29. Weber RS, Raad I, Frankenthaler R, et al. Ampicillin-sulbactam vs clindamycin in head and neck oncologic surgery. The need for gram-negative coverage. Arch Otolaryngol Head Neck Surg 1992;118:1159–1163.

30. Johnson JT, Kachman K, Wagner RL, et al. Comparison of ampicillin/sulbactam versus clindamycin in the prevention of infection in patients undergoing head and neck surgery. Head Neck 1997;19:367–371.

31. Johnson JT, Yu VL, Myers EN, et al. An assessment of the need for gram-negative bacterial coverage in antibiotic prophylaxis for oncological head and neck surgery. J Infect Dis 1987;155:331–333.

32. Rodrigo JP, Alvarez JC, Gomez JR, et al. Comparison of three prophylactic antibiotic regimens in clean-contaminated head and neck surgery. Head Neck 1997;19: 188–193.

33. Johnson JT, Myers EN, Thearle PB, et al. Antimicrobial prophylaxis for contaminated head and neck surgery. Laryngoscope 1984;94:46–51.

34. Robbins KT, Favrot S, Hanna D, et al. Risk of wound infection in patients with head and neck cancer. Head Neck 1990;12:143–148.

35. Johnson JT, Yu VL. Antibiotic use during major head and neck surgery. Ann Surg 1988;207:108–111.

36. Johnson JT, Yu VL, Myers EN, et al. Cefazolin vs moxalactam? A double-blind randomized trial of cephalosporins in head and neck surgery. Arch Otolaryngol Head Neck Surg 1986;112:151–153.

37. Burke JF. The effective period of preventive antibiotic action in experimental incisions and dermal lesions. Surgery 1961;50:161–168.

38. Classen DC, Evans RS, Pestotnik SL, et al. The timing of prophylactic administration of antibiotics and the risk of surgical-wound infection. N Engl J Med 1992;326:281–286.

39. Johnson JT, Schuller DE, Silver F, et al. Antibiotic prophylaxis in high-risk head and neck surgery: one-day vs. five-day therapy. Otolaryngol Head Neck Surg 1986;95:554–557.

40. Righi M, Manfredi R, Farneti G, et al. Short-term versus long-term antimicrobial prophylaxis in oncologic head and neck surgery. Head Neck 1996;18:399–404.

41. Fee WE Jr, Glenn M, Handen C, et al. One day vs. two days of prophylactic antibiotics in patients undergoing major head and neck surgery. Laryngoscope 1984;94:612–614.

42. Mustafa E, Tahsin A. Cefotaxime prophylaxis in major non-contaminated head and neck surgery: one-day vs. seven-day therapy. J Laryngol Otol 1993;107:30–32.

43. Carrau RL. Antibiotic Prophylaxis in cranical base surgery. Head and Neck 1991;13:311–317.

44. Carroll WR, Rosenstiel D, Fix JR, et al. Three-dose vs extended-course clindamycin prophylaxis for free-flap reconstruction of the head and neck. Arch Otolaryngol Head Neck Surg 2003;129:771–774.

45. Shapiro M. Perioperative prophylactic use of antibiotics in surgery: principles and practice. Infect Control 1982;3:38–40.

46. Mandell-Brown M, Johnson JT, Wagner RL. Cost-effectiveness of prophylactic antibiotics in head and neck surgery. Otolaryngol Head Neck Surg 1984;92:520–523.

47. Blair EA, Johnson JT, Wagner RL, et al. Cost analysis of antibiotic prophylaxis in clean head and neck surgery. Arch Otolaryngol Head Neck Surg 1995;121:269–271.

48. Burke JF. Preventing bacterial infection by coordinating antibiotic and host activity: a time-dependent relationship. South Med J 1977;70 Suppl 1:24–26.

49. Wittmann DH, Schein M. Let us shorten antibiotic prophylaxis and therapy in surgery. Am J Surg 1996;172:26S–32S.

50. Yee J, Dixon CM, McLean AP, et al. Clostridium difficile disease in a department of surgery. The significance of prophylactic antibiotics. Arch Surg 1991;126:241–246.

51. Brown BM, Johnson JT, Wagner RL. Etiologic factors in head and neck wound infections. Laryngoscope 1987;97:587–590.

52. Sorensen LT, Karlsmark T, Gottrup F. Abstinence from smoking reduces incisional wound infection: a randomized controlled trial. Ann Surg 2003;238:1–5.

53. Sorensen LT, Horby J, Friis E, et al. Smoking as a risk factor for wound healing and infection in breast cancer surgery. Eur J Surg Oncol 2002;28:815–820.

54. Allen DB, Maguire JJ, Mahdavian M, et al. Wound hypoxia and acidosis limit neutrophil bacterial killing mechanisms. Arch Surg 1997;132:991–996.

55. Hopf HW, Hunt TK, West JM, et al. Wound tissue oxygen tension predicts the risk of wound infection in surgical patients. Arch Surg 1997;132:997–1004; discussion 1005.

56. Kurz A, Sessler DI, Lenhardt R. Perioperative normothermia to reduce the incidence of surgical-wound infection and shorten hospitalization. Study of Wound Infection and Temperature Group. N Engl J Med 1996;334:1209–1215.

57. Sessler DI, Akca O. Nonpharmacological prevention of surgical wound infections. Clin Infect Dis 2002;35:1397–1404.

58. Johnson JT, Wagner RL, Schuller DE, et al. Prophylactic antibiotics for head and neck surgery with flap reconstruction. Arch Otolaryngol Head Neck Surg 1992;118:488–490.

59. Simons JP, Johnson JT, Yu VL, et al. The role of topical antibiotic prophylaxis in patients undergoing contaminated head and neck surgery with flap reconstruction. Laryngoscope 2001;111:329–335.

60. Pile JC. Evaluating postoperative fever: a focused approach. Cleve Clin J Med 2006;73 Suppl 1:S62–66.

61. Johnson J, Myers E. Management of Complications of Head and Neck Surgery. In: Myers E, Suen J, editors. Cancer of the Head and Neck. Philadelphia: W.B. Saunders Company; 1996. p. 693–711.

62. Seagle MB, Duberstein LE, Gross CW, et al. Efficacy of cefazolin as a prophylactic antibiotic in head and neck surgery. Otolaryngology 1978;86 (4 Pt 1):ORL-568–72.

63. Piccart M, Dor P, Klastersky J. Antimicrobial prophylaxis of infections in head and neck cancer surgery. Scand J Infect Dis Suppl 1983;39:92–6.

26

Wound Débridement

Gregory Schultz, PhD; Elizabeth Ayello, PhD; Harold Brem, MD

PHASES OF ACUTE WOUND HEALING

Acute wounds in skin normally heal by progressing through four distinct, but overlapping, phases of healing: *hemostasis, inflammation, repair,* and *remodeling* (Figure 1).[1–3] Wound healing is a complex process that involves several types of specialized cells, including platelets, neutrophils, macrophages, fibroblasts, epithelial cells, and vascular endothelial cells. The actions of these wound cells are regulated by the key proteins, including growth factors (Table 1), cytokines (Table 2), and chemokines (Table 3). Proteases, including the matrix metalloproteinases (MMPs), neutrophil elastase, and plasmin, play key roles in migration of epithelial cells and vascular endothelial cells and in removal of proteins in the extracellular matrix (ECM) damaged during injury (Table 4). In addition, the provisional wound matrix, which consists mainly of fibrin and fibronectin, actively influences the behavior of wound cells through interactions of the matrix proteins with the integrin receptors on wound cells. When all of these components function properly, injuries are repaired with scar tissue that approximates the original tissue structure.

Sequence of Molecular and Cellular Events in Healing Wounds

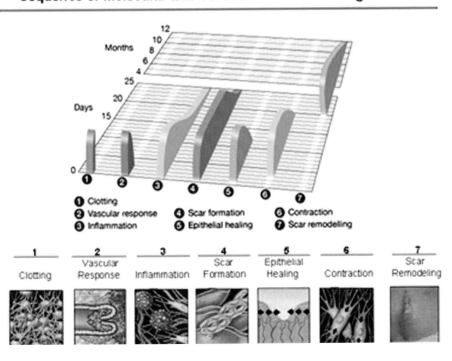

Figure 1. Sequence of molecular and cellular events in healing wounds.

Table 1 MAJOR GROWTH FACTOR FAMILIES INVOLVED IN REGULATING WOUND HEALING		
Growth Factor Family	**Cell Source**	**Actions**
Transforming growth factor (TGF)β TGF-β_1, TGF-β_2	Platelets Fibroblasts Macrophages	Fibroblast chemotaxis and activation ECM deposition Collagen synthesis TIMP synthesis MMP synthesis Reduces scarring Collagen Fibronectin
TGF-β_3 Platelet-derived growth factor (PDGF) PDGF-AA, PDGF-BB, VEGF	Platelets Macrophages Keratinocytes Fibroblasts	Activation of immune cells and fibroblasts ECM deposition Collagen synthesis TIMP synthesis MMP synthesis Angiogenesis
Fibroblast growth factor (FGF) Acidic FGF, basic FGF, KGF	Macrophages Endothelial cells Fibroblasts	Angiogenesis Endothelial cell activation Keratinocyte proliferation and migration ECM deposition
Insulin-like growth factor (IGF) IGF-I, IGF-II, insulin	Liver Skeletal muscle Fibroblasts Macrophages Neutrophils	Keratinocyte proliferation Fibroblast proliferation Endothelial cell activation Angiogenesis Collagen synthesis ECM deposition Cell metabolism
Epidermal growth factor (EGF) EGF, HB-EGF, TGF-α, amphiregulin, betacellulin Connective tissue growth factor (CTGF)	Keratinocytes Macrophages Fibroblasts Endothelial cells Epithelial cells	Keratinocyte proliferation and migration ECM deposition Mediates action of TGF-βs on collagen synthesis

ECM = extracellular matrix; HB = heparin-binding; KGF = keratinocyte growth factor; MMP = matrix metalloproteinase; TIMP = tissue inhibitor of metalloproteinases; VEGF = vascular endothelial growth factor.

Table 2 MAJOR CYTOKINES INVOLVED IN REGULATING WOUND HEALING		
Cytokine	**Cell Source**	**Biologic Activity**
Proinflammatory cytokines		
TNF-α	Macrophages	PMN margination and cytotoxicity, ± collagen synthesis; provides metabolic substrate
IL-1	Macrophages Keratinocytes	Fibroblast and keratinocyte chemotaxis, collagen synthesis
IL-2	T lymphocytes	Increases fibroblast infiltration and metabolism
IL-6	Macrophages PMNs Fibroblasts	Fibroblast proliferation, hepatic acute-phase protein synthesis
IL-8	Macrophages Fibroblasts	Macrophage and PMN chemotaxis, keratinocyte maturation
IFN-γ	T lymphocytes Macrophages	Macrophage and PMN activation; retards collagen synthesis and cross-linking; stimulates collagenase activity
Anti-inflammatory cytokines		
IL-4	T lymphocytes Basophils Mast cells	Inhibition of TNF, IL-1, IL-6 production; fibroblast proliferation, collagen synthesis
IL-10	T lymphocytes Macrophages Keratinocytes	Inhibition of TNF, IL-1, IL-6 production; inhibits macrophage and PMN activation

IFN = interferon; IL = interleukin; PMN = polymorphonuclear leukocyte; TNF = tumor necrosis factor.

Table 3 MAJOR CHEMOKINE FAMILIES INVOLVED IN REGULATING WOUND HEALING	
Chemokines	Cells Affected
α-Chemokines (CXC) with glutamic acid-leucine-arginine near the N-terminal	Neutrophils
Interleukin-8 (IL-8)	
α-Chemokines (CXC) without glutamic acid-leucine-arginine near the N-terminal	Activated T lymphocytes
Interferon-inducible protein of 10 kDa (IP-10)	
Monokine induced by interferon-γ (MIG)	
Stromal cell–derived factor 1 (SDF-1)	
β-Chemokines (CC)	Eosinophils
Monocyte chemoattractant proteins (MCPs): MCP-1, -2, -3, -4, -5	Basophils
Regulated upon activation normal T cell expressed and secreted (RANTES)	Monocytes
Macrophage inflammatory protein (MIP-1α)	Activated T lymphocytes
Eotaxin	
γ-Chemokines (C)	Resting T lymphocytes
Lymphotactin	
δ-Chemokines (CXXXC)	Natural killer cells
Fractalkine	

Table 4 MAJOR PROTEASES INVOLVED IN REGULATING WOUND HEALING		
Name	Pseudonym	Substrates
MMP-1	Interstitial collagenase	Type I, II, III, VII, and X collagens
	Fibroblast collagenase	
MMP-2	72 kDa gelatinase	Type IV, V, VII, and X collagens
	Gelatinase A	α₁-Protease inhibitor
	Type IV collagenase	
MMP-3	Stromelysin-1	Type III, IV, IX, and X collagens
		Type I, III, IV, and V gelatins
		Fibronectin, laminin and procollagenase
MMP-7	Matrilysin	Type I, III, IV, and V gelatins
	Uterine metalloproteinase	Casein, fibronectin, and procollagenase
MMP-8	Neutrophil collagenase	Type I, II, and III collagens
MMP-9	92 kDa gelatinase	Type IV and V collagens
	Gelatinase B	Type I and V gelatins
	Type IV collagenase	α₁-Protease inhibitor
MMP-10	Stromelysin-2	Type III, IV, V, IX, and X collagens
		Type I, III, and IV gelatins
		Fibronectin, laminin, and procollagenase
MMP-11	Stromelysin-3	Not determined
MMP-12	Macrophage	Soluble and insoluble elastin
	Metalloelastase	
MMP-14	Membrane type MMP-1 (MT-MMP-1)	Pro-MMP-2, gelatin, fibronectin
MMP-15	Membrane type MMP-2 (MT-MMP-2)	Pro-MMP-2, gelatin, fibronectin
TIMP-1	Tissue inhibitor of metalloproteinases 1	Inhibits all MMPs except MMP-14
TIMP-2	Tissue inhibitor of metalloproteinases 2	Inhibits all MMPs
TIMP-3	Tissue inhibitor of metalloproteinases 3	Inhibits all MMPs, binds pro-MMP-2 and pro-MMP-9
Elastase	Neutrophil elastase	Elastin; type I, II, III, IV, VIII, IX, and XI collagens; fibronectin; laminin; TIMPs
		Activates procollagenases, progelatinases, and prostromelysins
α₁-Protease inhibitor	α1-PI	Inhibits elastase
	α1-Antitrypsin	

MMP = matrix metalloproteinase.

The four phases of acute wound healing are as follows:

- *Hemostasis:* includes clotting and vascular response; establishes the fibrin provisional wound matrix, and platelets provide initial release of cytokines and growth factors in the wound
- *Inflammation:* mediated by neutrophils, and macrophages remove bacteria and denatured matrix components that retard healing and are the second source of growth factors and cytokines. Prolonged, elevated inflammation retards healing owing to excessive levels of proteases and reactive oxygen that destroy essential factors.
- *Proliferation:* includes scar formation, epithelial healing, and contraction; fibroblasts, supported by new capillaries, proliferate and synthesize disorganized ECM; basal epithelial cells proliferate and migrate over the granulation tissue to close the wound surface; myofibroblasts contract the new scar matrix
- *Remodeling:* fibroblast and capillary density decreases, and initial scar tissue is removed and replaced by ECM that is more similar to normal skin; ECM remodeling is the result of the balanced, regulated activity of proteases

Cellular functions during the different phases of wound healing are regulated by key cytokines, chemokines, and growth factors. Cell actions are also influenced by interaction with components of the ECM through their integrin receptors and adhesion molecules. MMPs produced by epidermal cells, fibroblasts, and vascular endothelial cells assist in migration of the cells, whereas proteolytic enzymes produced by neutrophils and macrophages remove denatured ECM components and assist in remodeling of initial scar tissue.

ABNORMAL HEALING RESULTS IN CHRONIC WOUNDS OR FIBROSIS

Pathologic conditions occur when healing fails to progress at an appropriate pace through all phases. Chronic wounds have been defined as wounds that have failed to proceed through an orderly and timely process to produce an anatomic and functional integrity or proceed through the repair process without establishing a sustained and functional result.[4] At the other end of the wound healing spectrum, excessive healing results from prolonged repair and inadequate remodeling phases, which produces pathologic conditions generally described as fibrosis.

CHRONIC WOUNDS AND FIBROSIS ARE MAJOR BURDENS FOR THE HEALTH CARE SYSTEM

The failure of wounds to heal normally, resulting in a chronic wound, is a major burden on the health care system in the United States.[5] It was estimated in 1998 that there were over 5 million chronic wounds (pressure ulcers, diabetic foot ulcers, venous ulcers, and arterial ulcers) in the United States annually.[6] The estimated costs associated with the estimated 1 to 1.7 million annual pressure ulcers was between $5 billion and $8.5 billion annually in the United States, with an estimated $5,457 per year per wound care patient.[7,8] An estimated 15% of patients with diabetes will develop a lower extremity ulcer during the course of their disease.[9] Despite the high cost of care, many patients with diabetes experience wounds that never heal, leading to the rapid increase in amputation rates in recent years.[9] Total direct and indirect costs of lower extremity amputations resulting from diabetic complications have been estimated at greater than $1 billion in 2000.[10] Venous ulcers are the most frequent type of chronic wound. The treatment of venous ulcers is often complicated by the refractory nature of these chronic wounds and the considerable morbidity and significant financial cost associated with them. An estimated 1 million Americans have venous ulcers,[11,12] with an annual cost of care as much as $1 billion.[13] Between 30 and 50% of venous ulcers fail to respond to standard therapy.[14] Therefore, a treatment modality that enhances wound healing could be beneficial for patients with chronic wounds.

Although the resolution of wound healing usually results in a normal scar without functional consequences, excessive scarring is a major health issue when scar resolution is unsuccessful, such as in burns, in traumatic injuries, or as a complication of many surgical procedures. Excessive scarring can result in major functional deficits, as well as changes in appearance that inhibit successful integration of patients into society. Excessive scarring characterizes many disease conditions in other organs, including the liver, lung, tendon, eye, and peritoneum, and thus constitutes a major national health problem. The hallmark of hypertrophic scarring is excess collagen production. Normal wound healing is a self-limited process whereby fibroblasts stop synthesizing ECM once sufficient matrix is deposited in the wound area. In pathologic scarring, however, instead of reverting to a quiescent phenotype or entering the apoptotic phase after completion of normal healing, fibroblasts continue synthesizing matrix components. Thus, the fibrotic process is usually not initiated as a primary pathologic event but often occurs after thermal injury, surgical incision, or other traumatic injuries.

The public most often associates hypertrophic scars with burn victims and the red, raised, massive scars often with contractures that distort the skin and usually cause limited motion and function of the arms, legs, and neck. The incidence of hypertrophic scars in burned children has been estimated to be about 30%.[15] However, hypertrophic scars also frequently develop in surgical incisions or traumatic lacerations in regions where the skin is under tension, such as midline chest incisions or the shoulder. Scars in areas not covered by clothing are often disfiguring; moreover, the psychological impact can greatly exceed the cost of treating the injury and is permanent. The major challenge in burn care today is dealing with the impact of scarring. Currently, the clinical options for preventing scar formation or reducing existing hypertrophic scars are very limited, consisting of intralesional corticosteroids, topical silicone sheeting (modest efficacy), and, for the most severe keloids, radiation therapy.[15,16] All other treatments are supported by anecdotal evidence only. Currently, no pharmacologic agents are available to modify scarring, except intralesional steroids, which are limited in their use by the pain of the injections, are limited by the dose to small scars, and have the potential for side effects of fat and dermal atrophy.

MOLECULAR AND CELLULAR PATHOLOGY OF CHRONIC WOUNDS

Given that all chronic wounds start as acute wounds, the key question is what causes acute wounds to fail to heal? Previous studies that analyzed fluids collected from chronic wounds found elevated levels of inflammatory cytokines,[17,18] elevated levels of proteases,[19–22] and low levels of growth factor activity compared with acute, healing wounds (Figure 2).[18,19,23,24] These observations led to the hypothesis that chronic wounds develop owing to prolonged inflammation in acute wounds, which produces elevated levels of proteinases that destroy growth factors, receptors, and ECM proteins that are essential for healing.[5,20,21,25] Furthermore, analysis of fibroblasts cultured from chronic wounds indicates that they frequently have reduced capacity to proliferate in response to specific growth factors.[26] If this hypothesis is correct, it follows that elevated levels of inflammatory cytokines and proteinases should decrease and

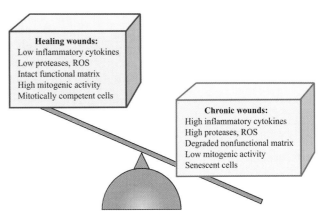

Figure 2. Imbalanced molecular environments of healing and chronic wounds. Reproduced with permission from Mast BA and Schultz GS.[19]

mitogenic activity should increase in fluids as chronic wounds begin to heal. Several studies have reported reduced levels of inflammatory cytokines and proteases and increased mitogenic activity in wound fluids as chronic wounds begin to heal.[17,22,27–31] These results support the concept that treatments that shift the molecular balance in chronic wounds to a pattern that resembles the molecular profile found in acute healing wounds will promote healing.

MOLECULAR AND CELLULAR PATHOLOGY OF FIBROSIS

Evidence strongly implicates that two growth factors, transforming growth factor β isoforms 1 and 2 (TGF-β_1 and TGF-β_2)[32–34] and connective tissue growth factor (CTGF), are the molecular signals that trigger the fibrotic process leading to scarring.[35–41] Most cell types associated with wound healing, such as fibroblasts, keratinocytes, and inflammatory and endothelial cells, secrete TGF-β protein and express TGF-β receptors.[42] TGF-β stimulates a host of fibroblast functions related to wound healing both in vitro and in vivo, including matrix synthesis, cytokine production, expression of cytokine receptors, proliferation, chemotaxis, differentiation, and apoptosis.[43] TGF-β-induced profibrotic molecular responses were abrogated by specific TGF-β inhibitors and antagonists.[44–47] In various animal models of fibrosis, injection of neutralizing antibodies to TGF-β,[48] overexpression of dominant negative receptors,[49] soluble receptors,[50] or Smad7, an endogenous inhibitor of TGF-β signaling,[51] all successfully reduced fibrosis. An important link between TGF-β and CTGF is that TGF-β upregulates synthesis of CTGF, and CTGF directly stimulates synthesis of ECM.[52,53] Furthermore, CTGF mediates the effects of TGF-β on ECM synthesis because neutralizing antibodies to CTGF or antisense oligonucleotides to CTGF totally block TGF-β upregulation of collagen synthesis.[52,53] Thus, therapeutic strategies selectively targeting TGF-β and CTGF should limit excessive scarring without producing major off-target side effects (Figure 3).

WOUND BED PREPARATION

Wound bed preparation is a concept for preparing acute or chronic wound beds for healing by removing the barriers to optimal healing, thereby accelerating endogenous healing or facilitating the effectiveness of other adjuvant therapies.[54] It was developed by a panel of 10 physicians, nurses, and basic scientists and published in a supplement issue of *Wound Repair and Regeneration* in 2003 (Table 5). Since then, the concept has rapidly emerged as a framework to guide treatment of acute and chronic wounds.[55,56] Given that chronic wounds do not undergo the ordered molecular and cellular processes of normal tissue repair, wound bed preparation is a systematic approach that focuses on all of the critical components, including débridement, bacterial balance, management of exudate, and epithelial cell migration at the edge of a wound. It also takes into account the overall health status of the patient and how this may impinge on the wound healing process. The ultimate aim is to ensure the formulation of

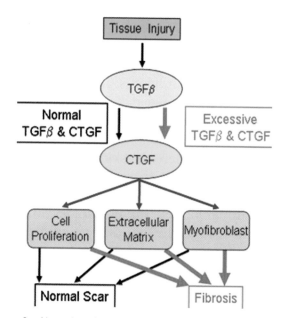

Figure 3. Normal synthesis of transforming growth factor β (TGF-β) and connective tissue growth factor (CTGF) in response to injury produces a normal scar, whereas prolonged, excessive synthesis causes fibrosis.

		Table 5 WOUND BED PREPARATION AND TIME		
Clinical Observations	Molecular and Cellular Problems	WBP Clinical Actions	Effects of Clinical Actions	Clinical Outcome
Tissue (nonviable or deficient)	Defective matrix and cell debris impair healing	Débridement (episodic or continuous) Autolytic, sharp, surgical, enzymatic, mechanical, or biologic Biologic agents	Restoration of wound base and functional extracellular matrix proteins	Viable wound base
Infection or inflammation	High bacteria counts or prolonged inflammation ↑ Inflammatory cytokines ↑ Proteases ↓ Growth factor activity	Remove infected foci Topical/systemic Antimicrobials Anti-inflammatories Protease inhibitors	Low bacteria counts or controlled inflammation ↑ Inflammatory cytokines ↑ Proteases ↓ Growth factor activity	Bacterial balance reduced inflammation
Moisture imbalance	Desiccation slows epithelial cell migration Excessive fluid causes maceration of wound	Apply moisture balancing dressings Compression, negative pressure, or other methods of removing fluid	Restore epithelial migration, desiccation avoided Edema, excessive fluid controlled, maceration avoided	Moisture balance
Edge (margin nonadvancing or undetermined)	Nonmigrating epidermal margin Nonresponsive wound cells and abnormalities in protease activities	Reassess cause, refer or consider corrective advanced therapies Débridement Bioengineered skin Skin grafts Adjunctive therapies	Migrating keratinocytes and responsive wound cells Restoration of appropriate protease profile in wound	Advancing epithelial margin

Adapted from Schultz GS et al.[54]
WBP = wound bed preparation.

good-quality granulation tissue, which will lead to complete wound closure either naturally or through skin products or grafting procedures.

WOUND BED PREPARATION: ONGOING DÉBRIDEMENT

Just as with acute wounds, efficient débridement is an essential step in wound bed preparation, but chronic wounds are likely to require an ongoing process of maintenance débridement rather than a single intervention. The underlying pathogenic abnormalities in chronic wounds cause a continual build-up of necrotic tissue, and regular débridement is necessary to reduce the necrotic burden to achieve healthy granulation tissue. Four general methods of débridement are available, each with its own advantages and limitations (Table 6). Those methods that are most efficient at removal of debris may, at the same time, be the most detrimental to fragile new growth (Table 6). Although débridement has long been regarded as a technique that

enhances wound closure, definitive proof that frequent débridement improved healing of chronic wounds was provided rather recently.[57] Débridement removes foreign bodies from the wound, an intervention that improves local host defense mechanisms and reduces active infection.[58] The removal of devascularized tissue, necrotic soft tissue, bone fascia, muscle, and ligament has a similar beneficial effect. Débridement also produces a more active wound and the release of tissue cytokines and growth factors.

DÉBRIDEMENT: NECROTIC OR CELLULAR BURDEN CONTROL

Débridement is a critical component of any plan to prepare the chronic wound bed for healing. Débridement addresses the "necrotic burden." The term *necrotic burden* is somewhat of a misnomer. Certainly, the goal of débridement is to remove obvious necrotic tissue. However, recent studies indicate that débridement may accomplish far more and, in some cases, should

Table 6 GENERAL CONSIDERATIONS FOR SELECTING A METHOD OF DéBRIDEMENT				
	Surgical and Sharp	Enzymatic	Autolytic	Mechanical
Advantages	Rapid	Selective removal of dead tissue	Safe	Inexpensive
	Local perfusion enhanced	Painless and bloodless	Selective	Easy to perform
	Low risk of infection	Attracts inflammatory cells and fibroblasts	No damage to surrounding skin	Rapid
	Can enhance formulation of granulation tissue	Enhances formation of granulation tissue	Painless	
		Minimal damage to healthy tissue		
Disadvantages	Trained clinician required	Expensive	Slow	Wet-to-dry procedures and whirlpool may damage fragile epithelial cells
	Painful	Care needed in application	Monitoring required	Maceration of surrounding skin
	Risk of bleeding	Possibility of inflammation		Irrigation may drive bacteria into soft tissue
	May damage tissue or nerves			Nonselective
				Painful

Table 7 RELATIVE ADVANTAGES OF DéBRIDEMENT METHODS				
Advantage	Autolytic	Surgical	Enzymatic	Mechanical
Speed	4	1	2	3
Tissue selectivity	3	2	1	4
Painful wound	1	4	2	3
Exudate	3	1	4	2
Infection	4	1	3	2
Cost	1	4	2	3

1 = most appropriate; 4 = least appropriate.

be continued slightly beyond the point of necrotic tissue removal. Perhaps a better term is *cellular burden* or removal of dead and senescent cells that stand in the way of healing.

As with other components of wound bed preparation, débridement decisions require that the health care provider think "out of the box" of the acute wound model. Several shifts in traditional thinking are required to answer clinical questions about débridement:

- *How does the clinician determine when further débridement is necessary and when to stop?* Débridement is not a singular (one-time) event. The wound is usually débrided at the initial visit but may require "maintenance débridement"[59] to maintain the wound bed in a state of "readiness to heal." Steed and colleagues found that diabetic foot ulcers were more likely to heal better with more frequent débridement (Figure 4).[57]

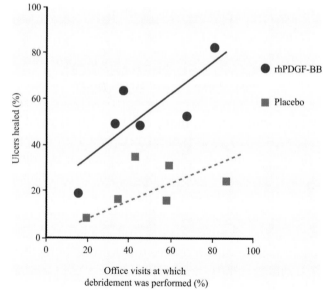

Figure 4. The incidence of complete healing increases with frequency of débridement in patients receiving recombinant human platelet-derived growth factor BB or placebo gel. When the frequencies of débridement are equal, the incidence of complete healing is approximately two to three times as high in patients receiving Regranex gel compared with that of patients receiving placebo gel. Reproduced with permission from Steed DL et al.[57]

- *How does the clinician know when to débride and when NOT to débride?* Most chronic wounds require some method of débridement. However, some wounds should not be débrided. For example, stable, noninfected heel ulcers with poor circulation should not be débrided unless they show signs of infection (fluctuance, edema, erythema, and drainage).[60] Know the patient's vascular status; you do not want to débride a wound that has inadequate circulation to heal. These wounds should be monitored daily.[60] Pyoderma gangrenosum may actually worsen with débridement.[61]

- *Which method of débridement should be used and in what situation?* A number of débridement methods are available for clinicians to use. These are discussed in more detail below. Several algorithms and charts are available to guide clinical decision making about débridement selection.

- *When should a primary care provider make a referral for immediate surgical débridement?* Some situations require immediate surgical débridement (eg, fulminate wound infection with sepsis and necrotizing fasciitis).

- *In most situations, time is not as critical, and there may be more than one "right way" to débride. How does the clinician select a débridement method (or combination of débridement methods) most appropriate for a given patient?* Using the *S.A.M.E. Clinical Guide to Débridement* may help clinicians select a primary, a secondary, and a maintenance débridement method from the options available (<u>S</u>urgical, <u>A</u>utolytic, <u>M</u>echanical, <u>E</u>nzymatic).[62]

TYPES OF DÉBRIDEMENT

The clinician can choose from several categories of débridement. These are surgical or sharp, mechanical, autolytic, enzymatic, and biologic (Figure 5). Although there has been a resurgence in biologic débridement using maggots, this chapter focuses on the four methods most commonly used in clinical settings.

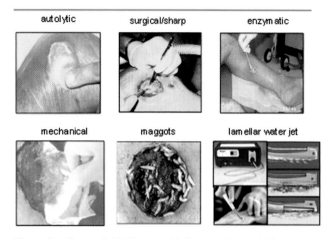

Figure 5. Types of débridement. Each type of wound débridement has advantages and disadvantages, but all types of débridement have the same objective of removing devitalized tissue that is an impediment to healing.

Surgical or Sharp Débridement

In this selective method of débridement, the clinician uses instruments to remove the necrotic tissue from the wound. Although lasers have been used, most clinicians employ scissors, scalpels, and forceps to accomplish surgical or sharp débridement. Individual skill plays a large role in the effectiveness of this treatment. Knowledge of underlying anatomy and proficiency with surgical instruments are essential. It is important to know when to refer the patient to the surgeon. Knowing what you are excising and when to stop is critical. Differentiating yellow slough from tendons can be challenging. If in doubt, do not cut!

When is surgical or sharp débridement indicated? Consider using this method whenever the goal is to quickly remove large amounts of necrotic tissue, the patient can tolerate this intervention, and facilities with skilled practitioners are available. When time is of the essence (as with infected wounds with systemic sepsis or necrotizing fasciitis), surgical débridement is the quickest and best way to remove necrotic tissue. Do not use this type of débridement for patients with clotting disorders or those taking anticoagulants as uncontrolled bleeding may occur. This method is usually painful, so premedicate with systemic analgesics and/or local anesthetics. Likewise, manage postprocedural pain accordingly. If large amounts of tissue are to be removed, débridement in the operating room under anesthesia may be preferable.

Mechanical Débridement

Mechanical débridement uses force to remove the necrotic tissue. This can include the use of irrigation fluids delivered by pulsed lavage, the agitation of water during whirlpool therapy, or the removal of tissue from wet-to-dry dressings. Mechanical débridement is considered a non-selective method of débridement as viable and nonviable tissue are both removed during the process. All of these methods have the potential for causing the patient episodic pain during the débridement process. Premedication of the patient is usually indicated prior to doing mechanical débridement. Whirlpool therapy requires the necessary equipment and the transportation of the patient to the location of the tank and therefore may not be available or practical in all settings. Risk of infection from cross-contamination and aerosolization are a danger and need to be considered. Pulse lavage requires training in the technique. Irrigation pressures should be between 4 and 15 psi.[60] Too high a pressure can drive debris or organisms deep into the tissue.

Wet-to-dry dressings are time consuming as they are done three times a day. Besides pain, maceration to surrounding wound skin is also a potential problem. Despite this, wet-to-dry dressings are one of the most frequently prescribed (and overused) methods of débridement in acute care settings.[46] Accurate technique is essential. If ordering this method, instruct staff to follow the clinical pointers found in Table 3.

One of the most controversial aspects of wet-to-dry dressings is which solution to use. Saline is safe and should be used in most situations. The Agency for Health Care Policy and Research (AHCPR) pressure ulcer treatment guidelines present data indicating that antiseptic solutions such as povidone-iodine, sodium hypochlorite (Dakin solution), hydrogen peroxide, and acetic acid damage cells needed for healing, such as fibroblasts.[60] Most of these studies were conducted in cell cultures. Some clinicians reason that for obviously infected wounds, preventing the spread of infection takes priority over protecting the few "healing cells" that manage to survive such a hostile wound environment. The goal at this point in time is preventing overwhelming infection, not healing. Dilute solutions of povidone-iodine, sodium hypochlorite, and acetic acid have been used as cleansing agents and soaking solutions for wet-to-dry and moist dressings. This is usually a temporary measure that is discontinued when the wound is débrided and cultured and appropriate antibiotics are initiated. A more recent in vivo study in wounded pigs compared the effects of various antimicrobial agents (5% mafenide acetate, 10% povidone-iodine, 0.25% sodium hypochlorite, 3% hydrogen peroxide, and 0.25% acetic acid) with a saline control. Positive and negative effects were observed for all agents; however, mafenide acetate (Sulfamylon) most effectively controlled bacterial counts while increasing angiogenesis, fibroblast proliferation, and dermal thickness in comparison with the control.[63] Drosou and colleagues recently completed a comprehensive review of the research available on antiseptic use in animal or human wounds.[64] They made the following conclusions:

Table 8 ACTIVITIES OF ENZYMATIC DéBRIDING AGENTS			
Fibrinolysin	DNAse	Papain	Bacterial Collagenase
Breaks down fibrin components of blood clots and fibrinous exudate	Acts on DNA of purulent exudate	Relatively ineffective alone, indiscriminate, and requires urea	Degrades native collagen and denatured collagen
pH range 4.5–5.5	pH range 7.0–8.0	pH range 3.0–12.0	pH range 6.0–8.0

DNA = deoxyribonucleic acid; DNAse = deoxyribonuclease.

- Antiseptics are often effective against a broader range of bacteria than antibiotics and are less likely to create resistant bacteria or patient sensitivities.
- Povidone-iodine produced mixed results. Bacterial counts were either decreased or unchanged. Healing increased in four human studies, decreased in four animal studies, and had no significant effect in six studies. Histologic evidence of tissue toxicity was noted with a 10% povidone-iodine solution.[65] Iodine sensitivity occurs in a small proportion of the population (0.73%).[66]
- Cadexomer iodine (available as an ointment or dressing) consists of hydrophilic beads of cadexomer starch, which release iodine slowly into the wound. Human studies consistently demonstrate decreases in bacterial counts and accelerations in wound healing.
- Hydrogen peroxide had little effect on wound healing or bacterial control, but its effervescent effect may be useful in cleaning or débriding wounds.
- Acetic acid usually decreased a variety of bacteria (including *Pseudomonas aeruginosa*, *Staphylococcus aureus*, and gram-negative rods) yet was not cytotoxic in the in vivo studies reviewed.
- Silver compounds have been effective in reducing bacterial loads, without adverse effects on wound healing. In fact, several in vivo studies show acceleration of wound healing.

The use of antiseptics in wounds remains an area of controversy. Slow-release cadexomer-iodine solutions and some of the newer silver dressings may provide the safest and most effective alternative for bacterial control and wound management.

Autolytic Débridement

Autolytic débridement can be accomplished by placing occlusive or semiocclusive moisture-retentive dressings (eg, hydrocolloids, transparent films) over the wound and allowing the natural wound fluids to soften eschar and the proteolytic enzymes within the wound fluid to digest and liquefy necrotic tissue. The dressing should be left in place for 2 to 3 days. When the dressing is removed, the wound should be irrigated with saline to remove liquefied debris.

Autolytic débridement (with hydrogels) may also soften a hard, dry eschar for easier mechanical or surgical débridement. This type of débridement is slow, requiring multiple dressing applications and irrigations over days or weeks; however, it is usually pain free and less stressful to the patient. It is not appropriate for infected wounds or very deep cavity wounds that require packing. The wound fluid under the dressing should be monitored closely; it may be tan colored. However, purulent drainage, unusual odor, inflammation, and increased pain are signs of infection that require immediate treatment. With signs of infection, autolytic débridement should be discontinued, a quicker method of débridement (usually surgical) should be used, and the infection should be treated. Failure to do so may result in serious wound infections and possibly sepsis. Immunocompromised and frail elderly patients should be monitored closely. They are at higher risk and may show more subtle signs of infection than the immunocompetent patient.

Enzymatic Débridement

Enzymatic débridement uses topical enzymes to remove necrotic tissue by digesting and dissolving the devitalized tissue in the wound bed. Some enzymes are selective and only recognize devitalized tissue.[59] Other enzymes are nonselective and therefore do not distinguish between viable and nonviable tissue. When using a nonselective enzyme, limit its application to the necrotic or slough tissue and avoid getting it on viable tissue such as the surrounding wound area.

Two widely used enzymatic débriding agents are currently available in the United States. One preparation contains papain and urea in a cream base, whereas the other is composed of collagenase in a petrolatum base. The papain-urea combination also comes in a formulation with chlorophyllin-copper complex.

Papain is a proteolytic enzyme derived from the fruit of *Carica papaya*. It is a nonspecific cysteine protease capable of breaking down a wide variety of necrotic tissue substrates.[66] Urea's role is to facilitate papain's proteolytic action by altering the structure of proteins.[67,68] The papain-urea combination has a pH range of activity of 3.0 to 12.0.[66] Hydrogen peroxide inactivates papain, so do not use it to clean the wound if this enzyme is being used. Heavy metal salts (eg, lead, silver, mercury) also may inactivate papain-urea, so their use should also be avoided. Store the drug at a controlled room temperature of 59 to 86°F (15–30°C). The manufacturer reports that some patients may experience a transient "burning" sensation with application of this product.

Collagenase, derived from *Clostridium histolyticum*, has optimal enzymatic activity in a pH range of 6 to 8. This corresponds to the pH range typically found in human wounds.[27] Some detergents and heavy metal ions (eg, silver, mercury) inactivate this product, so avoid using drugs such as silver sulfadiazine in conjunction with this enzyme. Avoid using metal ions or acidic solutions for cleaning the wound owing to the metal ion and low pH. Hydrogen peroxide, Dakin solution, and normal saline are compatible for use with collagenase. The manufacturer reports that some patients may experience a slight transient erythema in the surrounding tissue when this ointment is used and not confined to the wound area. Do not store this drug above 77°F (25°C).

When writing the order for these drugs, follow the manufacturer's recommendation for frequency of use. One enzyme has once-a-day application (collagenase); the other may need once- or twice-a-day application (papain-urea). Both suggest cross-hatching of hard eschar prior to application of the enzyme. Both drugs can be used with infected wounds.

Both enzymes have advantages and disadvantages. One enzyme preparation may be preferable in a given wound or at different times

in the same wound. In one in vitro study of the preparations' active ingredients, papain-urea digested fibrin (but not elastin), whereas the opposite was true of collagenase, which digested elastin but not fibrin.[69] Unfortunately, the clinical relevance of this is not clear as clinicians are often not able to identify the fibrin versus elastin tissue on a physical examination.

The papain-urea combination débrided necrotic tissue more quickly than collagenase in a prospective, randomized, nonblinded, clinical trial of 26 nursing home residents with pressure ulcers requiring débridement.[70] Despite the quicker time to débride, there was no evidence of faster healing in this study.

Two studies by Herman and one by Krieg suggested a fibrin/fibronectin-collagen segregation with the fibrin/fibronectin in the upper portion of the eschar and collagen in the lower portion.[71–73] This observation seems to lend credence to the belief that bacterial collagenase (which is more effective in digesting collagen and elastin) works from the bottom up and papain-urea preparations (which are more effective in digesting fibrin) work from the top down.[69] Clinically, what we may be seeing is a rapid removal of the upper portion of the eschar by papain-urea, whereas collagenase (when applied to a cross-hatched eschar) more effectively digests the lower (and less visible) portion of the eschar. Regardless of their respective sites of activity, healing rates were comparable in the clinical trial comparing collagenase and papain-urea.[70]

Papain urea produces more exudate from the enzymatic digestion, which may irritate the surrounding skin, requiring more frequent dressing changes.[74] The manufacturer's insert maintains that the product "is harmless to viable tissue" and cites "on-file data" as evidence. However, papain breaks down proteins containing cysteine residues. Most proteins, including growth factors, contain cysteine residues.[59] There is published (in vitro) research suggesting that papain-urea affects the biologic activity of recombinant human platelet-derived growth factor BB (rhPDGF-BB).[75] The study consisted of numerous biochemical evaluations of a variety of topically applied enzymatic débriders. All enzymes tested (with the exception of collagenase) proved to have some level of detrimental effect on the viability of the growth factor. Papain-urea may be most appropriate in situations in which large amounts of necrotic tissue must be débrided rapidly, important viable tissues (eg, tendons, large blood vessels) are not in direct contact with the agent, and the affected area is either insensate or any burning and pain can be effectively managed and becaplermin/rhPDGF-BB (Regranes) is not being used.[67,70]

Collagenase is a water-soluble proteinase that specifically attacks and breaks down collagen.[71,76] Although collagenase may débride obviously visible necrotic tissue more slowly than papain-urea, it is more selective in the number of substrates it digests;[69] does not affect cell viability in cell culture media, and carries less risk of pain or discomfort.

In chronic wounds, keratinocytes are not able to migrate over a wound covered by eschar or other necrotic debris and may proliferate at the edge of the wound, often creating a rolled edge and stalling healing. There is evidence that collagenase enhances keratinocyte migration over granulation tissue. In an early study evaluating the use of *C. histolyticum* for the débridement of dermal and pressure ulcers, the time required for complete débridement of the treated lesions averaged 10.5 days. Débridement was followed by gradual granulation and epithelialization, which generally proceeded at a faster rate than was expected in chronic dermal lesions of the type under treatment.[77] Subsequent studies have elucidated the cellular mechanisms involved in this clinical finding. A study by Grinnell and colleagues suggested that until the anchoring undenatured collagen fibers are severed, thereby allowing the necrotic plug to be removed, débridement cannot take place, granulation is slowed, and no supportive base is available for epithelialization.[78] Collagenase effectively digests intact, native (undenatured) collagen fibers,[69] allowing the necrotic plug to be removed. In cell cultures, collagenase increased human keratino-

cyte migration 3-fold and single cell motility up to 10-fold,[71] with bovine vascular endothelial cells increasing 5-fold.

Because of its specificity and selectivity, collagenase may also be preferable for "maintenance débridement."[67] Falanga suggested that collagenase may serve as a possible "pluripotential" wound bed preparation agent.[59] There is evidence that collagenase selectively reduces necrotic tissue and decreases bacterial burden,[79] increases chemotactic attraction of human fibroblasts,[80] can stimulate granulation tissue,[77,81] enhances the proliferation and migration of keratinocytes[71,82,83] and endothelial cells in cell cultures,[80] and may stimulate angiogenesis. Two clinical studies report significantly less pain with collagenase (when compared with control treatments) in 60 patients with diabetic foot ulcer and 79 patients with partial-thickness burn wounds.[79]

ALGORITHM ANNOTATION

This algorithm (Figure 6) provides decision points and preferred management pathways for débridement as part of an overall plan for wound bed preparation. It was developed by a national panel of wound care specialists in March 2001 using a consensus development approach. It may or may not represent individual viewpoints.

1. *Patient assessment.* Assess both the patient's overall health status and the wound. Determine the patient's and/or family's goals. Based on this analysis, decide with the patient and family whether the goal is to promote healing or to maintain the wound and the patient's comfort. In some situations (eg, palliative care), the goal might be to prevent further deterioration of the wound and maximize patient comfort by avoiding painful treatments. This is not always the case for palliative care patients. Some palliative care patients may benefit from more active treatment to promote healing. For example, some minimally invasive treatments may reduce wound size, drainage, and pain, thus improving quality of life. Weigh the risks and

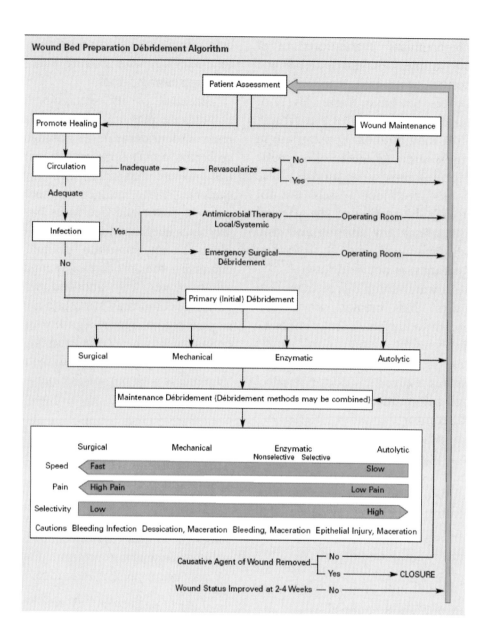

Figure 6.

benefits for the individual patient. If the wound maintenance option is chosen, continuously reassess the patient, the wound, and patient or family goals. In all cases, the patient, the wound, and the goals should be reexamined or reassessed on a periodic basis. Note that all decision nodes in the "promote healing" path return to patient assessment.

2. *Promote healing.* A decision to promote healing raises a number of clinical questions that are best answered using an interdisciplinary team approach. These include the following:

3. *Circulation.* Is there adequate circulation for healing? If yes, proceed to the next clinical decision node (infection). If circulation is not adequate for healing, determine if the patient is a candidate for revascularization. If revascularization is possible and the patient consents after risks and benefits are discussed, proceed to the operating room for revascularization. If revascularization is not an option, go to the wound maintenance decision node.

4. *Infection.* What is the level of bacterial burden? For *colonization* and *contamination*,

use routine cleansing and débridement methods. For *critical colonization* (bacteria impeding healing) or *local infection* (note classic and secondary signs of infection within the wound), more aggressive treatments should be added, such as local antimicrobial therapy (eg, topical antibiotics and local antibacterial agents such as dressings impregnated with silver or slow-release cadexomer iodine). Systemic antimicrobial therapy should be used for deeper infections not affected by topical agents. For fulminant infection spreading beyond the wound bed and presenting a risk of sepsis (or actual sepsis), emergency surgical débridement is required, assuming that the patient is a surgical candidate.

5. *Primary or initial débridement.* In the absence of severe infection, the clinician has time to consider the most appropriate method of primary débridement, given the choice of <u>S</u>urgical, <u>A</u>utolytic, <u>M</u>echanical, or <u>E</u>nzymatic method. Some clinicians consider these choices "pretty much the SAME." However, knowledge of wound characteristics, patient characteristics, the débridement method, and the biology of chronic wound healing will allow you to choose the best method to achieve goals for primary (initial) débridement.

6. *Maintenance débridement.* Débridement is no longer a "one-time" event. Maintenance débridement is now recommended to keep chronic wounds in a "state of readiness" for healing. Débridement methods vary on several factors, including speed, pain, and selectivity. Additionally, there are cautions with each method of débridement, such as bleeding, infection, desiccation, maceration, and epithelial injury. Consideration of these variables in conjunction with a comprehensive patient assessment is necessary to determine the most appropriate method for maintenance débridement.

The quick schematic representation at the end of the algorithm can guide clinicians in determining the optimal methods or combination of methods to use. This may change at different stages of healing and as the wound environment changes.

Maintenance débridement should be repeated until the causative agent of the wound is removed or controlled. The causative agent may be related to systemic disease (eg, diabetes) and/or visible wound conditions (eg, necrotic tissue, excess exudates). Although not visible to the naked eye, chronic wounds may contain high levels of inflammatory cytokines and proteases (MMPs), as well as senescent cells that fail to respond to growth factors. Maintenance débridement, as part of an overall plan of wound bed preparation, will address the biochemical burdens that impede healing.

Wound healing and closure are the desired outcome. Wound status should show improvement within 2 to 4 weeks of optimal treatment. If improvement is not noted, the clinician should go to the top of the algorithm and complete a patient assessment, following through with subsequent decision nodes within the algorithm.

Primary and maintenance débridement decisions may also be guided by answering the questions contained in the *S.A.M.E. Clinical Guide to Débridement*. The principle underlying the *S.A.M.E.* guide is that all débridement methods are NOT the same. By answering a series of questions based on patient and wound assessments, the clinician can select an appropriate method of initial or maintenance débridement for a given wound.

REFERENCES

1. Bennett NT, Schultz GS. Growth factors and wound healing: Part II. Role in normal and chronic wound healing. Am J Surg 1993;166:74–81.
2. Bennett NT, Schultz GS. Growth factors and wound healing: biochemical properties of growth factors and their receptors. Am J Surg 1993;165:728–37.
3. Lawrence WT. Physiology of the acute wound. Clin Plast Surg 1998;25:321–40.
4. Lazarus GS, Cooper DM, Knighton DR, et al. Definitions and guidelines for assessment of wounds and evaluation of healing. Arch Dermatol 1994;130:489–93.

5. Medina A, Scott PG, Ghahary A, Tredget EE. Pathophysiology of chronic nonhealing wounds. J Burn Care Rehabil 2005;26:306–19.

6. Tonnesen MG, Feng X, Clark RA. Angiogenesis in wound healing. J Investig Dermatol Symp Proc 2000;5:40–6.

7. Beckrich K, Aronovitch SA. Hospital-acquired pressure ulcers: a comparison of costs in medical vs. surgical patients. Nurs Econ 1999;17:263–71.

8. Xakellis GC, Frantz R. The cost of healing pressure ulcers across multiple health care settings. Adv Wound Care 1996;9:18–22.

9. Reiber GE, Boyko EJ, Smith DG. Lower extremity foot ulcers and amputations in diabetes. In: National Diabetes Data Group, editor. Diabetes in America. Bethesda (MD): National Institutes of Health; 1995. p. 409–27.

10. Hogan P, Dall T, Nikolov P. Economic costs of diabetes in the US in 2002. Diabetes Care 2003;26:917–32.

11. Ruckley CV. Socioeconomic impact of chronic venous insufficiency and leg ulcers. Angiology 1997;48:67–9.

12. Alguire PC, Mathes BM. Chronic venous insufficiency and venous ulceration. J Gen Intern Med 1997;12:374–83.

13. Phillips TJ, Dover JS. Leg ulcers. J Am Acad Dermatol 1991;25:965–87.

14. Kantor J, Margolis DJ. A multicentre study of percentage change in venous leg ulcer area as a prognostic index of healing at 24 weeks. Br J Dermatol 2000;142:960–4.

15. Mustoe TA, Cooter RD, Gold MH, et al. International clinical recommendations on scar management. Plast Reconstr Surg 2002;110:560–71.

16. Mustoe TA. Scars and keloids. BMJ 2004;328:1329–30.

17. Trengove NJ, Bielefeldt-Ohmann H, Stacey MC. Mitogenic activity and cytokine levels in non-healing and healing chronic leg ulcers. Wound Repair Regen 2000;8:13–25.

18. Harris IR, Yee KC, Walters CE, et al. Cytokine and protease levels in healing and non-healing chronic venous leg ulcers. Exp Dermatol 1995;4:342–9.

19. Mast BA, Schultz GS. Interactions of cytokines, growth factors, and proteases in acute and chronic wounds. Wound Repair Regen 1996;4:411–20.

20. Yager DR, Nwomeh BC. The proteolytic environment of chronic wounds. Wound Repair Regen 1999;7:433–41.

21. Nwomeh BC, Yager DR, Cohen IK. Physiology of the chronic wound. Clin Plast Surg 1998;25:341–56.

22. Trengove NJ, Stacey MC, Macauley S, et al. Analysis of the acute and chronic wound environments: the role of proteases and their inhibitors. Wound Repair Regen 1999;7:442–52.

23. Bucalo B, Eaglstein WH, Falanga V. Inhibition of cell proliferation by chronic wound fluid. Wound Repair Regen 1993;1:181–6.

24. Katz MH, Alvarez AF, Kirsner RS, et al. Human wound fluid from acute wounds stimulates fibroblast and endothelial cell growth. J Am Acad Dermatol 1991;25:1054–8.

25. Mast BA, Schultz GS. Interactions of cytokines, growth factors, and proteases in acute and chronic wounds. Wound Repair Regen 1996;4:411–20.

26. Agren MS, Eaglstein WH, Ferguson MW, et al. Causes and effects of the chronic inflammation in venous leg ulcers. Acta Derm Venereol Suppl (Stockh) 2000;210:3–17.

27. Trengove NJ, Langton SR, Stacey MC. Biochemical analysis of wound fluid from nonhealing and healing chronic leg ulcers. Wound Repair Regen 1996;4:234–9.

28. Rogers AA, Burnett S, Moore JC, et al. Involvement of proteolytic enzymes—plasminogen activators and matrix metalloproteinases—in the pathophysiology of pressure ulcers. Wound Repair Regen 1995;3:273–83.

29. Yager DR, Zhang LY, Liang HX, et al. Wound fluids from human pressure ulcers contain elevated matrix metalloproteinase levels and activity compared to surgical wound fluids. J Invest Dermatol 1996;107:743–8.

30. Ladwig GP, Robson MC, Liu R, et al. Ratios of activated matrix metalloproteinase-9 to tissue inhibitor of matrix metalloproteinase-1 in wound fluids are inversely correlated with healing of pressure ulcers. Wound Repair Regen 2002;10:26–37.

31. Bullen EC, Longaker MT, Updike DL, et al. Tissue inhibitor of metalloproteinases-1 is decreased and activated gelatinases are increased in chronic wounds. J Investig Dermatol 1995;104:236–40.

32. Border WA, Noble NA. Transforming growth factor B in tissue fibrosis. N Engl J Med 1994;331:1286–92.

33. Branton MH, Kopp JB. TGF-beta and fibrosis. Microbes Infect 1999;1:1349–65.

34. Blobe GC, Schiemann WP, Lodish HF. Role of transforming growth factor beta in human disease. N Engl J Med 2000;342:1350–8.

35. Lasky JA, Ortiz LA, Tonthat B, et al. Connective tissue growth factor mRNA expression is upregulated in bleomycin-induced lung fibrosis. Am J Physiol 1998; 275:L365–71.

36. Gupta S, Clarkson MR, Duggan J, Brady HR. Connective tissue growth factor: potential role in glomerulosclerosis and tubulointerstitial fibrosis. Kidney Int 2000;58:1389–99.

37. Ihn H. Pathogenesis of fibrosis: role of TGF-beta and CTGF. Curr Opin Rheumatol 2002;14:681–5.

38. Igarashi A, Nashiro K, Kikuchi K, et al. Connective tissue growth factor gene expression in tissue sections from localized scleroderma, keloid, and other fibrotic skin disorders. J Investig Dermatol 1996;106:729–33.

39. Ito Y, Aten J, Bende RJ, et al. Expression of connective tissue growth factor in human renal fibrosis. Kidney Int 1998;53:853–61.

40. Shi-wen X, Pennington D, Holmes A, et al. Autocrine overexpression of CTGF maintains fibrosis: RDA analysis of fibrosis genes in systemic sclerosis. Exp Cell Res 2000;259:213–24.

41. Paradis V, Dargere D, Vidaud M, et al. Expression of connective tissue growth factor in experimental rat and human liver fibrosis. Hepatology 1999;30:968–76.

42. Derynck R, Feng XH. TGF-beta receptor signaling. Biochim Biophys Acta 1997;1333:F105–50.

43. Varga J. Scleroderma and Smads: dysfunctional Smad family dynamics culminating in fibrosis. Arthritis Rheum 2002;46:1703–13.

44. Kubo M, Ihn H, Yamane K, Tamaki K. Up-regulated expression of transforming growth factor beta receptors in dermal fibroblasts in skin sections from patients with localized scleroderma. Arthritis Rheum 2001;44:731–4.

45. Yamamoto T, Takagawa S, Katayama I, Nishioka K. Anti-sclerotic effect of transforming growth factor-beta antibody in a mouse model of bleomycin-induced scleroderma. Clin Immunol 1999;92:6–13.

46. McCormick LL, Zhang Y, Tootell E, Gilliam AC. Anti-TGF-beta treatment prevents skin and lung fibrosis in murine sclerodermatous graft-versus-host disease: a model for human scleroderma. J Immunol 1999;163:5693–9.

47. Kaminski N, Allard JD, Pittet JF, et al. Global analysis of gene expression in pulmonary fibrosis reveals distinct programs regulating lung inflammation and fibrosis. Proc Natl Acad Sci U S A 2000;97:1778–83.

48. Ziyadeh FN, Hoffman BB, Han DC, et al. Long-term prevention of renal insufficiency, excess matrix gene expression, and glomerular mesangial matrix expansion by treatment with monoclonal antitransforming growth factor-beta antibody in db/db diabetic mice. Proc Natl Acad Sci U S A 2000;97:8015–20.

49. Reid RR, Mogford JE, Butt R, et al. Inhibition of procollagen C-proteinase reduces scar hypertrophy in a rabbit model of cutaneous scarring. Wound Repair Regen 2006;14:138–41.

50. Wang Q, Wang Y, Hyde DM, et al. Reduction of bleomycin induced lung fibrosis by transforming growth factor beta soluble receptor in hamsters. Thorax 1999;54:805–12.

51. Nakao A, Fujii M, Matsumura R, et al. Transient gene transfer and expression of Smad7 prevents bleomycin-induced lung fibrosis in mice. J Clin Invest 1999;104:5–11.

52. Duncan MR, Frazier KS, Abramson S, et al. Connective tissue growth factor mediates transforming growth factor beta-induced collagen synthesis: down-regulation by cAMP. FASEB J 1999;13:1774–86.

53. Blalock TD, Duncan MR, Varela JC, et al. Connective tissue growth factor expression and action in human corneal fibroblast cultures and rat corneas after photorefractive keratectomy. Invest Ophthalmol Vis Sci 2003;44:1879–87.

54. Schultz GS, Sibbald RG, Falanga V, et al. Wound bed preparation: a systematic approach to wound management. Wound Repair Regen 2003;11 Suppl 1:S1–28.

55. Schultz G, Mozingo D, Romanelli M, Claxton K. Wound healing and TIME; new concepts and scientific applications. Wound Repair Regen 2005;13 Suppl 1:S1–11.

56. Sibbald RG, Orsted H, Schultz GS, et al. Preparing the wound bed 2003: focus on infection and inflammation. Ostomy Wound Manage 2003;49:23–51.

57. Steed DL, Donohoe D, Webster MW, Lindsley L. Effect of extensive debridement and treatment on the healing of diabetic foot ulcers. Diabetic Ulcer Study Group. J Am Coll Surg 1996;183:61–4.

58. Elek SD. Experimental staphylococcal infections in the skin of man. Ann N Y Acad Sci 1956;65:85–90.

59. Falanga V. Wound bed preparation and the role of enzymes: a case for multiple actions of therapeutic agents. Wounds 2002;14:47–57.

60. Bergstrom N, Allman RM, Alvarez OM, et al. Treatment of pressure ulcers: clinical practice guideline. US Department of of Health and Human Services, Public Health Service, Agency for Health Care Policy and Research, Rockville, Maryland, 1994.

61. Chakrabarty A, Phillips TJ. Diagnostic dilemmas: pyoderma gangrenosum. Wounds 2002;14:302–5.

62. Ayello EA, Cuddigan JE. Conquer chronic wounds with wound bed preparation. Nurse Practitioner 2004;29:8–24.

63. Nanney LB, Bennett LL. Comparative evaluation of topical antiseptic/antimicrobial treatment on aspects of wound repair in the porcine model. Wounds 2002;14:14–9.

64. Drosou A, Falabella A, Kirsner R. Antiseptics on wounds: an area of controversy. Wounds 2003;15:149–66.

65. Severyn AM, Lejeune A, Rocoux G. Non-toxic antiseptic irrigation with chlorhexidine in experimental revascularization in the rat. J Hosp Infect 1991;17:197–206.

66. Niedner R. Cytotoxicity and sensitization of povidone-iodine and other frequently used anti-infective agents. Dermatology 1997;195 Suppl 2:89–92.

67. Sibbald RG. Topical antimicrobials. Ostomy Wound Manage 2003;49:14–8.

68. Miller JM. The interaction of papain, urea, and water-soluble chlorophyll in a proteolytic ointment for infected wounds. Surgery 1958;43:939–48.

69. Hebda PA, Lo C. Biochemistry of wound healing: The effects of active ingredients of standard debriding agents—papain and collagenase—on digestion of native and denatured collagenous substrates, fibrin and elastin. Wounds 2007;13:190–4.

70. Alvarez OM, Fernandez-Obregon A, Rogers RS, et al. A prospective, randomized comparative study of collagenase and papain-urea for pressure ulcer debridement. Wounds 2002;14:293–301.

71. Herman I. Stimulation of human keratinocyte migration and proliferation *in vitro*: insights into the cellular responses to injury and wound healing. Wounds 1996;8:33–41.

72. Herman IM. Extracellular matrix-cytoskeletal interactions in vascular cells. Tissue Cell 1987;19:1–19.

73. Krieg T. Collagen in the healing wound. Wounds 1995;7:5A–12A.

74. Hebda PA, Flynn KJ, Dohar JE. Evaluation of efficacy of enzymatic debriding agents for removal of necrotic tissue and promotion of healing in porcine skin wounds. Wounds 1998;10:83–96.

75. Gosiewska A, Yi CF, Brown L, Geesin JC. The effect of enzyme debriders on biological activity of recombinant human platelet-derived growth factor-BB, the active agent of Regranex gel. Wound Repair Regen 1998;6:A501.

76. Rao CN, Ladin DA, Liu YY, et al. Alpha 1-antitrypsin is degraded and non-functional in chronic wounds but intact and functional in acute wounds: the inhibitor protects fibronectin from degradation by chronic wound fluid enzymes. J Invest Dermatol 1995;105: 572–8.

77. Boxer AM, Gottesman N, Berstein H, Mandl I. Debridement of dermal ulcers and decubidi with collagenase. Geriatrics 1969;24:7–75.

78. Grinnell F, Toda K, Takashima A. Activation of keratinocyte fibronectin receptor function during cutaneous wound healing. J Cell Sci Suppl 1987;8: 199–209.

79. Hansbrough JF, Achauer B, Dawson J, et al. Wound healing in partial-thickness burn wounds treated with collagenase ointment versus silver sulfadiazine cream. J Burn Care Rehabil 1995;16:241–7.

80. Herman IM. Molecular mechanisms regulating the vascular endothelial cell motile response to injury. J Cardiovasc Pharmacol 1993;22 Suppl 4:S25–36.

81. Burgos A, Gimenez J, Moreno E, et al. Collagenase ointment application at 24-hour versus 28-hour intervals in the treatment of pressure ulcers. Clin Drug Investig 2000;19:399–407.

82. Pilcher BK, Dumin JA, Sudbeck BD, et al. The activity of collagenase-1 is required for keratinocyte migration on a type I collagen matrix. J Cell Biol 1997;137:1445–57.

83. Chen JD, Helmold M, Kim JP, et al. Human keratinocytes make uniquely linear phagokinetic tracks. Dermatology 1994;188:6–12.

27

Hyperbaric Oxygen and Wound Healing in the Head and Neck

John J. Feldmeier, DO

SPECIFIC THERAPY IN ITS CURRENT STATE

This chapter will discuss the role of hyperbaric oxygen in the management of problem wounds of the head and neck. The following topics are discussed:

1. History of hyperbaric medicine
2. Physiology and mechanisms of action of hyperbaric oxygen
3. Beneficial physiologic effects of hyperbaric oxygen in wound healing, including:

    a. Infection control
    b. Angiogenesis
    c. Epithelialization

4. The specific clinical applications of hyperbaric oxygen in the following specific pathologic sites are discussed:

    a. Osteoradionecrosis (ORN) treatment
    b. Osteoradionecrosis prevention
    c. Soft tissue radiation necrosis
    d. Necrotizing fasciitis
    e. Support of flaps and grafts
    f. Toxicity and side effects

SHORTCOMINGS

Hyperbaric oxygen is usually an adjunct to proper surgical intervention and appropriate antibiotic delivery and good local wound care. As a solo modality, it is unlikely to be successful in the treatment of problem wounds. As therapies go, hyperbaric oxygen has a fairly low likelihood of serious complications.

TREATMENT PEARLS

Hyperbaric oxygen is often described as a drug. As such, it must be given in adequate doses to be effective and should be delivered as part of a multidisciplinary management of problem wounds. A typical course of hyperbaric oxygen for radiation injury is 40 treatments, each consisting of 100% oxygen for 90 minutes at 2.0 to 2.5 atmospheres (atm) pressure. For failing flaps and necrotizing infections the course of treatment is typically shorter, often 5 to 10 treatments. For necrotizing infection, treatment is often delivered at pressures of 2.8 to 3.0 atm.

FUTURE PROMISE

A promising area for clinical trials would be the investigation of prophylactic delivery of hyperbaric oxygen. If reliable and reasonably simple biochemical or imaging assays could be developed to identify those likely at risk for radiation injury or infection or delayed wound healing, studies could be initiated to see if hyperbaric oxygen could reduce the likelihood of radiation necrosis, necrotizing infections, or delayed wound healing.

HISTORY OF HYPERBARIC MEDICINE

Hyperbaric or recompression chambers were originally developed to treat decompression sickness (commonly called "the bends") in divers or caisson workers. Caisson workers labor in a pressurized structure or chamber under water, with the increase in pressure holding the water out thus providing a dry working environment usually in the construction or excavation of tunnels or bridges. Commercial divers will work at considerable depths and accompanying pressures in the support of oil drilling operations or in salvage operations. Both types of worker are at risk for developing decompression sickness. This disorder is effectively treated by hyperbaric oxygen. In fact, this is the only definitive treatment.

In the early 1960s, Boerema and Brummelkamp in Holland began to investigate the application of hyperbaric oxygen to the treatment of various anaerobic infections. They showed a significant beneficial effect on clostridial myonecrosis (gas gangrene).[1] Beginning in the late 1960s and early 1970s, pioneer researchers such as Jefferson Davis in the United States Air Force and George Hart in the United States Navy began a formal investigation of hyperbaric oxygen therapy in a wide variety of disorders. Today, the Undersea and Hyperbaric Medical Society recognizes a total of 13 pathologic conditions or disease entities in which a convincing body of evidence supports its application.[2] These include:

1. Arterial or gas embolism (traumatic or iatrogenic)
2. Carbon monoxide poisoning
3. Clostridial myonecrosis and myositis (gas gangrene)
4. Crush injury, compartment syndrome and other acute ischemias
5. Decompression sickness
6. Wound-healing enhancement in problem wounds
7. Exceptional anemias
8. Intracranial abscess
9. Necrotizing soft tissue infections (necrotizing fasciitis)
10. Refractory osteomyelitis
11. Delayed radiation injuries (soft tissue and bony radiation necrosis)
12. Failing skin grafts and flaps
13. Thermal burns

Recently, the application of hyperbaric oxygen in chronic and advanced diabetic foot ulcers has undergone close scrutiny by the federal administrators of Medicare and Medicaid with the resultant approval for reimbursement for care by the Center for Medicare and Medicaid Services (CMS) for severe diabetic foot ulcers (Wagner's Grade III or higher).[3] Amputation rates have been shown to be decreased by hyperbaric oxygen. Many authors have reported efficacy for hyperbaric oxygen in the treatment of therapeutic radiation injuries, especially mandibular radiation necrosis. Other articles report efficacy in the treatment of patients with necrotizing fasciitis. Certain cases of chronic refractory osteomyelitis are amenable to treatment with hyperbaric oxygen as an adjunct to appropriate surgery and antibiotics. Hyperbaric oxygen has been applied to thermal burns as an adjunct to conventional treatments. Hyperbaric oxygen is also recommended to support compromised flaps and grafts (Figure 1).

HYPERBARIC OXYGEN: WHAT IT IS AND HOW IT WORKS

Hyperbaric oxygen therapy involves a patient entering into a pressure vessel, having the ambient pressure of that vessel increased and providing the patient with 100% oxygen to breathe at gas pressures typically of 1.5 atm or higher. Often, the ambient pressures are reported in atmospheres absolute (ATA) and includes the initial ambient pressure (usually close to 1 ATA depending on the altitude of the treating center) plus the increase in pressure. Most treatment protocols utilize pressures of 2.0 to 3.0 ATA ambient pressure (that is, 1 to 2 atm higher than the original pressure outside the chamber).

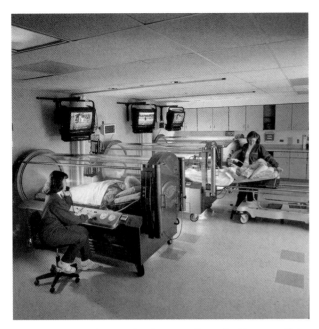

Figure 1. This photograph shows patients inside a multiplace hyperbaric chamber. They breathe oxygen by mask or oxygen hood.

Above 3.0 atm, oxygen toxicity manifested by grand mal seizure activity becomes common, even after short exposures, and for this reason, treatment pressures on 100% oxygen do not exceed 3.0 ATA. Two types of hyperbaric chambers are available. In the monoplace chamber, a single patient is treated, the entire chamber environment is pressurized with 100% oxygen and the patient breathes this oxygen. In the multiplace chamber, several patients are treated simultaneously. Because of potential fire or explosion hazards due to the large volumes of compressed gasses, multiplace chamber environments are pressurized with compressed air, and the patient receives 100% oxygen for inhalation by donning a mask or head tent device. In either case, the pharmacology and physiology are the same, although typically, patients are treated at higher pressures in the multiplace chamber (2.4 atm versus 2.0 atm in monoplace protocols for most indications). Most treatment sessions consist of 90 minutes to 2 hours of exposure to oxygen at the increased pressure. The most frequent treatment profile for decompression sickness and air embolism lasts for about 6 hours. Treatments are usually given once per day, although in emergency conditions, such as gas gangrene or necrotizing fasciitis, or in a rapidly deteriorating wound or failing flap, treatments may be given twice—even three times—daily. The total number of treatments may vary from one in certain emergency conditions to 40 or more for chronic disorders, including radiation injuries and chronic wounds, including diabetic ulcers.

Inspired oxygen pressures are increased from around 150 mm Hg at sea level to 1,520 mm Hg (2.0 ATA) and to 2,280 mm Hg (3.0 ATA) in the hyperbaric oxygen chamber. Patients with good respiratory function already have saturated or nearly saturated hemoglobin. The additional oxygen carrying capacity of the blood, which becomes the important mechanism for hyperbaric oxygen applied to wound-healing enhancement (and many other disorders), results from the additional oxygen, which is dissolved in plasma at high pressures. In 1960, Boerema and colleagues demonstrated that enough oxygen could be dissolved in the plasma to support life without hemoglobin.[4] They bled miniature pigs to an average hemoglobin level of 0.45 gm/dL and replaced the intravascular volume with plasma expanders. The animals were then placed in a hyperbaric chamber at 3.0 atm and kept alive for several hours with no perceptible decrement in their comfort or activity. Adequate oxygen was dissolved in the plasma to support the needs of the heart and brain for their metabolism. The solubility of oxygen in plasma is such that 2 cc of oxygen can be dissolved for every 100 cc of plasma when a patient breathes 100% oxygen at sea level pressure. At 3.0 atm in a hyperbaric chamber, 6 cc of oxygen can be dissolved and transported to the tissues for every 100 cc of plasma. This level of oxygen delivery is adequate to meet the metabolic needs of the brain and heart. This dissolved oxygen is essential to the efficacy of treating disorders such as carbon monoxide poisoning and exceptional anemias. In wound healing, it is this mechanism whereby additional oxygen can be delivered to a wound to support healing in hypoxic and ischemic circumstances. Arterial oxygen tensions have been shown to increase to about 1,400 mm Hg in individuals breathing 100% oxygen at 2.0 atm.

Hyperbaric oxygen has additional physiologic effects that can be therapeutic in certain pathologic circumstances. Trapped gases in the circulation or other body cavities respond according to ideal gas laws (Boyle's Law) and shrink with volume changes inversely proportional to the increase in ambient pressures. In decompression sickness and air embolism, this effect is especially important in reestablishing perfusion by reducing the volume of trapped and obstructing intravascular gas. Once the intravascular bubble is reduced in volume, it flows down the vascular tree to a smaller caliber vessel, and the blockade of perfusion is reduced to those tissues supplied by the smaller vessel and where collaterals are probably more plentiful. The inspiration of 100% oxygen also establishes a diffusion gradient whereby the inert gases in the bubble move out of the bubble, leading to its ultimate collapse and reestablishing circulation.

Hyperbaric oxygen also has a vasoconstrictive effect, which is sometimes useful in reducing edema. Concerns have been voiced that this vasoconstrictive effect might impair oxygen delivery by exacerbating ischemia. Tissue oxygen measurements have shown that the enhanced oxygen-carrying effect at hyperbaric pressures is the dominant effect providing increased oxygen delivery and overwhelming the vasoconstrictive effects.

Some authors have promoted topical oxygen as a safer and cheaper alternative and suggested that the results of such treatment were equivalent or even theoretically superior to systemic hyperbaric oxygen as described above. Feldmeier and colleagues reviewed the results of topical oxygen treatment and discussed the misleading literature that co-opts the systemic hyperbaric oxygen literature to support its use.[5] It is worth noting that the only truly randomized trial of topical oxygen, which was a study of diabetic foot ulcers, was a negative study and actually showed a trend of delayed healing in the topical oxygen group compared to control.

THE BENEFICIAL PHYSIOLOGIC EFFECTS OF HYPERBARIC OXYGEN IN WOUND HEALING

There really is no controversy regarding the need for adequate levels of oxygen in order to achieve successful wound closure. Investigators continue to address the essential role of oxygen in wound healing with an ever increasing understanding of the mechanisms whereby oxygen contributes to the complex cascade of biochemical events that must follow in sequence to achieve a healed wound. Oxygen plays a role by its influence on three major mechanisms needed for successful wound healing:

1. Control of infection
2. Angiogenesis and elaboration of growth factors
3. Epithelialization

Infection Control

During the initial inflammatory phase of wound healing, an important host response is the marshaling of immune responses in order to remove any bacterial contaminants from the wound environment. In chronic wounds, continued bacterial contamination often contributes to the wound's failure to heal. Hypoxic wounds are more subject to progressive infection, including the development of necrotizing infections and clostridial myonecrosis. In a hypoxic wound, hyperbaric oxygen intermittently increases oxygen tensions and enhances bacterial kill by enhanced leukocyte function. In the absence of molecular oxygen, neutrophils continue to phagocytose bacteria but do not effectively kill them because the various enzyme systems whereby neutrophils destroy bacteria are oxygen-dependent free radical systems.[6] Hyperbaric oxygen has also been shown to potentiate the effects of certain antibiotics, especially aminoglycosides and sulfonamides.[7]

A recent summary by Gottrup reviews the essential role of oxygen in wound healing in regard to infection control.[8] In this paper, the potential benefit of supplemental oxygen breathing at normal ambient pressures is also discussed.

Angiogenesis and Elaboration of Growth Factors

Another publication by Tandara and Mustoe summarizes the role of oxygen in the multiple interconnected events associated with wound healing, including the enhancement of angiogenesis as a prominent effect of adequate oxygen levels.[9] Oxygen is a known substrate for the synthesis and cross linkage of collagen. The concept of hyperbaric oxygen elevating tissue oxygen tensions, and its beneficial effect on collagen synthesis and release, have been promoted for some time as a mechanism of action by the advocates of its use. The successful release and cross-linking of collagen strands provides wounds with increased bursting strength and provides a supportive matrix for fragile budding capillaries. Recently, the all-important role of cytokines and up to now already identified growth factors has begun to be understood. Hyperbaric oxygen has been shown to enhance the activity of several growth factors important in wound healing, including vascular endothelial growth factor (VEGF) and platelet-derived growth factor (PDGF).[10] Marx and colleagues showed the beneficial effect of hyperbaric oxygen in enhancing angiogenesis in irradiated hypoxic tissues.[11] These demonstrations include a study of vascular density in a rabbit model wherein all animals were irradiated. The animals were divided into groups, and those receiving hyperbaric oxygen were found to have increased vascular density, with the number of vessels increasing in direct proportion to the hyperbaric oxygen treatment pressure. Marx and colleagues also demonstrated the enhanced vascular density after hyperbaric oxygen by comparing pre- and post-hyperbaric histologic specimens in patients receiving hyperbaric oxygen as treatment for their radiation-induced hypoxic osteoradionecrosis necrosis of the mandible.[12]

Very interesting recent work suggests that enhanced tissue oxygen levels provided by hyperbaric oxygen can increase the all-important VEGF levels, even without hypoxic drive.[10] The need for at least intermittent wound hypoxia to maximize the production of growth factors has been called into question by some wound-healing experts. Tandara and Mustoe do discuss the prominent role for hypoxia inducible factor-1 and a putative difference between chronic and acute wounding in terms of the effects of hypoxia.[9] The suggestion is made that hypoxia has a positive effect on healing in acute wounds and the totally opposite effect in chronic wounds.

Epithelialization

Epithelial migration from the edge of the wound is a process termed epiboly. Especially in chronic wounds closing by secondary intention, a base of vascular granulation tissue must be established before successful epithelial migration can occur. Keratinocytes initially establish a thin layer over the wound surface. As they migrate, they stimulate angiogenesis by releasing growth factors, including basic fibroblast growth factor (b-FGF) and VEGF.[13] The keratinocytes also release transforming growth factor-α , a chemoattractant and mitogen, and platelet derived growth factor (PDGF), which contributes to matrix formation. Contraction of the underlying connective tissue facilitates this process by decreasing the distance over which these cells must migrate.

Probably the most important effect of hyperbaric oxygen in enhancing epithelialization is the promotion of angiogenesis and development of the granulation tissue bed over which the keratinocytes can effectively migrate. Under study in at least two prominent wound research laboratories (University of California at San Francisco and Ohio State University) is the potential for enhancement of epithelial coverage as the result of increased oxygen delivery. There is some suggestion that even topically delivered 100% oxygen enhances the rate and success of epithelialization (H.W. Hopf, personal communication, June 2002).

CLINICAL APPLICATIONS OF HYPERBARIC OXYGEN IN VARIOUS WOUNDS OF THE HEAD AND NECK

Osteoradionecrosis

Since the 1970s, the application of hyperbaric oxygen in the treatment of mandibular osteoradionecrosis has been under study. Initial reports were mixed in terms of outcome. Hyperbaric oxygen was administered somewhat haphazardly without adequate surgical intervention.[14] In the late 1970s, Marx and Johnson, while at Wilford Hall USAF Medical Center in San Antonio, TX, developed a staging system for mandibular necrosis with a multidisciplinary treatment protocol that followed as a logical consequence of this staging system.[15] The Marx protocol embodies several important principles and, when utilized, should be applied in its entirety and not in a piecemeal fashion. A recent paper by Annane and colleagues purports to be the definitive randomized controlled trial in regard to the application of hyperbaric oxygen therapy to the treatment of mandibular necrosis.[16] The study is flawed, however, in that it did not provide for the surgical extirpation of necrotic bone. Marx and Johnson and Feldmeier and associates had already shown the absolute necessity of surgical extirpation of necrotic bone in the multidisciplinary management of osteoradionecrosis of the mandible or chest wall.[15,17]

Marx emphasizes several principles in applying hyperbaric oxygen in the treatment of mandibular osteoradionecrosis.[15] These include the emphasis on preoperative hyperbaric oxygen in order to improve the vascular status of tissues before surgical insult and the surgical removal of all necrotic bone, even if this necessitates a mandibular resection with resultant discontinuity defect.

In the Marx staging system, stage I ORN includes patients with chronically exposed necrotic and painful bone in whom only minor débridement is felt to be needed to eradicate the bony necrosis. In these patients, 30 daily predébridement hyperbaric oxygen treatments for 90 minutes on 100% oxygen are delivered. The original protocol involved hyperbaric treatments at 2.4 ATA, although some have adapted the protocol to 2.0 ATA in monoplace chambers. The minor débridement is accomplished next. If the patient is found to have more extensive necrotic bone after formal surgical débridement short of a discontinuity resection, he or she is advanced to stage II or III. Post-débridement, an additional 10 hyperbaric treatments with the same profile are given (Figure 2).

Stage II patients are those in whom the extent of necrosis is felt to require a larger and more formal débridement in the operating room. However, it is anticipated that, in these patients, a mandibular discontinuity procedure can be avoided. These patients have the same pre- and postoperative course of hyperbaric oxygen with the formal in-operating-room débridement occurring at 30 treatments. If the surgeon discovers that a mandibular resection is needed, the patient is advanced to management as a stage III patient.

Patients enter into treatment at stage III from the outset when they have certain serious manifestations, including pathologic fracture, cutaneous fistula, and/or extension of the necrotic process to the lower mandibular margin. In these patients and in those patients advanced to stage III, after the initial 30 preoperative treatments, the patients goes to the operating room for mandibular resection and external fixation.

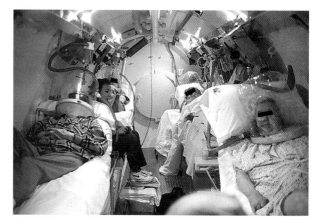

Figure 2. This photograph shows a monoplace hyperbaric chamber. The chamber environment is compressed with 100% oxygen and the patient breathes oxygen as the ambient gas.

The patient has 10 postoperative hyperbaric treatments. Usually after several weeks, the patient returns to undergo reconstruction. Myocutaneous flaps are employed if there are significant soft tissue deficits. The continuity of the mandible is reestablished by utilizing cadaveric cortical bone from a bone bank shaped into a tray to hold the patient's own corticocancellous bone usually harvested from the iliac crest. The procedure is done percutaneously to avoid bacterial contamination of the graft. The patient is kept in internal fixation until the graft has adequately ossified, usually about 6 weeks. Ten post-reconstruction hyperbaric oxygen treatments are given. Since the original development of the Marx protocol, microsurgical techniques have improved greatly, and free flaps using the fibula have been employed for mandibular reconstruction. Even when the reconstructive surgeon employs free flaps with microvascular anastomoses, the quality of the tissues constituting the recipient bed for the free flap can be improved to permit the more successful acceptance of those tissues used for reconstruction.

Marx reported his success in 268 patients treated according to his protocol for mandibular necrosis.[11] He achieved a remarkable 100% successful resolution in this group. Unfortunately, in order to achieve this success rate, 68% required treatment in stage III with mandibular resection and reconstruction. The validity of the Marx protocol is further established by the success that others, including community practitioners, have had in applying its principles and also achieving high success rates in the treatment of mandibular ORN.

A review of the hyperbaric oxygen (HBO_2) literature was accomplished by Feldmeier and Hampson.[18] It showed, a total of 14 publications reporting the experience of applying HBO_2 to mandibular necrosis. One very small randomized controlled trial by Tobey and Kelly is positive.[19] Only 12 patients were studied. These patients were randomized to 100% oxygen at 1.2 vs. 2.0 ATA. The authors state that those patients treated at 2.0 ATA "experienced significant improvement" compared to the group receiving

oxygen at 1.2 ATA. Unfortunately, the authors do not include much detail in regard to what constituted improvement, and no statistical analyses were done.

Besides the Tobey and Kelly trial, the rest of the publications are case series. Of these 13 publications, all show a positive outcome with HBO_2 except that of Maier and colleagues.[20] In this paper, hyperbaric oxygen was part of the overall treatment for ORN only after an initial attempt at surgical correction. No preoperative hyperbaric oxygen was given. As noted above, the more recent study by Ananne and colleagues was also a negative trial.[16] In both of these negative reports, the Marx protocol was not followed in its entirety.

A compilation of the results from the 14 studies reviewed by Feldmeier and Hampson demonstrates a positive therapeutic effect in 310 cases, or 83.6%.[18] Resolution would certainly be a more desirable endpoint. However, in many of the early reports, aggressive extirpation of necrotic bone or surgical reconstruction of bony discontinuity was not accomplished. As noted, Marx reported 100% resolution by adhering to the full multidisciplinary protocol. Marx also set as a criterion of success not only the resolution of necrosis but also the successful reestablishment of bony continuity and success in fitting the patient with a denture for cosmesis and mastication.

HYPERBARIC OXYGEN AS A PREVENTIVE MEASURE FOR ORN

Marx and colleagues accomplished a randomized trial comparing penicillin to HBO_2 prior to dental extractions with the intent of investigating the role for hyperbaric oxygen as a prophylactic strategy in the prevention of mandibular radiation necrosis in heavily irradiated mandibles.[21] Thirty-seven patients were enrolled in each group. ORN occurred in 11 of 37 (29.7%) of the penicillin group compared to only 2/37 (5.4%) in the HBO_2 group.

This protocol randomized only patients who had received a radiation dose of 6,800 centrigray or higher. The penicillin group received 1 million units of penicillin just prior to surgery, followed by 500 mg penicillin orally four times daily for 10 days. The HBO_2 group received 20 HBO_2 treatments before extractions and 10 HBO_2 treatments following extractions.

Two additional clinical reports confirm the Marx study.[22,23] In these studies, a total of 53 patients received hyperbaric oxygen in a similar fashion prior to dental extractions. When we combine patients in all three reports, we find an incidence of ORN in 4 of 90, or 4.5%, compared to about 30% in the Marx control group.

SOFT TISSUE RADIATION NECROSIS OF THE HEAD AND NECK

Laryngeal Radiation Necrosis

Radiation-induced laryngeal necrosis is an uncommon but serious complication of head and neck radiation. The incidence of laryngeal necrosis should be no more than 1% in a properly designed, dosed and fractionated course of radiation. Higher total doses, higher doses per individual treatment, and particle beam (neutron) irradiation increase the risk of laryngeal chondroradiation necrosis.

The hyperbaric oxygen treatment of chondroradiation necrosis of the larynx has been reported by three separate institutions.[24–26] Most of these patients had Chandler's grade III or IV necrosis and were at significant risk for laryngectomy. The usual recommendation for persistent laryngeal edema and necrosis is laryngectomy. In retrospective reviews, the vast majority of these patients harbor an occult tumor. Even when tumor-free, these patients have had no real option for successful treatment of their severe chondroradiation necrosis prior to the application of hyperbaric oxygen.

When the results from these three trials are combined, 29 of 35 patients were treated successfully with hyperbaric oxygen. Only 6 required laryngectomy. After hyperbaric oxygen, the others maintained a good quality voice and a patent airway.

Radiation Necrosis of Other Soft Tissues of the Head and Neck

Marx reported his experience in employing hyperbaric oxygen in the treatment of soft tissue radiation necrosis of the head and neck.[27] This report presents the results in a prospective controlled (but not strictly randomized) study applying hyperbaric oxygen to soft tissue radionecrosis. The control group was made up of patients who refused hyperbaric oxygen or for whom it was not logistically practical owing to the distance of a chamber from their homes. These two groups of patients were treated concurrently, and all other aspects of their treatment were identical. Eighty patients received hyperbaric oxygen, and 80 did not. The hyperbaric patients received 20 preoperative HBO_2 treatments followed by 10 postoperative treatments at 2.4 ATA.

These patients had surgery to include resection or flap reconstruction in heavily irradiated patients. Marx compared wound infection, wound dehiscence, and delayed wound healing. The incidence of complications in the HBO_2 group versus the control group was reported in the following fashion:

1. Wound infection: 6% versus 24%;
2. Wound dehiscence: 11% versus 48%; and
3. Delayed wound healing: 11% versus 55%.

No statistical analysis was done in the paper, but we can apply the Chi square test to these numeric results. When we do so, we obtain p values of .004, less than .0001 and less than .0001, respectively, for each of the above outcome measures.

Three additional reports of hyperbaric oxygen in the treatment of soft tissue injuries of the head and neck have been published. These are all case series of soft tissue radiation injuries of the head and neck (other than larynx). All detail a positive outcome in patients treated with HBO_2 for soft tissue radionecrosis of the head and neck. Davis and colleagues reported success in 15 of 16 patients treated for soft tissue radionecrosis of the head and neck.[28] Many of these patients suffered from large chronic soft tissue wounds. In 1997, Neovius and colleagues reported a series of 15 patients treated with hyperbaric oxygen for wound complications in irradiated patients.[29] A case controlled study was accomplished wherein the authors compared the hyperbaric group to a historical control group from their own institution. Eighty percent (12 of 15 patients) in the hyperbaric group healed completely, with improvement in two patients and no improvement in only one patient. In the historic control group, only 7 of 15 patients resolved. Two patients in the control group experienced life-threatening hemorrhage, and one of these bled to death.

Feldmeier and colleagues reported the successful application of prophylactic hyperbaric oxygen in the prevention of post-operative complications in patients undergoing surgical salvage for recurrence within a previously irradiated treatment field.[30] Typically, surgical complications are quite high when radical surgery is done in a previously radiated field. The incidence of serious complications including death is about 60%. With a short course of hyperbaric oxygen (median number of treatments 12; range 3 to 35) initiated as soon as possible after surgery, 87.5% of this group of 32 patients healed without serious complications. No deaths occurred in the immediate post-operative period.

NECROTIZING FASCIITIS

Necrotizing fasciitis is a deep severe progressive infection that spreads rapidly along fascial planes with resultant undermining and necrosis of the overlying skin.[31] It can affect virtually any part of the body. It is most common in the lower extremities. Its development often follows a traumatic insult such as a burn, an abrasion or an insect bite. In the head and neck, it often results from a tooth abscess. Organisms most frequently include streptococcal species and usually two or more organisms are involved. Many of these bacteria may be gas-producing. This syndrome is separate and distinct from gas gangrene or clostridial myonecrosis. Risk factors

for both its occurrence and severity include diabetes, peripheral vascular disease, and age over 50. The primary treatment is aggressive surgical débridement and systemic antibiotics. Mortality rates are high, even when aggressive surgical and pharmacologic treatments have been initiated. In several retrospective reviews, hyperbaric oxygen has been shown to reduce mortality.[32–35]

THERMAL BURNS

The application of hyperbaric oxygen in the treatment of thermal burns is somewhat controversial and is not widely applied. A review of this application was accomplished by Cianci and Slade.[36] The benefits of hyperbaric oxygen in reducing infection, in decreasing the need for fluid replacement, and in hastening the healing process are discussed. The authors in their review accomplish an evidence-based analysis. A total of 21 clinical publications are included. Only two of these reviewed papers (one a randomized controlled trial) fail to demonstrate an advantage for hyperbaric oxygen treatments. Three of the positive reports were randomized and controlled studies.

Reported advantages for the HBO_2-treated patients include decreased mortality, reduced healing time, reduced length of hospital stay, reduced time on ventilators, and reduced requirement for surgical débridement and grafting. Obviously, reports on burn treatment with hyperbaric oxygen have not been restricted to thermal injuries of the head and neck. However, the principles are applicable in this region just as they are elsewhere in the body and can be significant here, especially when a potential advantage is decreased scarring.[37]

FLAPS AND GRAFTS

Zamboni and Shah published a review of the application of hyperbaric oxygen to the preservation of skin grafts and flaps in compromised situations.[38] The authors clearly state that hyperbaric oxygen is not indicated in a normal setting where there is no impairment of perfusion. The authors go on to review the preclinical and clinical literature in regard to hyperbaric oxygen for flaps and grafts. In an earlier work, Zamboni discussed the use of hyperbaric oxygen applied to a variety of flaps, including free flaps, pedicle flaps, random flaps, irradiated wounds and flaps, composite flaps, and axial flaps.[39] In each of these, the author shows an advantage with hyperbaric oxygen treatment. Zamboni indicates that the advantages of hyperbaric oxygen in this application are the enhancement of collagen synthesis, the enhancement of angiogenesis, and favorable effects on the microcirculation. In the article by Zamboni and Shah, the authors discuss the effect of hyperbaric oxygen on ischemia reperfusion injury.[40] In models of flap ischemia, necrosis and adherence of neutrophils to vascular endothelium are significantly reduced with hyperbaric oxygen treatment.

TOXICITY AND SIDE EFFECTS

Sheffield and Sheffield published a 22-year experience of complications during hyperbaric oxygen therapy involving over 170,000 patient treatments in a busy multiplace hyperbaric practice.[40] The authors observed an incidence of 36 oxygen-induced seizures over this time period (1.7 per 10,000 exposures requiring removal from the chamber, and 0.4 seizures per 10,000 exposures addressed by removal from oxygen only).

The authors of this review report complications in several other organ systems. Otic barotrauma is unquestionably the most frequent complication and accounted for about 50% of all complications. Trauma to the middle ear is usually very minor and usually managed pharmacologically with decongestants. Pressure equalization tubes are placed for those patients who cannot equalize the pressure in the middle ear. Sinus barotraumas can occur but are very rare. Even more rare is barodontalgia, for which there is no specific treatment. Almost always, patients suffering from minor barotraumas to the ear, sinuses, or teeth will be able to reinitiate and

complete a course of hyperbaric treatment after a short interruption. Otic barotrauma was found to occur with a frequency of 83.4 events per 10,000 patient exposures. The most telling statistic is that, in 22 years time, only 39 patients refused to complete their treatment. Notably, in this report, no patient fatalities have occurred. Pott and colleagues reported a study that followed 18 hyperbaric oxygen patients for 6 weeks with weekly pulmonary function studies.[41] This report failed to demonstrate any decrement in pulmonary function.

Weaver and Churchill reported three patients with a cardiac history and reduced left cardiac output who experienced pulmonary edema after hyperbaric oxygen therapy.[42] One of these patients died as a result. The authors advise caution in the use of hyperbaric oxygen in patients with reduced cardiac output. Hyperbaric oxygen is likely to increase left ventricular afterload due to its vasoconstrictive effects. The authors note that this is a rare complication occurring in only 3 of more than 1,000 patients.

A common experience in patients receiving at least 20 hyperbaric treatments is a change in visual acuity towards myopia.[43] Interestingly, presbyopic patients perceive this as an improvement in vision. In any case, the visual acuity changes are virtually always temporary, and patients should be counseled that they should wait until their vision stabilizes before having new refraction and new corrective lenses made. This usually takes 6 weeks or less. The exact etiology of these refractive changes is not known.

REFERENCES

1. Kindwall EP. A history of hyperbaric medicine. In: Kindwall EP, editor. Hyperbaric Medicine Practice. Flagstaff: Best Publishing; 1995. p. 1–20.
2. Feldmeier JJ, editor. Hyperbaric oxygen 2003: indications and results: the hyperbaric oxygen therapy committee report. Kensington (MD): Undersea and Hyperbaric Medical Society; 2003.
3. Wang C, Lau J. Hyperbaric oxygen therapy in treatment of hypoxic wounds. Technology assessment. Agency for Healthcare Research and Quality. November 2, 2001.

4. Boerema I, Meyne NG, Brummelkamp WH, et al. Life without blood. A study of the influence of high atmospheric pressure and hypothermia on dilution of the blood. J Cardiovasc Surg 1960;1:133–46.

5. Feldmeier JJ, Hopf HW, Warriner RA 3rd, et al. UHMS position statement: topical oxygen for chronic wounds. Undersea Hyperb Med, 32:157–68.

6. Hohn DC. Oxygen and leukocyte microbial killing. In: Davis JC, Hunt TK, editors. Hyperbaric oxygen therapy. Bethesda (MD): Undersea Medical Society Inc.; 1977. p. 101–10.

7. Park M. Effects of hyperbaric oxygen in infectious diseases: basic mechanisms. In: Kindwall EP, Whelan HT, editors. Hyperbaric medicine practice. Flagstaff (AZ): Best Publishing Company; 1999. p. 205–43.

8. Gottrup F. Oxygen in wound healing and infection. World J Surg 2004;28:312–5.

9. Tandara AA, Mustoe TA. Oxygen in wound healing-more than a nutrient. World J Surg 2004;28:294–300.

10. Sheikh AY, Gibson JJ, Rollins MD, et al. Effect of hyperoxia on vascular endothelial growth factor levels in a wound model. Arch Surg 2000;135:1293–7.

11. Marx RE, Ehler WJ, Tayapongsak P, Pierce LW. Relationship of oxygen dose to angiogenesis induction in irradiated tissue. Am J Surg 1990;160:519–24.

12. Marx RE. Radiation injury to tissue. In: Kindwall EP, editor. Hyperbaric Medicine Practice. 2nd ed. Flagstaff (AZ): Best Publishing Company; 1999. p. 665–723.

13. Hunt TK, Hopf H, Hussain Z. Physiology of wound healing. Adv Skin Wound Care 2000;13 (Suppl 2):6–11.

14. Marx RE. Osteoradionecrosis of the jaws: review and update. HBO Rev 1984;5:78–126.

15. Marx RE, Johnson RP. Problem wounds in oral and maxillofacial surgery: the role of hyperbaric oxygen. In: Davis JC, Hunt TK, editors. Problem wounds: the role of hyperbaric oxygen. New York: Elsevier; 1988:65–123.

16. Annane D, Depondt J, Aubert P, et al. Hyperbaric oxygen therapy for radionecrosis of the jaw: a randomized placebo-controlled, double-blind trial from the ORN96 study group. J Clin Oncol 2004;22:4893–900.

17. Feldmeier JJ, Heimbach RD, Davolt DA, et al. Hyperbaric oxygen as an adjunctive treatment for delayed radiation injury of the chest wall: a retrospective review of 23 cases. Undersea Hyper Med 1995;22:383–93.

18. Feldmeier JJ, Hampson NB. A systematic review of the literature reporting the application of hyperbaric oxygen to the prevention and treatment of delayed radiation injuries: an evidence based approach. Undersea Hyperb Med 2002;29:4–30.

19. Tobey RE, Kelly JF. Osteoradionecrosis of the jaws. Otolaryngol Clin North Am 1979;12:183–6.

20. Maier A, Gaggl A, Klemen H, et al. Review of severe osteoradionecrosis treated by surgery alone or surgery with postoperative hyperbaric oxygenation. Br J Oral Maxillofac Surg 2000;38:173–6.

21. Marx RE, Johnson RP, Kline SN. Prevention of osteoradionecrosis: a randomized prospective clinical trial of hyperbaric oxygen versus penicillin. J Am Dent Assoc 1985;11:49–54.

22. Vudiniabola S, Pirone C, Williamson J, Goss ANN. Hyperbaric oxygen in the prevention of osteoradionecrosis of the jaws. Aust Dent J 1999;44:243–7.

23. David LA, Sandor GK, Evans AW, Brown DH. Hyperbaric oxygen therapy and mandibular osteoradionecrosis: a retrospective study and analysis of treatment outcomes. J Can Dent Assoc 2001;67:384–9.

24. Ferguson BJ, Hudson WR, Farmer JC. Hyperbaric oxygen for laryngeal radionecrosis. Ann Otol Laryngol 1987;96:1–6.

25. Feldmeier JJ, Heimbach RD, Davolt DA, Brakora MJ. Hyperbaric oxygen as an adjunctive treatment for severe laryngeal necrosis: a report of nine consecutive cases. Undersea Hyper Med 1993;20:329–35.

26. Filintisis GA, Moon RE, Kraft KL, et al. Laryngeal radionecrosis and hyperbaric oxygen therapy: report of 18 cases and review of the literature. Ann Otol Rhinol Laryngol 2000;109:554–62.

27. Marx RE. Radiation injury to tissue. In: Kindwall EP, editor. Hyperbaric medicine practice. 2nd ed. Flagstaff (AZ): Best Publishing Company; 1999. p. 665–740.

28. Davis JC, Dunn JM, Gates GA, Heimbach RD. Hyperbaric oxygen: a new adjunct in the management of radiation necrosis. Arch Otolaryngol 1979;105:58–61.

29. Neovius EB, Lind MG, Lind FG. Hyperbaric oxygen for wound complications after surgery in the irradiated head and neck: a review of the literature and a report of 15 consecutive cases. Head Neck 1997;19:315–322.

30. Feldmeier JJ, Newman R, Davolt DA, et al. Prophylactic hyperbaric oxygen for patients undergoing salvage for recurrent head and neck cancer following full course irradiation [abstract]. Undersea Hyperb Med 1998;22:10.

31. Freeman HP, Oluwole SF, Ganepola GAP, Dy E. Necrotizing fasciitis. Am J Surg 1981;142:377–83.

32. Bakker DJ. Pure and mixed aerobic and anaerobic soft tissue infections. HBO Rev 1985;6:65–96.

33. Zanetti CL. Necrotizing soft tissue infections and adjunctive hyperbaric oxygen. Chest 1988;92:70–1.

34. Korhonen K. Hyperbaric oxygen in acute necrotizing infections. With special reference to the effects on tissue gas tensions. Ann Chir Gynaecol 2000;89 (Suppl 214):7–36.

35. Stenberg AE, Larsson A, Gardlund B, et al. 13 cases of cervical necrotizing fasciitis-all patients survived. Surgery, antibiotics and hyperbaric oxygenation give the best results. Lakartidningen 2004;101(28–29):23336–41.

36. Cianci P, Slade JB. Thermal burns. In: Feldmeier JJ, editor. Hyperbaric oxygen 2003, indications and results: the hyperbaric oxygen therapy committee report. Kensington (MD): Undersea and Hyperbaric Medical Society; 2003. p. 109–19.

37. Mereola L, Piscitelli F. Considerations on the use of HBO in the treatment of burns. Ann Med Nav 1978;83:515–9.

38. Zamboni WA, Shah HR. Skin grafts and flaps (compromised). In: Feldmeier JJ, editor. Hyperbaric oxygen 2003, indications and results: the hyperbaric oxygen therapy committee report. Kensington (MD): Undersea and Hyperbaric Medical Society; 2003. p. 101–7.

39. Zamboni WA, Persons BL. Hyperbaric oxygen in plastic and reconstructive surgery. In: Bakker DJ, Cramer FS, editors. Hyperbaric Surgery, Flagstaff, AZ, Best Publishing. 2002. p. 397–416.

40. Sheffield PJ, Sheffield JC. Complication rates for hyperbaric oxygen therapy patients and their attendants: a 22 year analysis. In: Proceedings of the Fourteenth International Congress on Hyperbaric Medicine; 2003. p. 312–8.

41. Pott F, Westergaard P, Mortensen J, Jansen EC. Hyperbaric oxygen treatment and pulmonary function. Undersea Hyperb Med 1999;26:225–8.

42. Weaver LK, Churchill S. Pulmonary edema associated with hyperbaric oxygen therapy. Chest 2001;120:1407–9.

43. Clark J. Side effects and complications (of hyperbaric medicine). In: Feldmeier JJ, editor. Hyperbaric oxygen indications and results: the Hyperbaric Oxygen Therapy Committee report. Undersea and Hyperbaric Medical Society, Kensington MD. 2003. p. 137–41.

28

Blood Products in Wound Healing

Ryan M. Greene, MD, PhD; Benjamin Johnson, MD; Kevin O'Grady, BS, BA; Dean M. Toriumi, MD

The use of blood-derived products for wound management and healing has emerged as an important and useful resource in surgery. Following tissue injury, the body undergoes a programmed response which involves an intricate interaction of cellular components designed to repair the site of injury as quickly and effectively as possible. In addition to the body's own wound-healing capacities, additional methods of treatment utilizing blood-derived products have been developed in an effort to enhance the body's wound-healing properties. Two currently employed options that have been shown to enhance wound healing are fibrin tissue adhesives (FTA) and platelet-rich plasma (PRP). The safety and efficacy of these products, along with their associated growth factors, has been well-documented in the literature. In order to understand and appreciate the basis for using blood-derived products in wound healing, it is beneficial to have an appreciation for the mechanisms involved during the wound-healing process.

RESPONSE TO TISSUE INJURY

The body's response to tissue injury occurs in three overlapping phases: inflammation, proliferation, and remodeling. The inflammatory phase is initiated with platelet aggregation and results in subsequent hemostasis. Hemostasis is a complex process that involves the interaction of the subendothelium of disrupted blood vessels, platelets, and plasma proteins. Injury to tissues and their associated blood vessels leads to the initial formation of a platelet plug, mediated by adhesive proteins such as von Willebrand's factor. The formation of this initial platelet plug is unstable, and in time, the unstable clot converts to a more stable fibrin structure through a separate process. Formation of a fibrin clot is initiated by the exposure of tissue factor (TF) in the subendothelium following vessel injury. The TF binds and activates circulating factor VII to form a TF-factor VIIa complex. This activated complex then activates two additional factors, IX and X. Activated Xa then complexes with factor Va, calcium ions, and anionic phospholipid to form the prothrombinase complex. This complex activates prothrombin (factor II) to thrombin (factor IIa). Thrombin then cleaves large molecular weight fibrinogen units into smaller fibrin subunits. These subunits then polymerize in both an end-to-end and side-to-side fashion. Factor XIIIa, also activated by thrombin, enables the cross-linking of the polymerized subunits into a stable fibrin clot in the presence of calcium ions. (Figure 1).

Platelets also play an integral role in hemostasis and wound healing. Secretion of thromboxane and serotonin promotes hemostasis by causing vasoconstriction. Platelets also secrete histamine which increases vascular permeability to facilitate migration of polymorphonuclear (PMN) cells and monocytes to the site of injury. The appearance of PMNs and monocytes signals the onset of the proliferative phase of wound healing. Chemotactic growth factors recruit endothelial cells for the creation of new blood vessels (angiogenesis). The extracellular matrix is generated by fibroblasts that migrate to the injury

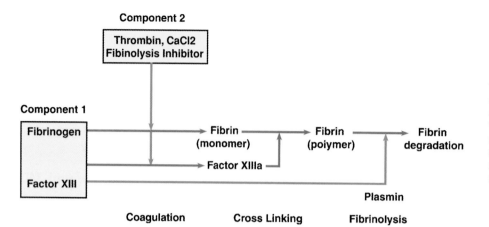

Figure 1. Fibrin tissue adhesives mimic the final common pathway of the coagulation cascade. In the presence of thrombin, calcium chloride and factor XIII, fibrinogen is converted to a fibrin polymer useful as an adhesive, sealant, or hemostatic agent. The rate of fibrin clot formation can be controlled by increasing or decreasing thrombin concentration.

site. Finally, epithelialization occurs from the cells along the periphery of the wound and gradually moves inward, resulting in the formation of a scar. The scar is altered by dynamic collagen lysis and synthesis in the remodeling phase.

A variety of cytokines and growth factors influence the healing and maturation of the wound. The cytokines serve to recruit cells and lead to cellular proliferation and differentiation, a topic that is beyond the scope of this chapter. Growth factors are also involved in similar roles. Platelet-derived growth factor (PDGF) is released from the alpha granules of platelets and aids in recruitment and activation of immune cells and fibroblasts. A topically applied B-chain isomer of PDGF (PDGF-BB) has been shown clinically to enhance wound strength and healing time, as well as improve wound healing in diabetic neuropathic ulcers.[1] The topical B-chain PDGF isomer has been approved by the United States Food and Drug Administration (FDA) for clinical use. Additionally, platelets release transforming growth factor-β (TGF-β), which promotes fibroblast maturation, migration, and extracellular matrix synthesis. Other growth factors, such as epidermal growth factor (EGF) and vascular endothelial growth factor (VEGF), are secreted by fibroblasts, endothelial cells, and immune cells to further enhance tissue injury repair.

The mechanism of wound healing is a complex process involving the intervention of clotting factors in conjunction with growth factors to achieve a common goal. Understanding this process gives insight into the scientific justification as to how and why fibrin tissue adhesive and platelet-rich plasma might enhance the wound-healing process.

FIBRIN TISSUE ADHESIVES

Whether used as an adhesive, sealant, hemostatic agent, or carrier for growth factors, fibrin tissue adhesives have gained widespread acceptance as important and useful adjuncts for a variety of surgical procedures. First used as a hemostatic by Bergel in 1909,[2] FTA has been used for a wide variety of surgical applications, including cardiovascular procedures,[3] cessation of cerebrospinal fluid leaks,[4-6] nerve anastomosis,[7] and stabilization of ossicles[8] and skin grafts. Additionally, FTA has been used as an adjunct to sutures in the sealing of vessels following vascular surgery and has proven effective in controlling bleeding in situations in which standard-of-care treatments are not an option.

Fibrin tissue adhesives have proven to be (1) safe for internal use, (2) biocompatible to host tissues, (3) biodegradable with minimal to no tissue reaction, (4) useful for a variety of surgical indications due to unique hemostatic, sealant, and adhesive properties, (5) readily available off the shelf, and (6) cost effective.[9] Additionally, depending on the intended use, fibrin tissue adhesives have been shown to be effective in preventing postoperative hematoma formation, decreasing surgical time, decreasing the need for drains, reducing tension on flaps, as well as decreasing patient recovery time following surgery.[10]

The properties of fibrin adhesives are based on the final common pathway of the coagulation cascade involving two plasma proteins, fibrinogen and thrombin. Fibrinogen is converted to its activated form, fibrin, in the presence of thrombin, calcium chloride, and factor XIII. Quality and tensile strength of the fibrin clot are dependent upon the source and concentration of the fibrinogen,[11,12] whereas the speed of polymerization from fibrinogen to fibrin is directly related to the thrombin concentration. The rate of fibrinolysis depends upon the extent of cross-linking of the fibrin clot and the host cellular response to the clot.

Fibrin tissue adhesives can be produced from autologous, single-donor homologous, or multiple-donor homologous sources. Autologous FTA is prepared from the patient's own blood products, thereby eliminating the risk of viral transmission from donor to recipient. However, the fibrinogen concentration from single-donor sources (approximately 15 to 30 mg/mL) is significantly less than that found in pooled commercial products (75 to 110 mg/mL). The lower fibrinogen concentration of the single-donor products yields a much lower binding strength. Additionally, the product is significantly less viscous than the higher–fibrinogen-concentration pooled-plasma products. The difference in fibrinogen concentration can have a significant effect on the efficacy of the given fibrin sealant, depending on the intended use. However, Man and colleagues reported achieving acceptable tensile strength with moderate fibrinogen concentrations using autologous fibrin sealant prepared intraoperatively.[10] They also noted that, with lower fibrinogen concentrations, less dense fibrin clots are produced which could theoretically improve access to platelets and improve wound healing. However, O'Grady and colleagues found that skin graft survival was not affected by fibrinogen concentration, but rather, wound healing was inhibited by application of a thick layer of fibrin sealant.[13] (Figure 2).

Most commonly, autologous preparations are achieved by cryoprecipitation. Currently, several devices are being developed to produce

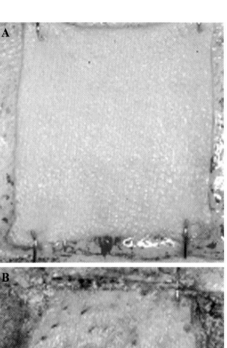
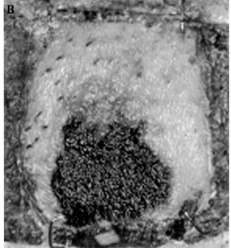
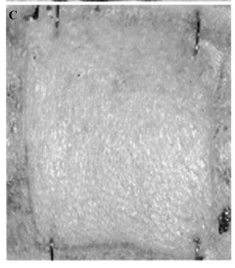

Figure 2. Freshly harvested 4 by 4 cm skin grafts placed over a thick layer of fibrin adhesive and stabilized with staples (*A*). Skin graft 4 weeks after placement on a wound bed treated with a thick layer of fibrin tissue adhesive (*B*). A larger area of tissue necrosis as well as areas of tissue discoloration and uneven healing were common in the thick adhesive group. Skin graft 4 weeks after placement on a wound bed treated with a thin layer of fibrin tissue adhesive (*C*). Smooth even healing is evident across the entire graft area.

autologous FTA from fresh plasma in as little as 30 minutes. However, its use has been limited due to the lengthy preparation time. Siedentop and colleagues performed a study comparing autologous, single-donor homologous, and multiple-donor homologous fibrin tissue adhesives on three different surfaces.[14] They found that the bonding power of the two homologous preparations, Vi-Guard (Melville Biologics, Inc., Melville, NY) and Tisseel (Immuno, Vienna, Austria), were significantly greater than the autologous preparations. The bonding strengths of Vi-Guard and Tisseel were comparable, except with pigskin, where Tisseel exhibited increased strength. Finally, preparation time was decreased in the homologous preparations (30 minutes) compared to the autologous products (45 to 90 minutes).

The pooled commercial product Tisseel, which was approved in Europe for clinical use in the 1970s, is produced by combining plasma from as many as 10,000 donors. The donors are screened in order to alleviate the potential of viral contaminants. Additionally, following extraction of fibrinogen from the pooled plasma, the product undergoes a viral inactivation process to destroy possible contaminants prior to use. Tisseel has been used in over 50 countries and in well over 1 million cases over the past two decades without a single reported case of viral transmission relating to seroconversion. Owing to this fact and significant testimony from the scientific and medical community on behalf of the potential benefits and minimal risks of the homologous pooled product, the FDA approved the commercial product for clinical use in the United States in 1998. It should be noted that the uses in facial plastic and reconstructive surgery are off-label indications. The convenient, "off the shelf" availability of Tisseel, in conjunction with the safety record presented over the past several decades should offer confidence to surgeons considering the use of FTA.

Cyanoacrylate tissue adhesives have tremendous bonding strength and have been shown to be useful for skin closure, but they are tissue toxic when used internally. On the other hand, fibrin tissue adhesives are safe for internal use, but their bonding strength is minimal compared to cyanoacrylates. The mechanical strength of a fibrin clot is dependent on a number of factors but is mainly a function of the fibrinogen concentration.[11,12] The adherent force of the clot at the site of application is not an attribute of the mechanical strength, but is rather a physiologic characteristic.[12] The mechanical strength and adherence have no correlation to hemostatic efficacy,[12] which is determined mainly by the concentration of thrombin. The clotting time of fibrinogen plateaus at a thrombin concentration of 20 U/mL is constant to 1,000 U/mL. With fibrin sealants, lower thrombin concentrations in the range of 4 to approximately 100 U/mL are often used when the surgeon requires or prefers some "working time" following application of the fibrin glue, such as is the case when securing skin grafts and flaps. Higher concentrations of thrombin yield rapid clot formation ideal for situations involving the sealing of tissues, or where rapid hemostasis of bleeding or oozing tissues is desired. At this point, there is no standard methodology for the measurement and reporting of mechanical properties of the clot and how they relate to hemostasis and sealing the wound.[15]

The multiple-donor homologous preparations are pooled to generate high concentrations of fibrinogen and factor XIII. Tisseel includes human thrombin and aprotinin as antifibrinolytic agents. The second-generation fibrin tissue adhesive Crosseal (Johnson & Johnson, New Brunswick, NJ) was approved by the FDA in 2003. Tisseel and Crosseal differ in the antifibrinolytic agents present in their formulations, with bovine aprotinin and tranexamic acid being added, respectively. Therefore, Tisseel should not be used in patients with a known hypersensitivity to bovine (factor V) protein.[16] On the other hand, Crosseal should be avoided in neurosurgery, where adverse neurologic symptoms may be encountered.[17]

Fibrin tissue adhesives can be applied using a dual cannula syringe, which involves two separate side-by-side channels. One channel expresses the fibrinogen component while the second component delivers the thrombin component. The device is effective in keeping the components separate until delivered to the desired location; however, this device deters adequate mixing of the two components, which is essential in order to achieve a well-formed fibrin clot. A second option of delivery is through the use of a dual-syringe applicator (eg, Duploject, Immuno AG, Vienna, Austria), which allows the fibrinogen and thrombin components to mix prior to delivery through a single needle cannula. This method allows for complete mixing between the two product components and results in a well developed fibrin clot. While this system is effective, it is difficult to control the thickness of application at a given site. At times, a thin layer of FTA is desired, such as in the case of securing skin grafts. In this case, an air-powered spray device (Tissomat, Immuno, Vienna, Austria), can be used. The device sprays each component from a separate port, with the components mixing in the air prior to reaching the desired field. This method of application is a highly effective method at both component mixing and at being able to control the amount of material delivered to a given site (Figure 3).[18]

Many studies have demonstrated the potential benefits of fibrin tissue adhesives in numerous areas of medicine, including craniofacial, maxillofacial, nerve anastomosis,[19,20] otologic surgery,[21] and cardiac surgery.[3] A number of investigations have involved the use of fibrin glue for the fixation of skin grafts.[13] The benefits reported from its use include improved hemostasis, improved graft adherence and take, as well as the potential for antibacterial effects.[22] There is also some scientific evidence that the use of fibrin glue may help to control scar formation when applied at the site of injury. Studies examining the effects of fibrin glue have stated that, for some indications, fibrin clots have been found to be undetectable on histologic and immunochemical section between 14 and 21 days post-application.[23,24] Wounds covered with fibrin also demonstrated decreased inflammation in an experimental dog model[25] and a reduction in skin graft contraction in a rat model.[26]

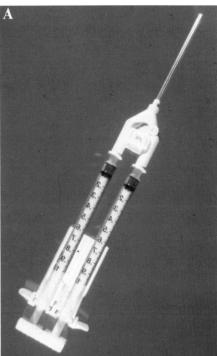

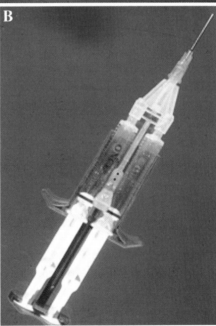

Figure 3. In a dual cannula syringe, the fibrinogen and thrombin components are delivered through distinct ports (*A*). The system allows for application of small volumes to precise locations without causing clotting in the cannula. Minimal mixing of the two components is achieved using this method of application. The fibrinogen and thrombin components are expressed through a common tip applicator (*B*). The device allows for controlled delivery of fibrin adhesive. The common needle port also allows for excellent product mixing during delivery. With the spray applicator, the two components are expressed through aerosolized spray tips, which are slightly angled toward each other (*C*). Delivery of fibrin adhesive using a spray applicator results in excellent mixing of the two components. Thickness of application can be controlled by the number of sprays to a given site.

The successful use of fibrin sealant in facial plastic and reconstructive surgery is well documented in the literature. Fibrin glue has been used in rhytidectomy, where application under skin flaps helps to obliterate dead space, promote hemostasis, decrease seroma formation, and possibly aid in neovascularization of the flap. One retrospective review showed that the overall incidence of postoperative hematomas following parotidectomy was 18% (six patients) in the non-fibrin tissue adhesive treated group and 6% (two patients) in the fibrin tissue adhesive treated group, although this was not significant.[27] A study by Fleming[28] demonstrated decreased hematoma formation with fibrin sealant application and decreased need for surgical drains following rhytidectomy. Postoperative drain output was also shown to be decreased by Marchac and Greensmith.[29] Fezza and colleagues performed a prospective nonrandomized study with fibrin sealant in patients undergoing rhytidectomy.[30] Drains were only placed in patients not receiving the tissue adhesive. They concluded that bruising and swelling were significantly decreased in the fibrin tissue adhesive group on the first postoperative day. They also reported a mean decrease in operative time with use of the tissue adhesive.

Fibrin tissue adhesive has been shown to be useful in a variety of other procedures in facial plastic and reconstructive surgery. Mandel used fibrin sealant as an alternative method of wound closure in blepharoplasty.[31] It has also been shown to be successful in fixation during endoscopy of the forehead.[32] One of the more unique applications was shown in rhinoplasty to correct or prevent a pollybeak deformity.[33] The authors hypothesized that fibrin glue would eliminate dead space and prevent hematoma formation to facilitate skin redraping. The supratip deformity was corrected successfully in all 30 patients treated with fibrin glue.

It is important to note that fibrin tissue adhesives will help achieve hemostasis even in the presence of inherited coagulation deficits and coagulopathies. Despite the benefits of tissue adhesives, some argue that the closure of the dead space produces a dense architecture that inhibits angiogenesis and vascular ingrowth.[13,34,35] In addition, these tissue adhesives are considered to be bioactively inert, since they do not possess growth factors or cytokines to recruit immune cells and fibroblasts that are essential in wound healing. The limitations noted with the use of fibrin adhesives relative to wound healing has aided the development of platelet-rich plasma, which provides a rich source of growth factors to accelerate the wound-healing process.

PLATELET-RICH PLASMA AND PLATELET GELS

Fibrin tissue adhesives are platelet-poor and thus do not significantly enhance the wound-healing response. Their primary roles are to obtain hemostasis and seal wounds and flaps. They do not offer the benefit of accelerated postoperative wound healing, since they lack the growth factors and cytokines found in platelets. Platelet-rich plasma, however, has a platelet concentration well above normal baseline and has been found to enhance tissue healing. Currently PRP is defined as a concentration of 1,000,000 platelets/microliter in a volume of 5 mL of plasma.[36]

Wound healing is a complex interaction among cells, proteins, and circulating factors. Many of these factors, such as von Willebrand's factor, TGF-β, platelet factor 4, interleukin-1, EGF, and PDGF are released by activated platelets. Many of these growth factors are chemoattractants and mitogens for immune cells and fibroblasts. PDGF has been shown to enhance wound healing in chronic wounds[37] and found to be absent in chronic, nonhealing wounds.[23] PDGF is a chemoattractant and mitogen for macrophages and fibroblasts. It also activates collagenase to assist in the remodeling stage of wound healing. TGF-β has also been shown to enhance wound healing in chronic wounds. Specifically, it stimulates collagen, proteoglycan, elastin, and fibronectin synthesis.[34]

Platelet gels consist of a concentrated PRP combined with thrombin and calcium chloride. They are prepared from autologous whole blood that is obtained in the immediate preoperative period. Differential centrifugation fractionates the whole blood into a concentrated PRP, prior to the addition of thrombin and calcium chloride. (Figure 4). Because they are autologous, there is no risk of viral transmission. Previous experiments have shown benefit with bone and soft-tissue healing using PRP with 1,000,000 cells/μL, and thus PRP is defined as a 5-mL volume of plasma at this concentration.[36] The increased cellularity allows it to be bioactive with enhanced tissue repair and regeneration. Finally, in contrast to the dense architecture produced by fibrin adhesives, the matrix created by platelet gels allows for the in-growth of capillaries, thereby promoting angiogenesis.

PRP has seven known growth factors: PDGF-AA, PDGF-BB, PDGF-AB, TGF-β1, TGF-β2, VEGF, and EGF. The relative concentrations of the growth factors found in vivo is maintained in the PRP harvesting procedure.[36] A study by Eppley and colleagues investigated the content of PRP, PDGF, TGF-β, VEGF, EGF, and insulin-like growth factor-1 (IGF-1).[38] The various growth factors were measured using an enzyme-linked immunosorbent assay (ELISA). The investigators determined that platelet concentration was increased eightfold compared to whole blood,

with a corresponding increase in the concentrations of all growth factors except for IGF-1. In addition, there was no increase in platelet activation during the concentration procedure.

Several new products are currently under design for the rapid and reliable production of PRP. Tabletop systems such as the SmartPReP Autologous Platelet Concentrate System (Harvest Technologies Corp, Plymouth, MA) and the Magellan Autologous Separator (Medtronic, Inc, Minneapolis, MN) are being refined for intraoperative use for rapid preparation of platelet-rich and platelet-poor plasma from a 20 to 120 cc sample of blood. (Figure 5) The system is designed to be used by operating room personnel without the need for an additional technician. Man and colleagues described the experience with a tabletop system as easy to use and highly effective in producing an autologous fibrin tissue adhesive or platelet gel.[10] Studies suggest that preparation of autologous products using such systems would be cost-effective compared to commercial products. In addition to other well-known applications, platelet gel has been used as an adjunct during liposculpture procedures to enhance longevity of the injected fat, as well as laser resurfacing procedures. The platelet gel is applied directly to the skin surface as a wound dressing resulting in faster healing with decreased erythema.

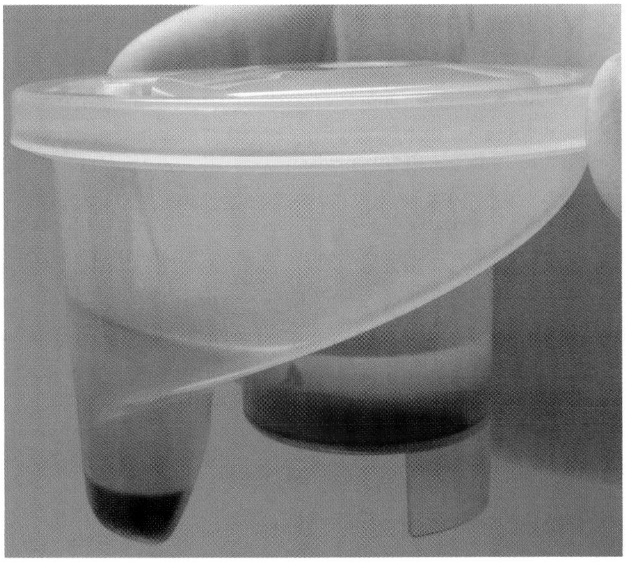

Figure 4. Platelet recovery chamber from Harvest Technologies (SmartPReP 2). Whole blood undergoes a dual spin and decanting process to capture concentrated platelets (left chamber at bottom). Platelet processing requires less than 15 minutes.

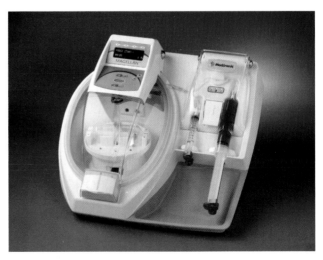

Figure 5. Magellan Autologous Separator (Medtronic, Inc, Minneapolis, MN), one of the products designed for rapid production of PRP.

Platelet gels have been shown to accelerate wound healing in a variety of other applications. They have been shown to accelerate the ingrowth of autologous grafts used for osteointegration and alveolar ridge augmentation during mandibular reconstruction.[36] Powell and colleagues also showed in a pilot study that platelet gels may prevent or decrease edema or ecchymosis in the early postoperative phase following rhytidectomy.[39] Despite these successes, more investigation is necessary to determine the specific applications for platelet gels in facial plastic surgery and wound healing.

RECOMBINANT PLATELET-DERIVED GROWTH FACTOR

As discussed previously, PDGF and TGF-β are important growth factors involved in wound healing. PDGF has been shown to enhance closure of open wounds,[40] stimulate fibroblasts for connective tissue remodeling, help initiate the synthesis of extracellular matrix components for wound remodeling, and promote angiogenesis and help maintain normal vascular maturation. PDGF is stored in alpha granules of circulating platelets and is released during injury. It is also released by macrophages, vascular endothelial cells, fibroblasts, epithelial cells, and vascular smooth muscle cells later in the wound-healing process.[41] As a result of these benefits, a recombinant human platelet-derived growth factor (PDGF-BB) called becaplermin (Regranex; Ortho-McNeil Pharmaceuticals, Raritan, NJ) was approved by the FDA in 1998 in the treatment of nonischemic diabetic neuropathic ulcers.[42,43] It has other uses as well, and has been shown to successfully treat a refractory dermal wound in previously irradiated skin.[44]

FUTURE CONSIDERATIONS

The process of wound healing involves the synergistic interaction of plasma proteins working in unison toward the common goal of wound repair. Scientific investigation continues to explore and elucidate the mechanisms involved in the wound-healing process. As new knowledge and understanding come to light, the potential for invention and subsequent treatment alternatives in the area of wound healing will arise.

Enhancements in wound healing may involve new methods of PRP delivery, novel modulated carrier devices that enable the controlled release of platelet factors yielding optimum healing results without excessive—or even moderate—scarring. Or perhaps new ways of producing platelet-rich or "platelet-precise" fibrin tissue adhesives that might "jump start" the healing process during the hemostasis phase will be developed. Independent of the paths pursued, it certainly appears that the use of platelet-rich plasma and its associated growth factors will be an integral part of developing a wound-healing strategy.

The ultimate goal in the pursuit of wound healing is understood, and that goal is to achieve repair at the site of injury to its pre-injury status. While this goal is certainly substantial, and may be difficult—if not impossible—to attain, it offers a target, as well as a measurement, that science and medicine can use to evaluate the progress toward new and improved healing modalities.

REFERENCES

1. Rumalla VK, Borah GL. Cytokines, growth factors, and plastic surgery. Plast Rectonstr Surg 2002;18:27–33.
2. Bergel S. Uber Wirkungen des Fibrins. Dtsch Med Wochenschr 1909;35:663–5.
3. Taylor LM. Introduction: does the evidence justify the routine use of fibrin sealants in cardiovascular surgery? Cardiovasc Surg 2003;11:3–4.
4. Ellis DA, Shaikh A. The ideal tissue adhesive in facial plastic and reconstructive surgery. J Otolaryngol 1990;19:68–72.
5. Lebowitz RA, Hoffman RA, Roland TJ, et al. Autologous fibrin glue in the prevention of cerebrospinal fluid leak following acoustic neuroma surgery. Am J Otol 1995;16:172–274.
6. Sierra DH, Nissen AJ, Welch J. The use of fibrin glue in intracranial procedures: preliminary results. Laryngoscope 1990;100:360–3.
7. Bento RF, Miniti A. Anastomoses of the intratemporal facial nerve using fibrin tissue adhesive. Ear Nose Throat J 1993;72:663–72.
8. Siedentop KH, Chung S, Park JJ, et al. Evaluation of pooled fibrin sealant for ear surgery. Am J Otol 1997;18:660–4.

9. Toriumi DM, O'Grady KM. Surgical tissue adhesives in otolaryngology-head and neck surgery. Otolaryngol Clin North Am 1994;27:203–9.

10. Man D, Plosker H, Winland-Brown JE. The use of autologous platelet-rich plasma (platelet gel) and autologous platelet-poor plasma (fibrin glue) in cosmetic surgery. Plast Reconstr Surg 2001;107:229–37.

11. Alving BM, Weinstein MJ, Finlayson JS, et al. Fibrin sealant: summary of a conference on characteristics and clinical uses. Tranfusion 1995;35:783–90.

12. Martinowitz U, Saltz R. Fibrin sealant. Curr Opin Hematol 1996;3:395–402.

13. O'Grady KM, Agrawal A, Bhattacharyya TK, et al. An evaluation of fibrin tissue adhesive concentration and application thickness on skin graft survival. Laryngoscope 2000;110:1931–5.

14. Siedentop KH, Park JJ, Shah AN, et al. Safety and efficacy of currently available fibrin tissue adhesives. Am J Otolaryngol 2001;22:230–5.

15. Busuttil RW. A comparison of antifibrinolytic agents used in hemostatic fibrin sealants. J Am Coll Surg 2003;197:1021–8.

16. Baxter Healthcare Corp. Tisseel VH [package insert} 2000.

17. American Red Cross. Crosseal fibrin sealant (human) [package insert] 2003.

18. Sierra DH, O'Grady K, Toriumi DM, et al. Modulation of mechanical properties in multiple-component tissue adhesives. J Biomed Mater Res 2000;52:534–42.

19. Gestring GF, Lerner R, Requena R. The sutureless microanastamosis. Vasc Surg 1983;17:364–7.

20. Smahel J, Meyer VE, Bachem U. Glueing of peripheral nerves with fibrin: experimental studies. J Reconstr Microsurg 1987;3:211–20.

21. Siedentop KH, Harris DM, Loewy A. Experimental use of fibrin tissue adhesive in middle ear surgery. Laryngoscope 1983;93:1310–3.

22. Currie LJ, Sharpe JR, Martin R. The use of fibrin glue in skin grafts and tissue-engineered skin replacements: a review. Plast Reconstr Surg 2001;108:1713–26.

23. Saltz R, Sierra D, Feldman D, et al. Experimental and clinical applications of fibrin glue. Plast Reconstr Surg 1991;88:1005–15.

24. Auger FA, Guignard R, Lopez Valle AC, et al. Role and innocuity of Tisseel, a tissue glue, in the grafting process and in vivo evolution of human cultured epidermis. Br J Plast Surg 1993;46:136–142.

25. Bornemisza G, Tarsoly E, Mido I. Restoration of skin defects with fibrin glue. Acta Chir Hung 1986;27:249.

26. Brown DM, Barton BR, Young VL, et al. Decreased wound contraction with fibrin glue-treated skin grafts. Arch Surg 1992;127:404–6.

27. Depondt J, Kova VN, Nasser T, et al. Use of fibrin glue in parotidectomy closure. Laryngoscope 1996;106:784–7.

28. Fleming I. Fibrin glue in facelifts. Facial Plast Surg 1992;8:79–88.

29. Marchac D, Greensmith AL. Early postoperative efficacy of fibrin glue in face lifts: a prospective randomized trial. Plast Reconstr Surg 2005;115:911–6.

30. Fezza JP, Cartwright M, Mack W. The use of aerosolized fibrin glue in face-lift surgery. Plast Reconstr Surg 2002;110:658–64.

31. Mandel MA. Minimal suture blepharoplasty: closure of incisions with autologous fibrin glue. Aesthetic Plast Surg 1992;16:269–72.

32. Marchac D, Ascherman J, Arnaud E. Fibrin glue fixation in forehead endoscopy: evaluation of our experience with 206 cases. Plast Reconstr Surg 1997;100:704–12.

33. Conrad K, Yoskovitch A. The use of fibrin glue in the correction of pollybeak deformity. Arch Facial Plast Surg 2003;5:522–7.

34. Bhanot S, Alex JC. Current applications of platelet gels in facial plastic surgery. Facial Plast Surg 2002;18:27–33.

35. Byrne DJ, Hardy J, Wood RA, et al. Effect of fibrin glues on the mechanical properties of healing wounds. Br J Surg 1991;78:841–3.

36. Marx RE. Platelet-rich plasma (PRP): what is PRP and what is not PRP? Implant Dent 2001;10:225–8.

37. Steed DL. Diabetic ulcer study group. Clinical evaluation of recombinant human derived growth factor for the treatment of lower extremity diabetic ulcers. J Vasc Surg 1995;21:71–81.

38. Eppley BL, Woodell JE, Higgins J. Platelet quantification and growth factor analysis from platelet-rich plasma: implications for wound healing. Plast Reconstr Surg 2004;114:1502–8.

39. Powell DM, Chang E, Farrior EH. Recovery from deep-plane rhytidectomy following unilateral wound treatment with autologous platelet gel: a pilot study. Arch Facial Plast Surg 2001;3:245–50.

40. Saba AA, Freedman BM, Gaffield JW, et al. Topical platelet-derived growth factor enhances wound closure in the absence of wound contraction: an experimental and clinical study. Ann Plast Surg 2002;49:62–6.

41. Lynch SE, Nixon JC, Colvin RB, et al. Role of platelet-derived growth factors in wound healing synergistic effects with other growth factors. Proc Natl Acad Sci U S A 1987;84:7696–700.

42. Steed DL. Modifying the wound healing response with exogenous growth factors. Clin Plast Surg 1998;25:397–405.

43. Wieman T. Clinical efficacy of becaplermin (rhPDGF-BB) gel. Am J Surg 1998;176 (Suppl 2A):74–9.

44. Hom DB, Manivel JC. Promoting healing with recombinant human platelet-derived growth factor-BB in a previously irradiated problem wound. Laryngoscope 2003;113:1566–71.

29

Growth Factors—Modulators of Wound Healing

Joseph A. Greco III, MD; Lillian B. Nanney, PhD

The very nature of wound healing remains both equally complex and fascinating. The process is one of the most fundamental entities for the survival of our species. The interplay between multiple cell lineages, cytokines, and the microenvironment can result in a spectrum of results, from complete healing to extensive failure to heal.

This chapter will focus on growth factors— key modulators of wound healing. Specifically, it will cover growth factor mechanisms that drive the healing process. Current wound-healing enhancement strategies for cytokines approved by the United States Food and Drug Administration (FDA) and for experimental formulations in multiple stages of development will be discussed. Growth factor therapy remains a vast area for potential breakthroughs. Robust initiatives from many groups continue to strive for the magic bullet that will expedite the process of wound healing.

GROWTH FACTORS AND WOUND HEALING

Growth factors have been referred to as the engines that drive wound healing.[1] The three stages or phases of wound repair (inflammation, proliferation, and remodeling) should be viewed as an overlapping spectrum as opposed to a rigid linear sequence of events (see Chapter 1). Growth factors are active in varying capacities, from the inciting injury to the final stages of maturation. The absolute presence of growth factors seems less important than their relative concentrations with respect to the other growth factors also present in the wound-healing milieu.[2] Moreover, growth-factor–mediated events are dependent on the presence of specific receptors. Growth factors act within a microenvironment filled with other cytokines, proteases, matrix precursors, free radicals, and microbes, all with the potential to modify their effects.

In addition to activity in all phases of wound healing, growth factors exhibit all three mechanisms of cell signaling—autocrine, paracrine, and endocrine.[3] This diversity of function allows for local, regional, and systemic effects, but their main function, intuitively, remains at the site of healing. To date, the use of growth factors as a therapeutic intervention has marginally outperformed the standards of optimal wound care, which include minimizing tissue trauma, aggressive débridement of necrotic tissue and cellular debris, and providing a moist, clean environment.[4,5]

An understanding of the potential clinical effectiveness from growth factor therapy must include a basic knowledge of the proteins individually, where each is produced and how each is believed to function. Most of our knowledge concerning growth factors comes from in vitro and animal research.[6] The exact expression, sequencing, what is known about the interplay between growth factors in the grand scheme of wound healing in vivo continues to remain sketchy.

GROWTH FACTORS: ORIGIN, FUNCTION, AND EVIDENCE FOR THERAPEUTIC USE

For the purpose of this chapter, we will focus on the following better characterized growth factors: platelet-derived growth factor (PDGF), keratinocyte growth factor (KGF), transforming growth factor-β (TGF-β), transforming growth factor-α (TGF-α) and epidermal growth factor (EGF), fibroblast growth factor (FGF), and vascular endothelial growth factor (VEGF). The cellular source, function, and commercially available products of each are summarized in Table 29-1.

In addition to providing a foundation of basic science, the evidence supporting each protein's clinical use as a wound-healing enhancer will be presented. It remains paramount to remember that under the current stipulations, a growth factor must augment wound healing above optimal standards in order to gain FDA approval as a Biologic Response Modifier.[4]

PDGF

Platelet derived growth factor belongs within a superfamily of growth factors.[7] PDGF exists as five isoforms based on the gene splicing of five unique protein chains—AA, BB, AB, CC, DD.[1,8] Platelets, as well as macrophages, endothelial cells, and keratinocytes, serve as sources of PDGF. After tissue injury, PDGF is released by degranulation of platelet alpha granules.[1,9] Two major PDGF receptors exist. Both receptor tyrosine kinases show a high degree of structural homology, although each has independent function and predilection for different isomers of PDGF.[10,11] At the inflammatory stage, the first effects after release include chemoattraction of neutrophils, other immune cells, and fibroblasts.[2] Once bound, the PDGF-receptor complex on fibroblasts causes replication and acts in concert

Table 29-1. SUMMARY OF GROWTH FACTOR SOURCE, FUNCTION, AND COMMERCIAL AVAILABILITY			
Growth Factor	Source	Function	Commercial Product.
PDGF: PDGF-AA, PDGF-BB, PDGF-AB, PDGF-CC, PDGF-DD	Platelets, macrophages, endothelial cells, keratinocytes	Chemotactic for neutrophils, macrophages, lympocytes, and fibroblasts; Mitogenic for fibroblasts; causes fibroblasts to produce collagen, hyaluronic acid and MMPs.	Becaplermin (rPDGF-BB) (Regranex, Ethicon Inc., Somerville, NJ) FDA-approved for diabetic neuropathic non-ischemic ulcers.
KGF: KGF-1, KGF-2	Fibroblasts, keratinocytes	Chemotactic and mitogenic for keratinocytes; Stimulate maturation and differentiation; NOT mitogenic for fibroblasts	Palifermin (rKGF-2) (Kepivance, Amgen Inc., Thousand Oaks, CA); FDA-approved for prevention/treatment of oral mucositis in patients undergoing chemotherapy for blood malignancies.
TGF-β: TGF-β1, TGF-β2, TGF-β3	Platelets, macrophages, fibroblasts, lymphocytes, endothelial cells	Chemotactic for neutrophils, macrophages, lymphocytes and fibroblasts; Stimulates keratinocytes and aids in angiogenesis; TGF-β1 & β2 strong inducers of collagen formation and implicated in excessive fibrosis; TGF-β3 implicated in scarless healing	Recombinant TGF-β3 (Juvista, Renovo, Manchester, UK) in Phase II trials; seeking indication for scar prevention.
FGF: acidic FGF, basic FGF, (multiple molecules in each isoform)	Macrophages, mast cells, lymphocytes, endothelial cells, fibroblasts	Chemotactic and mitogenic for fibroblasts and keratinocytes; plays a role in fibroblast proliferation, angiogenesis, and matrix deposition; Stimulates keratinocyte migration	CG531315-05 (rHuFGF-20) (Velafermin, CuraGen, Branford, CT) in Phase II trials, seeking indication similar to Kepivance for oral mucositis.
VEGF	Keratinocytes, fibroblasts, macrophages	Mitogenic for endothelial cells; increases vasopermeability; angiogenesis	Topical VEGF under development (Genentech, San Francisco, CA).
EGF: Similar to TGF-α	Keratinocytes, platelets, macrophages	Mitogenic for fibroblasts and keratinocytes; chemotactic for keratinocytes	

EGF = epidermal growth factor; FGF = fibroblast growth factor ; FDA = United States Food and Drug Administration; KGF = keratinocyte growth factor; MMP = matrix metalloproteinase; PDGF = platelet-derived growth factor ; TGF = transforming growth factor; VEGF = vascular endothelial growth factor.

with other growth factors to produce collagen secretion.[6] PDGF-receptor binding and signaling stimulates production of extracellular matrix precursors, such as fibronectin and hyaluronic acid, as well as matrix-metalloproteinases.[12]

Additionally, the different isoforms display unique functional differences from one another in vivo. Lepisto and colleagues studied a rat wound model and found evidence that, although the AB and BB isomers provoked healing tissue in the created wounds, AB seemed to elicit more collagen production from fibroblasts, whereas the BB isomer appeared largely mitogenic.[8]

PDGF, specifically the BB isomer, has been widely studied. In 1992 Robson and colleagues provided promising results by demonstrating that recombinant PDGF-BB (rPDGF-BB) accelerated wound healing in chronic ulcers. The group accomplished this by randomly assigning 20 patients with chronic dermal ulcers to receive placebo, 1, 10, or 100 μg/ml of rPDGF-BB applied topically for 28 days. At the end of the treatment period, they detected increased wound healing in the 100 μg/ml group based on depth and size of the defect. Histologic analysis revealed that the rPDGF-BB–treated wounds showed greater fibroblast presence and increased neovascularization. Additionally, the group also concluded that there was no delay in the normal sequence of wound healing in those patients receiving rPDGF-BB therapy.[13,14]

Another randomized control trial for diabetic-neuropathic wounds added evidence to support the use of PDGF-BB as a wound healing therapy. In a randomized, prospective study of 118 patients with diabetic ulcers that had been débrided and were not ischemic based on oxygen measurements in the wound bed, Steed reported that a statistically significant number of patients (48% compared to 25%, $p = .01$) achieved complete wound healing during the study duration (20 weeks).[15] Once analyzed, the results also showed no statistically significant difference in adverse events. Furthermore, the data also suggested that, not only did the wounds in the treatment group heal, those patients healed 35 days faster than the placebo cohort.

In 1998, a phase III, multicenter, randomized, placebo-controlled study of 382 patients with chronic non-healing diabetic neuropathic ulcers was published. The statistically significant results proved rPDGF-BB to be an effective therapeutic modality that increased the incidence of complete closure, and did so faster and with an equivalent adverse event profile compared to placebo.[16]

The consistent themes in these trials and other studies supported the eventual 1998 FDA approval of becaplermin (rPDGF-BB, trade name Regranex, Cthicon Inc., Somerville, NJ) for use on lower extremity diabetic neuropathic non-ischemic ulcers. In considering the approval of becaplermin, the FDA reviewed numerous studies, which included over 7,000 patients. When the data were analyzed, without exception there was a 10% increase in the rate of healing with use of becaplermin.[1]

KGF

Keratinocyte growth factor (KGF) is currently the most potent stimulator of keratinocyte migration.[1] This member of the fibroblast growth factor family, based on similar allele homology, exists as two known isomers—KGF-1 and KGF-2. It is produced predominantly by fibroblasts, but is also synthesized by endothelial cells.[9] Interestingly, the KGF receptor is mainly expressed on epithelial cells of epidermal origin only, whereas KGF itself is produced by cells with mesenchymal origin.[17] KGF is not abundantly present in normal human dermis, but its presence is strongly induced by dermal trauma. Following receptor binding to either skin keratinocytes or fibroblasts, additional KGF is produced and keratinocytes become increasingly proliferative. Additionally, receptor activation increases the intracellular production of enzymes to protect the keratinocyte from reactive oxygen species.[18] By functioning as a strong inducer of keratinocyte activity, KGF is vital in directing re-epithelialization of human wounds through keratinocyte differentiation.[3,17,19] Although

KGF is exceedingly similar to FGF, it has no mitogenic activity towards fibroblasts.[20]

KGF-2, also known as FGF-10, has been used in several animal models to improve wound healing, wound strength, and time to closure. In 1999, Xia and colleagues[17] used an ischemic rabbit ear ulcer model published earlier in the decade by Ahn and Mustoe[21] to study the effects of KGF-2 on ischemic ulcers in both young and aged rabbits. Several important results came from this study. First, KGF-2–treated ear wounds showed a statistically significant amount of neo-epithelialization compared to controls in young rabbits. This finding supports the use of KGF-2 in ischemic wounds. Furthermore, the extent of granulation tissue coverage in the wound-bed increased by 133% and 151% at doses of 5μg per wound and 15μg per wound, respectively.

Although the exact mechanism of endogenous KGF in normal wound healing is not completely understood, additional animal studies have been published that support KGF's role in normal healing in vivo. In their study, Brauchle and colleagues concluded that impaired wounds show downregulation of KGF messenger ribonucleic acid (mRNA).[22] Tagashira and colleagues, using a mouse model, found that KGF-2 mRNA was vastly induced as early as 1 day after injury.[23] The findings in these two publications support the hypothesis that regulated expression of KGF, as with other growth factors, is vital to the sequence that produces tissue healing. Moreover, Jimenez and Rampy showed statistically significant increases in breaking strength, epidermal thickness, and wound collagen content in KGF-2–treated incisional wounds in rats. The authors concluded that KGF-2 could enhance the healing of surgical wounds.[19]

Continued research postulated that KGF-2, applied topically, could stimulate faster re-epithelialization. Athymic rats received allografted human skin. The rats were treated with recombinant (r) KGF-1 or rKGF-2. Those receiving rKGF-2 showed accelerated re-epithelialization.[24] In 2001, Robson and colleagues expanded beyond the previously reported effects

of KGF-2.[25] His group reported the results of a large phase II, multicenter, randomized, double-blind, placebo-controlled trial of the use of manufactured rKGF-2 (repifermin) on venous stasis ulcers—wounds with notoriously slow re-epithelialization. Ninety-three patients with chronic venous stasis ulcers were enrolled in the study across 15 centers. They received control, 20μg/cm^2, or 60μg/cm^2 rKGF-2 sprayed topically twice a week for 12 weeks. Primary outcome measures were based on the percentage of wound closure at the end of the study interval. Although the results were only significant with subset analysis of smaller and less chronic wounds (≤ 15 cm^2 and ≤ 18 months), the data were sufficiently convincing for the undertaking of larger studies. Apparently, however, the sponsor ended the phase IIB trials because the data did not meet the primary end point of statistically better wound closure at 20 weeks.[3] Nevertheless, these large prospective trials serve as strong indicators of safety because there were no clinically or statistically significant differences in the adverse event profiles of placebo and repifermin.[25]

Another company, Amgen Inc., also manufactures rKGF-2 under the name palifermin (trade name Kepivance). In December 2004, this cytokine-based drug received FDA approval for use in preventing and treating oral mucositis in patients with blood-borne malignancies (ie leukemias and lymphomas) receiving chemotherapy and radiation. One of the first clinical research endeavors using palifermin in humans was a phase I trial reported by Meropol and colleagues.[26] The purpose of the study was to evaluate the maximum tolerable dose of palifermin, the safety profile, and, as secondary endpoints, the incidence of severe mucositis. Although the study was not designed specifically for evaluation of mucositis protection, the data showed enough of a trend to warrant further investigation.[26]

Subsequently, two large randomized studies have been published that directly contributed to the drug's FDA approval. In a phase III, randomized, placebo-controlled, double-blind, multicenter trial, 212 patients, 106 in each study arm, were given either a placebo or a palifermin (60μg/kg/day) intravenous injection for 3 days before total body irradiation, followed by etoposide chemotherapy. Severe (WHO grade 3 to 4) oral mucositis only developed in 63% of the treatment group, compared to 98% in the placebo group. These results were statistically significant. Furthermore, the safety profile of rKGF-2 was similar to placebo.[27] Based on these findings, Kepivance is rapidly becoming a widespread treatment option in the preventive management of oral mucositis in this group of cancer patients. A phase III clinical trial is currently under way to determine if the effects oral mucositis associated with hematologic malignancies also applies to oral mucositis stemming from head and neck cancers.

TGF-β

Transforming growth factor (TGF)-β has been studied over several decades. The literature on its structure, numerous functions, and possible clinical applications is voluminous. The TGF-β family of cytokines is considered to be exceedingly multifunctional, with numerous roles in the microenvironment of cell signaling, differentiation, and target gene activity.[28] Three known isomers have been characterized in wound repair—TGF-β1, TGF-β2, and TGF-β3. Almost all cells express serine-threonine kinase type I and II TGF-β1 receptors.[6,28] The exact function of TGF-β depends on the context, including the presence of other cytokines in the microenvironment, the cell it interacts with, and the state of differentiation of all the cell lineages involved in the specific signal process.[28–30]

Platelets, macrophages, fibroblasts, lymphocytes, and endothelial cells produce TGF-β. Some of the more noted effects of this family of growth factors are chemotaxis for neutrophils, macrophages, lymphocytes, and fibroblasts.[9,31] TGF-β1 and TGF-β2 also serve as strong inducers of extracellular matrix deposition and collagen formation.[28,32] In short, as noted earlier, TGF-β plays a role in many in vivo reactions related to inflammation and wound healing. Early studies

by Sporn, led him to postulate that TGF-β acts like a switch, or master growth factor, turning on or off various intercellular pathways.[30]

The literature contains a plethora of basic science and animal studies plus a few phase I and II trials attempting to elucidate potential clinical applications. Nevertheless, no recombinant formulation has been tested to date as a wound-healing modulator in prospective, randomized phase III trials.

TGF-β1 remains the most studied of the three isomers. Conflicting data exist in regard to its role as a wound-healing adjunct. On the favorable side, Beck and colleagues showed that topically delivered TGF-β1 could overcome the steroid-induced healing impairments in rats and rabbits.[33] The results showed that incisional wounds in the treatment group exhibited increased breaking strength. Furthermore, the data confirmed that, in ischemic ulcers on rat ears, TGF-β1 stimulated accelerated re-epithelialization compared to controls. By contrast, a more recent study applying TGF-β1 to ischemic wounds of aged rabbits demonstrated no enhancement of wound healing.[34] This finding is important in refuting attempts to extrapolate TGF-β1 use to the clinical arena, as the bulk of the wounds that would require treatment suffer from ischemia and chronicity.

The other side of the TGF-β debate focuses on literature that implicates TGF-β in scar formation, excessive granulation tissue, and fibrosis. Elevated TGF-β levels exist in medical conditions where excessive fibrosis is the pathologic hallmark.[31] Although studies connecting TGF-β1 and TGF-β2 to hypertrophic scarring and keloid formation have not been conclusive, data supporting this hypothesis have been published. One such small study conducted by Lee and colleagues demonstrated higher levels of TGF-β1 and TGF-β2 protein expression in keloid fibroblast cultures.[35]

In 1999, the data from a phase II, randomized, multicenter, placebo controlled trial comparing topical TGF-β2 to control in healing diabetic ulcers was presented by lead investigator Dr. Martin Robson.[36] All 177 patients in this randomized trial received optimal wound care (aggressive débridement, off-loading of weight for the affected limb, and compressive dressings). The treatment groups, which received optimal wound care plus TGF-β2 at varying strengths, showed a statistically significant improvement in wound closure for patients receiving the highest dose tested (5μg/cm^2). The data also demonstrated a trend in improvement in all dose groups and solidified the safety of TGF-β2.

Recently, increasing interest has been sparked by TGF-β3. A small randomized pilot study of 14 patients with chronic pressure ulcers treated with TGF-β3 done by Hirshberg and colleagues provided encouraging results in the ability of TGF-β3 to augment standard healing of chronic wounds.[37] Novartis, the company manufacturing a recombinant TGF-β3 formulation, sponsored a large phase III trial. The results apparently did not meet study goal endpoints and were not published.[1]

Ongoing work by Professor Mark Ferguson and colleagues with manufacturer Renovo, however, has demonstrated considerably positive results with the use of recombinant TGF-β3 (Juvista) in scar reduction and wound repair. In a study design using an intradermal injection at the time of operative wounding, visual comparisons and histologic evidence support improved wound healing, even in patients prone to scar formation. Several phase II trials have been completed in the United Kingdom, and similar protocols are under way in the U.S. aimed at substantiating these claims.[38] Regarding the ability of TGF-β isoforms to clinically and statistically enhance healing, the research world remains divided.

FGF

Fibroblast growth factor is a large family of proteins, including the first two isoforms discovered—acidic and basic FGF, also called FGF-1 and FGF-2, respectively. Two commonly studied members, FGF-7 and FGF-10, are also known as KGF-1 and KGF-2, as discussed previously.[9] One known receptor type has been identified that binds to all FGF isoforms with varying affinities. FGFs are released from multiple cell lineages, including macrophages, mast cells, T cells, endothial cells, and fibroblasts; they are known for their role in fibroblast proliferation, angiogenesis, and matrix deposition.[7,39,40]

As with all of the growth factors, animal models have yielded data that support the role of exogenous FGF supplementation in improving wound healing. An induced rat diabetes model demonstrated that a one-time injection (at the time of wounding) of basic FGF could increase the breaking strength of these wounds when compared to controls.[41] These findings suggested that basic FGF could overcome the deficiencies in the diabetic healing model. Likewise, Oda and colleagues demonstrated histologically increasing amounts of epithelialization and cell proliferation in rat palatal mucosal wounds treated with basic FGF at the time of injury.[42]

Promising data comparable to the studies cited above have fostered clinical trials in human subjects in attempts to support recombinant basic FGF as a wound-healing adjunct. In 1998, a large phase III, multicenter trial was completed in China that compared the effects of recombinant FGF to placebo in the healing of a multitude of wounds, including burns, operative defects, and chronic ulcers. The data indicated improvements in the quality and velocity of wound healing.[43]

In the United States, a large phase II, multicenter, randomized, double-blind, placebo-controlled trial of the safety and efficacy of CG53135-05 (recombinant human FGF-20, Velafermin, Cunagen Corp., Branford, CT) enrolled subjects to evaluate a single dose of Valefermin in the prevention of oral mucositis, one objective being to provide convincing data to gain FDA approval similar to the indication for Kepivance.

VEGF

Research over the last two decades has led to the widespread acceptance of vascular endothelial growth factor as the primary angiogenic growth factor. This cytokine is released in large amounts by keratinocytes, but is also produced by macrophages and fibroblasts.[7] More recently, it has also been shown to be secreted by platelets and peripherally circulating monocytes.[44,45] The main function of VEGF is to increase vascular permeability at the capillary level to allow the influx of inflammatory cells involved in the wound-healing paradigm into the location of tissue trauma. It is also quite mitogenic to existing endothelial cells, and as mentioned, is vital for angiogenesis.[46,47]

Hypoxia and cell disruption are well-known characteristics of tissue injury. These two features are also strong inducers of the up-regulation of VEGF and its receptor.[44] In wounds that do not heal (ones contaminated with gram negative bacteria delivering lipopolysaccharide), Power and colleagues showed a decrease in VEGF receptor expression on the endothelial cell membrane.[48] Additionally, these results were enhanced in a hypoxic environment. Curiously, in the absence of a lipopolysaccharide challenge, endothelial proliferation in response to VEGF was not affected.

Animal studies have been conducted with supplemental VEGF in wound healing. Although the literature is convincing concerning the role of VEGF in angiogenesis and that angiogenesis is vital in wound healing, it is not as concrete regarding the capacity of VEGF to enhance wound healing. Galiano and colleagues studied genetically diabetic mice that were surgically wounded.[49] The investigators made two wounds on the backs of each mouse. In the treatment group, each subject received 20µg of recombinant VEGF in one wound and vehicle only in the other. Control subjects received vehicle only in both wounds. The results showed significantly accelerated repair with VEGF therapy. Furthermore, the wounds treated only with vehicle on mice that also received VEGF contralaterally, showed improvements compared with the mice having no exposure to VEGF whatsoever. This demonstrated a potential systemic effect of VEGF therapy, which was confirmed by polymerase chain reaction analysis indicating increased presence of PDGF-BB and basic FGF. It seems plausible that the ability of VEGF to induce other growth factors was responsible for the positive effects of the study. Although encouraging results were ultimately observed, important confounding outcomes were also noted. VEGF-treated wounds exhibited excessive granulation tissue. Furthermore, the wounds looked immature and friable, and were not tested for breaking strength. Ultimately, the results were favorable only for time to heal and not for quality of healing.

Even so, VEGF still holds promise for wound-healing augmentation. Continued research focusing on ischemic wounds remains an active area of study, especially in the cardiac and peripheral vascular realms. Given VEGF's strong angiogenic properties, researchers have hopes that increasing its presence via direct application or through systemic up-regulation would increase new vessel formation in the wound bed. In studies as of this writing, it has been demonstrated that VEGF is present at supranormal levels in the plasma of patients with diabetes, atherosclerosis, and peripheral vascular disease. However, this does not correlate with increases in wound healing or increasing functional capillary density.[44,50,51] Moreover, since VEGF in and of itself does not directly stimulate re-epithelialization or matrix deposition it may well find a niche as a significant adjunctive treatment used in concert with other growth factors in hypoxic wounds.[1]

In another light, VEGF's role in tumorigenesis and the potential to block capillary neogenesis by downregulating VEGF production is under extensive study in various malignancies, including those in the head and neck. A multitude of clinical trials using a wide array of anti-VEGF combinations are enrolling patients. That said, a randomized trial or prospective human study using VEGF as a wound-healing enhancer has not yet reached the world literature.

EGF

Epidermal growth factor is a member of a very large, highly similar family of cytokines that includes TGF-α, heparin binding (HB)-EGF, amphiregulin and epiregulin. They all bind to EGF receptor types (ErbBs) that are found on nearly every cell in the body.[10,52] EGF is secreted in large amounts by epithelial cells and acts in an autocrine fashion.[53] In the skin these molecules are produced by keratinocytes, but in the wound-healing context, they are also released by platelets and macrophages into the wound environment.[7,9]

The potential for EGF augmentation of wound healing in human subjects was presented in the 1989 New England Journal of Medicine article by Brown and colleagues.[54] A prospective, randomized, double-blind trial of skin graft donor-site healing with topical EGF versus control was done that studied 12 patients with donor sites on each thigh. One of the wounds was treated with standard care of silver sulfadiazine alone. The other was treated with silver sulfadiazine plus topical EGF. The authors demonstrated a statistically significant rate of 100% healing with the addition of EGF in this severely burned patient population.

A few years later, Cohen and colleagues published another prospective study on 17 healthy subjects who volunteered to have split-thickness wounds created on both flanks in order to compare silver sulfadiazine to silver sulfadiazine plus EGF.[53] The results were not significant but did show a trend towards the EGF group. Additionally, trends towards enhancement of wound healing were shown in venous ulcers in 35 patients receiving recombinant EGF.[55] Failing to gain statistical significance in the primary endpoint, the study demonstrated a favorable safety profile and clinically appreciable wound improvement, although a lucrative position in the wound care market was never established.

GROWTH FACTORS: ROLES IN THE FACE AND NECK

Specific wound-healing models using growth factor supplementation for the face and neck are non-existent. Cutaneous ulcers in this region remain uncommon, but chronic wounds follow-ing trauma, operation, radiation, or epithelial ulcers (like ones from stomatitis) remain a persistent problem. Thus, skin healing augmentation strategies from other sites of the body are potentially applicable. As for direct application to the face and neck, the data on KGF-2 and the indication of its manufactured formulation, Kepivance, in preventing oral mucositis was presented earlier. At present, this is the sole FDA-approved use of a growth factor directly related to otorhinolaryngology.

What follows below is a miscellaneous mix of laboratory studies that may one day lead to clinical relevance for practicing physicians including those in otorhinolaryngology, dermatology, ophthalmology, and plastic surgery fields, who seek to favorably modulate wound-healing challenges within the head and neck region.

EGF has been shown in neonatal rats to enhance the ability of auditory epithelium to regrow hair cells following aminoglycoside toxicity.[56] Whether this finding applies to humans is unknown. Along similar lines, in vitro addition of FGF-1 enhances growth of spiral ganglion cells.[57] This discovery gives credence to the possibility of using FGF-1 in cochlear implantation as a means of protecting and/or supporting new ganglion cells.

As regards tympanic membrane perforations, EGF, FGF-2 and PDGF-AA have all shown improvement of healing parameters in animal models.[10,58,59] However, the experimental data have not been tested in any clinical trials.

Juvista, a recombinant TGF-β3 product described earlier, may gain approval as a pure growth factor enhancer for all surgically created wounds. If the promise of this product comes to fruition, this growth factor-based therapy will be add to the armamentarium of health care professionals aiming to augment wound repair.[62]

Over-expression of growth factor receptors has been implicated in the progression of squamous cell carcinomas in head and neck patients.[10] Among the receptors that have been studied, EGF receptors are the best characterized. Several anti-EGF receptor formulations (eg,

Herceptin, Genentech, San Francisco, CA) are currently in study as adjunctive chemotherapeutic agents. What remains unknown is the effect that blockade of the EGF pathway could have on healing of surgical wounds in such patients.

SHORTCOMINGS AND FUTURE DIRECTION OF GROWTH FACTOR THERAPY

In reviewing the vast amount of data for growth factor therapy, it is apparent that the shortcomings clearly delineate the future directions. Moreover, researchers are continually stumped by the fundamental principle that wound microenvironments are individualistic and definitively intricate. Such complexities render any approach to globally augment the wound-healing process intrinsically flawed and wrought with obstacles to overcome.

One of the main, widely recognized challenges of growth factor therapy has been the need to provide a sound delivery system that will sustain a therapeutic level of growth factor in the proper location.[9,60] At the same time, growth factor delivery must have temporal limitations that do not extend beyond the amount of time it takes to heal the wound. Without proper timing and method of delivery, potentially positive results may be missed.[1,9,60] One prospective vehicle is the microsphere-embedded gelatin sponge, which provides sustained but finite delivery and has shown positive results in several at least one study.[61]

Another shortcoming lies in the fact that most of the highly promising preclinical data furnished by models utilizing animals bred for their genetic similarity have not translated into clinical success. A potential rationale for this failure is the experimental use of young animals with acute wounds instead of aged animals with chronic wounds intrinsically hindered by senile collagen and tissue—the exact population in need of treatment.[1] Moreover, all studies compare the results demonstrated in treatment groups to controls. Validation of the results is based on the performance of both groups. If the control group underperforms compared to reasonable

expectations, the apparent advantage in healing in the experimental group is due to a faulty control and not to the therapuetic benefits of the studied intervention.

Several current products have caused a buzz in the wound-care world. Although scar reduction and fibrosis prevention have been an industry focus for quite some time, most products are either devices or anti-proliferative or cytotoxic agents. New optimism surrounds treatment approaches aimed at blocking growth factors via various mechanisms. One such therapy worth mentioning is Juvidex (Mannose-6-Phosphate, Renovo, Manchester, UK).[62] This treatment is a TGF-β1 antagonist. Juvidex is being tested in a phase II randomized trial to determine efficacy in scar reduction and safety profile. More information can be obtained on the manufacturer's Web site.[62]

As for the global future of growth factor therapy, one can speculate that, as with so many hot spots of medicinal intervention, the answer for 2008 and beyond is gene therapy. Targeting delivery of growth factor therapy into the wound microenvironment for a prescribed length of time is a very desirable proposition. An example of such a human trial encompasses this promise. Selective Genetics Inc. agreed to sponsor a phase I clinical trial led by primary investigator Dr. D. Mozingo utilizing PDGF-BB incorporated into a gene-activated matrix in an attempt to augment wound healing of diabetic ulcers. Using a PDGF-BB gene embedded in a deleted adenoviral vector, the study hopes to provide continuous PDGF-BB, a growth factor with proven efficacy in this study population, to further enhance wound healing.

Due to the inherent presence of multiple growth factors within the wound-healing milieu, the future possibilities using such recombinant proteins as supplements to tissue repair seem limitless. A select few recombinant growth factors (and their sponsor companies) have successfully navigated the lengthy pathway of translating knowledge gained at the lab bench into convincing human trials and FDA approval. Creative solutions to wound-healing problems abound and are only limited by the reality that drug or device development and clinical trials are expensive propositions.

REFERENCES.

1. Cross KJ, Mustoe TA. Growth factors in wound healing. Surg Clin North Am 2003;83:531–45, vi.
2. Pierce GF, Mustoe TA, Altrock BW, et al. Role of platelet-derived growth factor in wound healing. J Cell Biochem 1991;45:319–26.
3. Goldman R. Growth factors and chronic wound healing: past, present, and future. Adv Skin Wound Care 2004;17:24–35.
4. Pierce GF, Mustoe TA. Pharmacologic enhancement of wound healing. Annu Rev Med 1995;46:467–81.
5. Steed DL, Donohoe D, Webster MW, Lindsley L. Effect of extensive debridement and treatment on the healing of diabetic foot ulcers. Diabetic Ulcer Study Group. J Am Coll Surg 1996;183:61–4.
6. Steed DL. The role of growth factors in wound healing. Surg Clin North Am 1997;77:575–86.
7. Leong M, Phillips LG. Wound healing. In: Townsend CM, et al, editors. Sabiston textbook of surgery: the biologic basis of modern surgical practice. 17th ed. Philadelphia, PA: Elsevier Saunders; 2004. p. 183–207.
8. Lepisto J, Peltonen J, Vaha-Kreula M, et al. Selective modulation of collagen gene expression by different isoforms of platelet-derived growth factor in experimental wound healing. Cell Tissue Res 1996;286:449–55.
9. Rumalla VK, Borah GL. Cytokines, growth factors, and plastic surgery. Plast Reconstr Surg 2001;108:719–33.
10. Guntinas-Lichius O, Wittekindt C. The role of growth factors for disease and therapy in diseases of the head and neck. DNA Cell Biol 2003;22:593–606.
11. LaRochelle WJ, Jeffers M, McDonald WF, et al. PDGF-D, a new protease-activated growth factor. Nat Cell Biol 2001;3:517–21.
12. Witte MB, Barbul A. General principles of wound healing. Surg Clin North Am 1997;77:509–28.
13. Robson MC, Phillips LG, Thomason A, et al. Recombinant human platelet-derived growth factor-BB for the treatment of chronic pressure ulcers. Ann Plast Surg 1992;29:193–201.
14. Hom DB, Thatcher G, Tibesar R. Growth factor therapy to improve soft tissue healing. Facial Plast Surg 2002;18:41–52.
15. Steed DL. Clinical evaluation of recombinant human platelet-derived growth factor for the treatment of lower extremity diabetic ulcers. Diabetic Ulcer Study Group. J Vasc Surg 1995;21:71–81.
16. Wieman TJ, Smiell JM, Su Y. Efficacy and safety of a topical gel formulation of recombinant human platelet-derived growth factor-BB (becaplermin) in patients with chronic neuropathic diabetic ulcers. A phase III randomized placebo-controlled double-blind study. Diabetes Care 1998;21:822–7.
17. Xia YP, Zhao Y, Marcus J, et al. Effects of keratinocyte growth factor-2 (KGF-2) on wound healing in an ischaemia-impaired rabbit ear model and on scar formation. J Pathol 1999;188:431–8.
18. Beer HD, Gassmann MG, Munz B, et al. Expression and function of keratinocyte growth factor and activin in skin morphogenesis and cutaneous wound repair. J Investig Dermatol Symp Proc 2000;5:34–9.
19. Jimenez PA, Rampy MA. Keratinocyte growth factor-2 accelerates wound healing in incisional wounds. J Surg Res 1999;81:238–42.
20. Emoto H, Tagashira S, Mattei MG, et al. Structure and expression of human fibroblast growth factor-10. J Biol Chem 1997;272:23191–4.
21. Ahn ST, Mustoe TA. Effects of ischemia on ulcer wound healing: a new model in the rabbit ear. Ann Plast Surg 1990;24:17–23.
22. Brauchle M, Fassler R, Werner S. Suppression of keratinocyte growth factor expression by glucocorticoids in vitro and during wound healing. J Invest Dermatol 1995;105:579–84.
23. Tagashira S, Harada H, Katsumata T, et al. Cloning of mouse FGF10 and up-regulation of its gene expression during wound healing. Gene 1997;197:399–404.
24. Soler PM, Wright TE, Smith PD, et al. In vivo characterization of keratinocyte growth factor-2 as a potential wound healing agent. Wound Repair Regen 1999;7:172–8.
25. Robson MC, Phillips TJ, Falanga V, et al. Randomized trial of topically applied repifermin (recombinant human keratinocyte growth factor-2) to accelerate wound healing in venous ulcers. Wound Repair Regen 2001;9:347–52.
26. Meropol NJ, Somer RA, Gutheil J, et al. Randomized phase I trial of recombinant human keratinocyte growth factor plus chemotherapy: potential role as mucosal protectant. J Clin Oncol 2003;21:1452–8.
27. Spielberger R, Stiff P, Bensinger W, et al. Palifermin for oral mucositis after intensive therapy for hematologic cancers. N Engl J Med 2004;351:2590–8.
28. Sporn MB, Roberts AB. The transforming growth factor-betas: past, present, and future. Ann N Y Acad Sci 1990;593:1–6.
29. Letterio JJ, Roberts AB. Regulation of immune responses by TGF-beta. Annu Rev Immunol 1998;16:137–61.
30. Sporn MB. TGF-beta: 20 years and counting. Microbes Infect 1999;1:1251–3.
31. Border WA, Noble NA. Transforming growth factor beta in tissue fibrosis. N Engl J Med 1994;331:1286–92.
32. Kinbara T, Shirasaki F, Kawara S, et al. Transforming growth factor-beta isoforms differently stimulate proalpha2 (I) collagen gene expression during wound healing process in transgenic mice. J Cell Physiol 2002;190:375–81.
33. Beck LS, Deguzman L, Lee WP, et al. TGF-beta 1 accelerates wound healing: reversal of steroid-impaired healing in rats and rabbits. Growth Factors 1991;5:295–304.

34. Wu L, Xia YP, Roth SI, et al. Transforming growth factor-beta 1 fails to stimulate wound healing and impairs its signal transduction in an aged ischemic ulcer model: importance of oxygen and age. Am J Pathol 1999;154: 301–39.

35. Lee TY, Chin GS, Kim WJ, et al. Expression of transforming growth factor beta 1, 2, and 3 proteins in keloids. Ann Plast Surg 1999;43:179–84.

36. Robson CM, Steed DL, McPherson JM, Pratt BM. Use of transforming growth factor beta 2 in treatment of chronic foot ulcers in diabetic patients. 3rd Joint Meeting of the European Tissue Repair Society and the Wound Healing Society, 1999.

37. Hirshberg J, Coleman J, Marchant B, Rees RS. TGF-beta 3 in the treatment of pressure ulcers: a preliminary report. Adv Skin Wound Care 2001;14:91–5.

38. Renovo. Scar prevention and reduction – Juvista. 2005; [3 screens]. Available at: http://www.renovo.com/content.asp?c_id=9 (accessed June 21, 2006).

39. Kawai K, Suzuki S, Tabata Y, Nishimura Y. Accelerated wound healing through the incorporation of basic fibroblast growth factor-impregnated gelatin microspheres into artificial dermis using a pressure-induced decubitus ulcer model in genetically diabetic mice. Br J Plast Surg 2005.

40. Bikfalvi A, Savona C, Perollet C, Javerzat S. New insights in the biology of fibroblast growth factor-2. Angiogenesis 1998;1:155–73.

41. Phillips LG, Abdullah KM, Geldner PD, et al. Application of basic fibroblast growth factor may reverse diabetic wound healing impairment. Ann Plast Surg 1993;31: 331–4.

42. Oda Y, Kagami H, Ueda M. Accelerating effects of basic fibroblast growth factor on wound healing of rat palatal mucosa. J Oral Maxillofac Surg 2004;62:73–80.

43. Fu X, Shen Z, Chen Y. [Basic fibroblast growth factor (bFGF) and wound healing: a multi-centers and controlled clinical trial in 1024 cases]. Zhongguo Xiu Fu Chong Jian Wai Ke Za Zhi 1998;12:209–11.

44. Bates DO, Jones RO. The role of vascular endothelial growth factor in wound healing. Int J Low Extrem Wounds 2003;2:107–20.

45. Bottomley MJ, Webb NJ, Watson CJ, et al. Peripheral blood mononuclear cells from patients with rheumatoid arthritis spontaneously secrete vascular endothelial growth factor (VEGF): specific up-regulation by tumour necrosis factor-alpha (TNF-alpha) in synovial fluid. Clin Exp Immunol 1999;117:171–6.

46. Ferrara N, Davis-Smyth T. The biology of vascular endothelial growth factor. Endocr Rev 1997;18(1):4–25.

47. Nissen NN, Polverini PJ, Koch AE, et al. Vascular endothelial growth factor mediates angiogenic activity during the proliferative phase of wound healing. Am J Pathol 1998;152:1445–52.

48. Power C, Wang JH, Sookhai S, et al. Bacterial wall products induce downregulation of vascular endothelial growth factor receptors on endothelial cells via a CD14-dependent mechanism: implications for surgical wound healing. J Surg Res 2001;101:138–45.

49. Galiano RD, Tepper OM, Pelo CR, et al. Topical vascular endothelial growth factor accelerates diabetic wound healing through increased angiogenesis and by mobilizing and recruiting bone marrow-derived cells. Am J Pathol 2004;164:1935–47.

50. Lamah M, Mortimer PS, Dormandy JA. In vivo microscopic study of microcirculatory perfusion of the skin of the foot in peripheral vascular disease. Eur J Vasc Endovasc Surg 1999;18:48–51.

51. Blann AD, Belgore FM, McCollum CN, et al. Vascular endothelial growth factor and its receptor, Flt-1, in the plasma of patients with coronary or peripheral atherosclerosis, or Type II diabetes. Clin Sci (Lond) 2002;102: 187–94.

52. Schantz SP. Basic science advances in head and neck oncology: the past decade. Semin Surg Oncol 1995;11: 272–9.

53. Cohen IK, Crossland MC, Garrett A, Diegelmann RF. Topical application of epidermal growth factor onto partial-thickness wounds in human volunteers does not enhance reepithelialization. Plast Reconstr Surg 1995; 96:251–4.

54. Brown GL, Nanney LB, Griffen J, et al. Enhancement of wound healing by topical treatment with epidermal growth factor. N Engl J Med 1989;321:76–9.

55. Falanga V, Eaglstein WH, Bucalo B, et al. Topical use of human recombinant epidermal growth factor (h-EGF) in venous ulcers. J Dermatol Surg Oncol 1992;18: 604–6.

56. Zine A, de Ribaupierre F. Replacement of mammalian auditory hair cells. Neuroreport 1998;9:263–8.

57. Aletsee C, Volter C, Brors D, et al. [Effect of fibroblast growth factor-1 (FGF-1) on spiral ganglion cells of the mammalian cochlea]. Hno 2000;48:457–61.

58. Mondain M, Ryan A. Epidermal growth factor and basic fibroblast growth factor are induced in guinea-pig tympanic membrane following traumatic perforation. Acta Otolaryngol 1995;115:50–4.

59. Yeo SW, Kim SW, Suh BD, Cho SH. Effects of platelet-derived growth factor-AA on the healing process of tympanic membrane perforation. Am J Otolaryngol 2000;21:153–60.

60. Hom DB. Growth factors and wound healing in otolaryngology. Otolaryngol Head Neck Surg 1994;110:560–4.

61. Sakallioglu AE, Yagmurlu A, Dindar H, et al. Sustained local application of low-dose epidermal growth factor on steroid-inhibited colonic wound healing. J Pediatr Surg 2004;39:591–5.

62. Renovo. Scar prevention and reduction – Juvidex. 2005. [2 screens]. Available at: http://www.renovo.com/content.asp?c_id=10 (accessed June 22, 2006).

30

Vacuum Assisted Devices for Difficult Wounds of the Face and Neck

William T. Stoeckel, MD; Anthony J. DeFranzo, MD; Louis C. Argenta, MD; Joseph A. Molnar, MD, PhD

SPECIFIC THERAPY IN ITS CURRENT STATE:

Vacuum Assisted Closure (V.A.C. Therapy, Kinetic Concepts Inc., San Antonio, TX) consists of an open-cell polyurethane foam dressing that is sealed with an adherent dressing and connected to a vacuum pump to apply subatmospheric pressure. The device is useful in the management of difficult wounds of the head and neck as it aids the removal of wound fluid, decreases edema, promotes the formation of granulation tissue, modifies the inflammatory response, and minimizes bacterial counts in wounds. It is useful as an interim dressing prior to definitive closure or as an adjuvant therapy with flaps, skin grafts, or bioengineered skin substitutes. When used with skin grafts or skin substitutes, it allows for optimum contact with irregular surfaces, removes fluid that might interfere with vascularization, and prevents superficial shear forces to improve rates of engraftment. This device has even allowed direct skin grafting on properly prepared bone.

SHORTCOMINGS

While the V.A.C. Therapy unit has numerous applications for wounds of the face and neck, it does have limitations. The device cannot be used in direct contact with the nasal or oral airway and must be used with caution over the eyes and ears. In mobile areas such as the neck, it may be difficult to maintain a seal.

FUTURE PROMISE

Subatmospheric pressure therapy will have continued applications in treatment of wounds of the face and neck both by allowing the use of smaller procedures to accomplish closure or by augmenting the implementation of other techniques. Further engineering developments may allow use in difficult areas around airways and over mobile tissue.

Wounds of the face and neck provide an array of challenges for the reconstructive surgeon. The complexity of facial structures coupled with the importance of their function and aesthetics, makes wound repair an exciting but often difficult task. Paramount in these reconstructions is preservation and protection of critical underlying structures including the brain, major vessels, cranial nerves, and airway. Maintaining the intricate functions of mastication, facial expression, speech, respiration, glutition, vision, and olfaction is next in priority. Maintaining or rescuing facial aesthetics is a third, but equally important, objective. Reconstruction is further complicated by systemic factors such as concomitant injury, age, vascular compromise, and associated systemic illnesses that may limit or preclude major procedures. Such factors may present major timing considerations in reconstruction of this region.

CONVENTIONAL TREATMENT STRATEGIES

Fortunately, the local blood supply to the face and neck is robust. This has allowed evolution of a variety of local and regional solutions to face and neck wounds. Local flaps for reconstruction are well described in the literature and are a critical part of the training of the reconstructive surgeon. Larger defects often require regional tissue transfer, including the use of myocutaneous flaps of the neck and thorax. Advances in microsurgical techniques have widened the options for more complicated wounds and are often necessary for adequate tissue coverage. Free flaps, however, are still technically complex. They require extensive training and are significant metabolic insults in a debilitated patient. Problems with prolonged general anesthesia in an ill patient may contradict such procedures.

Skin grafting has been a mainstay treatment modality for wounds including those of the face and neck. Burn injuries and scar contractures are particularly well suited for skin graft reconstruction. Recent developments in synthetic skin substitutes have potentiated the value of skin grafting as a solution in such wounds. Often skin grafting is a solution in and of itself, but grafts are also commonly used in conjunction with other reconstructive techniques, including flaps and tissue rearrangement.

Many factors influence the success of the treatment options for face and neck wounds. The physical dimension of the wound clearly limits the options available with local flaps. Larger or deep wounds, especially those with exposed critical structures, may require the use of larger myocutaneous or free flaps. The operative management of large wounds should be considered thoughtfully, as there are inherent complications associated with the more extensive surgical procedures. Reducing the margins and depth of a wound prior to definitive repair may obviate the need for a more complex procedure

along with its associated potential for greater postoperative complications. With flaps and skin grafts, success rates are subject to the ability to prevent infection, minimize exudative fluid collections, and eliminate shearing forces to allow for optimal contact between donor and recipient surfaces. Each of these parameters is vastly improved with the use of topical negative pressure and the vacuum-assisted closure device.

VACUUM-ASSISTED CLOSURE

V.A.C. Therapy has become a first-line treatment for the promotion of wound healing. It has proven to be effective in the treatment of chronic and acute wounds, complications (such as dehiscence and infection), chemical and thermal burns, contaminated traumatic wounds, and exposed abdominal and thoracic cavity wounds. The physiologic mechanisms of action resulting in the acceleration of wound healing with subatmospheric pressure continue to be elucidated with current research studies. They have demonstrated V.A.C. Therapy to be effective in improving the wound environment and facilitating healing by multiple molecular, vascular, and cellular processes.[1]

Tissue Edema and Vascular Density

Tissue edema is a normal physiological response to injury, which can have deleterious effects on wound healing. Fluid pressure within the interstitial space can become greater than local capillary pressure, with a resultant decrease in microvascular perfusion. Removal of localized edema by subatmospheric pressure therapy can enhance blood flow by improving this pressure gradient between the interstitial space and capillary system. Studies have demonstrated a fourfold increase in blood flow using topical negative pressure therapy at -125 mm Hg in a porcine wound model.[2] Increased dermal blood flow in burn wounds has also been demonstrated with the use of topical subatmospheric pressure.[3]

Interstitial edema negatively affects the vascular density of a wound bed. An increase in fluid volume in a given region secondary to an inflammatory response coupled with a constant vascular supply results in a decrease in vascular density. In other words, when edema develops, a given number of capillaries become responsible for supplying nutrition to a greater volume of tissue. Removal of this excess fluid returns the vascular density to its original, more functional, state. The importance of vascular density is evidenced clinically when observing that wounds to the face heal more rapidly than those in the extremities. This is largely due to the superior vascular supply of the face and its overall high capillary density.

Inflammatory Control

In addition to promoting removal of excess fluid with restoration of a healthy interstitial fluid gradient, subatmospheric pressure therapy also serves to remove pro-inflammatory mediators from a wound bed.[1] Many cytokines, chemokines, proteolytic enzymes, and acute phase proteins found within wound fluid and serum inhibit wound healing. Collagenolytic enzymes, including matrix metalloproteinases (MMPs) which are found in high concentrations in chronic, non-healing wounds, have been shown to be removed effectively from wounds with the use of subatmospheric pressure.[4]

Infection Control

Wounds in the vicinity of the nose and mouth, and wounds that have been contaminated from other sources, are especially prone to infection. The increased blood flow to the wound elicited by topical negative pressure, and the removal of cellular debris and edema, decrease the potential for infection. Animal and human studies have demonstrated log factor decreases in wound bacterial concentrations over time with topical negative pressure. This technique allows the wound to be optimally clean with a bacterial count below 10^5 bacteria/gram tissue before attempts at definitive wound closure.

Cellular Response

When the V.A.C. sponge is compressed, there is a resultant deformation of the underlying tissue cells surrounding the wound. On a microscopic level, small blebs of tissue are pulled into the pore spaces within the sponge. The mechanical stress mediated at this foam interface has been shown to have direct effect on cellular mitotic activity.[1] The deformation of cells is known to create changes in molecular pathway stimulation, mitosis regulation, ion transport, second messenger release, protein synthesis control, and fibroblast activity.[1] The cellular promotion of angiogenesis has been demonstrated in several studies.[5–7] Specific gene groups important for tissue growth and cell proliferation have been shown to be upgraded. The decreased activity of these gene products, which include mitogen activated protein (MAP) kinases, interleukin (IL)-6, cyclin dependent kinase (CDK)4, immediate early protein, and IL enhancer binding protein, lead to increased fibroblast activity and collagen turnover. Tissue growth factors, including TGFβ-1 and vascular endothelial growth factor expression likewise have been shown to be enhanced.[8] Each of these processes have been implicated in the improvement of wound healing seen with topical negative pressure therapy.[9–12]

These mitosis-inducing changes in cell activity, the permanent removal of wound exudate while maintaining a moist environment, and the occlusive dressing's minimization of bacterial colonization are thought to be responsible for the stimulation of granulation tissue seen with V.A.C. Therapy in clinical studies.[13] Wounds can be expected to decrease in size as granulation tissue is promoted. This has made V.A.C. Therapy ideal for wound bed preparation, whether for future flap placement, skin grafting, delayed primary closure, or for accelerating healing by secondary intention.

Temporizing with V.A.C. Therapy

Many major wounds of the head and neck occur concomitantly with life-threatening injury. Often, the patient is so precarious that an extensive procedure to obtain wound closure is contraindicated. V.A.C. Therapy can be used in such cases as a temporizing measure acting as a bridge to definitive closure. The wound can be minimally débrided and the V.A.C device placed over the defect. In general, it is best to avoid placing it directly over the major vessels of the neck, particularly when they have been irradiated. In such cases, local muscle or soft tissue can be pulled over the vessel and the V.A.C. device applied over this tissue. The V.A.C. device is changed at 3-day intervals, usually at the bedside or concomitantly with other surgical procedures. When the wound is clean and the patient is stabilized, definitive reconstruction can proceed.

V.A.C. Therapy and Contused Wounds

Many wounds of the head and neck, particularly those following trauma, are contused and bruised. The margins between viable and nonviable tissue in such cases can be nebulous. Final optimal results are achieved when as much native tissue as possible is preserved. In such cases, minimal débridement and irrigation is performed and the V.A.C. device applied to the wound. The V.A.C. device is changed at 3-day intervals, and serial limited débridement of non-vital tissue carried on as needed. Many times, soft tissue that initially seems compromised will be found to be viable, thus possibly eliminating large time-consuming procedures.

V.A.C. Therapy and Treatment for Wound Complications

Often, wounds closed primarily, or with regional flaps, suffer dehiscence, infection, or loss of a portion of a flap. Such complications are often wounds surrounded by a zone of stasis where viability of the tissue remains in question. In such cases, only minimal débridement of obviously nonviable tissue is performed. The V.A.C. unit is applied to the dehisced wound; if infection is suspected, quantitative cultures are taken. The V.A.C. unit is then appropriately changed over a

period of time until the viable tissue level demarcates clearly. If the wound is infected, quantitative cultures are serially taken until a bacterial concentration of less than 10^5 bacteria/gram tissue is achieved.[14] The definitive reconstruction can then be performed with a high degree of success.

Patients with large lymphatic leaks, and even with chyle leaks, have been treated with the V.A.C. device. In these cases, leakage decreases with the accumulation of granulation tissue. The vast majority of wounds stabilize over a period of 7 to 10 days; definitive reconstruction can then be performed.

V.A.C. THERAPY AND FREE FLAPS

Microvascular free flaps are often the best or only choice for adequate reconstruction of extensive face and neck wound defects. Large craniofacial tumor resections and traumatic head and neck wounds account for most patients requiring microvascular surgical repair. There are multiple potential donor sites for such procedures including groin, latissimus dorsi, scapula, upper arm, and tensor fascia latae sources. Advances in microsurgical techniques have allowed for successful performance of these operations, but they remain technically challenging and not without postoperative complications. Perioperative infection, seroma formation, anastomotic leak, and microvascular occlusion secondary to thrombosis are the most commonly reported complications.

Topical negative pressure therapy in combination with the free flap increases the success rate of these flaps by several mechanisms. Occlusive dressings such as V.A.C. Therapy minimize secondary bacterial contamination and the development of infection. The removal of exudative fluid reduces or eliminates edema and minimizes seroma formation. It is also theorized that the topical negative pressure applied with a V.A.C. dressing exerts outward distracting forces on blood vessels and improves the patency of veins, particularly in the microvasculature.

In these cases, the V.A.C. device is placed directly over the microvascular flap, and pressures of 50 to 70 mm Hg are maintained for several days. The V.A.C. device may be removed and the flap checked as needed. V.A.C. Therapy has been used to salvage necrotic or floating free flaps in the head and neck. Usually enough granulation tissue can be developed from the viable portion of a free flap to cover the area that has been lost. This eliminates the need for a second procedure. Studies have demonstrated accelerated healing times, as well as successful salvage of compromised flaps, using topical negative pressure in animal models.[2] Clinically, microvascular flaps treated with V.A.C. Therapy have excellent outcomes.

V.A.C. THERAPY AND SKIN GRAFTING

The success (or take) of a skin graft depends upon an ability to survive several phases of healing and maturation. Initially, the graft must adhere to recipient tissue via the anchoring properties of a thin fibrin network, which stabilizes the graft as definitive revascularization occurs. For the first 2 to 3 days, the graft undergoes "plasmatic imbibition" in which recipient bed transudate is absorbed by capillary action into the grafted dermal blood vessels. Success in this time period ensures graft vessel patency, adequate graft nourishment, and desiccation prevention. It is critical to prevent shearing forces, infection, and accumulation of fluid between the graft and wound bed during this time to assume graft survival. If the graft avoids mechanical disruption, true neovascularization develops over the next 3 to 4 days. This occurs by the establishment of new vessel connections between the graft and recipient wound bed. New capillary ingrowth further provides a definitive blood supply and assumes graft survival.

Graft Contact and Shearing

The importance of preventing graft dislocation, especially during revascularization, has been well known and historically addressed with compression dressings and tie-over bolsters. Ideally,

constant and uniform tension and pressure over a skin graft provide the best environment to optimize successful take. Unfortunately, the irregular surfaces of many face and neck wounds appropriate for skin grafting make bolster and pressure dressings difficult to apply and unreliable. Even distribution of pressure over all areas of the graft often is impossible with these techniques. Motion of the patient while coughing, eating, or talking results in sheer forces that can compromise graft take. The V.A.C. dressing resolves the issue of applying uniform pressure and assures positive contact by providing continuous aspiration pressure over a graft, even when placed over irregular surfaces (Figure 1). This safeguard against shearing and dislocation allows the revascularization process to take place undisturbed.[15–17] Multiple studies have demonstrated an increased rate of graft take when the V.A.C. dressing is used in conjunction with skin grafting.

Bacterial Contamination and Fluid Egress

In addition to the avoidance of shearing forces and the prevention of the accumulation of intervening fluid collections, protection against

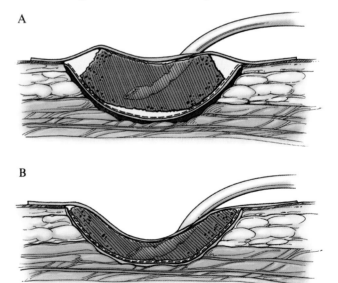

Figure 1. Skin graft treated with overlying V.A.C. dressing. The entire surface area of the graft has equally applied negative pressure allowing for maximal contact between the graft and recipient bed. Reproduced with permission from Schneider et al.[16]

bacterial contamination is critical to graft survival. Using V.A.C. Therapy to secure skin grafts also addresses these issues. The V.A.C. dressing is itself an occlusive dressing which primarily protects against bacterial contamination. Moreover, its continuous removal of wound exudative fluid minimizes seroma and hematoma formation, thereby secondarily eliminating a potential substrate for bacterial growth. Again, the elimination of interposed fluid collections ensures optimal contact between graft and recipient surfaces and allows both the dermal

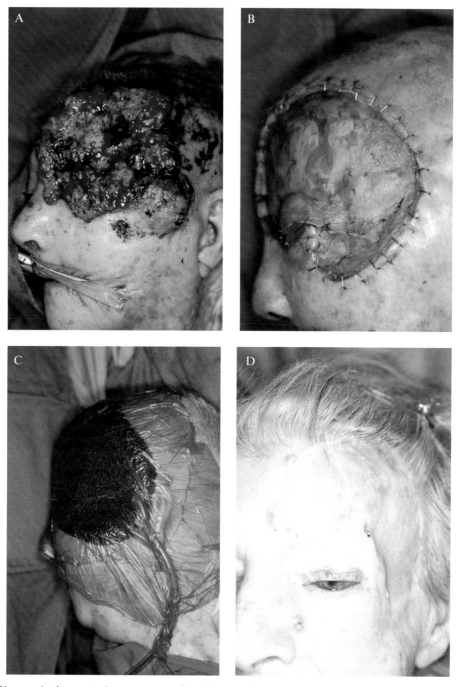

Figure 2.   Skin grafting repair of an extensive squamous cell carcinoma with good results using V.A.C. Therapy and the single-stage grafting technique. Eighty-nine-year-old female with extensive squamous cell carcinoma (*A*). After the lesion was excised, a portion of outer table of skull was removed to punctate bleeding (*B*). A skin graft was applied onto bone after placing a temporary tarsorrhaphy to the eyelid. Subatmospheric pressure system applied directly over skin graft (*C*). Stable skin graft at one year after surgery (*D*). Reproduced with permission from Molnar et al.[18]

and vascular connections to develop uninterrupted.

Grafting onto Exposed Bone

Wounds over the scalp can become problematic in burn, cancer, and trauma patients when full thickness skin loss leaves exposed skull requiring tissue coverage. Usually, local or distant flaps are the preferred choice of reconstruction of such

wounds; traditional skin grafting on exposed bone has been ineffective. In many cases, however, flap options are contraindicated by either comorbidities or tenuous overall patient condition. Removal of the outer table of the skull in such situations exposes the diploic space that, over time, granulates to form a wound bed with adequate vascularity for successful skin grafting. Until this technique was performed in conjunction with the V.A.C. dressing, a 1- to 2-week

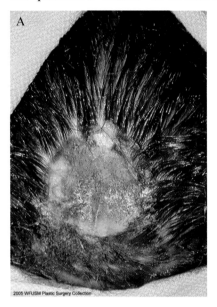
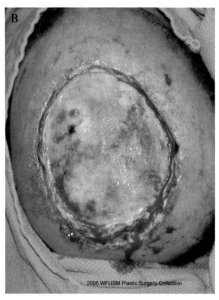
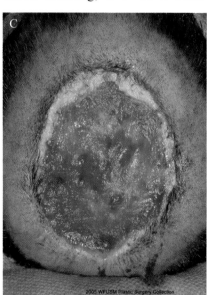
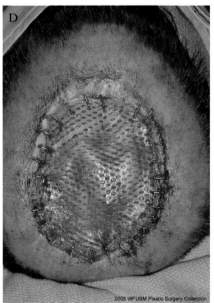
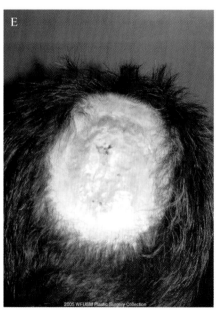

Figure 3. Electrical scalp injury which required débridement and assisted granulation tissue formation facilitated by the V.A.C. dressing. Forty-four-year-old male with 7,200-volt electrical injury to the skull (*A*). Outer table of skull removed after débridement of nonviable scalp; subatmospheric pressure system applied to encourage granulation (*B*). Integra was applied to neovascularized bed, and subatmospheric pressure system applied (*C*). Skin graft over vascularized Integra (*D*). Healed scalp at 3 months after injury (*E*). Reproduced with permission from Department of Plastic and Reconstructive Surgery.[21]

interval was necessary between the time of the diploic space exposure and the definitive grafting procedure to allow for appropriate granulation. The use of V.A.C. Therapy accelerates this process so that an adequate bed of granulation is formed in 6 to 8 days.

Over the past four years, it has become our practice to place a split thickness skin graft directly on the exposed diploë and then apply the V.A.C. dressing over the skin grafts (Figure 2). Successful take of the skin graft has been achieved in one procedure in most cases. Over time, enough soft tissue forms over the graft so that long term stability is achieved in most patients. Negative pressures of 75 to 125 mm Hg for 5 days are usually effective.[18]

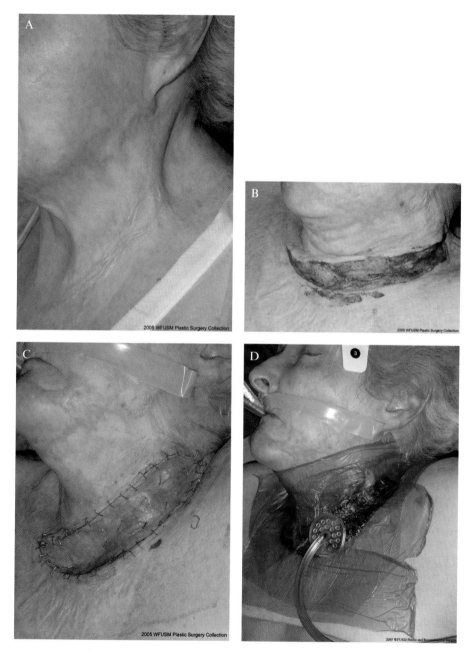

Figure 4. Burn scar contractures of anterior cervical skin effectively treated with V.A.C. Therapy. Sixty-eight-year-old female with scar contracture of the neck from burn injury (*A*). The scar was released and Integra placed (*B*). The subatmospheric pressure system was applied over the Integra for one week (*C*). A skin graft was applied over the Integra and the subatmospheric pressure system reapplied (*D*). Reproduced with permission from Department of Plastic and Reconstructive Surgery.[21]

V.A.C. THERAPY AND INTEGRA

Bioartificial skin substitutes, including Integra (Integra Life Sciences Corporation, Plainsboro, NJ), have been described as a temporary alternative to classic autograft or soft tissue coverage in difficult wound beds. Integra is a bilayer collagen template that can be applied to wounds with exposed bone, joints, or tendons. These defects formerly required coverage with vascularized flaps to ensure effective healing due to the compromised nature of their blood supply and propensity for bacterial contamination. Integra effectively covers these wounds and functions as an epidermal substitute until the dermal matrix becomes adequately vascularized. Once this is accomplished, the outer silicone layer can be removed, and traditional skin grafting can be performed onto the neodermis with excellent results. Colonization of the Integra usually takes 14 to 20 days, during which time the matrix is at risk for failure. Like skin grafting, the success and viability of Integra is directly related to preventing hematoma and seroma formation, eliminating shearing forces, and protecting against infection. Vacuum-assisted closure has been shown to enhance engraftment with Integra by accelerating its vascularization and improving

rate take.[19] The creation of many small puncture wounds in the silicone sheet allows the overlying V.A.C. sponge to remove fluid, improve approximation to underlying tissue and more rapidly facilitate colonization of the matrix. Functional cellular and vascular colonization usually occurs in 5 days. The skin graft can then be applied to the vascularized matrix and secured with a V.A.C. device. Results with this technique have been excellent (Figure 3 and Figure 4).

Keloid, Hypertrophic Scar, and Integra

Keloids and hypertrophic scarring can be difficult problems on the face and neck. A variety of nonsurgical approaches has been applied with similarly varying success. These include local injections, topical steroids, compressive dressings, silicon gel sheeting, cryotherapy, laser therapy, and electron beam irradiation. Simple excision with primary closure, skin grafting, and flap transfers also have been attempted in an array of multimodal combinations. Unfortunately, these high risk lesions are notoriously refractive to treatment, and recurrence is the norm. The reduced or absent hypertrophic scarring observed with the use of Integra in studies with postburn scar contractures[20] makes

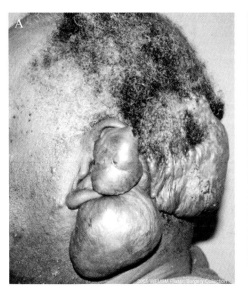
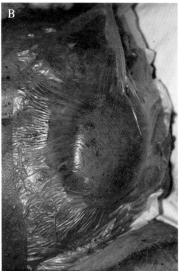
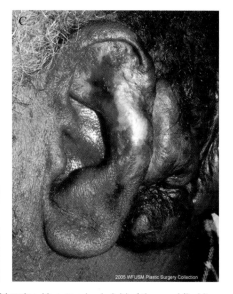

Figure 5. Keloid lesions excised and treated with Integra skin substitute. Fifty-seven-year-old male with extensive keloid of the ear (*A*). After excision of the keloid, a skin graft was placed. The subatmospheric pressure system was used to stabilize the skin graft (*B*). Stable skin graft at 6 weeks (*C*). Negative pressure therapy at therapeutic levels, typically −125 mm Hg, does not run the risk of tympanic membrane rupture. Reproduced with permission from Department of Plastic and Reconstructive Surgery.[21]

the dermal substitute an interesting alternative to traditional skin grafting or primary closure in patients with difficult keloid lesions. It is thought that the placement of Integra on the surgical wound beds from resected keloids may prevent recurrence (Figure 5). Early results with these techniques have been encouraging.

SUMMARY

Vacuum-assisted closure has been accepted as a means for treating difficult wounds, including those of the face and neck. Its use as a method to promote granulation tissue and prepare wounds for future definitive procedures is well documented. Its use as an adjuvant to other modalities of wound therapy, including flap coverage, skin grafting, and skin substitution, continues to show promise in current clinical research. It is by no means a panacea for all surgical wound problems and is not without its limitations, but V.A.C. Therapy should be strongly considered as an option for difficult wounds of the face and neck.

REFERENCES

1. Banwell P, Teot L. Topical negative pressure (TNP) focus group meeting: London UK; Txp communications. 2003. p. 1–232.
2. Morykwas MJ, Argenta LC, Shelton-Brown El, McGuirt W. Vacuum-assisted closure: a new method for wound control and treatment: animal studies and basic foundation. Ann Plas Surg 1997;38(6):553–62.
3. Banwell PE, Morykwas MJ, Jennings DA, et al. Dermal microvascular blood flow in experimental partial thickness burns: the effect of topical sub-atmospheric pressure. J Burn Care Rehabil 2000;21:s161.
4. Shi B, Chen SZ, Zhang P, Li JQ. Effects of vacuum-assisted closure (VAC) on the expressions of mMP-1,2,13 in human granulation wound. Zhonghua Zheng Xing Wai Ke Za Zhi 2003;19:279–81.
5. Ryan TJ, Barnhill RL. Physical factors and angiogenesis in development of the vascular system. Ciba Foundation Symposium 100. Pitman Books, London, pp80–94, 1983.
6. Ichioka S, Shibata M, Kosaki K, Sato Y, Harii K, Kamiya A. Effects of shear stress on wound-healing angiogenesis in the rabbit ear chamber. J Surg Res 1997;72(1):29–35.
7. Sumpio BE, Banes AJ, Levin LG, et al. Mechanical stress stimulates aortic endothelial cells to proliferate. J Vasc Surg 1987;6:252–256.
8. Kopp J, Hoff C, Rosenberg B, et al. Application of VAC therapy upregulates growth factor levels in diabetic foot ulcers. ETRS, 13th Annual meeting, Amsterdam September 2003.
9. Morykwas MJ, Camp M, Galvan MT, et al. Gene array analysis of stretched fibroblasts. ETRS 13th Annual Meeting: Amsterdam September, 2003.
10. Kessler D, Dethlefsen S, Haase I, et al. Fibroblasts in mechanically stressed collagen lattices assume a sythetic phenotype. J Biol Chem 2001;276:36575–85.
11. Kremers L, Kearns M, Hammon D, et al. Involvement of mitogen activated protein kinases (MAP kinases) in increased wound healing during sub-atmospheric pressure (SAP) treatment. ETRS 13th Annual Meeting Amsterdam, September, 2003.
12. Parsons M, Kessler E, Laurent GJ, et al. Mechanical load enhances procollagen processing in dermal fibroblasts by regulating levels of procollagen C-proteinase. Exp Cell Res 1999;252:319–31.
13. Morykwas MJ, Faler BJ, Pearce DJ, Argenta LC. Effects of varying levels of subatmospheric pressure on the rate of granulation tissue formation in experimental wounds in swine. Ann Plastic Surg 2001;47:547–51.
14. Banwell PE. Topical negative pressure therapy in wound care. J Wound Care 1999;8(2):79–84.
15. Isago T, Nozaki M, Kikuchi Y, et al. Skin graft fixation with negative-pressure dressings. J Dermatol 2003;30: 673–678.
16. Schneider AM, Morykwas MJ, Argenta LC. A new and reliable method of securing skin grafts to the difficult recipient bed. Plast Reconstr Surg 1998;102: 1195–8.
17. Gupta S, Gabriel A, Shores J. The perioperative use of negative pressure wound therapy in skin grafting. Ostomy Wound Manage 2004;50(4A Suppl):32–4.
18. Molnar JA, DeFranzo AJ, Marks MW. Single-stage approach to skin grafting the exposed skull. Plast Reconstr Surg 2000;105:174–7.
19. Molnar JA, DeFranzo AJ, Hadaegh A, et al. Acceleration of Integra incorporation in complex tissue defects with subatmospheric pressure. Plast Reconstr Surg 2004;113: 1339–46.
20. Hunt JA, Moisidis E, Haertsch P. Initial experience of Integra in the treatment of post-burn anterior cervical neck contracture. Br J Plast Surg 2000;53:652–8.
21. Department of Plastic and Reconstructive Surgery. A Collection of Images and Illustrations. Winston-Salem, NC: Wake Forest University School of Medicine.

31

Choice of Wound Dressings and Ointments

Christine D. Brown, MD; John A. Zitelli, MD

Over the last four decades, methods of managing wounds have changed dramatically. Perhaps the most striking change has been in the routine application of wound dressings. The development of the recent concept of moist wound healing has led to the creation of literally hundreds of different dressings. Selecting a dressing for a particular wound requires careful consideration of a number of factors. This chapter reviews the effects of antiseptics, antimicrobials, and wound dressings on the incidence of wound infection and on the process of wound healing. A set of guidelines is provided to help the reader decide what to apply topically to wounds and which dressing to select to achieve the best possible outcome in wound healing.

ANTISEPTICS

Antiseptics are chemical substances designed for application to intact skin in an effort to reduce bacterial contamination and infection, not for use in acute or chronic wounds. Regardless of the agent chosen, the most important principle of antisepsis, as acknowledged in definitive surgical texts, is to avoid placing solutions in wounds that cannot be tolerated in the conjunctival sac.[1,2] That is to say, antiseptics are meant for disinfection of intact skin up to the edges of a wound but not within it. It is a common misconception that antiseptics acceptable in terms of their microbicidal, resorptive, and allergenic properties are also permissible for disinfection of

wounds.[3] This misconception has been perpetuated by antiseptic manufacturers, despite the lack of US Food and Drug Administration (FDA) approval for the use of these agents on wounds.[4]

Because the risk-benefit ratio of antisepsis of contaminated wounds was never clearly established,[5] several studies were subsequently carried out. It became obvious that antiseptics provide little therapeutic benefit in treating either clean or contaminated wounds.[2,4,6-11] Their ineffectiveness arises from (1) inactivation by organic matter, such as clotted blood, serum, pus, and foreign debris, and (2) a multitude of deleterious effects on leukocytes, host defenses, and subsequent healing.

Antiseptics in therapeutic concentrations have been shown to be leukocytotoxic in both in vitro and in vivo assays.[6,12,13] In animal wound models treated with various antiseptics, the intensity and duration of inflammation are increased,[7,12,14,15] gross and histologic evidence of tissue necrosis is present, and endothelial damage and thrombosis are observed.[21] Antiseptics containing detergents (ie, scrub solutions) are particularly harmful to wounds.[6,7] Predictably, in vivo studies of both excisional and incisional full-thickness wounds exposed to antiseptics show a significantly higher infection rate over saline-treated controls.[5-7,16,17]

Antiseptics also have direct adverse effects on wound healing.[9,18-20] They retard both wound contraction[5,21] and epithelialization,[5,22] as well as decreased wound tensile strength.[22] In vitro cytotoxicity assays of human fibroblasts[12,22] and human keratinoctyes[23] corroborate these in vivo studies by showing a 50 to 100% cell mortality following exposure to antiseptics in therapeutic concentrations. Thus, the current recommendation based on the best evidence available in the literature is to avoid using antiseptics in open wounds and, instead, to use them for what they were originally intended, disinfection of intact skin.

Hydrogen peroxide deserves special attention only because it is the antiseptic most commonly used on wounds. Its bactericidal potency is minimal at best, however.[24,25] Hydrogen peroxide is ineffective in reducing infection in human appendectomy wounds.[10] The effervescence produced when hydrogen peroxide is applied to wounds is interpreted as visible evidence of its activity, but, in fact, the effervescence represents the rapid decomposition of hydrogen peroxide to oxygen and water by tissue catalases present in wounds.[26] Reliance on the effervescent quality of hydrogen peroxide to mechanically débride wounds comes at the expense of tissue toxicity. It can cause disruption of reepithelialization by producing bullae that may form under new epithelium.[20] Furthermore, this agent is toxic to fibroblasts even when diluted 1:100,[24] and it impairs the microcirculation of wounds.[21] Not surprisingly, hydrogen peroxide has been shown to delay wound healing in both animal and human wounds.[21]

Most recently, certain noble antimicrobial agents have been employed in the management of heavily contaminated traumatic or chronic wounds that exhibit delayed healing. Sustained low-level release of iodine has been proven to be highly effective against wound pathogens without impairing healing. An extensive literature review supports using cadexomer-iodine (Iodoflex, Smith & Nephew, United States, Worldwide) as a safe, effective, and economical treatment for these types of wounds.[27] Similarly, there has been a resurgence in sustained-release silver-impregnated dressings, stimulated by the emergence and escalation of bacteria resistant to multiple antibiotics. Pure ionic silver has a broad range of microbicidal activity against bacteria (including methicillin-resistant *Staphylococcus aureus* [MRSA] and vancomycin-resistant MRSA), fungi, and viruses and has no associated development of resistant organisms.[28] Also, it has superior antimicrobial activity and minimal toxicity in contrast with silver-containing compounds, such as silver sulfadiazine and silver nitrate, which can be proinflammatory and irritating to wounds.[29] Examples of silver-impregnated dressings are Aquacel Ag (Ag and hydrofiber) (Convatec, Deeside, United Kingdom) and Acticoat (Westaim Biomedical Inc, Fort Saskatchewan, AB).[30] Many others exist; however, those dressings that have sustained-release ionic silver concentrated on the surface perform the best.[31]

TOPICAL ANTIBIOTICS

Unlike antiseptics, topical antibiotics are both safe and effective in preventing wound infections. Several studies have demonstrated that topical antibiotics are toxic neither to human keratinocytes[32] nor to human fibroblasts.[12,24] They produce sustained, marked reductions in bacterial counts in open wounds.[7,23,33] Also, topical antibiotics reduce the incidence of infection in both animal and human wounds.[34] By protecting the surface of the wound from desiccation and necrotic or foreign debris, antibiotic ointments may reduce inflammation and infection, thereby facilitating wound repair.

Depending on the specific agent and vehicle, topical antibiotics may accelerate wound healing. In one study, bacitracin ointment U.S.P. (E. Fougera & Co., Melville, NY), mupirocin ointment 2% (Bactroban, GlaxoSmithKline Beecham, Research Triangle Park, NC), and Silvadene cream 1% (Hoechst Marion Roussel, Kansas City, MO) were shown to enhance reepithelialization and retard wound contraction in comparison with controls.[35] In another study, mupirocin accelerated healing by 8%, but the vehicle retarded healing by 5%.[36] In a third study, Neosporin ointment (Warner Wellcome, Morris Plains, NJ) promoted healing by 25%

compared with both the vehicle and the control. Silvadene cream and its vehicle both accelerated healing by 28% relative to the control.[9] Although it was concluded that the effects of topical antibiotics on wound healing are not purely antimicrobial, they may be safely used in acute or chronic wounds. They are the topical agents of choice for wound antisepsis.

In selecting an antibiotic ointment, it is helpful to consider the properties of an ideal topical antimicrobial agent[37]:

1. Wide range of antimicrobial effects
2. Minimum local and systemic toxicity
3. Minimal allergenicity
4. Infrequent emergence of resistant organisms

In terms of these characteristics, there are important differences to recognize among the topical antibiotics that are currently available.[23] Neomycin, for instance, is effective against staphylococci and most gram-negative bacilli, except *Pseudomonas aeruginosa* and obligate anaerobic bacteria. It is less effective against streptococci than staphylococci. Thus, neomycin is often combined with bacitracin, which inhibits both types of organisms and gram-positive bacilli. Polymyxin B, often used with neomycin and bacitracin (triple-antibiotic ointment), is active against aerobic gram-negative bacilli, including *P. aeruiginosa*, but not against gram-positive bacteria. Although *S. aureus* is still the single most commonly isolated pathogen, the gram-negative bacteria as a group make up the majority of pathogens found in surgical wounds.[38] Therefore, antibiotic combinations such as bacitracin and polymyxin B (Polysporin ointment, Warner Wellcome) provide an optimal spectrum of antimicrobial activity for prophylaxis against infection. It is important to recognize, however, that, occasionally, these agents may predispose patients to superinfection by *Candida* species, which can delay wound healing.[39]

Most of the topical antibiotic agents mentioned thus far could be considered ideal with respect to the potential for toxicity. The chief advantage of topical administration is the delivery of antimicrobial activity directly to the site of actual or potential contamination in a concentration greater than that safely achieved by systemic administration.[37] With few exceptions, these agents are very safe to use. For instance, the topical aminoglycosides neomycin and gentamicin (Garamycin, Schering Corporation, Kenilworth, NJ) should not be applied in the ear canal or over large denuded areas for extended periods because of the potential for ototoxicity and nephrotoxicity. Similar precautions exist for polymyxin B, which is also nephrotoxic and neurotoxic.[40] From a practical standpoint, toxicity can be minimized by using these agents only if they are likely to prove beneficial. Applying them to sutured wounds provides little benefit because significant contamination nearly always ceases with wound closure.[23] On the other hand, granulating and ischemic-type wounds are resistant to systemically administered antimicrobial drugs, and topical agents with an ability to penetrate tissue have a far greater likelihood of success in reducing infection.[41]

In selecting a topical antibiotic, it is important also to consider its potential for sensitization. Neomycin is notorious for inducing contact hypersensitivity reactions. Furthermore, cross-sensitization between neomycin and gentamicin has been reported, potentially eliminating the use of gentamicin in patients who are allergic to neomycin.[26] The frequency of sensitization to neomycin increases after repeated application of the antibiotic, especially when applied to dermatitic areas or to leg ulcers. Therefore, it is recommended to avoid using neomycin on surgical wounds, some of which may take weeks to heal.[19] In contrast, the incidence of contact allergy to bacitracin and polymyxin B is rare. It is interesting to note that in the majority of cases of bacitracin allergy, a neomycin-bacitracin ointment had been used. Consequently, it was postulated that neomycin may act as a cosensitizer in the development of allergy to bacitracin.[19] In the rare instance of bacitracin hypersensitivity, either mupirocin or erythromycin ointment (Ilotycin Ophthalmic Ointment,

Dista Products Col., Indianapolis, IN) is a reasonable alternative.[42] Another option for a topical antimicrobial with minimal toxicity and sensitization is zinc oxide. When applied on gauze, it has been shown to increase reepithelialization and decrease bacterial growth and inflammation.[43,44] Although not directly bactericidal, its antibacterial activity is mediated by local defenses.[45] Zinc oxide accelerates healing of both acute and chronic wounds possibly by increasing insulin-like growth factor 1.[46] Use of zinc oxide, like other noble antimicrobial agents, such as povidine-iodine and silver, obviates the problem of microbial resistance. In the future, we may see novel agents used in wounds, such as naturally occurring peptides that protect animals from infection by perforating microbial cell walls and causing death.[27]

The final criterion for an ideal topical antibiotic is that it should only rarely cause the emergence of resistant organisms. In reality, however, when topical antibiotics are used indiscriminately, especially in hospital settings, resistant organisms may emerge. This phenomenon has occurred after widespread administration of neomycin, gentamicin, and mupirocin.[23] Consequently, topical administration of gentamicin is discouraged because this antibiotic has important systemic uses. To avoid the problem of resistance, using topical antibiotics for only brief periods and in selected patients is recommended. Selecting a combination antibiotic ointment, such as Polysporin, may also reduce the risk of microbial resistance.[23]

In summary, topical antibiotics offer several advantages in the management of wounds:

1. Reduction of infection
2. Acceleration of reepithelialization
3. Maintenance of a moist environment
4. Prevention of tissue adherence to dressings

The use of neomycin is discouraged owing to frequent contact hypersensitivity, which can complicate wound healing. The preferred agent for wounds is Polysporin ointment, which only rarely causes contact allergic dermatitis and exerts all of the desirable effects of the topical antibiotic agents.

DRESSINGS

Since ancient times, a myriad of dressings have been employed to protect wounds and allow them to heal undisturbed. Not until 1962, however, was there solid scientific evidence that certain types of dressings could actually accelerate wound healing.[22,47] These dressings were called occlusive dressings because they occlude wounds, preventing evaporative loss of water and providing a moist environment for healing. Studies of their clinical effects show that they reduce pain, inflammation, infection, and scarring while enhancing reepithelialization and dermal repair.[14] Since the initial studies were published, countless numbers of occlusive dressings have flooded the market. With little knowledge of these dressings, one can easily become confused. The purpose of this discussion is to review the biologic effects, mechanisms of action, types, and clinical uses of occlusive dressings.

The first clinical observations of the effects of occlusive dressings on wounds reported that they could accelerate reepithelialization by 30 to 45% compared with air-exposed controls.[22,48] Later, it was reported that connective tissue is regenerated faster in occluded wounds.[49] The numbers of fibroblasts and inflammatory cells, however, are reduced, as is the breaking strength of occluded wounds.[50] Some authors have suggested that these findings possibly explain why there is less scar formation in occluded wounds.[50] Other authors have reported that occlusive dressings have no effect on wound contraction.[48] Initially, it was feared that the moist conditions created by occlusion would promote infection.[51] In fact, over the past decades, many studies have shown that fewer infections are associated with the use of occlusive dressings.[18,51]

Furthermore, a recently published meta-analysis of 12 randomized controlled trials comparing occlusive versus conventional dressings in 693 patients with 819 ulcers showed that

72% more ulcers healed completely with occlusive dressings.[52]

The exact mechanisms of action of occlusive dressings are not completely understood. Initially, it was thought that their beneficial effects on healing were the result of easier migration of epidermal cells in a moist environment.[13] In fact, the mitotic activity of epidermal cells is reduced by occlusion, suggesting that the observed acceleration of reepithelialization may be the result of enhanced migration and survival of keratinocytes.[14] Then several other mechanisms were proposed. One author suggested that the rate of reepithelialization may be related to greater wound-surface oxygen tension in occluded wounds[53]; however, other authors have been unable to confirm such a relationship. It has subsequently been shown that oxygen-permeable and oxygen-impermeable dressings are equivalent in terms of rates of reepithelialization.[13] Other authors have proposed that occlusive dressings may affect wound healing by enhancing the growth of microbial flora or by maintaining the electric potential between the wounded skin and surrounding skin.[18] More recently, the favored explanation is that occlusive dressings help contain various growth factors, such as platelet-derived growth factors, within the wound.[14,54] Numerous studies have since supported this hypothesis by demonstrating that acute wound fluid stimulates the growth of cells in vitro.

How occlusive dressings minimize bacterial infection of wounds is also not yet known. It has been suggested that occlusive dressings reduce infection by (1) acting as impermeable barriers to exogenous bacteria, (2) enhancing the viability of neutrophils and natural inhibitory substances in wound fluid, (3) reducing tissue desiccation and necrosis in the wound, (4) entrapping bacteria and debris, (5) absorbing excess wound exudates, and (6) releasing antimicrobial substances impregnated within their matrices.

The occlusive dressings are categorized according to their chemical composition into four main groups (Table 1): (1) polyurethane films, such as Op-site (Smith & Nephew) and Tegaderm (3M, Eagan, MN); (2) hydrocolloids, such as Duoderm (Convatec, Princeton, NJ); (3) hydrogels, such as Vigilon (Bard Home Health, Berkeley Heights, NJ); and (4) perforated plastic films with an absorptive pad backing, such as Band-Aid, (Johnson & Johnson, Skillman, NJ) and Telfa (Kendall Co., Chicago, IL). Newer composite dressings composed of two or more of these and other materials have been developed to maximize the advantages and minimize the drawbacks of occlusive dressings (Table 2). Although these dressings have been shown to accelerate healing in comparison with more traditional gauze dressings,[13,55,56] certain drawbacks should be recognized before one attempts to use them (Table 3).

The prototype of occlusive dressings is the semipermeable transparent adhesive polyurethane film dressing. It is reserved for superficial wounds, such as split-thickness graft donor sites, because it lacks absorptive capacity. Thus, fluid collection and leakage are frequent problems, especially if the dressing is used during the exudative phase of healing, in the first 7 to 10 days after wounding. To circumvent this problem, a combined dressing was devised of Tegaderm and Kaltostat (Ca Na alginate)

Table 1. PROPERTIES OF OCCLUSIVE DRESSINGS				
Property	Hydrocolloid	Polyurethane	Hydrogel	Telfa
Faster healing	+	+	+	+
Reduced pain	+	+	+	+
Absorbent	±	−	±	+
Adherent	+	+	−	−
Transparent	−	+	+	−
Excludes bacteria	+	±	−	−
Ease of application	+	−	+	+

Adapted from Eaglstein WH and Zitelli JA.[14,61]

Table 2. CHARACTERISTICS OF CURRENT DRESSINGS				
Dressing Type	Examples/Manufacturers	Features	Indications	Contraindications
Hydrocolloids Gel-forming agents, ie, gelatin, carboxymethylcellulose combined with elastomers and adhesives applied to a carrier, polyurethane foam, or film	Tegasorb, 3M Restore, Hollister Duoderm, Convatec Comfeel, Coloplast Hydrocol, Bertek Ultec, Kendall Replicare, Smith & Nephew Nuderm, Johnson & Johnson Invacare, 3M	Absorptive Gel forming Conformable Autolytic débridement Cushions Waterproof shield Moisture vapor permeable Low adhesion Nontransparent Change 1–5 d Easy to apply	Light to moderate exuding wounds Ulcers, venous, pressure, diabetic Necrotic wounds	Exposed muscle, tendon, bone infections Cancers Third-degree burns
Hydrogels	Vigilon, Bard	Highly absorbent	Partial-thickness wounds, dermabrasion, peels, laser resurfacing, burns, abrasions, dry necrotic wounds needing rehydration	Infection
Polyethylene oxide wafers (95% water) between polyethylene films	Nugel, Johnson & Johnson Tegagel, 3M Restore Hydrogel, Hollister Duoderm Hydroactive, Convatec ThinSite, Convatec Clearsite, ConMed Curagel, Kendall Aquasorb, DeRoyal Carrasyn, Carrington Lab Second Skin, Spenco ElastoGel, Southwest Tech Curasol, Health Point	Nonadherent Cooling, soothing Atraumatic Transparent Requires secondary dressing Frequent changes Requires antibiotic ointment		
Polyurethane foams	Allevyn, Smith & Nephew Sof-Foam, Britcair UK Lyofoam, Britcair UK Spyroflex, Britcair UK Mepilex, Mölnlycke (silicone-faced polyurethane foam) Cavicare (silicone foam stent for cavities)	Atraumatic Hydrophilic Highly absorbent Autodébridement Nonadherent center Adhesive border Cushions, protects Waterproof barrier backing Change in 1–5 d Used as a backing for many other dressing types	Moderate-heavy exuding wounds (ulcers various types) necrotic wounds	Dry wounds (might adhere)
Polyurethane films	Opsite, Smith & Nephew Tegaderm, 3M Blisterfilm, Kendall Polyskin, Kendall Bioclusive, Johnson & Johnson MeFilm, Mölnlycke Invacare, 3M	Semipermeable Gas permeable Antimicrobial barrier Waterproof Adhesive Nonabsorbent Decreases water vapor loss Change within 7 d Used as a backing for other dressing types Dressing may leak from lack of absorption	Superficial wounds only, split-thickness graft donor sites, abrasions, minor burns, shallow wounds Minor injuries	Heavy exuding wounds Deep cavities Infection Third-degree burns

Table 2. CONTINUED				
Dressing Type	**Examples/Manufacturers**	**Features**	**Indications**	**Contraindications**
Alginates Biodegradable dressings derived from seaweed; calcium salt of alginic acid combined with textile fiber	AlgisiteM, Smith & Nephew Kaltostat, Convatec Sorbsan, PharmaPlast Tegagel, 3M Seasorb Algosteril	Gel forming Hemostatic Requires moisture Highly absorptive Highly conformable Gas permeable Controls exudates by ion exchange (Ca, Na) Activates macrophages to make TNF-2, IL-6, IL-12 Nonadherent Atraumatic Biodegradable Rinsable with saline Change in 1–7 d	Moderate-heavy exuding wounds "Rope" for packing cavities, larger wounds Painful wounds Infected wounds Malodorous wounds, ulcers, pressure Split-thickness donor sites Second-degree burns Abrasions Blistering conditions Grafts	Dry wounds Necrotic wounds Gross infection
Composite hydrocolloid/ alginate	Coloplast/Sween, Johnson & Johnson Comfeel Plus, Johnson & Johnson Nuderm Alginate, Johnson & Johnson			
Hydrogel/alginate Contact layers	Saf-Gel, Convatec Telfa, Kendall Release, Johnson & Johnson Composition: perforated polyethylene sleeve encasing cotton	Nonadherent Low absorbency Allows for freedom to choose secondary dressing type, ointment type Change on strikethrough of secondary dressing, at least daily	Variety of wounds, mostly superficial, low exuding wounds, abrasions, lacerations, minor injuries, sutured wounds	Copious exuding viscous exudates can entrap this to cause maceration and inflammation of surrounding skin
	Mepitel, Mölnlycke Composition: soft silicone primary dressing	Nonadherent to wound, mild tackiness to seal wound (gentle adhesion), atraumatic Inhibits maceration Change in 2–7 d	Variety of wounds; mostly superficial, low exuding wounds, abrasions, lacerations, minor injuries, sutured wounds	
Contact layers	Tegapore, 3M Composition: woven porous polyamide net	Allows passage of exudates Transparent Nonadherent Can stay in place up to 14 d	Variety of wounds; mostly superficial, low exuding wounds, abrasions, lacerations, minor injuries, sutured wounds	
	Adaptic, Johnson & Johnson Composition: cellulose acetate/ petrolatum	Atraumatic Nonadherent Conforming-packing material Minimum pain Requires absorbent secondary dressing	Ulcers Acute surgical wounds Traumatic wounds First- and second-degree burns	

Table 2. CONTINUED				
Dressing Type	Examples/Manufacturers	Features	Indications	Contraindications
	Adaptic xeroform Composition: contains 3% bismuth tribromophinate Paratulle, Seton Healthcare group Composition: paraffin-impregnated gauze			Heavy-exuding wounds
	Sofratulle Composition: Paratulle plus framycetin (aminoglycoside)	For clinically infected wounds		
Silver-containing dressings	Acticoat, Smith & Nephew	Broad spectrum	High-risk, or infection-prone, or infected wounds	
	Composition: silver-impregnated polyethylene mesh/rayon/ polyester fabric	Antimicrobial, including MRSA and VRE		
		Fungi, viruses No reported resistant organisms Rapid sustained release of silver ions for 3–7 d		
	Actisorb, Johnson & Johnson		Malodorous infected wounds	
	Composition: silver-impregnated activated charcoal cloth Arglass, Unomedical Composition: alginate powder/ inorganic polymer/ionic silver Calgitrol, Biomedical Technologies Composition: silver alginate foam copolymer sheet Contreet Foam, Coloplast/Sween Composition: polyurethane foam/ ionic silver Contreet Foam, Coloplast/Sween Composition: polyurethane foam/ ionic silver Contreet Hydrocolloid, Coloplast/ Sween Composition: hydrocolloid/ionic silver Silveron, Argentum Medical Composition: ionic silver–plated knitted fabric Silvasorb, Medline Composition: polyacrylate–silver hydrophilic matrix Urgotal, SSD-Laboratories Urgo (Parema) Composition: SSD/carboxymethyl cellulose/paraffin polyester mesh			
Iodine	Iodoflex, Smith & Nephew Composition: cadexomer-iodine paste–impregnated gauze		Chronic exuding infected wounds, ulcers, diabetic, pressure	Iodine sensitivity Thyroid disease Renal failure

Table 2. CONTINUED				
Dressing Type	Examples/Manufacturers	Features	Indications	Contraindications
Cellulose/collagen	Promogran, Johnson & Johnson Composition: 45% oxidized cellulose, 55% collagen	Requires hydration and a secondary dressing Binds and inactivates metaproteases; binds and releases tissue growth factors	Chronic exuding wounds, surgical, traumatic wounds, partial-, full-thickness wounds, donor sites	Active vasculitis Collagen hypersensitivity Active infection Dry necrotic wounds
Collagen alginate	Fibracol, Johnson & Johnson Composition: 90% collagen, 10% alginate	Provides structure for cell growth; gel forming, soft, conformable, highly absorbent, autodébridement Nonadherent Absorbs exudates	Chronic exuding wounds; surgical, traumatic wounds; partial-, full-thickness wounds; donor sites	Active vasculitis Collagen hypersensitivity Active infection Dry necrotic wounds
Hydropolymer adhesive	Tielle, Johnson & Johnson Composition: polyurethane backing, wicking layer, hydropolymer foam	More absorptive than hydrocolloid, nonmelting, odorless; can leave in place 7 d	Mild-moderate exudative ulcers Surgical, débrided wounds Second-degree burns Donor/graft sites, acute wounds healing by second intention	

Adapted from Dressings Datacards and Thomas S.[31,63]

IL = interleukin; MRSA = methicillin-resistant *Staphyloccus aureus*; TNF = tumor necrosis factor; VRE = vancomycin risistant enterococci.

(Convatec), which very effectively absorbs excess exudates.[57] Kaltostat releases calcium ions and forms a gel that facilitates clotting and entraps bacteria and cellular debris. This type of dressing is meant only for moderately exudative wounds, such as deep surgical wounds, decubiti, chronic ulcers, and superficial burn wounds.[58]

Another problem of polyurethane film dressings is if the dressing is removed prematurely, the adhesive coating may strip off newly forming epidermis.[39,48,55] Therefore, it is recommended that these dressings be allowed to separate from the wound spontaneously or that a solvent be used to remove them from the wound. Alternatively, an antibiotic ointment may be used in conjunction with the dressing to prevent adherence to the wound.[39] Blister film (Kendall) is a dressing that lacks the adhesive coating in the center portion of the dressing; this design attempts to alleviate the problem of tissue adherence. The adhesive properties, although eliminating the need for tape, can create difficulty for the patient during application of the dressing.

The hydrocolloid dressings, such as Duoderm, are composed of gelling particles such as pectin, gelatin, and sodium carboxymethylcellulose, surrounded by a hydrophobic polymer such as a polyurethane film or foam. They are easy to apply, conformable, and waterproof. These dressings are designed for chronic wounds, such as venous stasis and diabetic and decubitus ulcers, because the gel produced contains enzymes, which cause débridement and stimulate the development of granulation tissue. They have the capacity to absorb fluid, which frequently leads to the production of a copious exudate in the first weeks of use. Patients must be warned of this possibility because, otherwise, it is commonly misinterpreted as a sign of infection. Because Duoderm is opaque, it must be removed to visualize the wound. Care must be taken as it is mildly adhesive and may reinjure the epidermis on its removal.[39]

The hydrogels, of which Vigilon is the prototype, are polyethylene oxide wafers containing 95% water that are sandwiched between two polyethylene semitransparent films. This

Table 3. ADVANTAGES AND DISADVANTAGES OF OCCLUSIVE DRESSINGS
Advantages
Rapid epithelialization
Reduced pain
Reduced inflammation
Reduced infection
Improved scar
Painless débridement
Stimulated granulation tissue
Waterproof
Provides a seal
Reduced dressing changes
Disadvantages
Expensive
Limited availability
Limited experience
Difficult to apply
Epidermal injury
Excess exudates
Fluid leakage
Hematoma
Seroma
Retarded regain of tensile strength
Requiring healthy borders

Adapted from Eaglstein WH.[14]

type of dressing is often used for partial-thickness wounds created from dermabrasions, peels, laser resurfacing, and burns because it is soothing and absorptive. Vigilon selectively permits the growth of gram-negative organisms; therefore, an antibiotic ointment is applied under it.[51] Because it is nonadherent, bacteria may gain entry at the sides of the dressing, and a secondary dressing is required to hold it in place. It requires more frequent changes than other types of dressings.

Over the past few years, a liquid adhesive bandage of medical-grade octylcyanoacrylate has gained popularity in the management of superficial wounds, including split-thickness graft donor sites, abrasions, lacerations, burns, incisions, and shave biopsy sites. Examples of this type of dressing include Dermabond (Ethicon, Sommerville, NJ) and Glustitch (Glustitch Inc., Delta British Columbia, Canada). These are FDA approved as topical wound closure devices. This material polymerizes with wound exudates, forming an occlusive dressing, and dries within 30 seconds into a thin, flexible, transparent, waterproof dressing. The advantages of these

dressings are the provision of immediate hemostasis, reepithelialization and cosmesis comparable to other occlusive dressings, decreased pain, inflammation, easy, economical use and care, and little, if any, infection owing to inherent antibacterial properties.[59,60]

Finally, the most commonly used commercial dressing, and the closest to the ideal dressing, is the perforated plastic film with an absorptive pad backing.[61] Unlike the dressings previously mentioned, this dressing is widely available and inexpensive. For small wounds, plastic strip bandages suffice; however, larger wounds require a nonadherent pad cut to fit the size of the wound and secured with, preferably, paper tape. Recently, two studies showed that polyethylene and hydrocolloid dressings are superior to the commercially available adhesive dressings in terms of healing, pain reduction, and cosmetic result of treated human superficial wounds.[11,62] In one of these studies, however, an antibiotic ointment was not used in conjunction with the plastic bandage dressing.[62] Furthermore, another study of shave biopsy wounds treated with either a polyurethane dressing or a plastic bandage dressing combined with bacitracin ointment showed no significant difference between the two dressings with regard to the rate of healing, infection, and pain.[25] The polyurethane dressing was found to be more convenient for the patients because it eliminated the necessity of daily dressing changes.

In summary, occlusive dressings allow wounds to heal more quickly and with less pain, inflammation, and, possibly, scarring. Their effects on reepithelialization depend on the timing of application of the dressing. They should be applied within 2 hours of wounding and kept in place for at least 24 hours.[18] Occlusive dressings alone should not be used on infected wounds. A nonadherent type of occlusive dressing is better to use on wounds with compromised epithelial edges to avoid reinjury of the epidermis.

WOUND MANAGEMENT GUIDELINES

We offer the following suggestions to optimize wound management:

1. Use antiseptics for disinfection of intact skin only.
2. For surgical procedures, select a method of wounding that minimizes tissue necrosis.
3. Apply topical antibiotics to the wound instead of antiseptics to prevent wound infection and accelerate healing.
4. Substitute tap water for hydrogen peroxide to cleanse wounds.
5. Use nonadherent occlusive dressings on wounds to prevent infection and accelerate healing.

Scrupulous aseptic technique combined with effective antisepsis should be followed to minimize infection and delay in wound healing. Antiseptics should be used on intact skin only, not in wounds. The surgical modality selected should be the most effective method that produces the minimum amount of tissue necrosis to avoid prolonged inflammation, infection, and delayed wound healing. Postoperative instructions for the patient should include (1) cleansing the wound daily with tap water instead of hydrogen peroxide; (2) applying a topical antibiotic, preferably Polysporin or bacitracin, to enhance healing and reduce bacterial infection; and (3) covering the wound with a nonadherent occlusive dressing to provide a moist environment, facilitating healing. We prefer Telfa pads and paper tape because they are inexpensive, readily available, and easy to apply. Furthermore, they offer many of the advantages of the other occlusive dressings (see Table 2) without disturbing the surrounding skin.

CHRONIC WOUND CARE

Although the focus of this article is on the management of acute wounds, a brief mention of chronic wound care is in order. With respect to wound care considerations, chronic wounds differ from acute wounds in two ways. First, there is a much higher incidence of bacterial colonization and infection in chronic wounds; therefore, more frequent and more liberal use of topical antibiotics and systemic antibiotics, in some cases, is required to promote healing. Second, necrotic tissue and debris are often present in chronic wounds and inhibit healing unless surgical débridement of this material is performed. Just as for acute wounds, tap water cleansings and nonadherent occlusive dressings are appropriate in the management of chronic wounds. Reepithelialization may occur more slowly in occluded chronic wounds, however, than in acute wounds treated with occlusive dressings.

CONCLUSION

Knowledge of those factors that may adversely affect wounds and adherence to the guidelines suggested above should minimize complications, such as infection and delayed healing, and make managing wounds an easier, more predictable, and more effective task.

REFERENCES

1. Lawrence WT. Cinical management of non-healing wounds. In: Cohen IK, Diegelman RF, Lindblad WT, editors. Wound healing: biochemical & clinical aspects. Philadelphia: WB Saunders; 1992. p. 541.
2. Schwartz SI, Shires GT, Spencer FL, editors. Principles of surgery. 5th ed. New York: McGraw-Hill; 1989. p. 320.
3. Viljanto J. Disinfection of surgical wounds without inhibition of normal healing. Arch Surg 1980;115:253.
4. Rodeheaver GT, Smith DL, Thacker G, et al. Mechanical cleansing of contaminated wounds with a surfactant. Am J Surg 1975;129:241.
5. Custer J, Edlich R. Studies in the management of the contaminated wound. Am J Surg 1971;121:572.
6. Becker G. Identification and management of the patient at high risk for wound infection. Head Neck Surg 1986;8: 205.
7. Bolton L, Olenlacz B, Constantine BO, et al. Repair and antibacterial effects of topical antiseptic agents in vivo. In: Maibach H, Lowe N, editors. Models in dermatology. Vol 1. Basel: Karger; 1985. p. 145.
8. Crossfil M, Hall R, London D. The use of chlorhexidine antisepsis in contaminated surgical wounds. Br J Surg 1969;56:906.
9. Geronemus RG, Mertz PM, Eaglstein WH. Wound healing: the effects of topical antimicrobial agents. Arch Dermatol 1979;115:1131.
10. Lau WY, Wong SH. Randomized prospective trial of topical hydrogen peroxide in appendectomy wound infections. Am J Surg 1981;142:393.

11. Nemeth AJ, Eaglstein WH, Taylor JR. Faster healing and less pain in skin biopsies treated with an occlusive dressing. Arch Dermatol 1991;127:1679.

12. Balin A, Leonig I, Carter DM. Effect of mupirocin on the growth and lifespan of human fibroblasts. J Invest Dermatol 1987;88:736.

13. Eaglstein WH. Occlusive dressings. J Dermatol Surg Oncol 1993;19:716.

14. Eaglstein WH. Experiences with biosynthetic dressings. J Am Acad Dermatol 1985;12:434.

15. Bryan CA, Rodeheaver GT. Search for a non-toxic surgical scrub solution for periorbital laceration. Ann Emerg Med 1984;13:317.

16. Faddis D, Daniel D, Boyes J. Tissue toxicity of antiseptic solutions. J Trauma 1977;17:895.

17. Gassett AR, Ishi Y. Cytotoxicity of chlorhexidine. Can J Ophthalmol 1975;10:98.

18. Eaglstein WH, Davis SC, Mehle AL, et al. Optimal use of an occlusive dressing to enhance healing. Arch Dermatol 1988;124:392.

19. Gette MT, Marks JG, Maloney ME. Frequency of postoperative allergic contact dermatitis to topical antibiotics. Arch Dermatol 1992;128:365.

20. Gruber RP, Vestnes L, Pardoc R. The effect of commonly used antiseptics on wound haling. Plast Reconstr Surg 1973;55:472.

21. Branemark PI, Ekholm R. Tissue injury caused by wound disinfectants. J Bone Joint Surg Am 1967;49A:48.

22. Hinman CD, Maibach H. Effect of air exposure and occlusion on experimental human skin wounds. Nature 1963;200:377.

23. Hirschmann JV. Topical antibiotics in dermatology. Arch Dermatol 1988;124:1691.

24. Lineweaver W, Howard R, Soucy D. Topical antimicrobial toxicity. Arch Surg 1985;120:267.

25. Phillips TJ, Kapoor AP, Ellerin T. A randomized prospective study of a hydroactive dressing vs conventional treatment after shave biopsy excision. Arch Dermatol 1993;129:859.

26. Reed BR, Clark RA. Cutaneous tissue repair: practical implications of current knowledge. II. J Am Acad Dermatol 1985;13:919.

27. Bowler PG, Duerden BI, Armstrong DG. Wound microbiology and associated approaches to wound management. Clin Microbiol Rev 2001;14:244–69.

28. Dowsett C. The use of silver based dressings in wound care. Nurs Stand 2004;19:56–60.

29. Caruso DM, Foster KN, Hermans MH, Rick C. Aquacel Ag 4 in the management of partial-thickness burns: results of a clinical trial. J Burn Care Rehabil 2004;25:89–97.

30. Jones SA, Bowler PG, Walker M, Parsons D. Controlling wound bioburden with a novel silver-containing hydrofiber dressing. Wound Repair Regen 2004;12:288–94.

31. Dressings Datacards, Available at: www.dressings.org (accessed May 17, 2006).

32. Tatnall FM, Leigh IM, Gibson JR. Comparative toxicity of antimicrobial agents on transformed human keratinocytes. J Invest Dermatol 1987;89:316.

33. Mack RM, Cantrell JR. Quantitative studies of bacterial flora on open skin wounds: the effect of topical antibiotics. Ann Surg 1967;166:886.

34. Waterman NG, Polland NT. Local antibiotic treatment of wounds. In: Maibach H, editor. Epidermal wound healing. Chicago: Yearbook Medical; 1972. p. 267.

35. Watcher M, Wheeland R. The role of topical antibiotics in the healing of full thickness wounds. J Dermatol Surg Oncol 1989;15:1188.

36. Mertz PM, Dunlop BW, Eaglstein WH. The effects of Bactroban ointment on epidermal wound healing in partial thickness wounds. In: Dobson R, Leyden JJ, Nobel WC, et al, editors. Bactroban. Princeton (NJ): Excerpta Medica; 1985. p. 211.

37. Polk H, Finn M. Chemoprophylaxis of wound infections. In: Simmon RL, Howard RJ, editors. Surgical infectious diseases. New York: Appleton-Century-Crofts; 1982. p. 471.

38. Sebben JE. Surgical antiseptics. J Am Acad Dermatol 1983;9:759.

39. Zitelli JA. Delayed wound healing with adhesive wound dressings. J Dermatol Surg Oncol 1984;10:709.

40. Physicians' desk reference. 47th ed. Montvale (NJ): Medical Economics Data; 1993. p. 813, 818, 2187.

41. Krizek TJ, Robson MC. Biology of surgical infection. Surg Clin North Am 1975;55:1261.

42. Katz MH, Alvarez BS, Kirsner RS, et al. Human wound fluid from acute wounds stimulates fibroblast and endothelial cell growth. J Am Acad Dermatol 1991;25:1054.

43. Agren MS, Soderberg TA, Reuterving CO, et al. Effect of topical zinc oxide on bacterial growth and inflammation in full-thickness skin wounds in normal and diabetic rats. Eur J Surg 1991;157:99–101.

44. Agren MS, Chrapil M, Franzen L. Enhancement of re-epithelialization with topical zinc oxide in porcine partial-thickness wounds. J Surg Res 1991;50:101–5.

45. Agren MS. Studies on zinc in wound healing. Acta Derm Venereol Suppl 1990;154:1–36.

46. Tarnow P, Agren M, Steenfos H, Jansson JO. Topical zinc oxide treatment increases endogenous gene expression of insulin-like growth factor-1 in granulation tissue from porcine wounds. Scand J Plast Reconstr Hand Surg 1994;28:255–9.

47. Winton GB, Salasche SJ. Wound dressings for dermatologic surgery. J Am Acad Dermatol 1985;13:1026.

48. Leipziger LS, Glushko V, DiBernardo B, et al. Dermal wound repair: role of collagen matrix implants and synthetic polymer dressings. J Am Acad Dermatol 1985;12:409.

49. Winter GD. Formation of scab and the rate of epithelialization of superficial wounds in the skin of the young domestic pig. Nature 1962;193:293.

50. Linsky CB, Rovee DT, Dow T. Effect of dressing on wound inflammation and scar tissue. In: Dineen P, Hildrick-Smith G, editors. The surgical wound. Philadelphia: Lea & Febiger; 1981. p. 191.

51. Mertz PM, Marshall DA, Eaglstein WH. Occlusive dressings to prevent bacterial invasion and wound infection. J Am Acad Dermatol 1985;12:662.

52. Singh A, Halder S, Menor GR, et al. Meta-analysis of randomized controlled trials on hydrocolloid occlusive dressing versus conventional gauze dressing in the healing of chronic wounds. Asian J Surg 2004;27(4): 326–32.

53. Silver IA. Oxygen tension and epithelialization. In: Maibach HI, Rovee DT, editors. Epidermal wound healing. Chicago: Yearbook Medical; 1972. p. 291.

54. Chen WY, Rogers AA, Hutchinson JJ, et al. Further characterization of biological properties of wound fluids—mitogenic and chemotactic properties. J Invest Dermatol 1991;96:566.

55. Alvarez OM, Mertz PM, Eaglstein WH. The effect of occlusive dressing on collagen synthesis and reepithelialization in superficial wounds. J Surg Res 1983;35: 142.

56. Many SH. A new primary wound dressing made of polyethylene oxide gel. J Dermatol Surg Oncol 1983;9: 153.

57. Disa JJ, Karek A, Smith JW, Qin-yin MD, et al. Evaluation of a combined calcium sodium alginate and bio-occlusive membrane dressing in the management of split-thickness skin graft donor sites. Ann Plast Surg 2001;46:405–8.

58. Ramos-e-Silva M, Ribciro deCastro MC. New dressings including tissue-engineered living skin. Clin Dermatol 2002;20:715–23.

59. Singh AJ, Mohammed M, Thode HC, McClain SA. Octylcyanoacrylate versus polyurethane for treatment of burns in swine: a randomized trial. Burns 2000;26: 388–92.

60. Singh AJ, Nable M, Carneah P, et al. Evaluation of a new liquid occlusive dressing for excisional wounds. Wound Repair Regen 2003;11:181–7.

61. Zitelli JA. Wound healing and wound dressings. In: Roenigk RK, Roenigk HR, editors. Dermatologic surgery: principles and practice. New York: Marcel Dekker; 1989. p. 97.

62. Woodley DT, Kim YH. A double-blind comparison of adhesive bandages with the use of uniform suction blister wounds. Arch Dermatol 1992;128:1354.

63. Thomas S. MRSA and the use of silver dressings: overcoming bacterial resistance. Available at: http://www.worldwidewounds.com/2004/november/Thomas/Introducing-Silver-Dressings (accessed May 17, 2005).

32

Adipose Tissue in Stem Cell Biology

Sunil S. Tholpady, MS, MD, PhD; Adam J. Katz, MD; Roy C. Ogle, PhD

DESCRIPTION OF PRESENT USE

Interest in the potential of adult stem cells generated from adipose tissue has grown exponentially as evidenced by the enormous proliferation of related publications in the last 4 years. Several reasons exist for the concentration of resources dedicated to understanding the biology of adipose-derived stem cells (ASCs). ASCs can be produced in nearly unlimited quantities when compared with bone marrow–derived stem cells (BMSCs), with much less donor-site morbidity. Further, the tissue extracted from liposuction or abdominoplasty is considered pathologic waste and has had little constructive use until now. ASCs derived from fat have shown themselves to be highly multipotential, giving rise to cells from all three germ layers. This multipotentiality is at least equivalent to that of other adult stem cells. Collection of these cells does not incur the political and moral costs of embryonic stem cells, and ASCs have already been shown to be safe in humans.

SHORTCOMINGS

This technology has several shortcomings, however. It is not known to what degree ASCs are multipotential, but it is thought that they may not be totipotent, as embryonic stem cells are. Another shortcoming is variability that exists at several levels, including person to person, site to site, freshly isolated cells versus cultured cells, and the method of isolation. Finally, the potential also exists for encouragement of tumor formation or depression of the immune system owing to ASC transfusion or implantation.

FUTURE PROMISE

Even considering these problems, enormous potential remains in future therapeutics centered on ASCs. At the most general level, they could function as the basic building blocks of damaged tissues. ASCs could also act as carriers of recombinant deoxyribonucleic acid (DNA) vectors, encoding several genes of interest. They also secrete a host of angiogenic and survival factors that could allow them to serve as support cells in the wound healing processes of several organs, including the brain, bone, heart, kidneys, and skin. Additionally, they possess immunomodulatory properties that could be useful to reduce transplant rejection, graft-versus-host disease, or autoimmune diseases. These benefits, coupled with the ability to extract, purify, manipulate, and reintroduce these cells in one patient encounter, could revolutionize treatment of several disparate illnesses.

INTRODUCTION

The term *stem cell* has entered the lexicon with such force that it is impossible to avoid some discussion. Two broad categories of stem cells exist: embryonic stem cells and adult stem cells. This chapter deals primarily with adult stem cells derived from adipose tissue, or adipose stem cells (ASCs). It is well known that stem cells may be used, at some point in the future, to provide adjunctive or curative modalities for diseases that have thus far escaped remediation. Exactly how this might happen, along with potential problems, is discussed below, in addition to a discussion of ASC multipotentiality in vitro and in vivo.

Stem cells were originally defined as a self-renewing multipotent entity capable of generating multiple cell types. This is true of embryonic stem cells, whose multipotentiality has been exploited in vitro to produce numerous cell types. This definition has been modified to some degree by referring to multipotential cells present in adults as stem cells. In this context, it refers to a cell with a more limited capacity for both self-renewal and differentiation. These cells have not yet been shown to be as multipotent as embryonic stem cells, nor are they immortal.

The prototypical and best studied adult stem cell is the bone marrow–derived mesenchymal stromal (or stem) cell (BMSC). Bone marrow had long been known to contain hematopoietic stem cells, but a separate stromal cell in the hematopoietic microenvironment existed that was more closely associated with the stromal component of marrow.[1] Under varying conditions, these cells could be forced to express gene products consistent with differentiation into bone, cartilage, muscle, tendon, cardiomyocytes, and neurons.[2–5] These differentiated cells were used with varying degrees of success to repair and regenerate tissue in a myriad of animal models.[6–9] A major limitation of this approach was that the volume of bone marrow that could be harvested for any particular use was usually miniscule when compared with the number of cells necessary to regenerate the injured tissue.

The excitement generated by BMSCs, as well as the recognition of their limitations, led to the exploration of alternative tissue sources and the possibility of niches containing undiscovered mesenchymal stem cells (MSCs). Studies had shown that adipose tissue harbored not only adipocytes but also endothelial cells, fibroblasts, preadipocytes, and pericytes. These cell types made up a stromal vascular fraction,[10] long thought to be the reserve for new adipocytes as

experiments had shown adipogenic conditions yielding conversion to adipocytes.[11–14] The application of a differentiative signal to cells contained within the stromal vascular fraction demonstrated the surprising and groundbreaking result that these mesenchymal cells were capable of differentiating into the same lineages as had previously been shown in BMSCs.[15,16]

SPECIFIC THERAPY IN ITS CURRENT STATE

In Vitro Differentiative Capacity

Adipose tissue is of mesodermal origin, except in the head and neck region, where it is neural crest derived, and transdifferentiation of ASCs to bone, cartilage, muscle, and fat does not cross germ layer boundaries. Differentiative methods used with ASCs are similar to those used in BMSCs, which are comparable to methods originally devised for differentiation of immortalized fibroblastic cell lines such as NIH3T3 cells.

Adipogenesis of ASCs requires the concerted actions of cyclic adenosine monophosphate (cAMP) agonists (isobutylmethylxanthine), hormones (insulin, dexamethasone), and anti-inflammatory agents (indomethacin).[15] Whereas complete differentiation can require 3 weeks, many cellular and molecular end points are present within the first week. The most intuitively relevant indicator is the presence of lipid-filled vacuoles. Lipid present within the cells starts as several small depots, which coalesce into a large unilocular lipid vesicle. By 3 weeks in culture, the cells are unable to counteract the buoyancy of the contained lipid and detach from tissue culture plates.[17]

Molecular markers of fatty differentiation already present within cells include aP2, lipoprotein lipase (LPL), and leptin. These markers are up-regulated with the addition of adipogenic media. Other markers are switched on during this time: peroxisome proliferator-activated response (PPAR)1 and GLUT4 at 1 and 2 weeks, respectively.[15]

Bony differentiation is similar in time course to adipogenesis but requires β-glycerophosphate, dexamethasone, and ascorbic acid.[18] Although these cells secrete matrix proteins and express genes indicative of a bony phenotype, the sequence of gene activation is unlike that encountered in normal physiology. ASCs in the undifferentiated state generate osteonectin, alkaline phosphatase, CBFA-1, CN1, RXR, VDR, parathyroid hormone receptors (PTHR), msx2, and c-fos. With the addition of osteogenic media, these cells also express osteocalcin, a marker for mature bone.[15,19]

Differentiation along chondrogenic lineages requires a specific culture technique known as micromass culture, in which cells are plated at high numbers in a limited volume.[20] This effectively forces cells to adhere to one another and create a ball of cells. Matrix proteins present in cartilage are secreted by this expanding ball of differentiating chondrocytes in the presence of insulin, transferrin, selenium, transforming growth factor β1, ascorbic acid-2-phosphate, and dexamethasone. Uninduced cells are capable of expressing biglycan and decorin, but only induced cells express collagen II, aggrecan (at 7 days), and collagen X (at 2 weeks).[15,21]

The differentiation of ASCs to myocytes has one of the lowest yields of any other type. Only a small percentage of cells are capable of fusion, producing multinucleated cells that contain genes normally expressed by myocytes.[15,22] This process takes significantly longer as well; 6 weeks is needed to observe these rare cells. MyoD, myogenin, and myosin heavy chains are all induced with the addition of myogenic media.[15,22]

Perhaps the most intriguing differentiative protocol involves the transmutation of ASCs into neural-like cells. The methods by which this can be accomplished were first described in BMSCs.[5] Reducing agents such as β-mercaptoethanol and butylated hydroxyanisole[5] and agents increasing cAMP[23] were shown to produce cells of neuronal morphology in less than 6 hours of exposure. MSCs up-regulated expression of neuron-specific enolase, neurofilament M, and trkA while down-regulating nestin, a protein expressed by neuronal precursor stem cells.[5,23] These observations were furthered and expanded by several groups working in ASCs.[17,24–26]

The final appearance of differentiated and undifferentiated cells in vitro is shown in Figure 1. Note the varied morphologies present when exposing the same cell to varying environments. These milieus are listed in Table 1.

The differentiative properties of these cells are not limited to the above-mentioned phenotypes. Cardiomyocytes,[27,28] hepatocytes,[29] and endothelial cells[30–32] are other lineages that have been successfully generated with ASCs. The potential of these cells to regenerate tissue in vivo remains to be seen.

In Vivo Behavior

Because of the recent discovery of ASCs, in vivo applications of the technology are not as well developed as are those in stem cells from other locations. The preliminary uses of these cells in vivo will most likely be dependent on the availability of easy to use, low-risk

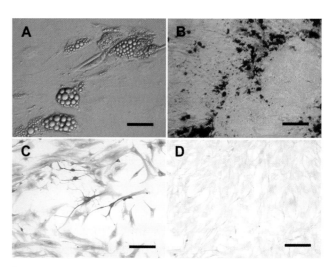

Figure 1. Adipocyte- (A), osteoblast- (B), and neuron- (C) differentiated adipose stem cells (ASCs). Control ASCs are pictured in D. Notice the elongated fibroblastic appearance of ASCs in the undifferentiated state (D). Lipid-filled vacuoles present in adipocytes (A) after 4 weeks. von Kossa's staining of osteoblasts demonstrates mineral deposition in B. Neurite-like branching of ASCs exposed to neurogenic media (C) stains positively for neurofilament M, whereas undifferentiated cells (D) do not. Reproduced with permission from Tholpady SS et al.[17] (×10 original magnification)

Table 1 METHODS OF IN VITRO ADIPOSE STEM CELL DIFFERENTIATION TO SELECTED PHENOTYPES			
Differentiated Phenotype	Basal Media	Media Supplements	Differentiative Time
Control	DMEM + 10% FBS		
Adipocytes	DMEM + 10% FBS	1 μM dex, 500 μM IBMX, 200 μM indomethacin, 10 μM insulin[15]	3 wk
Osteoblasts	DMEM + 10% FBS	0.01 μM VD3, 10 mM β-GP, 50 μM ASAP[19]	3 wk
Chondrocytes	DMEM + 1% FBS	50 nM ASAP, 10 ng/mL TGF-β_1, 6.25 μg/mL insulin[17]	3 wk
Myocytes	DMEM + 10% FBS + 5% HS	50 μM hydrocortisone[15]	6 wk
Neurons	DMEM	1–10 mM β-ME[16]; 1 μM hydrocortisone, 200 μM BHA, 5 mM KCl, 2 μM valproic acid, 10 μM forskolin, 5 g/mL insulin[77]	6 h
Hepatocytes	60% DMEM-LG/40% MCDB-201/ITS	10^{-9} M dex, 10^{-4} ASAP, 0.1% DMSO, 10 ng/mL rhEGF, 10 ng/mL rhHGF, 10 ng/mL rhOSM[29]	4 wk
Cardiomyocytes	MethoCult GF M3534,[28] DMEM + 10% FCS[27]	Rat cardiomyocyte extract[27]	3–4 wk,[28] 3 wk[27]

ASAP = ascorbate 2-phosphate; BHA = butylated hydroxyanisole; dex = dexamethasone; DMEM = Dulbecco's Modified Eagle's Medium; DMSO = dimethylsulfoxide; FBS = fetal bovine serum; FCS = fetal calf serum; β-GP = β-glycerophosphate; HS = horse serum; IBMX = isobutylmethylxanthine; ITS = insulin, transferrin, selenium; LG = low glucose; β-ME = β-mercaptoethanol; NCS = newborn calf serum; rhEGF = recombinant human epidermal growth factor; rhHGF = recombinant human hepatocyte growth factor; rhOSM = recombinant human oncostatin M; TGF-β_1 = transforming growth factor β_1; VD3 = 1,25-dihydroxyvitamin D_3.

applications and/or the perceived need for novel, innovative technological solutions for disease (Figure 2).

Bone engineering fits the first of these qualifications in that there are several sensitive and specific assays with which to quantitate bone healing. One such assay involves loading cells of interest onto hydroxyapatite–tricalcium phosphate (HA-TCP) cubes and implanting them in vivo to measure osteoid formation in the implant. Cubes loaded with ASCs were shown to create osteoid, whereas cell-free cubes were incapable of generating osteoid.[33]

Although the study above was one of the first to demonstrate the potential usefulness of these cells in skeletal engineering applications, there is an even more important point to be recognized. The cells that were implanted were undifferentiated, so signals from the HA-TCP and the in vivo environment induced the undifferentiated cells to produce osteoid. Another study employing undifferentiated cells in a cranial critical-size defect (CSD) yielded similar results.[34] Here, adult ASCs derived from mouse subcutaneous tissue were cultured in vitro for several weeks and then placed on apatite-coated polylactic-co-glycolic acid constructs. These cell-polymer constructs were then reimplanted into circular CSDs created in mouse calvaria. ASCs were capable of

creating bone and mineralizing the area of repair, although not as well as osteoblasts.[34]

The lower risk of ASC implantation for bone repair applications has allowed for one study to date in humans. A 7-year-old girl who suffered from severe traumatic calvarial fractures and defects complicated with chronic infection was treated using ASCs. Autologous ASCs, mixed with cryopreserved skull fragments in fibrin glue and sandwiched between two macroporous resorbable polymeric sheets, were used.[35] The ASCs were harvested and reimplanted during the same procedure as the bone graft placement. Complete bony coverage was achieved using this method. It can be deduced that the ASCs that were implanted did not hinder bone regeneration, even though these were undifferentiated. To what extent they were capable of mediating bone differentiation and repair is unknown because both bone fragments and fibrin are osteoconductive and osteoinductive.[36] The knowledge that ASCs can be implanted without deleterious effects is vital to future human clinical research.

Although human trials determining safety and efficacy of implanted ASCs do not exist yet for injured tissue types other than bone, a few studies exist in which experimentally injured animals were treated with ASCs. In the brain, a

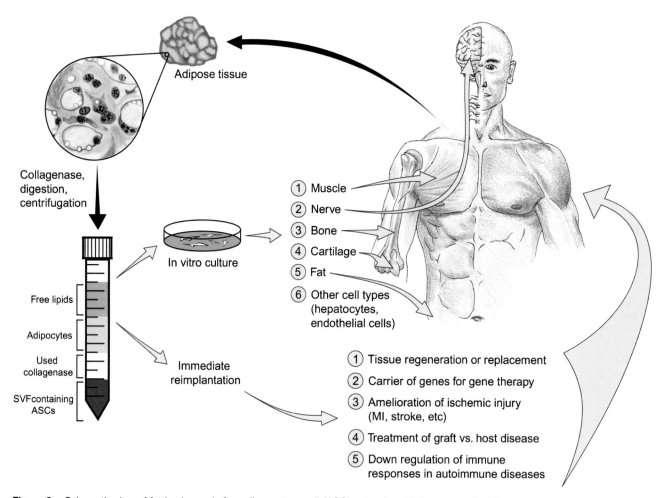

Figure 2. Schematic view of fat in vivo and after adipose stem cell (ASC) extraction. Various uses of ASCs are diagrammed.

simple yet highly effective method to induce injury is through controlled occlusion of the middle cerebral artery. This ischemic insult causes significant damage to areas of the brain supplied by this vessel. Repair and amelioration of deficits can be determined functionally, providing a quantitative assessment of the utility of a particular treatment. One study has been performed in mice to establish the value of implanted ASCs in injured animals. Naive cells and cells exposed to brain-derived neurotrophic factor in vitro were transplanted into the ventricles of animals with middle cerebral artery occlusion. Both groups of cells were capable of migrating into the brain and engrafting into host tissue, with concomitant expression of glial fibrillary acidic protein (GFAP) and microtubule associated protein 2 (MAP2), two nerve-specific genes. Interestingly, ASCs demonstrated a greater propensity to migrate in tissue that was injured along white matter tracts. Animals treated in this manner were observed to have significant functional recovery.[37]

Differentiation protocols have been devised for the conversion of ASCs to hepatocytes, and implantation of ASCs into animals with a hepatic injury yields results similar to those of brain injury models. Cells are capable of migrating and tracking to a site of injury and expressing tissue-specific markers.[29,38]

Bone marrow rescue is another newly discovered property of ASCs. In one study, lethally irradiated mice were able to reconstitute blood-forming elements after injection with ASCs.[39] Donor ASCs were found in the blood, spleen, and bone marrow of animals that survived the procedure. These results indicate one of two possibilities: either the population of cells used contained hematopoietic progenitors or the cells were capable of supporting endogenous hematopoietic recovery.

SHORTCOMINGS

Are ASCs Truly Stem Cells?

As stated before, stem cells were originally defined as having an unlimited capacity for self-renewal, as well as the ability to differentiate and give rise to any tissue type present within a given organism. This is accepted as true for embryonic stem cells, but less evidence exists for the totipotentiality of ASCs. Protocols that trigger differentiation in embryonic stem cells do not necessarily have the same effect in adult stem cell lines, including ASCs. Currently, there does not appear to be the same potential present in adult stem cells as there is in embryonic stem cells.

Multiple unanswered questions exist regarding ASC differentiation to target cell types. Although ASCs can be coerced to express genetic markers and cellular behaviors reminiscent of a given cell or tissue type, it is not known whether the resultant cell is capable of assuming the behavior of the original cell in vivo. Studies show that the patterns of gene expression that occur during differentiation do not correspond to those proceeding throughout development. It is possible that such differences will become important as ASCs are implanted for tissue regenerative purposes.

Differentiation to certain types, notably nerve-like cells, has also been questioned. Studies originally performed in BMSCs displayed the neurogenic consequences on contact of these cells with reducing agents and antioxidants. These finding have recently been qualified such that the cells may not be undergoing neural differentiation; rather, the observed morphologic changes are a stress response just before cell death. Several lines of evidence support this conclusion. There is no perceptible change in gene expression patterns on differentiation as cells do not up-regulate important neural genes when differentiated. Cells placed in differentia-tive media too long will detach from plates and die.[40,41]

An additional controversy exists as to the fate of cells implanted into animals. A few studies suggest that instead of transdifferentiating into the tissue in which engraftment takes place, cells may actually fuse with host cells.[42,43] Many experimental designs take advantage of differences between transplanted ASCs and host tissue (human ASCs in mouse tissue, male ASCs containing a Y chromosome in female mice) to detect the implanted cells after necropsy. However, cell fusion would allow hybrid cells to carry human antigens or a Y chromosome while still not being truly representative of an in vivo differentiative event. The possibility of this event requires techniques that can detect it in vivo.

Are ASCs a Homogeneous Population of Cells?

ASCs are most likely not a homogeneous population of cells as cells have been sorted and subdivided with cell surface markers into populations with unique properties. These studies show that cells can be subdivided according to CD34, a marker of hematopoietic progenitor cells, and CD31, which marks leukocytes, platelets, and endothelial cells. $CD34^-CD31$ cells show the characteristics of ASCs so far discussed, whereas $CD31^+$ cells are quiescent.[30,44]

Given that the cells derived from a harvest are heterogeneous, other factors exist that can contribute to variability, which may account for differences between reported results and efficacy in animal experiments. These are the site of harvest variability, interperson variability, isolation method variability, and culture condition variability. Adipose tissue can differ depending on the site from which it is harvested. Evidence has long existed supporting site-specific differences in adipocyte behavior.[45–48] Differences between subcutaneous fat and visceral fat are most commonly studied.

Interperson differences are accompanied by intraperson differences in ASCs' multipotentiality. Two recognized sources of person-to-person variation are age and sex differences.[45,49,50] A negative correlation exists between proliferative activity and age in subcutaneous ASCs.[45] This is not an unexpected result because increasing age can reduce cell life span. ASCs derived from mice also show a sex-specific difference in that female ASCs show a greater up-regulation of fat-related genes on differentiation to fat than their male counterparts.[49] The correlation of this finding to other differentiative pathways remains to be discovered. Patients vary in relation to what genes are expressed in total harvested ASC populations. In one study, gene expression profiles from ASCs from three patients showed 66% concordance among nearly 200 genes studied (Figure 3).[51]

It is also possible that the method of isolation will change the populations studied. Although the first published reports regarding ASCs were made using cells taken from liposuction speci-

mens, our laboratory group has routinely gathered cells predominantly from waste abdominoplasty tissue. We have found that cells from either method have the capacity to differentiate into any of the cell types listed above. However, differences have started to reveal themselves when cells are analyzed using total cell population studies using flow cytometry. Flow cytometry is an expedient method by which a heterogeneous mixture of cells can be quickly profiled and sorted according to expression of cell surface markers. Our results match the results of other groups, with a few important exceptions. These differences could be due to method, but there is also another explanation. During liposuction, an intense inflammatory reaction is instigated in the body.[52,53] This may lead to a cascade of proinflammatory events and mobilization of various cell types. During longer procedures, these cells may travel to sites of injury and be collected in the liposuction aspirate.

This effect in liposuction is distinct from events that occur during abdominoplasty, where blood flow is cut off from the fat to be removed. The cells later gathered from this tissue may not contain the same profile of cells seen during liposuction. Although we have tested differentiation to bone, fat, cartilage, muscle, and nerve, it is possible that differentiation to endothelial cells and hematopoietic cell types could differ depending on the collection method.

One other source of cell variability derives from the differences between the in vivo versus the in vitro environment. Some studies have discovered that cells in culture behave differently from cells that are freshly isolated.[44] The change from a three-dimensional environment to a two-dimensional culture situation ostensibly entails changes in cellular morphology and metabolism but also more subtly changes in gene expression.

Our laboratory group has noticed that the nerve-specific β_3-tubulin is present in undifferentiated cells but does not appear until after 3 days in culture. As expected, cells before this threshold point do not express the protein. Microarray experiments detailing genome-wide

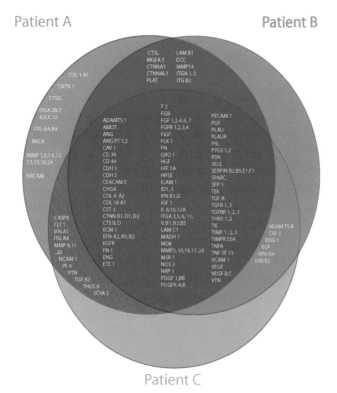

Figure 3. Venn diagram detailing the similarities and differences in adipose stem cell (ASC) populations among three patients undergoing gene profiling for survival and angiogenic genes. Note that whereas most genes are expressed by all three patients, a few genes are expressed by two or only one. Such differences may be responsible for differences in the phenotypic behavior of ASCs. Adapted with permission from Katz AJ et al.[51]

expression patterns have shown a similar trend. Cells that are freshly isolated and placed in culture for 1 day are significantly different from cells in culture just 4 days later, expressing genes that are reflective of multiple tissue types.

Is There Any Danger in Implanting ASCs into Humans?

Although dangers exist with ASC harvest and reimplantation, procedures as invasive and risky are performed routinely in medical centers worldwide. Experience with such procedures has led to knowledge of the incidence, management, and minimization of adverse events. However, two unique theoretical problems may arise with ASC implantation.

BMSCs have been known for several years to have immunomodulatory capabilities. They do not express class II major histocompatibility complex or B7 costimulatory proteins, and this is thought in part to lead to their ability to evade an immune response.[54–56] This property extends even further as BMSCs are capable of inhibiting lymphocytic proliferation and activation,[57,58] as well as altering secreted cytokine profiles of dendritic cells, T cells, and natural killer cells.[59] ASCs have also been shown to have this immunomodulatory capacity.[60]

Immune response modulation may be responsible for the result of a recent study that raised the possibility that BMSCs may be capable of supporting cancer growth. In this series of experiments, B16 melanoma cells were injected alone or with primary allogeneic BMSCs. Melanoma cells alone formed no tumors, but B16 melanoma cells injected subcutaneously simultaneously with BMSCs (either subcutaneously or intravenously) demonstrated rapid and sustained tumor growth in allogeneic animals.[61] It is obvious that such an experiment would never be replicated in humans; however, a similar situation may be possible in clinical settings because autologous primary ASCs have been used in humans.[35] It remains to be answered whether ASCs are capable of potentiating immunosurveillance of tumor cells. In other

words, will implantation of cells cause cryptic cancers to become more pronounced, or is the effect solely related to allogeneic cells, as were present in the previous study? Questions relating to the possibility of these cells encouraging tumor growth undoubtedly require further research.

BMSCs are also known to home to the sites of chronic inflammation or injury; the skin,[62,63] kidney,[64,65] and lung[66,67] are only a few examples. A recent study has shown homing of BMSCs to gastric sites in a mouse model of *Helicobacter pylori* infection.[68] In this elegant study, infected mice were irradiated, and their bone marrow was replaced with the marrow of mice expressing β-galactosidase, an easily traceable marker. BMSCs from transplanted marrow were found to migrate to gastric mucosa. Additionally, BMSCs contributed to a majority of glands that showed high-grade gastrointestinal intraepithelial neoplasia, a direct precursor of gastric adenocarcinoma, within 1 year.[68]

It is not known to what extent ASCs are recruited and migrate to areas of inflammation or injury. This study demonstrates, however, that cells closely related to ASCs are capable of transforming into entities with undesirable properties. Further research dealing with the possibility of ASCs undergoing metaplastic processes should be considered.

FUTURE PROMISE

The imminent benefits of ASCs are easily observable and readily predictable. Notwithstanding many of the weaknesses and potential risks of the technology, ASCs have clear advantages over almost every other stem cell. ASCs are present in great abundance and easily obtainable, with little donor-site morbidity.

Cell harvests from adipose tissue yield quantities of autologous cells that are unsurpassed. To put this statement in perspective, it is possible to extract 400,000 ASCs per milliliter of processed liposuction aspirate.[69] Volumes of 100 mL are routinely, quickly, and safely removed through liposuction from patients, optimally yielding 40 million cells. Liposuction is the most commonly performed aesthetic procedure, with a large postoperative patient base through which the long-term risks of the procedure, although small, are known. Additionally, adipose tissue removed through liposuction or abdominoplasty is usually discarded as waste.

Once removed, potential uses for ASCs are limited only by the potential applications. Initially, risk-reward ratios will dictate uses similar to those already described in bone.[35] Replacement of tissue that has been damaged—cartilage, bone, or fat—that entails a low risk will be tried first. Optimization of implantation conditions will need to be addressed to indicate whether cells should be undifferentiated or differentiated for implantation. Because these primary cells are also useful as carriers of genes,[70–74] they will also be used for mesenchymal tissue engineering.

As more is learned about their ability to home to sites of injury, ASCs will be used for injuries that are not as well defined as bony or cartilaginous defects. Ischemic injuries of the heart or brain, cirrhosis, end-stage renal disease, or any disease in which dysfunctional tissue coexists with normal tissue at the cellular level would be amenable to therapies in which ASCs would be injected systemically and later expected to migrate to sites of injury.

Reperfusion injury associated with extremity reattachment or free flap movement may also be supplementally treated with ASC infusions. An ischemic hindlimb model in the mouse has been treated with ASCs, with resulting increases in capillary density and blood flow. Additionally, ASCs were incorporated into the vessels of the limb.[75] Because of the similarity of the underlying pathogenesis between ischemic limbs and flap movements, it may be beneficial to treat with ASCs.

The mechanism of deficit amelioration in this case would probably be twofold: differentiation of ASCs to target tissue and support of existing tissue by secretion of proangiogenic and prosurvival cytokines. ASCs have already been shown to differentiate into target cells on implantation into animal models in bone and brain. ASCs also secrete potent cytokines known to induce angiogenesis and inhibit cell death.[31] Instead of differentiating into the target tissue, ASCs may promote health in already existent cells.

Perhaps the most counterintuitive use of ASCs may be their allogeneic use. The immuno-modulatory reaction provoked by these cells could possibly be useful for down-regulating graft-versus-host disease (GVHD). This has already been done with MSCs[76]; a 9-year-old child was infused with allogeneic MSCs for refractory GVHD after blood stem cell transplantation for acute lymphoblastic leukemia. One year after treatment, the authors reported that he is well, with minimal residual disease.

Use of ASCs for down-regulation of unwanted immune responses need not be limited to infusion of cells after the onset of rejection. Injection of donor ASCs before or during transplantation may become a standard of therapy in the future. Such a strategy may augment take of transplanted organs and decrease the symptoms seen in these patients. Similarly, autoimmune diseases may also be amenable to treatment with ASC transfusions.

The most immediate promise of ASCs, however, is the idea of the bedside autograft. Simple local anesthesia could be used to extract enough adipose tissue to garner millions of cells. Currently being developed are "black box" devices into which harvested fat can be placed, with the output being transplantation-ready ASCs. Such a device, used at the bedside, could greatly enhance the accessibility and use of ASCs for a variety of illnesses.

REFERENCES

1. Friedstein AJ, Petrakova KV, Kurolesova AI, et al. Heterotopic of bone marrow. Analysis of precursor cells for osteogenic and hematopoietic tissues. Transplantation 1968;6:230–47.
2. Pittenger MF, Mackay AM, Beck SC, et al. Multilineage potential of adult human mesenchymal stem cells. Science 1999;284:143–7.
3. Grigoriadis AE, Heersche JN, Aubin JE. Differentiation of muscle, fat, cartilage, and bone from progenitor cells present in a bone-derived clonal cell population: effect of dexamethasone. J Cell Biol 1988;106(6):2139–51.

4. Mackay AM, Beck SC, Murphy JM, et al. Chondrogenic differentiation of cultured human mesenchymal stem cells from marrow. Tissue Eng 1998;4:415–28.

5. Woodbury D, Schwarz EJ, Prockop DJ, et al. Adult rat and human bone marrow stromal cells differentiate into neurons. J Neurosci Res 2000;61:364–70.

6. Young RG, Butler DL, Weber W, et al. Use of mesenchymal stem cells in a collagen matrix for Achilles tendon repair. J Orthop Res 1998;16(4):406–13.

7. Bruder SP, Kraus KH, Goldberg VM, et al. The effect of implants loaded with autologous mesenchymal stem cells on the healing of canine segmental bone defects. J Bone Joint Surg Am 1998;80:985–96.

8. Bruder SP, Kurth AA, Shea M, et al. Bone regeneration by implantation of purified, culture-expanded human mesenchymal stem cells. J Orthop Res 1998;16(2):155–62.

9. Fukuda K. Use of adult marrow mesenchymal stem cells for regeneration of cardiomyocytes. Bone Marrow Transplant 2003;32(Suppl 1):S25–7.

10. Rodbell M. Metabolism of isolated fat cells. J Biol Chem 1964;239:375–80.

11. Hauner H, Loffler G. Adipose tissue development: the role of precursor cells and adipogenic factors. Part I: adipose tissue development and the role of precursor cells. Klin Wochenschr 1987;65:803–11.

12. Loffler G, Hauner H. Adipose tissue development: the role of precursor cells and adipogenic factors. Part II: the regulation of the adipogenic conversion by hormones and serum factors. Klin Wochenschr 1987;65:812–7.

13. Poznanski WJ, Waheed I, Van R. Human fat cell precursors: morphologic and metabolic differentiation in culture. Lab Invest 1973;29:570–6.

14. Deslex S, Negrel R, Vannier C, et al. Differentiation of human adipocyte precursors in a chemically defined serum-free medium. Int J Obes 1987;11:19–27.

15. Zuk PA, Zhu M, Mizuno H, et al. Multilineage cells from human adipose tissue: implications for cell-based therapies. Tissue Eng 2001;7:211–28.

16. Zuk PA, Zhu M, Ashjian P, et al. Human adipose tissue is a source of multipotent stem cells. Mol Biol Cell 2002; 13:4279–95.

17. Tholpady SS, Katz AJ, Ogle RC. Mesenchymal stem cells from rat visceral fat exhibit multipotential differentiation in vitro. Anat Rec 2003;272:398–402.

18. Halvorsen YC, Wilkison WO, Gimble JM. Adipose-derived stromal cells—their utility and potential in bone formation. Int J Obes Relat Metab Disord 2000; 24 Suppl 4:S41–4.

19. Halvorsen YD, Franklin D, Bond AL, et al. Extracellular matrix mineralization and osteoblast gene expression by human adipose tissue-derived stromal cells. Tissue Eng 2001;7:729–41.

20. Erickson GR, Gimble JM, Franklin DM, et al. Chondrogenic potential of adipose tissue-derived stromal cells in vitro and in vivo. Biochem Biophys Res Commun 2002;290:763–9.

21. Huang JI, Zuk PA, Jones NF, et al. Chondrogenic potential of multipotential cells from human adipose tissue. Plast Reconstr Surg 2004;113:585–94.

22. Mizuno H, Zuk PA, Zhu M, et al. Myogenic differentiation by human processed lipoaspirate cells. Plast Reconstr Surg 2002;109:199–209; discussion 10–1.

23. Deng W, Obrocka M, Fischer I, et al. In vitro differentiation of human marrow stromal cells into early progenitors of neural cells by conditions that increase intracellular cyclic AMP. Biochem Biophys Res Commun 2001;281(1):148–52.

24. Safford KM, Hicok KC, Safford SD, et al. Neurogenic differentiation of murine and human adipose-derived stromal cells. Biochem Biophys Res Commun 2002;294: 371–9.

25. Ashjian PH, Elbarbary AS, Edmonds B, et al. In vitro differentiation of human processed lipoaspirate cells into early neural progenitors. Plast Reconstr Surg 2003; 111:1922–31.

26. Safford KM, Safford SD, Gimble JM, et al. Characterization of neuronal/glial differentiation of murine adipose-derived adult stromal cells. Exp Neurol 2004;187:319–28.

27. Gaustad KG, Boquest AC, Anderson BE, et al. Differentiation of human adipose tissue stem cells using extracts of rat cardiomyocytes. Biochem Biophys Res Commun 2004;314:420–7.

28. Planat-Benard V, Menard C, Andre M, et al. Spontaneous cardiomyocyte differentiation from adipose tissue stroma cells. Circ Res 2004;94:223–9.

29. Seo MJ, Suh SY, Bae YC, et al. Differentiation of human adipose stromal cells into hepatic lineage in vitro and in vivo. Biochem Biophys Res Commun 2005;328:258–64.

30. Martinez-Estrada OM, Munoz-Santos Y, Julve J, et al. Human adipose tissue as a source of Flk-1(+) cells: new method of differentiation and expansion. Cardiovasc Res 2005;65:328–33.

31. Rehman J, Traktuev D, Li J, et al. Secretion of angiogenic and antiapoptotic factors by human adipose stromal cells. Circulation 2004;109:1292–8.

32. Planat-Benard V, Silvestre JS, Cousin B, et al. Plasticity of human adipose lineage cells toward endothelial cells: physiological and therapeutic perspectives. Circulation 2004;109:656–63.

33. Hicok KC, Du Laney TV, Zhou YS, et al. Human adipose-derived adult stem cells produce osteoid in vivo. Tissue Eng 2004;10:371–80.

34. Cowan CM, Shi YY, Aalami OO, et al. Adipose-derived adult stromal cells heal critical-size mouse calvarial defects. Nat Biotechnol 2004;22:560–7.

35. Lendeckel S, Jodicke A, Christophis P, et al. Autologous stem cells (adipose) and fibrin glue used to treat widespread traumatic calvarial defects: case report. J Craniomaxillofac Surg 2004;32:370–3.

36. Urist MR. Bone: formation by autoinduction. Science 1965;150:839–99.

37. Kang SK, Lee DH, Bae YC, et al. Improvement of neurological deficits by intracerebral transplantation of human adipose tissue-derived stromal cells after cerebral ischemia in rats. Exp Neurol 2003;183:355–66.

38. Kim DH, Je CM, Sin JY, et al. Effect of partial hepatectomy on in vivo engraftment after intravenous

administration of human adipose tissue stromal cells in mouse. Microsurgery 2003;23:424–31.

39. Cousin B, Andre M, Arnaud E, et al. Reconstitution of lethally irradiated mice by cells isolated from adipose tissue. Biochem Biophys Res Commun 2003;301:1016–22.

40. Neuhuber B, Gallo G, Howard L, et al. Reevaluation of in vitro differentiation protocols for bone marrow stromal cells: disruption of actin cytoskeleton induces rapid morphological changes and mimics neuronal phenotype. J Neurosci Res 2004;77:192–204.

41. Lu P, Blesch A, Tuszynski MH. Induction of bone marrow stromal cells to neurons: differentiation, trans-differentiation, or artifact? J Neurosci Res 2004;77:174–91.

42. Ying QL, Nichols J, Evans EP, et al. Changing potency by spontaneous fusion. Nature 2002;416:545–8.

43. Terada N, Hamazaki T, Oka M, et al. Bone marrow cells adopt the phenotype of other cells by spontaneous cell fusion. Nature 2002;416:542–5.

44. Boquest AC, Shahdadfar A, Fronsdal K, et al. Isolation and transcription profiling of purified uncultured human stromal stem cells: alteration of gene expression following in vitro cell culture. Mol Biol Cell 2005;16(3):1131–41.

45. Van Harmelen V, Rohrig K, Hauner H. Comparison of proliferation and differentiation capacity of human adipocyte precursor cells from the omental and subcutaneous adipose tissue depot of obese subjects. Metabolism 2004;53:632–7.

46. Bruun JM, Lihn AS, Madan AK, et al. Higher production of IL-8 in visceral vs. subcutaneous adipose tissue. Implication of nonadipose cells in adipose tissue. Am J Physiol Endocrinol Metab 2004;286:E8–13.

47. Bakker AH, Van Dielen FM, Greve JW, et al. Preadipocyte number in omental and subcutaneous adipose tissue of obese individuals. Obes Res 2004;12:488–98.

48. Tchkonia T, Giorgadze N, Pirtskhalava T, et al. Fat depot origin affects adipogenesis in primary cultured and cloned human preadipocytes. Am J Physiol Regul Integr Comp Physiol 2002;282:R1286–96.

49. Ogawa R, Mizuno H, Watanabe A, et al. Adipogenic differentiation by adipose-derived stem cells harvested from GFP transgenic mice-including relationship of sex differences. Biochem Biophys Res Commun 2004;319:511–7.

50. Sen A, Lea-Currie YR, Sujkowska D, et al. Adipogenic potential of human adipose derived stromal cells from multiple donors is heterogeneous. J Cell Biochem 2001;81:312–9.

51. Katz AJ, Tholpady A, Tholpady SS, et al. Cell surface and transcriptional characterization of human adipose-derived adherent stromal (hADAS) cells. Stem Cells 2005;23:412–23.

52. Kenkel JM, Brown SA, Love EJ, et al. Hemodynamics, electrolytes, and organ histology of larger-volume liposuction in a porcine model. Plast Reconstr Surg 2004;113:1391–9.

53. Lipschitz AH, Kenkel JM, Luby M, et al. Electrolyte and plasma enzyme analyses during large-volume liposuction. Plast Reconstr Surg 2004;114:766–75.

54. Tse WT, Pendleton JD, Beyer WM, et al. Suppression of allogeneic T-cell proliferation by human marrow stromal cells: implications in transplantation. Transplantation 2003;75:389–97.

55. Maitra B, Szekely E, Gjini K, et al. Human mesenchymal stem cells support unrelated donor hematopoietic stem cells and suppress T-cell activation. Bone Marrow Transplant 2004;33:597–604.

56. Le Blanc K. Immunomodulatory effects of fetal and adult mesenchymal stem cells. Cytotherapy 2003;5:485–9.

57. Krampera M, Glennie S, Dyson J, et al. Bone marrow mesenchymal stem cells inhibit the response of naive and memory antigen-specific T cells to their cognate peptide. Blood 2003;101:3722–9.

58. Gotherstrom C, Ringden O, Tammik C, et al. Immunologic properties of human fetal mesenchymal stem cells. Am J Obstet Gynecol 2004;190:239–45.

59. Aggarwal S, Pittenger MF. Human mesenchymal stem cells modulate allogeneic immune cell responses. Blood 2005;105:1815–22.

60. Puissant B, Barreau C, Bourin P, et al. Immunomodulatory effect of human adipose tissue-derived adult stem cells: comparison with bone marrow mesenchymal stem cells. Br J Haematol 2005;129:118–29.

61. Djouad F, Plence P, Bony C, et al. Immunosuppressive effect of mesenchymal stem cells favors tumor growth in allogeneic animals. Blood 2003;102:3837–44.

62. Borue X, Lee S, Grove J, et al. Bone marrow-derived cells contribute to epithelial engraftment during wound healing. Am J Pathol 2004;165:1767–72.

63. Badiavas EV, Abedi M, Butmarc J, et al. Participation of bone marrow derived cells in cutaneous wound healing. J Cell Physiol 2003;196:245–50.

64. Gupta S, Verfaillie C, Chmielewski D, et al. A role for extrarenal cells in the regeneration following acute renal failure. Kidney Int 2002;62:1285–90.

65. Poulsom R, Forbes SJ, Hodivala-Dilke K, et al. Bone marrow contributes to renal parenchymal turnover and regeneration. J Pathol 2001;195:229–35.

66. Theise ND, Henegariu O, Grove J, et al. Radiation pneumonitis in mice: a severe injury model for pneumocyte engraftment from bone marrow. Exp Hematol 2002;30:1333–8.

67. Kotton DN, Ma BY, Cardoso WV, et al. Bone marrow-derived cells as progenitors of lung alveolar epithelium. Development 2001;128:5181–8.

68. Houghton J, Stoicov C, Nomura S, et al. Gastric cancer originating from bone marrow-derived cells. Science 2004;306:1568–71.

69. Aust L, Devlin B, Foster SJ, et al. Yield of human adipose-derived adult stem cells from liposuction aspirates. Cytotherapy 2004;6:7–14.

70. Dragoo JL, Choi JY, Lieberman JR, et al. Bone induction by BMP-2 transduced stem cells derived from human fat. J Orthop Res 2003;21:622–9.

71. Edwards PC, Ruggiero S, Fantasia J, et al. Sonic hedgehog gene-enhanced tissue engineering for bone regeneration. Gene Ther 2005;12:75–86.

72. Morizono K, De Ugarte DA, Zhu M, et al. Multilineage cells from adipose tissue as gene delivery vehicles. Hum Gene Ther 2003;14:59–66.

73. Gamradt SC, Lieberman JR. Genetic modification of stem cells to enhance bone repair. Ann Biomed Eng 2004;32: 136–47.

74. Gimble JM. Adipose tissue-derived therapeutics. Exp Opin Biol Th 2003;3:705–13.

75. Miranville A, Heeschen C, Sengenes C, et al. Improvement of postnatal neovascularization by human adipose tissue-derived stem cells. Circulation 2004;110:349–55.

76. Le Blanc K, Rasmusson I, Sundberg B, et al. Treatment of severe acute graft-versus-host disease with third party haploidentical mesenchymal stem cells. Lancet 2004; 363:1439–41.

INDEX